Cell Membrane Nanodomains

From Biochemistry to Nanoscopy

Cell Membrane Nanodomains

From Biochemistry to Nanoscopy

Edited by
Alessandra Cambi • Diane S. Lidke

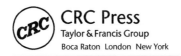
CRC Press
Taylor & Francis Group
Boca Raton London New York

CRC Press is an imprint of the
Taylor & Francis Group, an **informa** business

CRC Press
Taylor & Francis Group
6000 Broken Sound Parkway NW, Suite 300
Boca Raton, FL 33487-2742

First issued in paperback 2021
First issued in hardback 2019

© 2015 by Taylor & Francis Group, LLC
CRC Press is an imprint of Taylor & Francis Group, an Informa business

No claim to original U.S. Government works

ISBN 13: 978-1-03-223674-2 (pbk)
ISBN 13: 978-1-4822-0989-1 (hbk)

Library of Congress Cataloging-in-Publication Data

Cell membrane nanodomains : from biochemistry to nanoscopy / editors, Alessandra Cambi and Diane S. Lidke.
   p. ; cm.
   Includes bibliographical references and index.
   ISBN 978-1-4822-0989-1 (alk. paper)
   I. Cambi, Alessandra, editor. II. Lidke, Diane S., editor.
   [DNLM: 1. Cell Membrane--ultrastructure. 2. Cell Communication--physiology. 3. Membrane Lipids--metabolism. 4. Membrane Lipids--physiology. 5. Nanostructures. QU 350]

QP552.M44
572'.696--dc23
   2014017885

Visit the Taylor & Francis Web site at
http://www.taylorandfrancis.com

and the CRC Press Web site at
http://www.crcpress.com

Contents

SECTION I Protein and Lipid Nanodomains

SECTION II   Advanced Ensemble Imaging Techniques

SECTION III   Expanding the Fluorescence Toolbox

SECTION IV Nanoscopy

Preface

An emerging concept in cell biology is that spatially defined subcellular compartments on the cell membrane (lipid nanodomains, cytoskeleton-induced membrane corrals, signaling nanoplatforms, etc.) influence the diffusion, location, and interactions between multiple molecular components in a dynamic fashion. Yet, little is known about the underlying mechanisms that control membrane organization at the nanoscale. Thus, a major drive in this lively research field is to bring understanding on how such discrete membrane nanoscale interactions are capable of finely modulating cellular signaling and physiological responses. Over the last few years, enormous developments in imaging technologies, new optical probes, and genetic engineering have allowed the rapid emergence of single-molecule fluorescence techniques and their application to biological imaging. Of particular relevance is the development of various superresolution nanoscopy techniques capable of reaching nanometer resolution by optical means (highlighted as the method of the year by *Nature Methods* in 2008). These techniques now provide unprecedented details on the spatial and temporal heterogeneities of nanoscale biological processes and are just starting to reshape our understanding of molecular organizations and interactions in cells and tissues.

In preparing this book, we brought together a collection of works where the application of these novel imaging techniques revealed new concepts in biology. The contributors are experts from the optical nanoscopy and microscopy fields, membrane biophysicists, biochemists, and cell biologists. In Section I, there is a broad description of membrane organization. These include the seminal work on lipid partitioning in model systems and the roles of proteins in membrane organization. Section I also considers how lipids and membrane compartmentalization can regulate protein function and signal transduction. In the remaining sections of the book, we focused on recent advancements in imaging techniques and tools that will allow for further advancements in our understanding of signaling nanoplatforms. In Section II, we highlight several diffraction-limited imaging techniques that allow for measurements of protein distribution/clustering and membrane curvature in living cells. Of course, fluorescence microscopy is nothing without fluorescent probes. Section III summarizes the current state of the field with chapters describing new fluorescent proteins, novel Laurdan analyses, and the toolbox of labeling possibilities with organic dyes. Since superresolution optical techniques have been crucial to advancing our understanding of cellular structure and protein behavior, we end this book with technologies that are enabling the visualization of lipids, proteins, and other molecular components at unprecedented spatiotemporal resolution. Chapters in Section IV explain the ins and outs of the rapidly developing high- or super resolution microscopy field, including new methods and data analysis tools that pertain exclusively to these techniques.

This integration of membrane biology and advanced imaging techniques emphasizes the interdisciplinary nature of this exciting field. We hope that the array of contributions from leading world experts will provide a valuable tool for those interested in the visualization of signaling nanoplatforms by means of cutting-edge optical microscopy tools.

MATLAB® is a registered trademark of The MathWorks, Inc. For product information, please contact:

The MathWorks, Inc.
3 Apple Hill Drive
Natick, MA 01760-2098 USA
Tel: 508-647-7000
Fax: 508-647-7001
E-mail: info@mathworks.com
Web: www.mathworks.com

Acknowledgments

The editors thank all of the authors who contributed to this book. We are grateful for their expertise, time, and dedication that have made it possible to bring this book to completion. We thank Christopher Valley and Patrick Cutler for cover images. We also acknowledge the financial support from the following: the Netherlands Organisation for Scientific Research (NWO), Meervoud subsidy to AC; the European Commission's Seventh Framework Programme (FP7-ICT-2011-7) under grant agreement no. 288263 (NanoVista); the New Mexico Spatiotemporal Modeling Center (NIH P50GM085273); and the Human Frontier Science Program (RGY0074/2008 and RGP0027/2012).

Finally, we dedicate this book to our postdoc mentors, Dr. Thomas Jovin and Dr. Donna Arndt-Jovin, who sparked in us the excitement for using fluorescence microscopy to study cellular processes. We are ever grateful for their inspiring mentorship and will continue to be excited by the unexpected results.

Editors

Alessandra Cambi earned a PhD in biology from the University of Camerino (Italy) in 2000 and a PhD in medical sciences (cum laude) from Radboud University Nijmegen (the Netherlands) in 2005. During the first PhD, under the supervision of Prof. Dr. Alberto Vita and Paolo Natalini, she investigated the enzyme cytidine deaminase, while during the second PhD, under the supervision of Prof. Dr. Carl G. Figdor, she studied how the nanoscale organization of the adhesion receptor LFA-1 and the pathogen-recognition receptor DC-SIGN regulates their function. As a long-term EMBO postdoctoral fellow, she moved to the Max Planck Institute for Biophysical Chemistry in Göttingen (Germany) in Thomas Jovin's group, where she applied ligand-coated quantum dots to mimic virus binding and uptake by antigen-presenting cells. In 2006, Dr. Cambi obtained a VENI postdoctoral fellowship from the Dutch Scientific Organization (NWO) and returned to Radboud University Medical Center in Nijmegen as junior group leader. In 2008, she was awarded a Young Investigator grant from the Human Frontier Science Program in collaboration with Diane S. Lidke (University of New Mexico, USA) and became a permanent staff member. Awarded a MEERVOUD subsidy from NWO in 2009, she became an assistant professor and since July 2011 she also has a part-time appointment at the University of Twente in the Nanobiophysics Laboratory. Dr. Cambi is currently an associate professor and group leader of the Nano-Immunology group, a young interdisciplinary team that studies the nanoscale organization and dynamics of membrane receptors exploiting high-resolution microscopy.

Diane S. Lidke earned a PhD in biophysical sciences and medical physics from the University of Minnesota in 2002. She was a postdoctoral fellow at the laboratory of Thomas Jovin at the Max Planck Institute for Biophysical Chemistry (Göttingen, Germany), where she developed the use of quantum dot ligands for live-cell imaging. In 2005, Dr. Lidke became an assistant professor in the Pathology Department at the University of New Mexico (UNM). At UNM, she continues applying fluorescence microscopy and biophysical techniques to the study of cell signal transduction, with an emphasis in the spatiotemporal regulation of signaling molecules in allergy and cancer. In 2008, she was awarded a Young Investigator grant from the Human Frontier Science Program in collaboration with Alessandra Cambi (Radboud University Nijmegen, the Netherlands). In 2009, she received the National Science Foundation (NSF) Faculty Early Career Development Award, NSF's most prestigious awards in support of junior faculty who exemplify the role of teacher-scholars through outstanding research and excellence in education. In 2011, Dr. Lidke was the recipient of the Biophysical Society's Margaret Oakley Dayhoff Award that is given to a woman who holds very high promise or has achieved prominence while developing the early stages of a career in biophysical research.

Contributors

Luis A. Bagatolli
Membrane Biophysics and Biophotonics
  Group
MEMPHYS—Center for Biomembrane
  Physics
Department of Biochemistry and
  Molecular Biology
University of Southern Denmark
Odense, Denmark

Štefan Bálint
ICFO—Institut de Ciències Fotòniques
Barcelona, Spain

Facundo D. Batista
Lymphocyte Interaction Lab
London Research Institute
Cancer Research United Kingdom
London, United Kingdom

Alexis Bergsma
Van Andel Institute Graduate School
Grand Rapids, Michigan

Marcel P. Bruchez
Department of Chemistry
Molecular Biosensor and Imaging
  Center
and
Department of Biological Sciences
Carnegie Mellon University
Pittsburgh, Pennsylvania

Andreas Bruckbauer
Lymphocyte Interaction Lab
London Research Institute
Cancer Research United Kingdom
London, United Kingdom

Ünal Coskun
Laboratory of Membrane Biochemistry
Paul Langerhans Institute Dresden,
  Faculty of Medicine Carl Gustav
  Carus
TU Dresden
Dresden, Germany

and

German Center for Diabetes Research
  (DZD)

Yves De Koninck
Institut universitaire en santé mentale
  de Québec
and
Département de Psychiatrie et
  Neurosciences
Université Laval
Québec City, Québec, Canada

and

Department of Pharmacology and
  Therapeutics
and
Alan Edwards Center for Research of
  Pain
McGill University
Montréal, Québec, Canada

Miguel A. Del Pozo
Integrin Signaling Laboratory
Vascular Biology and Inflammation
  Department
Centro Nacional de Investigaciones
  Cardiovasculares (CNIC)
Madrid, Spain

Michelle A. Digman
Laboratory for Fluorescence Dynamics
Department of Biomedical Engineering
University of California
Irvine, California

Memed Duman
Institute for Biophysics
Johannes Kepler University Linz
Linz, Austria

and

Institute of Science, Nanotechnology
    and Nanomedicine Division
Hacettepe University
Ankara, Turkey

Asier Echarri
Integrin Signaling Laboratory
Vascular Biology and Inflammation
    Department
Centro Nacional de Investigaciones
    Cardiovasculares (CNIC)
Madrid, Spain

Christian Eggeling
MRC Human Immunology Unit
Weatherall Institute of Molecular
    Medicine
University of Oxford
Oxford, United Kingdom

Sharon Eisenberg
Program in Cell Biology
The Hospital for Sick Children
Toronto, Ontario, Canada

Christoph Feest
Lymphocyte Interaction Lab
London Research Institute
Cancer Research United Kingdom
London, United Kingdom

Yan Fu
Section on Biophotonics
National Institute of Biomedical
    Imaging and Bioengineering
National Institutes of Health
Bethesda, Maryland

Maria F. Garcia-Parajo
ICFO—Institut de Ciències Fotòniques
and
ICREA—Institucio Catalana de
    Recerca i Estudis Avancats
Barcelona, Spain

Subhasri Ghosh
Institute for Stem Cell Biology and
    Regenerative Medicine
Bangalore, India

Antoine G. Godin
Department of Physics
McGill University
Montreal, Québec, Canada

and

Institut universitaire en santé mentale
    de Québec
Québec City, Québec, Canada

Enrico Gratton
Laboratory for Fluorescence
    Dynamics
Department of Biomedical
    Engineering
University of California
Irvine, California

Sergio Grinstein
Division of Cell Biology
Hospital for Sick Children
and
Keenan Research Centre of the Li Ka
    Shing Knowledge Institute
St. Michael's Hospital
Toronto, Ontario, Canada

Michal Grzybek
Laboratory of Membrane Biochemistry
Paul Langerhans Institute Dresden,
    Faculty of Medicine Carl Gustav
    Carus
TU Dresden
Dresden, Germany

and

German Center for Diabetes Research
    (DZD)

Erich Gulbins
Institute for Virology and
    Immunobiology
University of Wuerzburg
Wuerzburg, Germany

and

Institute for Molecular Biology
University of Duisburg-Essen
Essen, Germany

Theresia Gutmann
Laboratory of Membrane Biochemistry
Paul Langerhans Institute Dresden,
    Faculty of Medicine Carl Gustav
    Carus
TU Dresden
Dresden, Germany

and

German Center for Diabetes Research
    (DZD)

Peter Hinterdorfer
Institute for Biophysics
and
Christian Doppler Laboratory for
    Nanoscopic Methods in Biophysics
Johannes Kepler University Linz
and
Center for Advanced Bioanalysis
Upper Austrian Research
Linz, Austria

Alf Honigmann
Department of NanoBiophotonics
Max-Planck Institute for Biophysical
    Chemistry
Göttingen, Germany

Adam D. Hoppe
Department of Chemistry and
    Biochemistry
South Dakota State University
Brookings, South Dakota

Melike Lakadamyali
ICFO—Institut de Ciències Fotòniques
Barcelona, Spain

Shalini T. Low-Nam
Department of Chemistry and
    Biochemistry
South Dakota State University
Brookings, South Dakota

Josef Madl
Institute for Biophysics
Johannes Kepler University Linz
Linz, Austria

Carlo Manzo
ICFO—Institut de Ciències Fotòniques
Barcelona, Spain

Satyajit Mayor
National Centre for Biological Sciences
and
Institute for Stem Cell Biology and
    Regenerative Medicine
Bangalore, India

Cindy K. Miranti
Laboratory of Integrin Signaling and
    Tumorigenesis
Van Andel Research Institute
Grand Rapids, Michigan

Mathieu Mivelle
ICFO—Institut de Ciències Fotòniques
Barcelona, Spain

Ole G. Mouritsen
Department of Physics, Chemistry, and
    Pharmacy
MEMPHYS—Center for Biomembrane
    Physics
University of Southern Denmark
Odense, Denmark

Nora Müller
Institute for Virology and
    Immunobiology
University of Würzburg
Würzburg, Germany

Robert P.J. Nieuwenhuizen
Quantitative Imaging Group
Faculty of Applied Sciences
Delft University of Technology
Delft, the Netherlands

Anna Oddone
ICFO—Institut de Ciències Fotòniques
Barcelona, Spain

George H. Patterson
Section on Biophotonics
National Institute of Biomedical
    Imaging and Bioengineering
National Institutes of Health
Bethesda, Maryland

Laurent Potvin-Trottier
Department of Physics
McGill University
Montreal, Québec, Canada

Benjamin Rappaz
Department of Physics
McGill University
Montreal, Québec, Canada

Bernd Rieger
Quantitative Imaging Group
Faculty of Applied Sciences
Delft University of Technology
Delft, the Netherlands

Saumya Saurabh
Department of Chemistry
Molecular Biosensor and Imaging
    Center
Carnegie Mellon University
Pittsburgh, Pennsylvania

Sibylle Schneider-Schaulies
Institute for Virology and
    Immunobiology
University of Würzburg
Würzburg, Germany

Gerhard J. Schütz
Institute of Applied Physics
Vienna University of Technology
Vienna, Austria

Sjoerd Stallinga
Quantitative Imaging Group
Faculty of Applied Sciences
Delft University of Technology
Delft, the Netherlands

Johnny Tam
ICFO—Institut de Ciències Fotòniques
Barcelona, Spain

Martin ter Beest
Department of Tumor Immunology
Nijmegen Centre for Molecular Life
    Sciences
Radboud University Medical Center
Nijmegen, the Netherlands

Geert van den Bogaart
Department of Tumor Immunology
Nijmegen Center for Molecular Life
    Sciences
Radboud University Medical Center
Nijmegen, the Netherlands

Annemiek B. van Spriel
Department of Tumor Immunology
Radboud Institute for Molecular Life
    Sciences
Radboud University Medical Center
Nijmegen, the Netherlands

Thomas S. van Zanten
ICFO—Institut de Ciències Fotòniques
Barcelona, Spain

Ione Verdeny Vilanova
ICFO—Institut de Ciències Fotòniques
Barcelona, Spain

Paul W. Wiseman
Department of Physics
and
Department of Chemistry
McGill University
Montreal, Québec, Canada

Rong Zhu
Institute for Biophysics
Johannes Kepler University Linz
Linz, Austria

Section I

Protein and Lipid Nanodomains

1 Giant Unilamellar Vesicles (GUVs) as a Laboratory to Study Mesoscopic Lipid Domains in Membranes

Luis A. Bagatolli and Ole G. Mouritsen

CONTENTS

1.1 MEMBRANE DOMAINS: A HISTORICAL OVERVIEW

There is a substantial literature from the 1970s, often overlooked by many present workers, on the physical chemistry of lipid bilayer systems, which have laid the foundation for studying lateral organization and lipid domains in membranes (for a critical review, see Ref. 1). Early evidence that lipids could laterally segregate in model membrane systems under certain conditions and form different lipid domains with particular structural characteristics (i.e., different lateral packing) was reported in 1970 by Phillips et al.,[2] who assessed, using differential scanning calorimetry (DSC), the lateral mixing of different glycerophospholipid species; in 1973 by Shimshick and McConnell,[3] who explored lipid lateral phase separation by using electron paramagnetic resonance (EPR); in 1974 by Grant et al.,[4] who observed lipid domains by freeze-fracture electron microscopy; and in 1976 by Lentz et al.,[5] who demonstrated nonideal mixing among different glycerophospholipids containing saturated and unsaturated chains using fluorescence anisotropy. Detailed nuclear magnetic resonance (NMR) studies of sphingomyelin (SM) in bilayers by Schmidt et al.[6] in 1977 prompted the hypothesis that sphingolipids might form microdomains in biological membranes. Also in 1977, Gebhardt et al.[7] considered the lipid compositional heterogeneity in natural membranes and predicted that lipid lateral segregation might arise under particular environmental conditions such as those that mimic a physiological state. In a similar manner, Marcelja[8] in 1976 and Sackmann[9] in a classical review from 1984 anticipated the possible role of different membrane regions induced by lipid–protein interactions as a physical basis for membrane-mediated processes. This discussion was repeatedly addressed on several occasions by various researchers.[10–13] Yet, the view of the main structural/dynamical features of biological membranes was profoundly influenced and to a significant extent biased by the fluid mosaic model proposed in 1972 by Singer and Nicolson.[14] The fluid mosaic model, which to date is the most influential model for biological membranes, supports the idea of lipids forming a more or less randomly organized bidimensional fluid matrix where proteins perform their distinct functions. Although lipid-mediated lateral heterogeneity in membranes was simultaneously described during the 1970s, this feature was not considered in the Singer and Nicolson model.

To account for lipid-mediated lateral heterogeneity and its influence on the supramolecular properties of biological membranes, alternative models have been proposed. For example, the "plate model" introduced in 1977 by Jain and White[15] proposed that separation of ordered regions from disordered (fluid) regions occurs in biological membranes as a natural consequence of specific intermolecular interactions and lattice deformation. At the same time, Israelachvili proposed another model to account for the need of membrane proteins and lipids to adjust to each other.[16] This insight paved the way for "the mattress model" proposed by Mouritsen and Bloom in 1984[17] who suggested that, in membranes, proteins and lipids display interactions with a positive Gibbs energy content attributed to a fundamental hydrophobic matching condition imposed between the lipid bilayer thickness and the hydrophobic span of integral membrane proteins. Mismatch between lipids and proteins in this model would be a source for lateral heterogeneity and lipid-mediated indirect protein–protein interactions owing to capillary forces. A model accounting for the importance of the cytoskeleton and the glycocalyx on membrane organization was developed by Sackmann in 1995.[18]

Regrettably, many important physical aspects accounted for in the abovementioned models have been largely ignored, and the outlook introduced by the fluid mosaic model still prevails.[19,20] In fact, it has been suggested that the fluid mosaic model of membranes has been successful because it does not bias the reader strongly, allowing for broad interpretations of new experimental data and novel theoretical concepts.[19,21] For instance, considerable effects associated with the membrane transbilayer structure and the associated lateral pressure profile,[22] curvature stress,[23] instabilities toward nonlamellar symmetries,[24] as well as coupling between internal membrane structure and hydrophobic matching[17] are generally not taken into account when basic membrane-related phenomena are addressed (ion channels, pumps, and hydrophobic second messenger, to mention a few) although there are some notable exceptions.[25]

The most popular model to date that takes into account lipid-mediated lateral heterogeneity came with the "raft" hypothesis. This hypothesis has its origin in observations reported by Simons and van Meer in 1988.[26] These authors envisage the formation of lipid domains in cellular membranes (asymmetric separation of sphingolipids and glycerophospholipids) as the first event during the sorting process in epithelial cells. This was subsequently refined by claiming the existence of microdomains (named "rafts") enriched in sphingolipids (e.g., SM) and cholesterol in plasma membranes. These domains would be associated with specific proteins involved in cellular functions such as intracellular lipid traffic and cell signaling.[27] This refinement referring to physical membrane structure was partly based on original observations in model membrane systems reported by Ipsen et al. in 1987,[28] showing that under particular conditions, cholesterol in lipid bilayers generates the coexistence of liquid-disordered (ld) and liquid-ordered (lo) lamellar phases. The lo phase would combine free lipid-acyl-chain rotational and lipid-molecule translational diffusion (as found in the fluid liquid crystalline phases) with a low proportion of *gauche* rotamers in the hydrocarbon chains (i.e., high acyl-chain order rather than low order), as is usually found in the solid-ordered (so, or gel) phases.[28] The history of the lo phase has recently been reviewed.[29,30]

In one way or another, it is clear that the raft hypothesis extends the mosaic nature of the membrane proposed in the Singer and Nicolson model to now include functionally important distinct—but *fluid* as prescribed in the Singer and Nicolson model—lateral domains, selective in terms of *both* protein and lipid components. In other words, the generic view of the fluid mosaic model seems to continue to prevail and no reference is made to several fundamental physical features of the membrane as those mentioned above.

Since 1997, the raft hypothesis has become extremely popular among researchers from a wide range of biology-related fields. In fact, the paper from Simons and Ikonen[27] has originated literally thousands of projects and publications in multiple areas of cell biology, biochemistry, molecular biology, neuroscience, and biophysics. For example, rafts have been referred to as constitutive elements of cellular plasma membranes, generalized to a wide variety of different membranes (although compositional differences with plasma membranes are observed), and claimed to exist in a sort of lo phase (although in most cases, there is no quantitative experimental evidence to sustain this). Generally, membranes with mixtures of cholesterol and lipid species with high low melting points are tacitly assumed in their phase diagram to possess phase-separated regions involving an lo phase. Whether or not this updated version of the fluid mosaic model represents a realistic connection with the structure and dynamics of biological membranes,[19,20] it is clear that the idea of rafts has revitalized the debate about the existence and functional implications of domains in natural membranes.

1.2   LATERAL STRUCTURE AND DYNAMICS OF LIPID BILAYERS

1.2.1   FORMATION OF MEMBRANE DOMAINS

Because of the cooperative nature of the molecular interactions between lipids and with their environment, in particular water, these molecules self-assemble and laterally organize in the plane of a bilayer membrane in a nonuniform and nonrandom fashion. In other words, the reason for the formation of a particular membranous structure, its thermodynamic phases, and the transitions between these phases is the cooperative phenomena caused by the manybodyness of the system.[19] Bilayers under equilibrium conditions have a number of phase transitions. The most relevant in the context of lipid-domain formation is the so-called main transition, which takes the membrane from a solid phase with conformationally ordered lipid-acyl chains (solid-ordered, so) to a liquid phase with conformationally disordered lipid acyl chains (ld).[31] The main transition is a first-order phase transition but thermodynamics allows the phase equilibria in multicomponent systems under certain conditions to develop into specific critical-point behavior. Critical points are characterized by long-range correlations in fluctuations in the molecular state of lipids (e.g., molecular area, chain length, etc.) occurring in the plane of the membrane. This behavior has been reported, for example, when cholesterol is incorporated in model membranes composed of phospholipids.[28,32] Critical behavior is best described in terms of the so-called correlation length (or coherence length). The correlation length defines the range over which lipids, via their interactions, effectively can "sense" each other's molecular state (i.e., position in space, lipid-chain order, orientation, composition).[19,33] Therefore, the correlation length measures the range of fluctuations in the molecular state of lipids in the bilayer plane and is one way of quantifying the spatial extension of possible lipid domains. For example, the main transition is strongly influenced by lateral density fluctuations in the membrane and hence the correlation length becomes particularly large near this transition.

Lipid domains caused by fluctuations should be considered dynamic entities that come and go and which have lifetimes that depend on their size and the prevailing thermodynamic conditions. This type of domain formation, which is fundamentally different from formation of thermodynamic phases, has been referred to as dynamic heterogeneity.[34] The lateral bilayer heterogeneity in terms of lipid domains also implies changes in the macroscopic bilayer properties, for example, lateral compressibility, bending rigidity, permeability, binding affinity for various solutes, and the way the bilayer mediates the interaction and organization of membrane proteins and peptides. Obviously, being dynamic, the domains need not be sharply defined, and a certain gradual variation in the lipid bilayer properties is expected upon crossing a domain boundary. Other types of lateral membrane organization may arise on scales all the way from nanometers to micrometers, for example, out-of-plane protrusions, undulations, bending modes, and large-scale shape fluctuations.

Lateral phase equilibria in multicomponent lipid membranes imply the existence of regions of macroscopic phase separation in the plane of the membrane. These can be assessed by, for example, bulk thermodynamic and scattering techniques or indirectly by spectroscopic probes.[35] In some cases, the phases can be observed and identified by imaging techniques such as fluorescence microscopy or atomic force microscopy (AFM). It is often found that even simple lipid mixtures seem not to relax to global phase equilibrium and only finite-size domains develop rather than global thermodynamic phases. This is particularly the case when it comes to the small-scale structure and microheterogeneity in the nanometer-to-micrometer range.[36] Particularly, nanometer-scale structure is experimentally difficult to access by direct and noninvasive methods, for example, neutron scattering,[37] mostly because the small-scale structure is often dynamic and changes in time. However, recently, a breakthrough has been reported in the use of neutron diffraction to quantitatively assess small-scale structure in binary lipid-cholesterol membranes in the lo phase.[38,39] The experiments revealed the existence of highly ordered lipid domains in equilibrium with a disordered matrix. The lipids in these domains were found to be in a lo state and thought to be saturated with cholesterol molecules.

In summary, and as discussed in more detail elsewhere,[19] the molecular interactions in membranes can lead to the formation of a highly nonrandom and nontrivial lateral organization of biological membranes. First, proteins anchored to the cytoskeleton can provide effective fences or corrals that lead to transient or permanent membrane domains.[18] Second, phase separation can occur under particular conditions and lead to large areas of different molecular composition. Finally, the molecular interactions between the membrane constituents (cooperative phenomena) can possibly lead to critical behavior, associated with significant fluctuations in local membrane structure and composition, thereby generating distinct membrane domains on different time and length scales. In order to judge which physical phenomena are relevant in a particular situation, membrane diversity (composition, lipid/protein ratio) and dynamics (e.g., molecular turnover) need to be carefully taken into account.

1.2.2   MODEL SYSTEMS AND SOME EXPERIMENTAL TECHNIQUES

Since the 1970s, major research efforts have been presented to elucidate lipid domains in model membranes. In particular, studies of phase transitions and phase coexistence in artificial lipid mixtures are numerous and have involved a wide range of techniques, such as fluorescence spectroscopy,[5,40–42] infrared spectroscopy, EPR,[43] NMR,[44,45] DSC,[46–48] X-ray-related techniques,[49–51] and neutron scattering,[50] as well as computer simulations.[52–55]

Among different options,[56] perhaps one of the most popular membrane model systems are liposomes. These freestanding bilayer models discovered by A.D. Bangham[57] in the 1960s are classified with respect to their size (small and large, but also giant; see Section 1.3) and the number of lipid lamellae (unilamellar, oligolamellar, and multilamellar).[56,58] Liposome studies generally involve aqueous suspensions consisting of small unilamellar vesicles (SUVs; mean diameter, 30–50 nm), large unilamellar vesicles (LUVs; mean diameter, 100 nm), and multilamellar vesicles (MLVs), which are the most popular model systems. The composition of these membranes can range from single lipid components to mixtures of lipids (synthetic or natural lipid extracts), both with and without membranes proteins, including in some cases closed vesicles obtained from native biological membranes. Preparation of these model membranes is straightforward and different protocols are reported in the existing literature (for a comprehensive review, see Ref. 56).

Lately, strategies involving imaging techniques offer new complementary information to that obtained with the traditional bulk-sample approaches mentioned above. Although there are cases where it is possible to apply classical biophysical techniques to study cellular membranes, the data interpretation is generally obscured by the compositional complexity of native membranes. Generally, these classical biophysical techniques lack spatially resolved information at the level of *single* membranes, a quality that can be provided by microscopy-related techniques (e.g., AFM and fluorescence microscopy). For example, imaging strategies such as fluorescence microscopy can be applied similarly in cells and some membrane models (e.g., GUVs and planar supported membranes) offering good possibilities to infer experimental correlations between these different experimental systems.

1.3 DIRECT VISUALIZATION OF LIPID DOMAINS IN GUVs USING FLUORESCENCE MICROSCOPY

1.3.1 GIANT UNILAMELLAR VESICLES AND FLUORESCENT DYES FOR MICROSCOPY EXPERIMENTS

GUVs have become popular objects as a versatile laboratory to study lateral membrane structure. One of the reasons is that the dimensions of GUVs (mean diameter, ~30 μm) are larger than the intrinsic resolution limit of light microscopy–related techniques (~250 nm radial in the visible light range), allowing observation of structural details in membrane organization practically above ~300 nm. The particular size of GUVs permits experiments to be carried out at the level of single vesicles on the same length scale as some natural membrane systems (cell plasma membrane, for example) or alternatively exploring curvature effects by pulling tubes using micropipettes.[59] Since the experiments are performed at the level of single vesicles, heterogeneity in shape and size or the presence of multilamellar vesicles, often complicating studies of vesicle suspensions, is ruled out. Modern laser-scanning confocal microcopy imaging allows for sectioning images of a selected liposome in a stack of two-dimensional images from which a three-dimensional image can be reconstructed as illustrated in Figure 1.1.

One of the first studies using GUVs and optical microscopy derives from the early 1980s, where the micropipette aspiration technique was adapted and developed by the group of Evans[60–62] to study mechanical properties of lipid membranes using compositionally simple GUVs (i.e., composed of single phospholipid species or mixtures with cholesterol). Interestingly, it was not until 1999 that a wider application of fluorescence microscopy–related techniques was applied to GUVs, although some seminal experiments on GUVs using fluorescence microscopy was reported in the late 1980s from the group of Glaser.[63] One of the significant aspects in using giant vesicles as model systems is the ability to control membrane composition as well as distinct environmental conditions. Although original studies on membranes' lateral structure were restricted to GUVs composed of single lipids or mixtures with few lipid components,[64–79] it is also possible to form giant vesicles from natural lipid

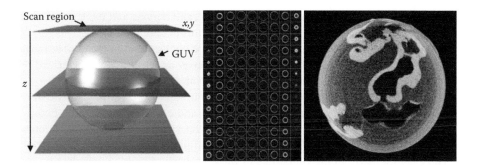

FIGURE 1.1   Laser-scanning fluorescence confocal microscopy of a GUV (left), showing consecutive sections (fluorescent images) along the axial direction (middle). This stack of fluorescent images is used to reconstruct a three-dimensional picture of the GUV (right). The GUV composition is POPC/ceramide/cholesterol 2:1:1 mol and the vesicle diameter is 30 μm.

extracts[67,80–84] and native membranes.[80,85–87] Additionally, GUVs containing membrane proteins can also be generated.[86,88–94]

Many different protocols have been reported in the literature for preparation of GUVs.[86,89,91,95–103] This plethora of methods may likely reflect a lack of understanding of the mechanisms underlying giant vesicle formation. Most (but not all) of these protocols are based on two main experimental methods: the gentle hydration method, originally described by Reeves and Dowben,[98] and the electroformation method introduced by Angelova and collaborators.[96,103] Of these two experimental protocols, the electroformation method has the advantage because it provides a more homogeneous population of GUVs, with sizes between 5 and 100 μm in diameter.[104,105] More recently, an approach based on inverted emulsions of lipids,[102,106] methods involving microfluidics,[100] or gel-assisted formation of GUVs[101,107] have opened a very interesting alternative to produce giant vesicles. These methods allow for easy control of lipid composition, incorporation of substances in the GUVs' lumen, and, importantly, formation of asymmetric membranes,[100,102] something that it is not possible to achieve by electroformation or gentle hydration methods when the starting point includes mixtures of lipids in organic solvents or small vesicles whose bilayers are compositionally symmetric. It has been shown, however, that asymmetry in some cases can be generated after GUV electroformation, for example, a simple method using mβCD-mediated lipid exchange was reported to modify the composition of the outer leaflet of the GUV bilayer leading to asymmetric GUVs.[108] Regarding native membranes, Montes et al. showed that asymmetry is maintained in GUVs produced from red blood cell membranes[86] by subjecting erythrocyte ghosts to electroformation. Also, Baumgart et al. showed that the formation of GUVs composed of asymmetric innate plasma membranes is possible by inducing blebbing in live cells.[87] Additional information about the giant vesicle field can be found in an excellent review by Menger and Keiper[109] and a book completely devoted to giant vesicles edited by Luisi and Walde.[110]

A large pool of choices of amphiphilic fluorescent probes is presently available to facilitate fluorescence microscopy experiments. Taking into account the partitioning properties between coexisting membrane regions and the capability of the probes to respond to environmental changes, this pool of fluorescent dyes can be split into two families. The first family includes probes excited in the visible range (used in wide-field and confocal fluorescence microscopy) that are characterized by exhibiting uneven partitioning between coexisting membrane regions.[65,69,71,111–113] Examples are amphiphilic derivatives of rhodamines, fluoresceins, dialkylcarbocyanines (DiI, DiO), dialkylaminostyryls (DiA), and coumarins, including bodipy, perylene, and naphtopyrene. The partitioning properties of this family of fluorescence probes have been used as criteria to assign lipid phases in GUVs.[113] However, changes in the partitioning properties of these probes are highly dependent on the chemical composition of the local membrane domain and not necessarily on the phase state.[65,77,113] A practical solution to avoid artifacts is the use of complementary methods such as fluorescence correlation spectroscopy (FCS),[69,71] where the diffusion of the probe can be measured to report on the lateral packing of a given membrane region. The second family of probes includes environmentally sensitive membrane dyes and polarity-sensitive probes. These molecules are generally UV-fading probes, rendering them less useful for conventional fluorescence microscopy experiments since the extent of photobleaching is high and therefore it is often technically difficult to obtain reliable fluorescence images. However, an alternative method to exploit these types of fluorophores in GUV experiments is to use multiphoton excitation fluorescence microscopy, where the 6-dodecanoyl-2-dimethylaminonaphthalene (LAURDAN) probe is a good example.[113–118] Perhaps one of the most remarkable features of these probes (particularly the ones that have a fatty acid-like structure, i.e., DPH, LAURDAN, and parinaric acid) is the fact that they show an even distribution in membranes displaying phase coexistence, allowing simultaneous spatially resolved information on fluorescence parameters (spectral shift, polarization, or lifetimes) from the whole membrane. Other recently reported polarity-sensitive probes are 3-hydroxyflavone derivatives,[119] C-LAURDAN,[120] and di-4-ANEPPDHQ.[121] These probes not only show different emission spectra depending on the membrane phase but also exhibit an even probe distribution in membranes displaying lateral phase separation.

Finally, it is important to point out that potential detrimental effects of fluorescent reporters on the supramolecular properties of membranes are always an issue raised when GUV data are discussed. Recently, it has been shown for some fluorophores (even at concentrations up to 2% mol with respect to total lipid) that the mechanical properties of the model membranes are not affected compared with membranes devoid of probes.[122] In any case, this is an important aspect, and control experiments to check potential artifacts are highly recommended.[123]

1.3.2 FLUORESCENCE MICROSCOPY STUDIES OF GUVs

A seminal study involving membranes and fluorescence microscopy was reported by McConnell et al. in 1984.[124] This work first reports on the visualization and physical characterization of lipid domains in monomolecular lipid films composed of DPPC at the air–water interface. This lipid monolayer is doped with a lipid-like fluorescent probe. Upon compression, the probe preferentially distributes into one of the two particular regions developed in the film in a particular lateral pressure interval. This phenomenon allowed the authors to obtain fluorescence images of the lipid film at different lateral pressures and to characterize the physical behavior of these distinct membrane regions. However, this very appealing experimental strategy was not applied to free-standing membranes until 1988 where Haverstick and Glaser reported on the first visualization of membrane patches in GUVs using wide-field fluorescence microscopy.[63] These authors directly visualized Ca^{2+}-induced membrane domains in several types of GUVs composed of either mixtures of unsaturated diacylphosphatidylcholines/diacylphosphatidylethanolamines/diacylphosphatidic acid, natural lipid extracts from erythrocyte membranes, or directly on membranes from intact erythrocyte ghosts.[63,125] Nevertheless, it was not until 1999–2001 that seminal papers appeared in the literature using confocal fluorescence microscopy techniques (laser-scanning confocal fluorescence microscopy combined with FCS or two-photon excitation fluorescence microscopy using polarity sensitive probes) to demonstrate membrane lateral heterogeneity in GUVs composed of single phospholipids, phospholipid binary mixtures, and ternary lipid mixtures containing phospholipids, sphingolipids, and cholesterol, at different temperatures and composition.[64,65,67,68,71,77] These papers showed for the first time images of different micrometer-sized lipid domains in bilayers, including dynamical information from the coexisting membrane regions.[64,65,67,77] The presence of distinct membrane domains was related to the coexistence of equilibrium thermodynamic phases, that is, so/ld or lo/ld. Particular features of these domains were pointed out to be their shape (elongated, flower shape, snowflake-like, and circular, to mention a few) and their size dependence on lipid composition and temperature.[64,65,67,68,71,77] Additionally, in all cases reported from GUVs, the domains were found to span the lipid bilayer. That this observation cannot be generalized to all types of lipid bilayer systems was demonstrated by the finding that lipid domains in supported planar membranes can be decoupled; that is, domains can form independently in the two leaflets of the bilayer owing to the interaction with the substrate.[126–128]

Several studies exploring membrane-domain coexistence were recently reported using similar approaches, particularly involving wide-field fluorescence microscopy as an alternative technique.[73] Most of these studies explored "canonical" raft mixtures, generally composed of unsaturated phospholipids, single or natural mixtures of SM, and cholesterol (though in some cases, SM has been replaced by DPPC).[66,70,73,74,112,113] Other studies involved mixtures containing other sphingolipids (ceramides and cerebrosides), phospholipids, and cholesterol.[78,129,130] It is noteworthy that the experimental data involving fluorescence microscopy and GUVs have offered a new alternative to construct lipid phase diagrams.[69,73,112] Finally, the partitioning of particular membrane proteins (e.g., those relevant to the raft hypothesis) into membranes displaying lo/ld phase coexistence has also been explored using GUVs subjected to fluorescence microscopy.[87,88,90,93]

In order to illustrate the imaging capabilities of fluorescence microscopy of GUVs, Figure 1.2a–c provides a gallery of images for three representative binary lipid mixtures and Figure 1.2d–f provides similar images for three representative ternary lipid mixtures.

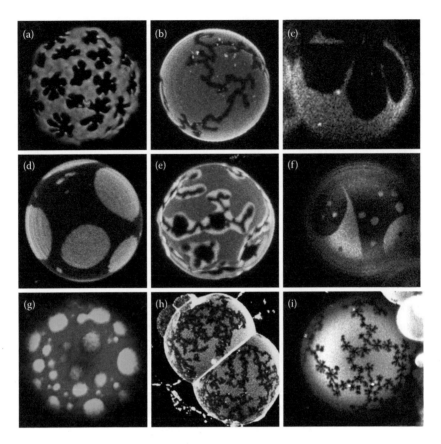

FIGURE 1.2   Gallery of GUV images (false color representation). The images are grouped in rows according to their compositional complexity. The first row shows binary mixtures: (a) egg-sphingomyelin (SM)/egg-ceramide 9:1 mol, (b) C_{12}-SM/C_{12}-ceramide-1-phosphate 9:1 mol, and (c) DLPC/DAPC 1:1 mol. The second row shows ternary mixtures: (d) DOPC/DPPC/cholesterol 2:2:1 mol, (e) POPC/cerebroside/cholesterol 2:1:1 mol, and (f) DOPC/SM/cholesterol 1:1:1 mol. The third row shows natural membranes: (g) native lung surfactant from pig, (h) skin lipids from stratum corneum membranes (the ratio between ceramides/cholesterol/fatty acid is ~1:0.9:0.4 mol), and (i) polar lipid fraction E from archaebacteria. The mean diameter of the different vesicles is approximately 25 μm. The fluorescent probes used were DiIC18 (a, b, e, and h), LAURDAN (f and i), DiIC18/Bodipy-PC (d and g), and Rhodamine-PE (c).

1.4   REPRESENTATIVE EXAMPLES ON GUVs/ FLUORESCENCE MICROSCOPY STUDIES

1.4.1   EQUILIBRIUM THERMODYNAMIC STUDIES

GUV experiments have been used to construct phase diagrams for different lipid mixtures.[69,73,112] Most of the reported data used fluorescent images of GUVs obtained under fluorescence wide-field illumination,[73] and only in a single case was information on the probe's diffusional characteristics exploited.[69] The data utilized for the construction of the phase diagram consist of partial images of GUVs (not fully three-dimensional) in which the visual appearance or vanishing of micron-sized lipid domains is observed for a given lipid composition at selected temperatures. However, the lateral resolution limit of fluorescence microscopes precludes detection of possible nanoscopic lipid domains (below ~300 nm). In this respect, questions have been raised about the accuracy in describing the complete phase diagram of different lipid mixtures using this approach. Indeed, some discrepancies have been noted for the phase diagram of ternary mixtures of palmitoyl-SM/POPC/cholesterol obtained from fluorescence microscopy[74] and fluorescence spectroscopy experiments, respectively (e.g., Förster resonance energy transfer experiment in LUVs).[35,131]

Recently, some novel image analysis protocols have been tested to analyze data obtained from fluorescence microscopy experiments involving GUVs. These protocols allow quantitative information on morpho-topological parameters from GUVs displaying phase coexistence. For example, Fidorra et al.[132] reported a novel analytical procedure for measuring the surface areas of coexisting lipid domains in GUVs. The method is based on three-dimensional image processing. The procedure involves deconvolution and further segmentation of the obtained images (fluorescence image stacks of GUVs), followed by reconstruction in three dimensions of the surface of the GUVs, permitting information to be extracted on domain area and perimeter, at the level of single vesicles.[132] Obtaining area fractions at different compositions allowed scrutiny of the thermodynamic lever rule from an already known phase diagram. In the work of Fidorra et al.,[132] the lever rule was validated for 10–15 randomly selected DLPC/DPPC GUVs per molar fraction, using domain-area fractions. These experiments confirm a correspondence of the observation of membrane domains with equilibrium thermodynamic phases. In a comparable way, Juhasz et al.[133] showed that the lever rule also applies to GUVs composed of DOPC/DPPC/cholesterol using fluorescence microscopy, showing a correlation with tie lines already obtained using NMR experiments. Recently, Husen et al.[134] demonstrated that the data obtained from fluorescence microscopy can be analyzed using refined image analysis approaches[135] to obtain information on the orientation and length of tie lines in ternary mixtures containing cholesterol, without the necessity to use tie-line information obtained by other methods. This idea has also been explored by Bezlyepkina et al. for mixtures of DOPC/eSM/cholesterol.[136]

All these observations support the fact that GUVs are indeed reliable model systems for performing equilibrium thermodynamic studies of membranes provided the proper steps are taken during the preparation procedure and the acquisition of the images, that is, particularly limiting light exposure and checking for oxidation if unsaturated lipids are used in the samples.[123]

1.4.2 SPECIALIZED BIOLOGICAL MEMBRANES

Imaging techniques have consistently failed to reveal large-scale laterally segregated structures in the plasma membranes of living cells. For example, micron-sized membrane domains enriched in glycosylphosphatidylinositol-anchored proteins (considered one of the major "raft components" in the so-called raft hypothesis) have not been seen using conventional fluorescence microcopy[137] (except if coalescence is promoted by antibody cross-linking, for example). These observations suggest that membrane domains may be much smaller than those found in artificial membrane systems and hence undetectable by the limited resolution of conventional optical microscopy and extremely dynamic or simply fast compositional fluctuations. However, the rich compositional diversity and associated physical characteristics of natural membranes enable, in some cases, the observation of micrometer-sized structures as illustrated in Figure 1.2g–i.

A visual correlation between cholesterol-containing ternary mixtures (DOPC/DPPC/Chol) with a peculiar type of natural membrane, viz, pulmonary surfactant bilayer, has been reported using laser-scanning confocal and multiphoton excitation fluorescence microscopy.[80,83] This material, which contains an important amount of DPPC (~40 mol% weight), cholesterol, and unsaturated lipids, including a low fraction of membrane proteins (~10% in weight), shows coexistence of two different liquid-like domains at physiological temperatures.[80,83,138] It is inferred that a relatively slow molecular turnover may exist in this membrane upon secretion from pneumocyte type II cells. Therefore, local equilibrium conditions are prone to prevail, allowing correlation of these domains with equilibrium thermodynamic phases (of the type of lo/ld phase coexistence). Among other observations, studies on lung surfactants demonstrate that removal of cholesterol, but not removal of hydrophobic proteins, from this material significantly alters the observed membrane lateral structure.[80] Interestingly, for studies performed with lung surfactant from mice, the molar ratios obtained from mass spectrometry experiments between MPS saturated and unsaturated phospholipids and cholesterol (39:43:18 mol) coincide with a region in the DOPC/DPPC/cholesterol phase diagram where ld/lo-like phase coexistence occurs.[83] The coexistence of liquid domains observed in native pulmonary surfactants at physiological temperatures has been linked with functional properties of this material.[80] In particular, it was reported that upon extraction of cholesterol, the spreading capabilities associated with the function of lung surfactant were impaired, suggesting that liquid immiscibility may be a requirement for optimal lung surfactant function. All these observations, which to a large extent are based on studies of GUVs with the natural material, indicate that pulmonary surfactant could be one of the first membranous systems reported where the coexistence of specialized membrane domains may exist as a structural basis for its function.[80]

Finally, another interesting example of the possible existence of coexisting thermodynamic lipid phases in biological membranes pertains to skin stratum corneum lipid membranes. These membranes are composed of saturated ceramides with very long chains, cholesterol, and long-chain free fatty acids (lacking glycerophospholipids and SM). In experiments using excised pig, mice, and human skin, it was shown that these membranes display a gel-like character, being one of the very few functional biological membranes exhibiting this type of membrane organization.[139–142] Hydrated bilayers, (freestanding) giant structures composed of lipid mixtures extracted from human skin, were directly visualized using fluorescence microscopy techniques.[143] At skin physiological temperatures (28°C–32°C), the state of these hydrated bilayers corresponds microscopically (radial resolution limit, 300 nm) to a single gel phase at pH 7. However, coexistence of two distinct micrometer-sized gel-like lipid domains is observed between pH 5 and 6, and no fluid phase is observed at the pH range explored (5 to 8). This observation suggests that the proton activity gradient existing in the stratum corneum could distinctly influence the physical properties of the extracellular lipid matrix, affecting membrane lateral structure and stability. Again, in this case, local equilibrium conditions may be asserted, since a slow molecular turnover is expected after the membranes reach the stratum corneum (upon secretion from specialized cells as lamellar bodies, similar to that described for lung surfactant membranes).

1.5   CHALLENGES AND FUTURE PERSPECTIVES

GUVs have established themselves as one of the more versatile laboratories for studying lateral membrane structure under highly controlled conditions using a range of fluorescence microscopy techniques. Special fluorescent probes with distinct spectroscopic properties report back not only on lateral organization but also on structural properties of lipid domains. The GUVs can be formed both by simple lipid mixtures and by lipid and protein material from natural membranes, allowing for comparison between simple and more complex models of biological membranes. Some advances have been made recently regarding resolving issues of finite-size effects and to which extent GUVs can represent the thermodynamic state of membranes.[132–134] A major challenge has been and still is to take the study of GUVs beyond the stage of "pretty pictures." Advanced image analysis involving image deconvolution and faithful quantitative reconstruction of curved two-dimensional areas on the three-dimensional liposomes has shown the way.[132,135] A major shortcoming of fluorescence microscopy imaging of GUVs is the inherent spatial resolution dictated by the diffraction limit of visible light. Sophisticated super-resolution techniques and fast image recording, for example, stimulated emission depletion microscopy,[144] may eventually be part of the solution to this challenge.

Most of the membrane systems that have been studied by fluorescence imaging of GUVs strive to image the systems as close as possible to thermodynamic equilibrium. Some studies have revealed dynamics of phase separation and the time evolution of the domain patterns.[73,145] Still, the most exciting challenge would be to use GUVs to study biologically functioning and active membranes under fully controlled conditions to study the interplay between protein function and the lateral organization of membranes. A recent study of GUVs incorporated with actively ion-pumping Na^+,K^+-ATPase revealed that the impact of the lipid–protein interactions on the nonequilibrium mechanics of the GUV is very substantial in terms of membrane softening,[94] an effect that may turn out to be reflected in the lateral organization of the different lipid species and the protein in the plane of the bilayer.

ACKNOWLEDGMENT

This work was supported in part by a grant from the Danish Research Councils (11-107269).

REFERENCES

1. Mouritsen, O. G. "Lipidology and Lipidomics—Quo Vadis? A New Era for the Physical Chemistry of Lipids." *Phys Chem Chem Phys* 13, no. 43 (2011): 19195–205.
2. Phillips, M. C., B. D. Ladbrooke, and D. Chapman. "Molecular Interactions in Mixed Lecithin Systems." *Biochim Biophys Acta* 196, no. 1 (1970): 35–44.
3. Shimshick, E. J., and H. M. McConnell. "Lateral Phase Separation in Phospholipid Membranes." *Biochemistry* 12, no. 12 (1973): 2351–60.
4. Grant, C. W., S. H. Wu, and H. M. McConnell. "Lateral Phase Separations in Binary Lipid Mixtures: Correlation between Spin Label and Freeze-Fracture Electron Microscopic Studies." *Biochim Biophys Acta* 363, no. 2 (1974): 151–8.
5. Lentz, B. R., Y. Barenholz, and T. E. Thompson. "Fluorescence Depolarization Studies of Phase Transitions and Fluidity in Phospholipid Bilayers. 2 Two-Component Phosphatidylcholine Liposomes." *Biochemistry* 15, no. 20 (1976): 4529–37.
6. Schmidt, C. F., Y. Barenholz, and T. E. Thompson. "A Nuclear Magnetic Resonance Study of Sphingomyelin in Bilayer Systems." *Biochemistry* 16, no. 12 (1977): 2649–56.
7. Gebhardt, C., H. Gruler, and E. Sackmann. "On Domain Structure and Local Curvature in Lipid Bilayers and Biological Membranes." *Z Naturforsch C* 32, no. 7–8 (1977): 581–96.
8. Marcelja, S. "Lipid-Mediated Protein Interaction in Membranes." *Biochim Biophys Acta* 455, no. 1 (1976): 1–7.
9. Sackmann, E. "Physical Basis for Trigger Processes and Membrane Structures." In *Biological Membranes*, edited by D. Chapman, 105–43. London: Academic Press, 1984.
10. Op den Kamp, J. A. "Lipid Asymmetry in Membranes." *Annu Rev Biochem* 48 (1979): 47–71.
11. Thompson, T. E., and T. W. Tillack. "Organization of Glycosphingolipids in Bilayers and Plasma Membranes of Mammalian Cells." *Annu Rev Biophys Biophys Chem* 14 (1985): 361–86.
12. Träuble, H. "Membrane Electrostatics." In *Structure of Biological Membranes*, edited by S. Abrahamsson and I. Pascher, 509–50. New York: Plenum, 1976.
13. Vaz, W. L. C., and P. F. F. Almeida. "Phase Topology and Percolation in Multi-Phase Lipid Bilayers: Is the Biological Membrane a Domain Mosaic?" *Curr Opin Struc Biol* 3 (1993): 482–8.
14. Singer, S. J., and G. L. Nicolson. "The Fluid Mosaic Model of the Structure of Cell Membranes." *Science* 175, no. 23 (1972): 720–31.
15. Jain, M. K., and H. B. White III. "Long-Range Order in Biomembranes." *Adv Lipid Res* 15 (1977): 1–60.
16. Israelachvili, J. N. "Refinement of the Fluid-Mosaic Model of Membrane Structure." *Biochim Biophys Acta* 469, no. 2 (1977): 221–5.
17. Mouritsen, O. G., and M. Bloom. "Mattress Model of Lipid–Protein Interactions in Membranes." *Biophys J* 46, no. 2 (1984): 141–53.
18. Sackmann, E. "Biological Membranes. Architecture and Function." In *Handbook of Biological Physics*, edited by R. Lipowski and E. Sackmann, 1–63. Amsterdam: Elsevier, 1995.
19. Bagatolli, L. A., J. H. Ipsen, A. C. Simonsen, and O. G. Mouritsen. "An Outlook on Organization of Lipids in Membranes: Searching for a Realistic Connection with the Organization of Biological Membranes." *Prog Lipid Res* 49, no. 4 (2010): 378–89.
20. Bagatolli, L. A. "Membrane Domains and Their Relevance to the Organization of Biological Membranes." In *Comprehensive Biophysics*, edited by L. Tamm, 16–36. Amsterdam: Academic Press, 2012.
21. Mouritsen, O. G., and O. S. Andersen, eds. In *Search of a New Biomembrane Model. Biol Skr Dan Vid Selsk* 49, 1–214, 1998.

22. Cantor, R. S. "The Lateral Pressure Profile in Membranes: A Physical Mechanism of General Anesthesia." *Biochemistry* 36, no. 9 (1997): 2339–44.

23. Miao, L., U. Seifert, M. Wortis, and H. G. Dobereiner. "Budding Transitions of Fluid-Bilayer Vesicles: The Effect of Area-Difference Elasticity." *Phys Rev E Stat Phys Plasmas Fluids Relat Interdiscip Topics* 49, no. 6 (1994): 5389–407.

24. Seddon, J. M., and R. H. Templer. "Polymorphism of Lipid-Water Systems." In *Handbook of Biological Physics*, edited by R. Lipowsky and E. Sackmann, 97–160. Amsterdam: Elsevier, 1995.

25. Lundbaek, J. A., S. A. Collingwood, H. I. Ingolfsson, R. Kapoor, and O. S. Andersen. "Lipid Bilayer Regulation of Membrane Protein Function: Gramicidin Channels as Molecular Force Probes." *J R Soc Interface* 7, no. 44 (2010): 373–95.

26. Simons, K., and G. van Meer. "Lipid Sorting in Epithelial Cells." *Biochemistry* 27, no. 17 (1988): 6197–202.

27. Simons, K., and E. Ikonen. "Functional Rafts in Cell Membranes." *Nature* 387, no. 6633 (1997): 569–72.

28. Ipsen, J. H., G. Karlstrom, O. G. Mouritsen, H. Wennerstrom, and M. J. Zuckermann. "Phase Equilibria in the Phosphatidylcholine-Cholesterol System." *Biochim Biophys Acta* 905, no. 1 (1987): 162–72.

29. Mouritsen, O. G. "The Liquid-Ordered State Comes of Age." *Biochim Biophys Acta* 1798, no. 7 (2010): 1286–8.

30. Rheinstädter, M. C., and O. G. Mouritsen. "Small-Scale Structure in Fluid Cholesterol-Lipid Bilayers." *Curr Opin Colloid Int Sci* 18 (2013): 440–7.

31. Mouritsen, O. G. *Life—as a Matter of Fat. The Emerging Science of Lipidomics*. Berlin, Heidelberg: Springer Verlag, 2005.

32. Veatch, S. L., O. Soubias, S. L. Keller, and K. Gawrisch. "Critical Fluctuations in Domain-Forming Lipid Mixtures." *Proc Natl Acad Sci U S A* 104, no. 45 (2007): 17650–5.

33. Honerkamp-Smith, A. R., P. Cicuta, M. D. Collins et al. "Line Tensions, Correlation Lengths, and Critical Exponents in Lipid Membranes near Critical Points." *Biophys J* 95, no. 1 (2008): 236–46.

34. Mouritsen, O. G., and K. Jorgensen. "Dynamic Lipid-Bilayer Heterogeneity: A Mesoscopic Vehicle for Membrane Function?" *Bioessays* 14, no. 2 (1992): 129–36.

35. Goni, F. M., A. Alonso, L. A. Bagatolli et al. "Phase Diagrams of Lipid Mixtures Relevant to the Study of Membrane Rafts." *Biochim Biophys Acta* 1781, no. 11–12 (2008): 665–84.

36. Mouritsen, O. G., and K. Jorgensen. "Dynamical Order and Disorder in Lipid Bilayers." *Chem Phys Lipids* 73, no. 1–2 (1994): 3–25.

37. Pencer, J., T. T. Mills, N. Kucerka, M. P. Nieh, and J. Katsaras. "Small-Angle Neutron Scattering to Detect Rafts and Lipid Domains." *Methods Mol Biol* 398 (2007): 231–44.

38. Armstrong, C. L., D. Marquardt, H. Dies et al. "The Observation of Highly Ordered Domains in Membranes with Cholesterol." *PLoS One* 8, no. 6 (2013): e66162.

39. Armstrong, C. L., M. A. Barrett, L. Toppozini et al. "Co-Existence of Gel and Fluid Domains in Single-Component Phospholipid Membranes." *Soft Matter* 8 (2012): 4687–94.

40. Parasassi, T., M. Loiero, M. Raimondi, G. Ravagnan, and E. Gratton. "Absence of Lipid Gel-Phase Domains in Seven Mammalian Cell Lines and in Four Primary Cell Types." *Biochim Biophys Acta* 1153, no. 2 (1993): 143–54.

41. Almeida, P. F., W. L. Vaz, and T. E. Thompson. "Lateral Diffusion and Percolation in Two-Phase, Two-Component Lipid Bilayers. Topology of the Solid-Phase Domains in-Plane and across the Lipid Bilayer." *Biochemistry* 31, no. 31 (1992): 7198–210.

42. Schram, V., H. N. Lin, and T. E. Thompson. "Topology of Gel-Phase Domains and Lipid Mixing Properties in Phase-Separated Two-Component Phosphatidylcholine Bilayers." *Biophys J* 71, no. 4 (1996): 1811–22.

43. Shimshick, E. J., and H. M. McConnell. "Lateral Phase Separations in Binary Mixtures of Cholesterol and Phospholipids." *Biochem Biophys Res Commun* 53, no. 2 (1973): 446–51.

44. Arnold, K., A. Losche, and K. Gawrisch. "31p-NMR Investigations of Phase Separation in Phosphatidylcholine/Phosphatidylethanolamine Mixtures." *Biochim Biophys Acta* 645, no. 1 (1981): 143–8.

45. Blume, A., R. J. Wittebort, S. K. Das Gupta, and R. G. Griffin. "Phase Equilibria, Molecular Conformation, and Dynamics in Phosphatidylcholine/Phosphatidylethanolamine Bilayers." *Biochemistry* 21, no. 24 (1982): 6243–53.

46. Mabrey, S., and J. M. Sturtevant. "Investigation of Phase Transitions of Lipids and Lipid Mixtures by Sensitivity Differential Scanning Calorimetry." *Proc Natl Acad Sci U S A* 73, no. 11 (1976): 3862–6.

47. van Dijck, P. W., A. J. Kaper, H. A. Oonk, and J. de Gier. "Miscibility Properties of Binary Phosphatidylcholine Mixtures. A Calorimetric Study." *Biochim Biophys Acta* 470, no. 1 (1977): 58–69.

48. Maggio, B. "Geometric and Thermodynamic Restrictions for the Self-Assembly of Glycosphingolipid-Phospholipid Systems." *Biochim Biophys Acta* 815, no. 2 (1985): 245–58.

49. Caffrey, M., and F. S. Hing. "A Temperature Gradient Method for Lipid Phase Diagram Construction Using Time-Resolved X-Ray Diffraction." *Biophys J* 51, no. 1 (1987): 37–46.

50. Kucerka, N., J. F. Nagle, J. N. Sachs et al. "Lipid Bilayer Structure Determined by the Simultaneous Analysis of Neutron and X-Ray Scattering Data." *Biophys J* 95, no. 5 (2008): 2356–67.

51. Mills, T. T., S. Tristram-Nagle, F. A. Heberle et al. "Liquid-Liquid Domains in Bilayers Detected by Wide Angle X-Ray Scattering." *Biophys J* 95, no. 2 (2008): 682–90.

52. Jorgensen, K., and O. G. Mouritsen. "Phase Separation Dynamics and Lateral Organization of Two-Component Lipid Membranes." *Biophys J* 69, no. 3 (1995): 942–54.

53. Meinhardt, S., R. L. Vink, and F. Schmid. "Monolayer Curvature Stabilizes Nanoscale Raft Domains in Mixed Lipid Bilayers." *Proc Natl Acad Sci U S A* 110, no. 12 (2013): 4476–81.

54. Almeida, P. F. "A Simple Thermodynamic Model of the Liquid-Ordered State and the Interactions between Phospholipids and Cholesterol." *Biophys J* 100, no. 2 (2011): 420–9.

55. Amazon, J. J., S. L. Goh, and G. W. Feigenson. "Competition between Line Tension and Curvature Stabilizes Modulated Phase Patterns on the Surface of Giant Unilamellar Vesicles: A Simulation Study." *Phys Rev E Stat Nonlin Soft Matter Phys* 87, no. 2 (2013): 022708.

56. Bagatolli, L. A. "Lipid Membrane Technology." In *Encyclopedia of Applied Biophysics*, edited by H. Bohr, 711–40. Berlin: Wiley-VCH, 2009.

57. Bangham, A. D., and R. W. Horne. "Negative Staining of Phospholipids and Their Structural Modification by Surface-Active Agents as Observed in the Electron Microscope." *J Mol Biol* 8 (1964): 660–8.

58. Lasic, D. D., and D. Papahadjopoulos. "Liposomes Revisited." *Science* 267, no. 5202 (1995): 1275–6.

59. Callan-Jones, A., B. Sorre, and P. Bassereau. "Curvature-Driven Lipid Sorting in Biomembranes." *Cold Spring Harb Perspect Biol* 3, no. 2 (2011): a004648.

60. Evans, E., and R. Kwok. "Mechanical Calorimetry of Large Dimyristoylphosphatidylcholine Vesicles in the Phase Transition Region." *Biochemistry* 21, no. 20 (1982): 4874–9.

61. Evans, E., and D. Needham. "Physical-Properties of Surfactant Bilayer-Membranes—Thermal Transitions, Elasticity, Rigidity, Cohesion, and Colloidal Interactions." *J Phys Chem* 91, no. 16 (1987): 4219–28.

62. Kwok, R., and E. Evans. "Thermoelasticity of Large Lecithin Bilayer Vesicles." *Biophys J* 35, no. 3 (1981): 637–52.
63. Haverstick, D. M., and M. Glaser. "Visualization of Ca^{2+}-Induced Phospholipid Domains." *Proc Natl Acad Sci U S A* 84, no. 13 (1987): 4475–9.
64. Bagatolli, L. A., and E. Gratton. "Two-Photon Fluorescence Microscopy Observation of Shape Changes at the Phase Transition in Phospholipid Giant Unilamellar Vesicles." *Biophys J* 77, no. 4 (1999): 2090–101.
65. Bagatolli, L. A., and E. Gratton. "A Correlation between Lipid Domain Shape and Binary Phospholipid Mixture Composition in Free Standing Bilayers: A Two-Photon Fluorescence Microscopy Study." *Biophys J* 79, no. 1 (2000): 434–47.
66. Baumgart, T., S. T. Hess, and W. W. Webb. "Imaging Coexisting Fluid Domains in Biomembrane Models Coupling Curvature and Line Tension." *Nature* 425, no. 6960 (2003): 821–4.
67. Dietrich, C., L. A. Bagatolli, Z. N. Volovyk et al. "Lipid Rafts Reconstituted in Model Membranes." *Biophys J* 80, no. 3 (2001): 1417–28.
68. Feigenson, G. W., and J. T. Buboltz. "Ternary Phase Diagram of Dipalmitoyl-PC/Dilauroyl-PC/Cholesterol: Nanoscopic Domain Formation Driven by Cholesterol." *Biophys J* 80, no. 6 (2001): 2775–88.
69. Kahya, N., D. Scherfeld, K. Bacia, B. Poolman, and P. Schwille. "Probing Lipid Mobility of Raft-Exhibiting Model Membranes by Fluorescence Correlation Spectroscopy." *J Biol Chem* 278, no. 30 (2003): 28109–15.
70. Kahya, N., D. Scherfeld, and P. Schwille. "Differential Lipid Packing Abilities and Dynamics in Giant Unilamellar Vesicles Composed of Short-Chain Saturated Glycerol-Phospholipids, Sphingomyelin and Cholesterol." *Chem Phys Lipids* 135, no. 2 (2005): 169–80.
71. Korlach, J., P. Schwille, W. W. Webb, and G. W. Feigenson. "Characterization of Lipid Bilayer Phases by Confocal Microscopy and Fluorescence Correlation Spectroscopy." *Proc Natl Acad Sci U S A* 96, no. 15 (1999): 8461–6.
72. Veatch, S. L., and S. L. Keller. "Organization in Lipid Membranes Containing Cholesterol." *Phys Rev Lett* 89, no. 26 (2002): 268101.
73. Veatch, S. L., and S. L. Keller. "Separation of Liquid Phases in Giant Vesicles of Ternary Mixtures of Phospholipids and Cholesterol." *Biophys J* 85, no. 5 (2003): 3074–83.
74. Veatch, S. L., and S. L. Keller. "Miscibility Phase Diagrams of Giant Vesicles Containing Sphingomyelin." *Phys Rev Lett* 94, no. 14 (2005): 148101.
75. Veatch, S. L., I. V. Polozov, K. Gawrisch, and S. L. Keller. "Liquid Domains in Vesicles Investigated by Nmr and Fluorescence Microscopy." *Biophys J* 86, no. 5 (2004): 2910–22.
76. Sot, J., L. A. Bagatolli, F. M. Goñi, and A. Alonso. "Detergent-Resistant, Ceramide-Enriched Domains in Sphingomyelin/Ceramide Bilayers." *Biophys J* 90 (2006): 903–14.
77. Bagatolli, L. A., and E. Gratton. "Two Photon Fluorescence Microscopy of Coexisting Lipid Domains in Giant Unilamellar Vesicles of Binary Phospholipid Mixtures." *Biophys J* 78, no. 1 (2000): 290–305.
78. Fidorra, M., L. Duelund, C. Leidy, A. C. Simonsen, and L. A. Bagatolli. "Absence of Fluid-Ordered/Fluid-Disordered Phase Coexistence in Ceramide/Popc Mixtures Containing Cholesterol." *Biophys J* 90, no. 12 (2006): 4437–51.
79. Bali, R., L. Savino, D. Ramirez, N. Tsvetkova, L. A. Bagatolli, F. Tablin, J. H. Crowe, and C. Leidy. "Macroscopic domain formation during cooling in the platelet plasma membrane: An issue of low cholesterol content." *Biochim. Biophys. Acta* 1788, no. 6 (2009): 1229–37.
80. Bernardino de la Serna, J., J. Perez-Gil, A. C. Simonsen, and L. A. Bagatolli. "Cholesterol Rules: Direct Observation of the Coexistence of Two Fluid Phases in Native Pulmonary Surfactant Membranes at Physiological Temperatures." *J Biol Chem* 279, no. 39 (2004): 40715–22.

81. Nag, K., J. S. Pao, R. R. Harbottle et al. "Segregation of Saturated Chain Lipids in Pulmonary Surfactant Films and Bilayers." *Biophys J* 82, no. 4 (2002): 2041–51.

82. Bagatolli, L. A., E. Gratton, T. K. Khan, and P. L. Chong. "Two-Photon Fluorescence Microscopy Studies of Bipolar Tetraether Giant Liposomes from Thermoacidophilic Archaebacteria Sulfolobus Acidocaldarius." *Biophys J* 79, no. 1 (2000): 416–25.

83. Bernardino de la Serna, J., S. Hansen, Z. Berzina et al. "Compositional and Structural Characterization of Monolayers and Bilayers Composed of Native Pulmonary Surfactant from Wild Type Mice." *Biochim Biophys Acta* 1828, no. 11 (2013): 2450–9.

84. Kubiak, J., J. Brewer, S. Hansen, and L. A. Bagatolli. "Lipid Lateral Organization on Giant Unilamellar Vesicles Containing Lipopolysaccharides." *Biophys J* 100, no. 4 (2011): 978–86.

85. Ruan, Q., M. A. Cheng, M. Levi, E. Gratton, and W. W. Mantulin. "Spatial-Temporal Studies of Membrane Dynamics: Scanning Fluorescence Correlation Spectroscopy (SFCS)." *Biophys J* 87, no. 2 (2004): 1260–7.

86. Montes, L. R., A. Alonso, F. M. Goni, and L. A. Bagatolli. "Giant Unilamellar Vesicles Electroformed from Native Membranes and Organic Lipid Mixtures under Physiological Conditions." *Biophys J* 93, no. 10 (2007): 3548–54.

87. Baumgart, T., A. T. Hammond, P. Sengupta et al. "Large-Scale Fluid/Fluid Phase Separation of Proteins and Lipids in Giant Plasma Membrane Vesicles." *Proc Natl Acad Sci U S A* 104, no. 9 (2007): 3165–70.

88. Bacia, K., C. G. Schuette, N. Kahya, R. Jahn, and P. Schwille. "Snares Prefer Liquid-Disordered over 'Raft' (Liquid-Ordered) Domains When Reconstituted into Giant Unilamellar Vesicles." *J Biol Chem* 279, no. 36 (2004): 37951–5.

89. Girard, P., J. Pecreaux, G. Lenoir et al. "A New Method for the Reconstitution of Membrane Proteins into Giant Unilamellar Vesicles." *Biophys J* 87, no. 1 (2004): 419–29.

90. Kahya, N., D. A. Brown, and P. Schwille. "Raft Partitioning and Dynamic Behavior of Human Placental Alkaline Phosphatase in Giant Unilamellar Vesicles." *Biochemistry* 44, no. 20 (2005): 7479–89.

91. Kahya, N., E. I. Pecheur, W. P. de Boeij, D. A. Wiersma, and D. Hoekstra. "Reconstitution of Membrane Proteins into Giant Unilamellar Vesicles Via Peptide-Induced Fusion." *Biophys J* 81, no. 3 (2001): 1464–74.

92. Koster, G., M. VanDuijn, B. Hofs, and M. Dogterom. "Membrane Tube Formation from Giant Vesicles by Dynamic Association of Motor Proteins." *Proc Natl Acad Sci U S A* 100, no. 26 (2003): 15583–8.

93. Kahya, N. "Targeting Membrane Proteins to Liquid-Ordered Phases: Molecular Self-Organization Explored by Fluorescence Correlation Spectroscopy." *Chem Phys Lipids* 141, no. 1–2 (2006): 158–68.

94. Bouvrais, H., F. Cornelius, J. H. Ipsen, and O. G. Mouritsen. "Intrinsic Reaction-Cycle Time Scale of Na+,K+-Atpase Manifests Itself in the Lipid–Protein Interactions of Nonequilibrium Membranes." *Proc Natl Acad Sci U S A* 109, no. 45 (2012): 18442–6.

95. Akashi, K., H. Miyata, H. Itoh, and K. Kinosita Jr. "Preparation of Giant Liposomes in Physiological Conditions and Their Characterization under an Optical Microscope." *Biophys J* 71, no. 6 (1996): 3242–50.

96. Angelova, M. I., and D. S. Dimitrov. "Liposome Electroformation." *Faraday Discuss Chem Soc* 81 (1986): 303–11.

97. Moscho, A., O. Orwar, D. T. Chiu, B. P. Modi, and R. N. Zare. "Rapid Preparation of Giant Unilamellar Vesicles." *Proc Natl Acad Sci U S A* 93, no. 21 (1996): 11443–7.

98. Reeves, J. P., and R. M. Dowben. "Formation and Properties of Thin-Walled Phospholipid Vesicles." *J Cell Physiol* 73, no. 1 (1969): 49–60.

99. Pott, T., H. Bouvrais, and P. Meleard. "Giant Unilamellar Vesicle Formation under Physiologically Relevant Conditions." *Chem Phys Lipids* 154, no. 2 (2008): 115–9.

100. Richmond, D. L., E. M. Schmid, S. Martens et al. "Forming Giant Vesicles with Controlled Membrane Composition, Asymmetry, and Contents." *Proc Natl Acad Sci U S A* 108, no. 23 (2011): 9431–6.

101. Horger, K. S., D. J. Estes, R. Capone, and M. Mayer. "Films of Agarose Enable Rapid Formation of Giant Liposomes in Solutions of Physiologic Ionic Strength." *J Am Chem Soc* 131, no. 5 (2009): 1810–9.

102. Pautot, S., B. J. Frisken, and D. A. Weitz. "Engineering Asymmetric Vesicles." *Proc Natl Acad Sci U S A* 100, no. 19 (2003): 10718–21.

103. Angelova, M. I., S. Soleau, P. Meleard, J. F. Faucon, and P. Bothorel. "Preparation of Giant Vesicles by External AC Electric-Fields—Kinetics and Applications." *Trends Colloid Interface Sci VI* 89 (1992): 127–31.

104. Bagatolli, L. A., T. Parasassi, and E. Gratton. "Giant Phospholipid Vesicles: Comparison among the Whole Lipid Sample Characteristics Using Different Preparation Methods: A Two Photon Fluorescence Microscopy Study." *Chem Phys Lipids* 105, no. 2 (2000): 135–47.

105. Düzgünes, N., L. A. Bagatolli, P. Meers, Y. K. Oh, and R. M. Straubinger. "Fluorescence Methods in Liposome Research." In *Liposomes: A Practical Approach* (2nd Edition), edited by V. Weissig and V. Torchilin, 105–47. Oxford: Oxford University Press, 2003.

106. Pautot, S., B. J. Frisken, and D. A. Weitz. "Production of Unilamellar Vesicles Using an Inverted Emulsion." *Langmuir* 19, no. 7 (2003): 2870–9.

107. Weinberger, A., F. C. Tsai, G. H. Koenderink et al. "Gel-Assisted Formation of Giant Unilamellar Vesicles." *Biophys J* 105 (2013): 154–64.

108. Chiantia, S., P. Schwille, A. S. Klymchenko, and E. London. "Asymmetric GUVs Prepared by MβCD-Mediated Lipid Exchange: An FCS Study." *Biophys J* 100, no. 1 (2011): L1–3.

109. Menger, F. M., and J. S. Keiper. "Chemistry and Physics of Giant Vesicles as Biomembrane Models." *Curr Opin Chem Biol* 2, no. 6 (1998): 726–32.

110. Luisi, P. L., and P. Walde, eds. *Giant Vesicles, Vol. 6, Perspectives in Supramolecular Chemistry*. Chichester: John Wiley & Sons, 2000.

111. Baumgart, T., G. Hunt, E. R. Farkas, W. W. Webb, and G. W. Feigenson. "Fluorescence Probe Partitioning between Lo/Ld Phases in Lipid Membranes." *Biochim Biophys Acta* 1768, no. 9 (2007): 2182–94.

112. Veatch, S. L., and S. L. Keller. "Seeing Spots: Complex Phase Behavior in Simple Membranes." *Biochim Biophys Acta* 1746, no. 3 (2005): 172–85.

113. Bagatolli, L. A. "To See or Not to See: Lateral Organization of Biological Membranes and Fluorescence Microscopy." *Biochim Biophys Acta* 1758, no. 10 (2006): 1541–56.

114. Celli, A., S. Beretta, and E. Gratton. "Phase Fluctuations on the Micron-Submicron Scale in Guvs Composed of a Binary Lipid Mixture." *Biophys J* 94, no. 1 (2008): 104–16.

115. Parasassi, T., E. Gratton, W. M. Yu, P. Wilson, and M. Levi. "Two-Photon Fluorescence Microscopy of Laurdan Generalized Polarization Domains in Model and Natural Membranes." *Biophys J* 72, no. 6 (1997): 2413–29.

116. Gaus, K., E. Gratton, E. P. Kable et al. "Visualizing Lipid Structure and Raft Domains in Living Cells with Two-Photon Microscopy." *Proc Natl Acad Sci U S A* 100, no. 26 (2003): 15554–9.

117. Bagatolli, L. A. "Laurdan Fluorescence Properties in Membranes: A Journey from the Fluorometer to the Microscope." In *Fluorescent Methods to Study Biological Membranes*, edited by Y. Mely and G. Duportail, 3–36. Heidelberg-New Springer, 2013.

118. Golfetto, O., E. Hinde, and E. Gratton. "Laurdan Fluorescence Lifetime Discriminates Cholesterol Content from Changes in Fluidity in Living Cell Membranes." *Biophys J* 104, no. 6 (2013): 1238–47.

119. M'Baye, G., Y. Mely, G. Duportail, and A. S. Klymchenko. "Liquid Ordered and Gel Phases of Lipid Bilayers: Fluorescent Probes Reveal Close Fluidity but Different Hydration." *Biophys J* 95, no. 3 (2008): 1217–25.

120. Kim, H. M., H. J. Choo, S. Y. Jung et al. "A Two-Photon Fluorescent Probe for Lipid Raft Imaging: C-Laurdan." *Chembiochem* 8, no. 5 (2007): 553–9.

121. Jin, L., A. C. Millard, J. P. Wuskell et al. "Characterization and Application of a New Optical Probe for Membrane Lipid Domains." *Biophys J* 90, no. 7 (2006): 2563–75.

122. Bouvrais, H., T. Pott, L. A. Bagatolli, J. H. Ipsen, and P. Meleard. "Impact of Membrane-Anchored Fluorescent Probes on the Mechanical Properties of Lipid Bilayers." *Biochim Biophys Acta* 1798, no. 7 (2010): 1333–7.

123. Morales-Penningston, N. F., J. Wu, E. R. Farkas et al. "GUV Preparation and Imaging: Minimizing Artifacts." *Biochim Biophys Acta* 1798, no. 7 (2010): 1324–32.

124. McConnell, H. M., L. K. Tamm, and R. M. Weis. "Periodic Structures in Lipid Monolayer Phase Transitions." *Proc Natl Acad Sci U S A* 81, no. 10 (1984): 3249–53.

125. Haverstick, D. M., and M. Glaser. "Visualization of Domain Formation in the Inner and Outer Leaflets of a Phospholipid Bilayer." *J Cell Biol* 106, no. 6 (1988): 1885–92.

126. Jensen, M. H., E. J. Morris, and A. C. Simonsen. "Domain Shapes, Coarsening, and Random Patterns in Ternary Membranes." *Langmuir* 23, no. 15 (2007): 8135–41.

127. Keller, D., N. B. Larsen, I. M. Moller, and O. G. Mouritsen. "Decoupled Phase Transitions and Grain-Boundary Melting in Supported Phospholipid Bilayers." *Phys Rev Lett* 94, no. 2 (2005): 025701.

128. Lin, W. C., C. D. Blanchette, T. V. Ratto, and M. L. Longo. "Lipid Asymmetry in DLPC/DSPC-Supported Lipid Bilayers: A Combined AFM and Fluorescence Microscopy Study." *Biophys J* 90, no. 1 (2006): 228–37.

129. Blanchette, C. D., W. C. Lin, T. V. Ratto, and M. L. Longo. "Galactosylceramide Domain Microstructure: Impact of Cholesterol and Nucleation/Growth Conditions." *Biophys J* 90, no. 12 (2006): 4466–78.

130. Fidorra, M., T. Heimburg, and L. A. Bagatolli. "Direct Visualization of the Lateral Structure of Porcine Brain Cerebrosides/POPC Mixtures in Presence and Absence of Cholesterol." *Biophys J* 97, no. 1 (2009): 142–54.

131. de Almeida, R. F., L. M. Loura, A. Fedorov, and M. Prieto. "Lipid Rafts Have Different Sizes Depending on Membrane Composition: A Time-Resolved Fluorescence Resonance Energy Transfer Study." *J Mol Biol* 346, no. 4 (2005): 1109–20.

132. Fidorra, M., A. Garcia, J. H. Ipsen, S. Hartel, and L. A. Bagatolli. "Lipid Domains in Giant Unilamellar Vesicles and Their Correspondence with Equilibrium Thermodynamic Phases: A Quantitative Fluorescence Microscopy Imaging Approach." *Biochim Biophys Acta* 1788, no. 10 (2009): 2142–9.

133. Juhasz, J., F. J. Sharom, and J. H. Davis. "Quantitative Characterization of Coexisting Phases in DOPC/DPPC/Cholesterol Mixtures: Comparing Confocal Fluorescence Microscopy and Deuterium Nuclear Magnetic Resonance." *Biochim Biophys Acta* 1788, no. 12 (2009): 2541–52.

134. Husen, P., L. R. Arriaga, F. Monroy, J. H. Ipsen, and L. A. Bagatolli. "Morphometric Image Analysis of Giant Vesicles: A New Tool for Quantitative Thermodynamics Studies of Phase Separation in Lipid Membranes." *Biophys J* 103, no. 11 (2012): 2304–10.

135. Husen, P., M. Fidorra, S. Hartel, L. A. Bagatolli, and J. H. Ipsen. "A Method for Analysis of Lipid Vesicle Domain Structure from Confocal Image Data." *Eur Biophys J* 41, no. 2 (2012): 161–75.

136. Bezlyepkina, N., R. S. Gracia, P. Shchelokovskyy, R. Lipowsky, and R. Dimova. "Phase Diagram and Tie-Line Determination for the Ternary Mixture DOPC/eSM/Cholesterol." *Biophys J* 104, no. 7 (2013): 1456–64.

137. Lingwood, D., and K. Simons. "Lipid Rafts as a Membrane-Organizing Principle." *Science* 327, no. 5961 (2010): 46–50.

138. Bernardino de la Serna, J., G. Oradd, L. A. Bagatolli et al. "Segregated Phases in Pulmonary Surfactant Membranes Do Not Show Coexistence of Lipid Populations with Differentiated Dynamic Properties." *Biophys J* 97, no. 5 (2009): 1381–9.

139. Carrer, D. C., C. Vermehren, and L. A. Bagatolli. "Pig Skin Structure and Transdermal Delivery of Liposomes: A Two Photon Microscopy Study." *J Control Release* 132, no. 1 (2008): 12–20.
140. Bloksgaard, M., S. Bek, A. B. Marcher et al. "The Acyl-CoA Binding Protein Is Required for Normal Epidermal Barrier Function in Mice." *J Lipid Res* 53, no. 10 (2012): 2162–74.
141. Iwai, I., H. Han, L. den Hollander et al. "The Human Skin Barrier Is Organized as Stacked Bilayers of Fully Extended Ceramides with Cholesterol Molecules Associated with the Ceramide Sphingoid Moiety." *J Invest Dermatol* 132, no. 9 (2012): 2215–25.
142. Bloksgaard, M., V. Svane-Knudsen, J. A. Sorensen, L. Bagatolli, and J. Brewer. "Structural Characterization and Lipid Composition of Acquired Cholesteatoma: A Comparative Study with Normal Skin." *Otol Neurotol* 33, no. 2 (2012): 177–83.
143. Plasencia, I., L. Norlen, and L. A. Bagatolli. "Direct Visualization of Lipid Domains in Human Skin Stratum Corneum's Lipid Membranes: Effect of pH and Temperature." *Biophys J* 93, no. 9 (2007): 3142–55.
144. Klar, T. A., E. Engel, and S. W. Hell. "Breaking Abbe's Diffraction Resolution Limit in Fluorescence Microscopy with Stimulated Emission Depletion Beams of Various Shapes." *Phys Rev E Stat Nonlin Soft Matter Phys* 64, no. 6 Pt 2 (2001): 066613.
145. Staneva, G., M. Seigneuret, H. Conjeaud, N. Puff, and M. I. Angelova. "Making a Tool of an Artifact: The Application of Photoinduced Lo Domains in Giant Unilamellar Vesicles to the Study of Lo/Ld Phase Spinodal Decomposition and Its Modulation by the Ganglioside GM1." *Langmuir* 27, no. 24 (2011): 15074–82.

2 An Active Basis for the Nanoscopic Organization of Membrane Components in Living Cell Membranes

Subhasri Ghosh and Satyajit Mayor

CONTENTS

2.1   INTRODUCTION

2.1.1   COMPOSITIONAL HETEROGENEITY IN THE PLASMA MEMBRANE

In 1972, Singer and Nicolson proposed the fluid mosaic model of the plasma membrane of a eukaryotic cell. This was based on an equilibrium picture of interactions between membrane components, where the fluid bilayer composed of lipids acts as a "solvent" for proteins. Although not expressed explicitly, this conception of the membrane precludes any long-range order or large-scale lateral heterogeneities.[1] However, given the compositional diversity of membrane components (up to at least 1000 lipid and protein species), it would not be entirely unrealistic to assume the existence of a mosaic-like pattern of proteins and lipids based on random fluctuations of the local concentration of individual molecular species.

At the same time, the inherent asymmetry in the lipid distribution of the two leaflets of the plasma membrane was already recognized (reviewed in Ref. 2). The outer leaflet is rich in sphingomyelin (SM) and phosphatidylcholine (PC), while the inner leaflet has significantly more phosphatidylethanolamine (PE) and almost all the phosphatidylserine (PS) and phosphatidylinositol phosphates (PIPs). Membrane-resident enzymes such as scramblases and flippases have been postulated to be involved in actively maintaining this lipid asymmetry.[3] Glycosylphosphatidylinositol-anchored proteins (GPI-APs) and glycosphingolipids are present only in the outer leaflet while prenylated proteins are present exclusively in the inner leaflet. This asymmetry is dictated by their synthetic origins, that is, luminal assembly for the GPI-APs and cytoplasmic attachment for the prenylated proteins.[4,5]

2.1.2   THE LIPID RAFT HYPOTHESIS AND DETERGENT-RESISTANT MEMBRANES

The notion of functional lateral heterogeneities in the plasma membrane arose from compelling cell biological observations,[6] which necessitated a reconsideration of the fluid mosaic model. The observation that, in many polarized cells, GPI-APs and glycosphingolipids are enriched in the apical plasma membrane compared to the basolateral surface led to the conceptualization of "lipid rafts"[7] as a platform for lateral segregation of certain lipids and proteins forming distinct functional domains in cell membranes. Following on from this observation, detergent-resistant membrane (DRM) fractions of polarized cells were shown to be enriched in apically sorted glycosphingolipids, GPI-APs, and cholesterol and depleted of basolaterally targeted proteins.[8] This in turn led to the suggestion that apically sorted cargos form DRMs, which could serve as sorting platforms. Finally, this led to the hypothesis that lipid rafts were the equivalent of DRMs.

Cholesterol depletion was shown to cause loss of DRM components, emphasizing the role of lipids in forming these molecular aggregates. At the same time, biophysical studies on artificial membranes (Section 2.1.3) provided a physicochemical justification for lipid–lipid immiscibility as a driving mechanism for the generation of these lateral asymmetries. Concurrently, chemical or antibody-mediated cross-linking of several different GPI-APs or the raft resident protein CD44 led to copatching of Src family tyrosine kinases and G-proteins in the inner leaflet, thereby implicating lipid rafts as signaling platforms.[9,10]

2.1.3 LEARNING FROM MODEL MEMBRANES

Model membranes, composed of varying ratios of purified lipids such as cholesterol, SM, and phospholipids, have been used to study self-organization of lipid molecules (reviewed in Ref. 11). In a simplified system where the compositional ratio of the ternary lipid mixture closely resembled the ratio in plasma membrane, coexistence of both liquid-ordered (l_o) and liquid-disordered (l_d) phases occur. The l_o phase is characterized by enrichment of cholesterol and phospholipids with saturated acyl chains compared to the l_d phase. Cholesterol molecules aid tighter packing of the saturated acyl chains by stacking interactions as compared to the unsaturated acyl chains, thereby causing differential packing in l_o and l_d domains. The size of phase-segregated domains observed in artificial membranes depends on the physicochemical parameters in the experiment. The association of GPI-APs (e.g., Thy-1) and glycosphingolipids (e.g., GM1) with lipid rafts was explained in terms of preferential association of their predominantly saturated acyl tails with l_o domains formed in ternary mixture model membranes or brush-border membrane extract.[12] Similar observations of phase segregation into optically resolvable domains was made in plasma membrane vesicles or blebs at temperatures below 25°C but not at 37°C.[13] Furthermore, l_o domains exhibit a propensity to remain insoluble in cold nonionic detergents, a property that immediately correlated with DRMs derived from intact cells. These results suggested that equilibrium thermodynamic principles of phase separation of lipids, which lead to compositional heterogeneities in model membranes, may be manifest in cell membranes.

2.1.4 QUESTIONING THE EQUATION OF FUNCTIONAL RAFTS WITH DRMs

A clear indication that all was not well with the simple correlation between lipid domains in cells and DRMs in fact came from studies in artificial membranes where, using isothermal titration calorimetry, Heerklotz and coworkers showed the preexisting organization of lipids in the bilayer is drastically perturbed during detergent addition.[14] Correlative microscopy studies during the process of creating DRMs from live cell membranes also showed that the preexisting organization of lipids in membranes cannot be equated to the membrane remnants derived from DRMs.[15] Thus, the simple correlation of lipid rafts (as functional segregation of lipidic species) and DRMs began breaking down. Furthermore (Section 2.4), in vivo observations of nanoscale molecular complexes having functionally regulated assembly on live cell membranes clearly indicate that an equilibrium framework of lipid–lipid interactions as a mechanism of formation of plasma membrane heterogeneities is an oversimplification.

2.2 VISUALIZING LIPID RAFTS IN LIVING CELLS

2.2.1 ILLUSIVE OR ELUSIVE?

In contrast to the macroscopic phase segregation easily observed in artificial membranes, visualizing lipid rafts in live cell membranes has remained a challenging task for the membrane biologist.[16,17] Much of the early work on exploring the organization of membrane components was done ignoring the consequences of multivalent reagents such as clustering antibodies.[18,19] Cross-linking by primary and secondary antibodies induces formation of visible patches of raft components, and hence, one must consider that these methods may create long-lived clusters or highlight stable assemblies without revealing any native, preexisting organization. GPI-APs labeled with fluorescent primary antibodies showed a relatively uniform distribution contrasting with the cross-linked patches obtained with the use of potentially multivalent strategies, at the limit of optical resolution in live and even in improperly fixed cell membranes.[20,21] This suggested that preexisting organization of native lipid rafts, if they existed, would have to be smaller than 250 nm, the resolution of optical light microscopy. Indeed, studies involving nonperturbing techniques already indicated that GPI-APs are clustered in domains smaller than 70 nm[22] and indeed could form small molecular-scale oligomeric assemblies.[23] These contrasting results fueled doubts about the very existence of segregated molecular entities or lipid rafts on the live cell membrane.[16]

2.2.2 ELECTRON MICROSCOPY

A robust methodology with resolution at the nanometer scale is electron microscopy (EM), but it is limited by its application on fixed cells. Immunogold EM studies of several membrane lipids or lipid-anchored proteins, such as gangliosides and GPI-APs on the outer leaflet and signaling proteins of the Ras family in the inner leaflet, have revealed nanoscale assemblies.[24,25] Analysis of their spatial patterns on either side of the same plasma membrane sheet showed partial overlap of raft domains in the two leaflets but with different scales of clustering. Immunogold EM of the IgE immune receptor in the native state and after cross-linking mediated activation have revealed a reorganization at the nanoscale of clusters of 2–3 molecules to >20 molecules, with concomitant redistribution of downstream inner leaflet–anchored signaling molecules.[26,27] These studies implicated that lipid rafts could be thought of as nanoscale molecular assemblies.

2.2.3 PROXIMITY METHODS

To probe into nanoscale membrane complexes without perturbing their native organization or the physiological status of the plasma membrane, biophysical methods using optical tools would be ideal. Estimating Forster resonance energy transfer (FRET) efficiency between donor and acceptor fluorophores turned out to be a critical and powerful experimental tool in elucidating the puzzle of membrane complexes. FRET reports on the proximity of two fluorescently labeled species at a scale

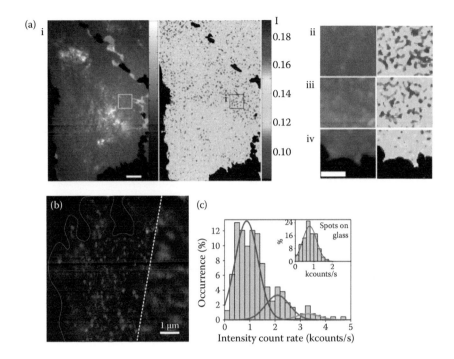

FIGURE 2.1   Nanoscale organization of GPI-anchored proteins. (a) (i) Intensity and fluorescence anisotropy images showing the plasma membrane distribution of folate receptor (a GPI-AP) on the live cell membrane at high spatial resolution. The plasma membrane shows local heterogeneity in the extent of GPI-AP nanoclustering indicated by the fluorescence anisotropy map obtained from the lamella (ii–iii) or the tip of the lamellipodia (iv). The scale bar represents 8 μm (i) and 4 μm (ii–iv). (Adapted from Goswami D et al., *Cell*, 135, 1085–97, 2008.) (b) GPI-AP distribution on the monocyte plasma membrane shows nanoscale complexes when imaged by NSOM (left) as compared to confocal microscopy (right). (c) Intensity distribution of GPI-AP punctae reveals 70% monomers with the rest clustered in dimers, trimers, and a small fraction of higher-order oligomers. (Adapted from van Zanten T S et al., *PNAS*, 106, 18557–62, 2009.)

of 5–10 nm with high sensitivity as the efficiency drops by the sixth power of intermolecular distance. Using a specialized kind of FRET microscopy where the extent of FRET between like fluorophores (i.e., homo-FRET) is detected by measuring fluorescence emission anisotropy,[28] dynamic nanoclusters of GPI-APs (Figure 2.1) on the live cell membrane have been observed.[22,29] Using time-resolved FRET measurements, similar nanoscale complexes of GPI-APs and epidermal growth factor receptor were identified by another research group.[30]

2.2.4   SUPER-RESOLUTION METHODS

The recent development of super-resolution imaging modes combining techniques to manipulate the photophysical properties of fluorophores, shaping of excitation sources, and extensive computational analysis of image data revealed structural details at a resolution of tens of nanometers. Combining photoactivation and image localization microscopy with pair correlation analysis, Sengupta et al. mapped the nanoscale organization of a range of membrane proteins such as GPI-APs, VSVG, and signaling adaptors Lyn and Lat, essentially varying in their mode of anchoring.[31] Employing dSTORM imaging, another super-resolution localization technique involving switching between dark and fluorescent states of a fluorophore, the nanoscale organization of B-cell receptor molecules and coreceptor CD91 was observed on the plasma membrane.[32] Near-field scanning optical microscopy (NSOM) is a super-resolution technique that can report on the number of molecules in membrane domains.[33] Using this technique, the nanoscale organization, dynamics, and redistribution of GPI-APs and integrins in the plasma membrane of resting or stimulated immune cells have been elucidated (Figure 2.1b).[34,35]

2.2.5 DIFFUSION MEASUREMENTS

Over the past decades, several techniques have been deployed to observe the dynamics of membrane components in order to decipher the nature of their surrounding environment. Fluorescence recovery after photobleaching experiments revealed higher immobile fractions of GPI-APs with reduced diffusion when compared to a generic membrane lipid; a behavior that was dependent on the presence of membrane cholesterol and actin activity.[9] High-speed single-particle tracking (SPT) of raft components such as GPI-APs and glycosphingolipids revealed that these molecules exhibit transient trapping in membrane domains 50–100 nm in size unlike nonraft lipids with unsaturated acyl chains.[36–38] Another SPT study where 40-nm colloidal gold particles clustering approximately six molecules of CD59 (a GPI-AP) were tracked showed stimulation-induced temporary arrest of lateral diffusion (STALL), a transient state where the recruitment of PLCγ, Gαi2, and Lyn to these clusters led to the activation of IP3-Ca^{2+} signaling cascade.[39]

Fluorescence correlation spectroscopy (FCS), a powerful technique for measuring molecular diffusion and the nature of its environment, has been typically applied as a single-point, optically resolved measurement and later adapted to super-resolution imaging modalities. Careful choice of the model to fit the raw FCS data (from single-point measurements or from image series) followed by a comparison with the "diffusion laws" defined by phenomenological simulations for membrane molecules not only can differentiate between free, hindered, and hop diffusion but also can estimate the size of the confinement zones.[40,41] FCS in a stimulated emission depletion (STED) microscope has been used effectively to probe the organization of membrane components on a suboptical scale.[42] In this technique, the diffraction-limited excitation volume of the excitation laser is restricted using a coaxial, donut-shaped, red-shifted laser that depletes excited-state fluorophores to the ground state in the periphery of the excitation spot. The extent of depletion, and thereby the sub-diffraction illumination volume, depends on the power of the depletion laser, which must be carefully tuned keeping the vitality of the cells in mind. By STED-FCS, the diffusion of "raft" lipids was measured from a spot size of 40 nm laterally and compared to that of a general phosphoglycerolipid. The raft components showed transient trapping for 10–20 ms in cholesterol-sensitive nanoscale domains.[42]

Together, these diverse methodologies and model systems reveal a complex and often contradictory picture of the organization of membrane components but ascertained that native rafts can be nanoscale transient assemblies.

2.3 FUNCTIONAL RELEVANCE OF NANOCLUSTERS OF MEMBRANE MOLECULES

A large variety of membrane molecules are clustered in nanoscale domains whose size, molecular densities, formation, and localization vary with cellular responses, exemplified here by the classical raft-resident GPI-APs. Several classes of membrane molecules such as receptors, enzymes, adhesion molecules, and surface antigens are GPI anchored, where the anchor itself dictates the cellular function and fate of these molecules. It was observed that folate uptake by folate receptor (a GPI-AP) is functionally impaired if the GPI anchor is replaced by a transmembrane domain.[43] The GPI anchor seems to be essential for directing the endocytosis of GPI-APs by a clathrin- and dynamin-independent route.[44] Moreover, upon perturbation of their native organization by antibody-mediated cross-linking, both the endocytic mode and intracellular trafficking of GPI-APs are altered.[18,29]

Functional cross talk between membrane nanoscale complexes was observed to occur when binding of ligand to integrin nanoclusters led to the reorganization of GPI-AP nanoclusters creating signaling-competent domains on the T-cell membrane.[34] The nanoclustered organization of Ras-GTP, an inner leaflet-anchored signaling molecule, is important for maintaining the fidelity of initiating the mitogen-activated protein kinase signaling cascade.[45]

2.4 CHARACTERISTICS OF NANOCLUSTERS ON THE PLASMA MEMBRANE

It is interesting to note that GPI-APs and Ras molecules, both lipid-anchored plasma membrane molecules, show concentration-independent nanoclustered organization of similar stoichiometries. Ras molecules are maintained as a constant fraction (~40%) of nanoclusters where each cluster consists of six to eight molecules.[46] Similarly, ~30–40% of GPI-APs are nanoclustered with two to four molecules per cluster (Figure 2.1c).[29,34] To understand the distribution and dynamics of GPI-AP nanoclusters on mammalian cell membranes, homo-FRET has served as a powerful tool. Briefly, homo-FRET (FRET between similar fluorophores such as GFP) can be estimated by measuring the extent of depolarization in the fluorescence emission as a direct consequence of FRET between fluorophores that are excited by plane polarized excitation light.[47] The quantity "fluorescence anisotropy" is a mathematical measure of the fluorescence emission polarization. The method and its application on several different microscopy platforms (discussed elsewhere) have allowed ourselves and others to visualize the spatial distribution and the temporal dynamics of nanoclusters of many membrane[28] and cytoplasmic components.[48]

2.4.1 Spatial Heterogeneity in GPI-AP Organization

The distribution of GPI-AP nanocluster-enriched domains is nonrandom, and over a large concentration range, a constant fraction of nanoclusters to monomers is maintained. Cholesterol depletion or actin perturbations lead to loss of GPI-AP nanoclusters.[49] The local heterogeneity is evident from high-resolution fluorescence anisotropy images of the cell membrane (Figure 2.1a). Microvilli and edges of ruffles show high anisotropy, indicating a lack of nanoclusters, while flat lamella show low anisotropy, indicating an enrichment of nanoclusters (Figure 2.1a, ii–iv); these are confirmed by time-resolved anisotropy measurements that report on the extent of FRET.[29] The role of the membrane-apposed cortical acto-myosin mesh in driving the nanoclustering of GPI-APs was revealed from observing the bleb expansion and retraction cycle. A bleb during the expansion phase lacks a visible actin cortex and also lacks nanoclusters of GPI-APs, which start to reform during the bleb retraction phase powered by regrowth of the acto-myosin-based contractile cortex.[49]

2.4.2 Dynamics of Nanoscale Organization

The dynamics of GPI-AP nanocluster formation was probed by fluorescence intensity and anisotropy recovery after photobleaching experiments in a microphotolysis-type assay.[49] This assay was designed to report on the kinetics of nanoclustering over a range of temperatures or under conditions where specific inhibitors were added to perturb the activity of cortical acto-myosin. In brief, this assay revealed that GPI-AP nanoclusters show second scale clustering dynamics along with a crossover from almost negligible dynamics to fast remodeling kinetics at temperatures higher than 24°C. This temperature dependence was associated in part with an increase in acto-myosin activity.[49]

Here, the readers should note that exogenously incorporated short acyl chain fluorescent lipids showed random distribution and concentration-dependent nanoclustering on the plasma membrane. This suggests that the organizational characteristics of GPI-APs are unique to their molecular nature, possibly reflecting a sensitive and specific interaction with an "active" templating machinery. Thus, the regulated, nonequilibrium, nanoscale clustering of molecules like GPI-APs compelled a questioning of the notion of membrane organization by thermodynamic equilibrium phase segregation and prompted a probing of the nature of the membrane-associated active machinery.

2.5 AN EXPLANATION FOR ACTIN-COUPLED NANOSCALE MEMBRANE ORGANIZATION

2.5.1 Evoking a Theoretical Framework

To explain the nanoscale dynamics as well as the atypical spatial distribution of the GPI-APs in connection to cortical actin dynamics, the existence of a highly dynamic pool of filamentous actin tangentially disposed against the plasma membrane was proposed (see Section 2.6.2 for some circumstantial evidence).[50] A first-principles, coarse-grained theory that looks at the collective behavior of this two-species actin "material" from the perspective of physics of active hydrodynamics[51] provides a potential explanation for the nanoscale organization and dynamics of membrane molecules governed by the degree of interaction with the actin filaments. The concentration and orientation of the short filaments can be analytically derived from hydrodynamic equations describing their orientation and local concentration over a range of active temperatures.[50] The solutions provide us with a picture where aster-like patterns form and disassemble in the plane of the membrane, creating a nanoscale patterning machinery capable of generating forces and currents (Figure 2.2a). Membrane

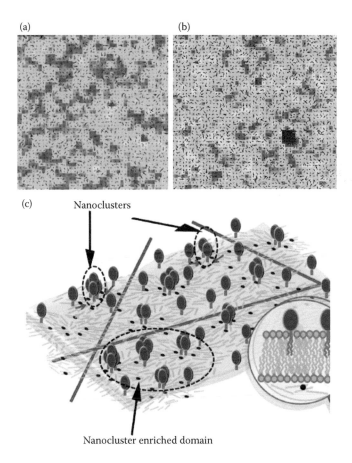

FIGURE 2.2 Plasma membrane as an active composite with the dynamic actin. (a) Snapshot representing the pseudocolored local orientation ordering and density of dynamic actin filaments (black arrows) in the rapidly remodeling regime. (b) Passive particle density map (pseudocolored) obtained as a result of advection along the active filaments (black arrows) showing clustering at the core of aster-like formation. (Adapted from Gowrishankar K et al., *Cell*, 149, 1353–67, 2012.) (c) Cartoon represents the "active" mechanism of nanoscale organization of membrane molecules (e.g., GPI-APs depicted in purple) where the membrane-apposed patterning machinery is composed of short, dynamic actin filaments (yellow) driven by myosin motors (black) to form aster-like patterns amid the larger actin mesh (brown).

molecules that can interact with these filaments may be advected along them, leading to their trapping and clustering into nanoscale complexes (Figure 2.2).

2.5.2   CLASSIFICATION OF MEMBRANE MOLECULES ON THE BASIS OF THEIR INTERACTION WITH DYNAMIC ACTIN

Membrane molecules could be coupled to the dynamic actin filaments either directly, owing to the presence of cytoplasmic actin binding motifs on transmembrane proteins, or indirectly, via actin-binding adaptor proteins associating with cytoplasmic tails of membrane proteins or with the inner leaflet lipids.[52] Thus, on the basis of the nature and the effect of the interaction of membrane molecules with the underlying dynamic actin filaments, the theoretical framework allowed a classification of membrane molecules into three broad categories: inert, passive, and active. *Inert molecules* are those that do not bind to the dynamic actin but couple hydrodynamically with the static mesh (e.g., short tail lipid molecules in the outer leaflet of the plasma membrane). *Passive molecules* are those that bind (directly or indirectly) to the dynamic actin but cannot influence the nature or dynamics of actin. GPI-APs show signatures of being in this class, as their spatiotemporal dynamics is highly sensitive to cortical acto-myosin activity but has not been observed to influence the acto-myosin machinery. *Active molecules* are those whose membrane organization is influenced by actin, and in turn, these molecules also influence the creation, coupling, or dynamics of the active actin filaments. Prime examples of such active molecules are integrins,[34] T-cell receptors,[53] and acetylcholine receptors,[54] which not only recruit molecules involved in cortical acto-myosin remodeling but also are organized in microclusters by actin-dependent processes.

This picture provides a broad explanatory framework to understand the behavior of a variety of membrane molecules and also makes useful predictions about non-equilibrium density fluctuations of "passive" particles that are borne out by experiment.[50] This suggested that GPI-APs are possibly reporting on large fluctuations in the underlying patterns created by the hypothesized dynamic actin filaments.

2.6   PROBING THE NATURE OF CORTICAL ACTIN

2.6.1   THE STABLE CORTICAL ACTIN MESH

A static picture of the actin-based cortex underlying the plasma membrane has emerged from electron tomography of the rapidly frozen plasma membrane skeleton[55] as well as from super-resolution imaging methods.[56] These studies have revealed a cross-linked network of actin filaments creating a membrane-associated meshwork. However, this cellular cortex is not a static structure as it can be remodeled by specific signals to generate various actin-based surface specializations such as microvilli, filopodia, lamellipodia, ruffles, phagocytic cups, and endocytic pits satisfying diverse functional needs.[57] The dynamics of the cortical actin has been studied by several high-resolution microscopy modalities revealing the meshwork restructuring occurring over timescales of seconds to minutes, which can influence dynamics of membrane molecules at the micron scale.[58–60]

2.6.2 DYNAMIC ACTIN FILAMENTS!

In order to probe the existence of highly dynamic, short, filamentous actin amid the static cortical mesh, we resorted to imaging the spatial and subsecond temporal dynamics of F-actin tagged with the actin filament binding domain of utrophin (GFP-Utr-AFBD) in live cells.[61] Single-molecule particle tracking (SMPT) of GFP-Utr-AFBD in a total internal reflection fluorescence microscope revealed short-lived actin filaments apposed to the plasma membrane. Most importantly, the occurrence of these F-actin structures is highly sensitive to low doses of drugs that perturb the actin polymerization–depolymerization kinetics. FCS-based diffusion measurements of the cortical actin labeled similarly resonated the results from the SMPT experiments by revealing a slow diffusing component that was confirmed to be arising from F-actin only.[50] Thus, these results support the basic assumption of the theoretical framework (Section 2.5.1) that short dynamic actin filaments at the cell cortex exist. In conjunction with the experimental verification of the prediction that the local dynamics of these filaments will be reflected onto the behavior of membrane molecules capable of advecting along them, we have set the foundations for an active mechanism of nanoscale complex formation.

2.7 CONNECTING CORTICAL ACTIN TO EXOPLASMIC PLASMA MEMBRANE COMPONENTS

From several examples of cellular function such as the formation of cell protrusions or membrane invaginations, the ability of the cortical actin to associate with the plasma membrane and deform the same is evident. The mode of association between the membrane components and actin can be direct or indirect depending on the interacting molecules in question.[52] For exoplasmic components such as GPI-APs, a transbilayer lipid tail-based domain coupling mechanism could be translating the influence of the dynamic actin filaments across the leaflets. This hypothesis is supported by experimental observations in model membranes mimicking the outer and inner leaflet composition of the plasma membrane, demonstrating the role of cholesterol and saturated fatty acyl chains of lipids in inducing lipid segregation in both leaflets through transbilayer coupling.[2,62] These domains may locally enrich certain lipid species capable of recruiting members of the actin binding or nucleation-promoting factor family thus setting up a link to the cortical cytoskeleton.[52]

2.7.1 LINKING ACTIN TO THE INNER LEAFLET LIPIDS

The lipid compositional asymmetry between the two leaflets of the plasma membrane is marked by the enrichment of negatively charged lipid species such as PE, PS, and PIPs, most of which are essential for maintaining functional interactions with membrane-to-cortical cytoskeleton linkers, modulators of acto-myosin dynamics and signaling proteins.[63,64] Cofilin activity, and thus the local actin remodeling machinery, is regulated by binding to PIPs (among other mechanisms), which have been elucidated as an important arm of the membrane–cytoskeleton cross talk involved in cell migration. Interactions with the inner leaflet lipids are usually mediated by specific lipid binding motifs such as PH, PX, C2, and FYVE domains to name a few, where the binding regulates not only the localization of the proteins but often their state of activity as well. The significance of these interactions may be further elucidated by the case of the migrating cell where local enrichment of specific PIPs between the front and rear ends of the cell orchestrates the activity of several acto-myosin regulators that drive the motility engine.[65]

2.7.2 ASSOCIATION OF DYNAMIC ACTIN WITH MEMBRANES

Specific nucleators or actin modulators associated with the plasma membrane can be hypothesized to generate short dynamic actin filaments in proximity of the membrane. Rho GTPases, which are upstream activators of nucleation-promoting factors and actin nucleators, carry posttranslational lipid modifications that allow them to insert into the membrane and preferentially associate with the lipid rafts, thereby redirecting actin remodeling.[66] Several groups have demonstrated that such short filamentous actin may be associating with intracellular membranes such as with the Golgi complex. The presence of clusters of short actin filaments associating with tropomyosins near the Golgi membranes was detected in immuno-electron micrographs.[67] The rapidly remodeling nature of this acto-myosin machinery was implicated from studies showing that cargo sorting and vesicle formation from Golgi membranes were affected by perturbing nucleators such as formins, depolymerizing agents such as cofilin, and unconventional myosin motors.[68–71] Myosin 1c has been suggested to be a raft-associated motor maintaining membrane–actin connections required for GPI-AP recycling, macropinocytosis, and cell shape changes.[72] In a rather interesting work where actin remodeling by malaria parasites in infected red blood cells was being investigated, actin filaments smaller than 100 nm were imaged by cryoelectron tomography near the cell membrane of uninfected RBCs.[73]

2.8 CONCLUSION

Summarizing a large body of work from many investigators including ourselves, a picture where the plasma membrane may be visualized as a composite of the bilayer and the actin cortex seems to be the most reasonable explanation for the gamut of observations made on the properties of its constituents. The living cell membrane does not appear to be a well-equilibriated mix of molecules as evoked by the fluid mosaic model, but instead is a structurally defined yet fluid platform where molecular heterogeneity is actively maintained. Uncovering the existence and unusual dynamics of nanoscale membrane domains in live cells has forced a questioning of the equilibrium picture of molecular aggregation. Studies on lipid-tethered proteins have indeed helped paint a compelling picture of the plasma membrane where nanoscale clustering is principally driven by the spatiotemporal patterning of a membrane-apposed dynamic acto-myosin machinery composed of short filaments of actin (Figure 2.2c). It is likely that this framework will provide a general way to understand the organization of most of the components in the membrane and their relationship to the external and internal milieu that the plasma membrane serves to create a barrier against.

REFERENCES

1. Singer, S J, and G L Nicolson. "The Fluid Mosaic Model of the Structure of Cell Membranes." *Science (New York, N.Y.)* 175 (1972): 720–31.
2. Kiessling, V, C Wan, and L K Tamm. "Domain Coupling in Asymmetric Lipid Bilayers." *Biochimica et Biophysica Acta* 1788 (2009): 64–71.
3. Daleke, D L. "Regulation of Transbilayer Plasma Membrane Phospholipid Asymmetry." *Journal of Lipid Research* 44 (2003): 233–42.
4. Chatterjee, S, and S Mayor. "The GPI-Anchor and Protein Sorting." *Cellular and Molecular Life Sciences: CMLS* 58 (2001): 1969–87.
5. Orlean, P, and A K Menon. "GPI Anchoring of Protein in Yeast and Mammalian Cells, Or: How We Learned to Stop Worrying and Love Glycophospholipids." *Journal of Lipid Research* 48 (2007): 993–1011.
6. Simons, K, and G van Meer. "Lipid Sorting in Epithelial Cells." *Biochemistry* 27, (1988): 6197–202.
7. Simons, K, and E Ikonen. "Functional Rafts in Cell Membranes." *Nature* 387 (1997): 569–72.
8. Brown, D A, and J K Rose. "Sorting of GPI-Anchored Proteins to Glycolipid-Enriched Membrane Subdomains During Transport to the Apical Cell Surface." *Cell* 68 (1992): 533–44.
9. Oliferenko, S, K Paiha, T Harder et al. "Analysis of Cd44-Containing Lipid Rafts: Recruitment of Annexin II and Stabilization by the Actin Cytoskeleton." *The Journal of Cell Biology* 146 (1999): 843–54.
10. Simons, K, and D Toomre. "Lipid Rafts and Signal Transduction." *Nature Reviews. Molecular Cell Biology* 1 (2000): 31–9.
11. Simons, K, and W L C Vaz. "Model Systems, Lipid Rafts, and Cell Membranes." *Annual Review of Biophysics and Biomolecular Structure* 33 (2004): 269–95.
12. Dietrich, C, Z N Volovyk, M Levi, N L Thompson, and K Jacobson. "Partitioning of Thy-1, GM1, and Cross-Linked Phospholipid Analogs into Lipid Rafts Reconstituted in Supported Model Membrane Monolayers." *Proceedings of the National Academy of Sciences of the United States of America* 98 (2001): 10642–7.
13. Baumgart, T, A T Hammond, P Sengupta et al. "Large-Scale Fluid/Fluid Phase Separation of Proteins and Lipids in Giant Plasma Membrane Vesicles." *Proceedings of the National Academy of Sciences of the United States of America* 104 (2007): 3165–70.
14. Heerklotz, H, H Szadkowska, T Anderson, and J Seelig. "The Sensitivity of Lipid Domains to Small Perturbations Demonstrated by the Effect of Triton." *Journal of Molecular Biology* 329 (2003): 793–9.
15. Mayor, S, and F R Maxfield. "Insolubility and Redistribution of GPI-Anchored Proteins at the Cell Surface after Detergent Treatment." *Molecular Biology of the Cell* 6 (1995): 929–44.
16. Munro, S. "Lipid Rafts: Elusive or Illusive?" *Cell* 115 (2003): 377–88.
17. Mayor, S, and M Rao. "Rafts: Scale-Dependent, Active Lipid Organization at the Cell Surface." *Traffic (Copenhagen, Denmark)* 5 (2004): 231–40.
18. Rothberg, K G, Y Ying, J F Kolhouse, B A Kamen, and R G W Anderson. "The Glycophospholipid-Linked Folate Receptor Internalizes Folate without Entering the Clathrin-Coated Pit Endocytic Pathway." *The Journal of Cell Biology* 110 (1990): 637–49.
19. Rothberg, K G, Y-S Ying, B A Kamen, and R G W Anderson. "Cholesterol Controls the Clustering of the Glycophospholipid-Anchored Membrane Receptor for 5-Methyltetrahydrofolate." *The Journal of Cell Biology* 111 (1990): 2931–8.
20. Mayor, S, K G Rothberg, and F R Maxfield. "Sequestration of GPI-Anchored Proteins in Caveolae Triggered by Cross-Linking." *Science* 264 (1994): 1948–51.
21. Tanaka, K A K, K G N Suzuki, Y M Shirai et al. "Membrane Molecules Mobile Even after Chemical Fixation." *Nature Methods* 7 (2010): 865–6.

22. Varma, R, and S Mayor. "GPI-Anchored Proteins Are Organized in Submicron Domains at the Cell Surface." *Nature* 394 (1998): 798–801.

23. Friedrichson, T, and T V Kurzchalia. "Microdomains of GPI-Anchored Proteins in Living Cells Revealed by Crosslinking." *Nature* 394 (1998): 802–5.

24. Prior, I A, C Muncke, R G Parton, and J F Hancock. "Direct Visualization of Ras Proteins in Spatially Distinct Cell Surface Microdomains." *The Journal of Cell Biology* 160 (2003): 165–70.

25. Fujita, A, J Cheng, M Hirakawa et al. "Gangliosides GM1 and GM3 in the Living Cell Membrane Form Clusters Susceptible to Cholesterol Depletion and Chilling." *Molecular Biology of the Cell* 18 (2007): 2112–22.

26. Wilson, B S, J R Pfeiffer, and J M Oliver. "Observing FcεRI Signaling from the inside of the Mast Cell Membrane." *The Journal of Cell Biology* 149 (2000): 1131–42.

27. Wilson, B S, J R Pfeiffer, Z Surviladze, E A Gaudet, and J M Oliver. "High Resolution Mapping of Mast Cell Membranes Reveals Primary and Secondary Domains of FcεRI and LAT." *The Journal of Cell Biology* 154 (2001): 645–58.

28. Ghosh, S, S Saha, D Goswami, S Bilgrami, and S Mayor. "Dynamic Imaging of Homo-FRET in Live Cells by Fluorescence Anisotropy Microscopy." *Methods in Enzymology* 505 (2012): 291–327.

29. Sharma, P, R Varma, R C Sarasi et al. "Nanoscale Organization of Multiple GPI-Anchored Proteins in Living Cell Membranes." *Cell* 116 (2004): 577–89.

30. Bader, A N, E G Hofman, J Voortman et al. "Homo-FRET Imaging Enables Quantification of Protein Cluster Sizes with Subcellular Resolution." *Biophysical Journal* 97 (2009): 2613–22.

31. Sengupta, P, T Jovanovic-Talisman, D Skoko et al. "Probing Protein Heterogeneity in the Plasma Membrane Using Palm and Pair Correlation Analysis." *Nature Methods* 8 (2011): 969–75.

32. Mattila, P K, C Feest, D Depoil et al. "The Actin and Tetraspanin Networks Organize Receptor Nanoclusters to Regulate B Cell Receptor-Mediated Signaling." *Immunity* 38 (2013): 461–74.

33. Lange, F D, A Cambi, R Huijbens et al. "Cell Biology Beyond the Diffraction Limit: Near-Field Scanning Optical Microscopy." *Journal of Cell Science* 114 (2001): 4153–60.

34. van Zanten, T S, A Cambi, M Koopman et al. "Hotspots of GPI-Anchored Proteins and Integrin Nanoclusters Function as Nucleation Sites for Cell Adhesion." *Proceedings of the National Academy of Sciences of the United States of America* 106 (2009): 18557–62.

35. Jan, G, C Eich, J A Torreno-Pina et al. "Lateral Mobility of Individual Integrin Nanoclusters Orchestrates the Onset for Leukocyte Adhesion." *Proceedings of the National Academy of Sciences of the United States of America* 109 (2012): 4869–74.

36. Dietrich, C, B Yang, T Fujiwara, A Kusumi, and K Jacobson. "Relationship of Lipid Rafts to Transient Confinement Zones Detected by Single Particle Tracking." *Biophysical Journal* 82 (2002): 274–84.

37. Schütz, G J, G Kada, V Ph Pastushenko, and H Schindler. "Properties of Lipid Microdomains in a Muscle Cell Membrane Visualized by Single Molecule Microscopy." *The EMBO Journal* 19 (2000): 892–901.

38. Kusumi, A, Y M Shirai, I Koyama-Honda, K G N Suzuki, and T K Fujiwara. "Hierarchical Organization of the Plasma Membrane: Investigations by Single-Molecule Tracking vs. Fluorescence Correlation Spectroscopy." *FEBS Letters* 584 (2010): 1814–23.

39. Suzuki, K G N, T K Fujiwara, M Edidin, and A Kusumi. "Dynamic Recruitment of Phospholipase C γ at Transiently Immobilized GPI-Anchored Receptor Clusters Induces IP3-Ca2+ Signaling: Single-Molecule Tracking Study 2." *The Journal of Cell Biology* 177 (2007): 731–42.

40. Wawrezinieck, L, H Rigneault, D Marguet, and P-F Lenne. "Fluorescence Correlation Spectroscopy Diffusion Laws to Probe the Submicron Cell Membrane Organization." *Biophysical Journal* 89 (2005): 4029–42.

41. Di Rienzo, C, E Gratton, F Beltram, and F Cardarelli. "Fast Spatiotemporal Correlation Spectroscopy to Determine Protein Lateral Diffusion Laws in Live Cell Membranes." *Proceedings of the National Academy of Sciences of the United States of America* 110 (2013): 12307–12.

42. Sandhoff, K, C Eggeling, C Ringemann et al. "Direct Observation of the Nanoscale Dynamics of Membrane Lipids in a Living Cell." *Nature* 457 (2009): 1159–62.

43. Ritter, T E, O Fajardo, H Matsue, R G Anderson, and S W Lacey. "Folate Receptors Targeted to Clathrin-Coated Pits Cannot Regulate Vitamin Uptake." *Proceedings of the National Academy of Sciences of the United States of America* 92 (1995): 3824–8.

44. Sabharanjak, S, P Sharma, R G Parton, and S Mayor. "GPI-Anchored Proteins Are Delivered to Recycling Endosomes Via a Distinct Cdc42-Regulated, Clathrin-Independent Pinocytic Pathway." *Developmental Cell* 2 (2002): 411–23.

45. Harding, A S, and J F Hancock. "Using Plasma Membrane Nanoclusters to Build Better Signaling Circuits." *Trends in Cell Biology* 18 (2008): 364–71.

46. Plowman, S J, C Muncke, R G Parton, and J F Hancock. "H-Ras, K-Ras, and Inner Plasma Membrane Raft Proteins Operate in Nanoclusters with Differential Dependence on the Actin Cytoskeleton." *Proceedings of the National Academy of Sciences of the United States of America* 102 (2005): 15500–5.

47. Weber, G. "Dependence of the Polarization of the Fluorescence on the Concentration." *Transactions of the Faraday Society* 50 (1954): 552–60.

48. Altman, D, D Goswami, T Hasson, J A Spudich, and S Mayor. "Precise Positioning of Myosin VI on Endocytic Vesicles in Vivo." *PLoS Biology* 5 (2007): e210.

49. Goswami, D, K Gowrishankar, S Bilgrami et al. "Nanoclusters of GPI-Anchored Proteins Are Formed by Cortical Actin-Driven Activity." *Cell* 135 (2008): 1085–97.

50. Gowrishankar, K, S Ghosh, S Saha et al. "Active Remodeling of Cortical Actin Regulates Spatiotemporal Organization of Cell Surface Molecules." *Cell* 149 (2012): 1353–67.

51. Kruse, K, J F Joanny, F Julicher, J Prost, and K Sekimoto. "Asters, Vortices, and Rotating Spirals in Active Gels of Polar Filaments." *Physical Review Letters* 92 (2004): 1–4.

52. Doherty, G J, and H T McMahon. "Mediation, Modulation, and Consequences of Membrane-Cytoskeleton Interactions." *Annual Review of Biophysics* 37 (2008): 65–95.

53. Varma, R, G Campi, T Yokosuka, T Saito, and M L Dustin. "T Cell Receptor-Proximal Signals Are Sustained in Peripheral Microclusters and Terminated in the Central Supramolecular Activation Cluster." *Immunity* 25 (2006): 117–27.

54. Dai, Z, X Luo, H Xie, and H B Peng. "The Actin-Driven Movement and Formation of Acetylcholine Receptor Clusters." *The Journal of Cell Biology* 150 (2000): 1321–34.

55. Morone, N, T Fujiwara, K Murase et al. "Three-Dimensional Reconstruction of the Membrane Skeleton at the Plasma Membrane Interface by Electron Tomography." *The Journal of Cell Biology* 174 (2006): 851–62.

56. Xu, K, H P Babcock, and X Zhuang. "Dual-Objective Storm Reveals Three-Dimensional Filament Organization in the Actin Cytoskeleton." *Nature Methods* 9 (2012): 185–8.

57. Chhabra, E S, and H N Higgs. "The Many Faces of Actin: Matching Assembly Factors with Cellular Structures." *Nature Cell Biology* 9 (2007): 1110–21.

58. Ponti, A, A Matov, M Adams et al. "Periodic Patterns of Actin Turnover in Lamellipodia and Lamellae of Migrating Epithelial Cells Analyzed by Quantitative Fluorescent Speckle Microscopy." *Biophysical Journal* 89 (2005): 3456–69.

59. Vallotton, P, S L Gupton, C M Waterman-Storer, and G Danuser. "Simultaneous Mapping of Filamentous Actin Flow and Turnover in Migrating Cells by Quantitative Fluorescent Speckle Microscopy." *Proceedings of the National Academy of Sciences of the United States of America* 101 (2004): 9660–5.

60. Andrews, N L, K A Lidke, J R Pfeiffer et al. "Actin Restricts FcεRI Diffusion and Facilitates Antigen-Induced Receptor Immobilization." *Nature Cell Biology* 10 (2008): 955–63.

61. Burkel, B M, G Von Dassow, and W M Bement. "Versatile Fluorescent Probes for Actin Filaments Based on the Actin-Binding Domain of Utrophin." *Cell Motility and the Cytoskeleton* 64 (2007): 822–32.

62. Wan, C, V Kiessling, and L K Tamm. "Coupling of Cholesterol-Rich Lipid Phases in Asymmetric Bilayers." *Biochemistry* 47 (2008): 2190–8.

63. Saarikangas, J, H Zhao, and P Lappalainen. "Regulation of the Actin Cytoskeleton-Plasma Membrane Interplay by Phosphoinositides." *Physiological Reviews* 90 (2010): 259–89.

64. Hartman, M A, D Finan, S Sivaramakrishnan, and J A Spudich. "Principles of Unconventional Myosin Function and Targeting." *Annual Review of Cell and Developmental Biology* 27 (2011): 133–55.

65. Swaney, K F, C-H Huang, and P N Devreotes. "Eukaryotic Chemotaxis: A Network of Signaling Pathways Controls Motility, Directional Sensing, and Polarity." *Annual Review of Biophysics* 39 (2010): 265–89.

66. Ridley, A J. "Rho GTPases and Actin Dynamics in Membrane Protrusions and Vesicle Trafficking." *Trends in Cell Biology* 16 (2004): 522–9.

67. Percival, J M, J A I Hughes, D L Brown et al. "Targeting of a Tropomyosin Isoform to Short Microfilaments Associated with the Golgi Complex." *Molecular Biology of the Cell* 15 (2004): 268–80.

68. Almeida, C G, A Yamada, D Tenza et al. "Myosin 1b Promotes the Formation of Post-Golgi Carriers by Regulating Actin Assembly and Membrane Remodelling at the Trans-Golgi Network." *Nature Cell Biology* 13 (2011): 779–89.

69. Zilberman, Y, N O Alieva, S Miserey-Lenkei et al. "Involvement of the Rho-mDia1 Pathway in the Regulation of Golgi Complex Architecture and Dynamics." *Molecular Biology of the Cell* 22 (2011): 2900–11.

70. Salvarezza, S B, S Deborde, R Schreiner et al. "LIM Kinase 1 and Cofilin Regulate Actin Filament Population Required for Dynamin-Dependent Apical Carrier Fission from the Trans-Golgi Network." *Molecular Biology of the Cell* 20 (2009): 438–51.

71. Blume, J V, J M Duran, E Forlanelli et al. "Actin Remodeling by ADF/Cofilin Is Required for Cargo Sorting at the Trans-Golgi Network." *The Journal of Cell Biology* 187 (2009): 1055–69.

72. Brandstaetter, H, J Kendrick-Jones, and F Buss. "Myo1c Regulates Lipid Raft Recycling to Control Cell Spreading, Migration and Salmonella Invasion." *Journal of Cell Science* 125 (2012): 1991–2003.

73. Cyrklaff, M, C P Sanchez, N Kilian, C Bisseye, J Simpore, F Frischknecht, and M Lanzer. "Hemoglobins S and C Interfere with Actin Remodeling in Plasmodium Falciparum-Infected Erythrocytes." *Science* 334 (2011): 1283–6.

3 Functional Role of Membrane Lipids in EGF Receptor Dynamics and Regulation

Michal Grzybek, Theresia Gutmann, and Ünal Coskun

CONTENTS

3.1 INTRODUCTION

Receptor tyrosine kinases (RTKs) serve as cell surface receptors for peptide ligands and are central for regulating processes such as cell proliferation, apoptosis, migration, and differentiation. RTK signaling pathways lead to diverse cellular responses although converging on a relatively confined set of highly conserved core signaling processes.[1,2] Our knowledge of RTK signaling networks advances with increasing pace, but our understanding of how specific cell fate decisions are orchestrated lags behind and deterministic modeling of RTK signaling is missing so far. Surprisingly, the fact that crucial initial activation steps occur at the membrane itself is still greatly underestimated, although accumulating evidence suggests a functional role of membrane lipids directly involved in regulating receptor signaling.[3–5]

The epidermal growth factor receptor (EGFR) is a member of a subfamily of four closely related RTKs: EGFR (ErbB1), HER2 (ErbB2), HER3 (ErbB3), and HER4 (ErbB4). According to the canonical model of RTK signaling, inactive EGFR monomers dimerize upon ligand binding, leading to the activation of the intracellular tyrosine kinase domain and hence transphosphorylation of several tyrosine and serine residues, which serve as docking sites for downstream effector proteins that propagate the activation signal inside the cell. Aberrant EGFR activation is implicated in pathophysiological conditions, such as cancer and neurodegenerative diseases.[6] Ligand binding also induces rapid receptor endocytosis and trafficking to early endosomes from where the receptor can be routed for degradation or recycling.[7,8] The initiated signaling cascade results eventually in one of the many responses regulated by the activation of EGFR.[6] The mechanisms governing the different responses are regulated at various stages, for example, ligand diversity as well as concentration, affinity of ligand binding, receptor dimerization partners, receptor density, posttranscriptional regulation, and subcellular localization. A challenging regulatory mechanism that has received comparatively little attention is the regulation of receptor signaling by the membrane microenvironment and specific protein–lipid interactions. In the following, we review our current understanding of the EGFR as a model RTK in regard to its ligand-induced activation and resulting conformational transitions, the effect of its lipidic environment at the plasma membrane, and its intracellular localization upon endocytosis.

3.2   LIGAND BINDING

Apart from EGF, the EGFR also recognizes other ligands, i.e., transforming growth factor-α, heparin binding EGF-like growth factor,[9] betacellulin,[10] amphiregulin,[11] and epiregulin.[12] Under physiological conditions, EGFR-expressing cells are exposed to a wide range of local ligand concentrations varying from a low to a high nanomolar range.[7] For over two decades, ligand binding has been thought to induce dimerization, but the precise activation mechanism of the full-length receptor remains elusive.[13,14] Particularly puzzling was the finding that cell surface EGFRs have promiscuous, vastly different affinities for the same EGF ligand, i.e., high affinity ($K_D \sim 0.3$ nM) and low affinity ($K_D \sim 2$ nM),[15,16] as inferred from concave-up Scatchard plots, indicating either heterogeneity of binding sites, distinct receptor populations, or negative cooperativity in ligand binding. Initially, this duality of ligand binding was believed to result from a differential ligand association with distinct receptor populations, i.e., low- and high-affinity receptors, or from two distinct binding sites present on the EGFR.[17,18] However, the concept of two independent binding sites is difficult to reconcile with X-ray structures of the ligand-stabilized dimeric receptor, which reveal symmetrical binding sites for both ligands.[19,20] The majority of EGFRs present at the plasma membrane are in the low-affinity state and only a minor fraction (2–5%) is present in the high-affinity state.[15] Most single-molecule experiments indicate higher amounts of high-affinity receptors than equilibrium binding data do, suggesting a negative-feedback loop involved in EGF binding, implying that cells might respond to EGF stimulation by converting high-affinity receptors to the low-affinity state. These two receptor classes are structurally distinct as they are distinguishable by different antibodies.[21,22] Their actual role is not solved yet, but high-affinity EGFRs are thought to regulate the early responses of EGFR activation such as inositol phosphate production or calcium release from intracellular stores, as has been shown by inhibition of the high-affinity site by either monoclonal antibodies or phosphorylation of EGFR by protein kinase C.[21–23] Ligand-dependent activation of only 1% of all cell surface EGFRs is sufficient to trigger a calcium wave response in EGFR-overexpressing A431 epidermoid carcinoma cells.[24] Conversely, the reduction of low-affinity receptors by the 2e9 antibody, which specifically blocks EGF binding of the low-affinity EGFR population, does not inhibit this early cell response to EGF.[21] Additionally, EGF concentrations that activate either only high-affinity receptors or both high- and low-affinity receptors induce differential signaling routes in cells.[25] Activated high- and low-affinity receptors might reside at different sites in the plasma membrane as indicated by their differing endocytic routes, clathrin-mediated and clathrin-independent, respectively.[7] The molecular mechanisms regulating their structural differences, membrane localization, and trafficking remain poorly understood.

Previous reports with fluorescently labeled EGF suggested the presence of a minor fraction of ligand-independent preformed EGFR dimers.[26,27] Förster resonance energy transfer (FRET) studies in quiescent A431 cells indicate those pre-existing dimers or oligomers representing the high-affinity functional subclass.[26] The presence of preformed dimers was confirmed in follow-up studies[24,28] by direct visualization of EGFR distribution, either by expressing GFP-tagged receptors in metabolizing cells[29] or by the use of Fab fragments directed against the ectodomain of EGFR.[30] In summary, these data suggested that the binding sites of the dimeric receptor would represent the high-affinity sites while the EGFR monomers would represent the low-affinity sites. In this model, however, positive cooperativity in ligand binding would be expected, for which experimental data are controversial.[15] The concept is at the moment best explained by a model involving negative cooperativity in an aggregating system:[31] high-affinity binding occurs to the first site on the receptor dimer, whereas low-affinity binding occurs to the second site on the dimer as well as to the monomer. This model is supported by a study of cells expressing increasing levels of EGFR-GFP using simultaneous fitting of binding isotherms and by obtaining values for the monomer–dimer equilibrium constants, which, for wild-type EGFRs, corresponded to ~50,000 receptors per cell.[31] It has been demonstrated that changes in receptor expression density within the physiological range modulate the outcome of a signaling stimulus. This model was validated, as dimerization-defective mutated receptors (Y246D-EGFR) exhibit a single class of binding sites. Therefore, it is assumed that binding of EGF to its receptor is positively linked with dimer assembly but shows negative cooperativity within the dimer.[32] This provides a framework for understanding secondary dimer formation and lateral signaling in the EGFR family.

3.3   FROM STRUCTURE TO FUNCTION

Our understanding of ligand binding and EGFR dimerization is strongly based on data from protein crystal structures.[33] The discovery of ligand-dependent dimerization initially led to the assumption that the ligand itself contributes to the formation of the dimerization interface,[26,34] as observed for other receptors.[1] However, X-ray structures of doubly liganded ectodomain dimers point to an EGFR dimerization interface, which is exclusively formed by the receptor itself without ligand involvement.[19,20] Additional crystal structures of the unliganded EGFR ectodomain,[35] which adopts a so-called tethered conformation, together with the solution structure of the liganded monomeric EGFR ectodomain[36] allowed conceptualizing the molecular mechanism of ligand-dependent EGFR dimerization.[37,38] Further insights were gained from the crystal structure of the monomeric HER2 ectodomain,[39] which displays an extended conformation and is believed to resemble the ligand-bound EGFR monomer. In the current model, the ectodomain (consisting of four subdomains DI, DII, DIII, and DIV) adopts an autoinhibited tethered conformation, where the dimerization domains (DII and DIV) are involved in stabilizing the actual tether (Figure 3.1). Limited fluctuations occur between the tethered and ligand-free, opened (extended) conformation, which is stabilized by the presence of the ligand. In the extended conformation, the dimerization sites on domains II and IV are exposed and therefore may be involved in the intermolecular associations. From a series of crystal structures of the *Drosophila* EGFR extracellular region, Alvarado et al. showed how the first ligand binding event induces the formation of an asymmetric EGFR ectodomain dimer with only one ligand bound.[40] The unoccupied site in this dimer is structurally restrained, leading to a reduced affinity for binding of the second ligand, and thus negative cooperativity.[40] This would explain the characteristics of cell surface EGFRs upon EGF binding; however, the crystal structures of doubly liganded human EGFR ectodomain are fully symmetrical.[19,20] Putting together the

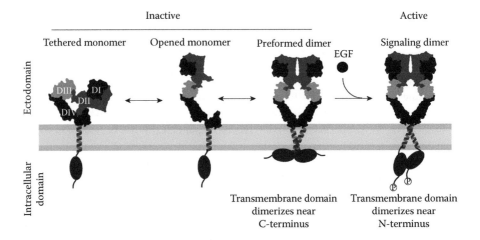

FIGURE 3.1 Schematic representation of EGFR activation. The monomeric EGFR is thought to exist predominantly as a monomer, fluctuating between a tethered and a "possible" extended conformation. The tether is stabilized by interaction of DII and DIV, and this interaction needs to be broken for the structure to open up. In the opened conformation, the dimerization arms at DII and DIV are supposed to be exposed and available for engaging a partner. In the absence of a ligand, the receptor can form preformed inactive dimers, which are characterized by dimerization of the transmembrane domains at their C-termini and formation of a symmetric dimer in their kinase domain part. Ligand binding, either to the monomeric or to the dimeric receptor, drives the formation of the active signaling dimer, which is characterized by dimerization of the transmembrane helices near their N-termini and formation of asymmetric kinase domain dimers.

bits and pieces of various structures, one could build an almost complete model of ligand-driven dimerization and activation, but it still does not explain the nature of the high-affinity EGFR population as no structures for either unliganded or singly liganded human receptor dimers are available.

Ligand-driven dimerization that leads to receptor activation not only involves interactions within the ectodomain but also leads to a mutual association within the intracellular domains of the EGFR, resulting eventually in autophosphorylation of several tyrosine and serine residues. Biochemical studies clearly demonstrated that the intracellular domain is involved in the dimerization process,[41–43] and deletion of this domain produced low-affinity receptors at the cell surface.[18] How the dimerization and activation processes could be decoupled from each other cannot be answered to date, as crystallization of a full-length receptor has not been achieved. Crystal structures of kinase domain dimers not only provided information about kinase domain activation but also shed light on the formation of active and inactive dimers.[41,42] The presented data suggest a mechanism that allows the transition of the kinase domain from a symmetric dimer structure to an asymmetric one, representing a switch from an inactive to an active dimeric kinase domain (Figure 3.1). Most importantly, these data imply a mechanism in which the extracellular domains block the intrinsic ability of the transmembrane and cytoplasmic domains to dimerize and activate upon ligand binding.[41,43] This mechanism could be verified by comparing the activation of the full-length to the truncated EGFR.[44] In contrast to the full-length receptor, the expression of the transmembrane helix and the intracellular module together suffice for constitutive activity even at low receptor densities. Therefore, ligand binding and receptor dimerization should be considered as mechanistically distinguishable events, and the presence of ligand-free dimers in the plasma membrane does not automatically imply their kinase activity.[45] In comparison, insulin or insulin-like growth factor receptors are present on the cell surface as covalent dimers, yet they still need to bind their respective ligands, which allosterically regulate the kinase domain activation.[46] To understand how ligand binding is coupled to the conformational changes in the ectodomain and to the kinase domains across the membrane, the receptor structure needs to be studied in a more holistic way. Single-particle electron microscopy (EM) analysis of nearly full-length EGFR was the first attempt to look at this process.[47,48] The ectodomain of unliganded monomeric EGFR was found to display a tethered conformation as predicted previously. Interestingly, however, the relative orientation between the ectodomain and kinase domain is variable, and thus, these domains appeared to be uncoupled. In the liganded dimeric receptor, the asymmetric kinase dimer was coexisting with a symmetric kinase dimer and a monomeric kinase assembly. The coupling of the activated receptor ectodomain conformations to multiple kinase domain arrangements suggests an unexpected variability and complexity in transmembrane signal propagation, implying a significant role of the juxtamembrane and cytoplasmic environment in regulating receptor function. These studies are limited as they do not reveal the coupling and transition mechanisms at the molecular scale. To bypass this limitation, a number of atomistic molecular dynamics (MD) simulations were used, the majority of which have very short timescales of a few nanoseconds. So far, only one study was done on an extensive timescale of nearly 5 μs,[49] for the first time indicating that, in ligand-bound dimers, the extracellular domains adopt conformations that favor dimerization of the transmembrane helices near their N-termini and formation of asymmetric (active) kinase dimers. In this configuration, the doubly liganded ectodomains stand upright on the membrane. In contrast, in the ligand-free dimer (or ligand-free monomer), the ectodomains lie flat on the membrane. Moreover, in ligand-free dimers, the extracellular domains favor C-terminal dimerization of the transmembrane helices and formation of symmetric (inactive) kinase dimers. The authors predict a significant regulatory role of the membrane, as electrostatic interactions of EGFR's intracellular module with the phosphatidylserine lipids used in these studies were critical in maintaining this coupling. Comparison of the MD simulations with low-resolution structures obtained by single-particle EM analysis exposed several discrepancies and triggered new questions about the mechanism of EGFR activation.[47,49] Although the tethered structure of the ectodomain in the ligand-free monomer can be distinguished in the EM analysis, the spatial distribution differs significantly from the MD simulations. Here, the ectodomain protrudes from the membrane, whereas in the MD simulations, the ectodomain lies flat on the membrane. The first view is also supported by FRET studies, which predict that the distance of the EGFR N-terminus (DI) to the membrane should be 6–8 nm.[50,51]

One explanation for this discrepancy might be that the low-resolution images were taken from molecules solubilized in detergent micelles not representing the compositional complexity and functionality of the biological membrane. This is most likely since the observed number of different conformations for the doubly liganded EGFR suggests high flexibility of the structures, which makes it difficult to imagine how ligand binding would be coupled to EGFR activation. Here, it needs to be emphasized that EGFR solubilized in detergent micelles show only low-affinity ligand binding, therefore not exhibiting negative cooperativity.[52] On the contrary, the MD simulations were built de novo from high-resolution crystal structures based on receptors with stabilized conformations prior to or during the crystallization process.[49]

3.4 LIPIDS AND EGFR SIGNALING

The idea that the lipid environment might have a modulatory function on receptor activity is not new; however, early studies addressing such questions have not found their way through to the current cell-signaling canon.[3,52–54] The lipid composition of a membrane defines its biophysical properties such as thickness, lateral pressure, and fluidity.[55] The discovery of lipid rafts and their role in plasma membrane compartmentalization and modulation of cell signaling has substantially changed our perception of membranes.[56,57] This model takes account of functional lipid–lipid and lipid–protein interactions and nanodomains with distinct biochemical and biophysical properties that directly influence protein function upon association. With the advancement of lipid mass spectrometry, the compositional diversity and complexity of the membrane lipid bilayer can be assessed in a quantitative manner.[58] An increasing number of high-resolution structures of membrane proteins display lipids as an integral part of their structure, indicating the relevance of specific lipid–protein interactions for structural stability and protein function (non-annular lipids).[3,59,60]

The regulation of RTKs by lipids has implications for various functional aspects such as ligand binding and autophosphorylation.[4]

The most abundant lipid in the mammalian plasma membrane is cholesterol, which constitutes up to 45 mol% of all plasma membrane lipids,[61,62] modulating fundamental membrane properties such as fluidity and lateral heterogeneity.[63–65] Acute depletion of cholesterol with methyl-β-cyclodextrin increases cell surface EGF binding by 40% via a mechanism that does not involve externalization of receptors from an internal pool. Cholesterol depletion furthermore leads to a two- to fivefold stimulation of EGFR autophosphorylation in vivo, without altering the rate of receptor dephosphorylation.[66,67] Signaling of the EGFR and of other RTKs is modulated by changes in cellular cholesterol content, implying that receptor localization or association to lipid rafts might be of functional importance.[68] Raft localization was suggested on the basis of EM,[66] fluorescence lifetime imaging microscopy,[69] and near-field scanning optical microscopy[70] studies. The raft-targeting determinants are localized in the EGFR ectodomain, as receptors lacking this domain do not associate with rafts. By contrast, receptors lacking the entire cytoplasmic domain or receptors in which the transmembrane domain was exchanged for that of the non-raft LDL receptor still localized to lipid rafts. The precise localization of the raft association motif has never been achieved, and it has been suggested that there might be more than one.[71] Since the EGFR ectodomain has been shown to interact with glycolipids[72] and as the extraction of cholesterol does not affect the nanoscale colocalization of GM1 with the EGFR,[69] a colocalization mechanism based on specific and direct glycolipid–receptor interaction is discussed. In this respect, glycolipid–receptor interactions could provide a "wetting" effect, enabling the receptor to be specifically targeted to raft domains.[57,73]

Single-molecule analysis using number and brightness measurements of EGFR–EGFP showed that acute depletion of cholesterol by methyl-β-cyclodextrin increases receptor dimerization/oligomerization, while cholesterol loading inverts this process. Interestingly, low or high levels of cholesterol directly correlate with the increased or decreased ligand-driven activation of the EGFR, respectively.[29,66] The depletion of membrane cholesterol has also been reported to induce ligand-independent EGFR activation.[74] It is important to note that extraction of cholesterol induces a wide range of cellular alterations such as phosphoinositide turnover and actin cytoskeleton rearrangements.[75–77] Therefore, complementary in vitro studies with reconstituted receptors in proteoliposomes are required to assess, in a controlled manner, the effects of specific lipid–protein interactions on receptor regulation.[78] Upon reconstitution in liposomes containing only 5 mol% of cholesterol, the EGFR undergoes ligand-independent kinase activation, while in the presence of 25 mol% of cholesterol, the receptor is activated only after ligand binding and in a dose-dependent manner. The underlying mechanism might relate to the increased fluidity and decreased average thickness of the cholesterol-poor bilayer, in which the transmembrane and juxtamembrane domains (JMDs) of EGFR might sustain increased flexibility, facilitating the formation of active EGFR dimers. In contrast, high cholesterol levels increase the average membrane thickness and might therefore restrict the flexibility of the transmembrane domain and thus the intra- and extracellular membrane proximal fragments. This hypothesis would be in good agreement with EM single-particle analysis of detergent-solubilized receptors showing flexibility and uncoupling of the EGFR extracellular and intracellular domains.[47]

Gangliosides are the most complex glycolipids in mammalian cells and contain negatively charged oligosaccharides with one or more sialic acid residues, which extend well beyond the surfaces of the cell membranes. Exogenous addition of the ganglioside GD1a increases both the number of high-affinity receptors and EGF-induced cell proliferation.[79] Conversely, the ganglioside GM3 has been repeatedly reported (for more than 30 years) to have inhibitory effects on cell growth through an unknown mechanism that decreases the EGFR kinase activity.[54,80] The overexpression of enzymes required for GM1 synthesis (which in turn decreases GM3 levels) results in enhanced cell proliferation in response to EGF.[81,82] Whether these effects were based on direct lipid–protein interactions could not be answered unambiguously in the cellular context. The confirmation that GM3 allosterically inhibits the kinase domain activity of the EGFR was furnished by reconstituting the EGFR in proteoliposomes. Although the ganglioside does not interfere with ligand binding or ligand-driven dimerization, the presence of GM3 in membranes with high cholesterol leads to a complete abrogation of ligand-induced EGFR kinase activation.[78] Moreover, the inhibition was highly specific since neither lactosylceramide, which is the precursor of GM3, nor GM2 showed any similar effect. Although it is suggested that GM3 inhibits EGFR tyrosine kinase through binding to N-linked glycan-presenting multivalent GlcNAc termini on the EGFR, a molecular mechanism and the precise sites where GM3 (or any other glycolipid) and the receptor interact are missing. Tunicamycin treatment of cells, which blocks N-glycosylation of proteins, abolishes GM3 susceptibility of EGFR, supporting the possibility of an involvement of N-linked glycans.[83] It remains unclear though whether this interaction is solely based on glycan–glycan interaction between the glycolipid and EGFR glycosylation sites or whether protein glycosylation is only required for maintenance of a specific EGFR conformation that enables interaction of GM3 with the receptor ectodomain.

In a recent study, the b-series disialoganglioside GD3, for which GM3 acts as a precursor, is reported to be directly responsible for sustaining the expression of EGFR and its downstream signaling to maintain the self-renewal capability of neural stem cells.[84] GD3-synthase knock-out mice exhibit a decreased self-renewal capability of neural stem cells, which was accompanied by reduced levels of EGFR expression and accelerated rates of EGFR degradation after EGF stimulation.[84]

The molecular mechanism through which predimerized receptors are kept in an inactive conformation remains enigmatic but recent data hint toward direct interactions between the intracellular domain and the plasma membrane in regulating this process. The positively charged JMD binds to the negatively charged phosphatidylserines (PSs) of the inner leaflet, as does the positive surface of the kinase domain,[49,85,86] which is predicted to prevent the two kinase domains from aberrant interactions, even in preformed dimers or oligomers. The EGFR would escape such an inhibition only at high expression levels when the amount of negatively charged lipids is not enough to sustain such inhibition.[49] The finding that the kinase domain of EGFR is active in solution but inhibited when bound to the membrane additionally supports this hypothesis.[44] PS is the major negatively charged phospholipid in the inner leaflet of the plasma membrane, but the presence of phosphatidic acid (PA) and phosphorylated phosphatidylinositols (PIPs), though less abundant than PS, might also contribute to this process. Upon bilayer binding, the JMD region produces a local positive electrostatic potential that attracts and sequesters $PI(4,5)P_2$, even in the presence of excess amounts of monovalent acidic lipids, as demonstrated using FRET and following PLCγ activity.[86] It is assumed that the release of calcium to the cytoplasm would initiate binding of Ca^{2+}/calmodulin to the JMD, which would retract this fragment from the membrane and support the formation of the active signaling EGFR dimers after EGF binding.[85] In this model, however, it remains puzzling how the formation of the first active dimers would take place if the intracellular calcium wave is initiated after EGFR activation, though only as little as 1% of plasma membrane EGFR need to be activated for the calcium response to appear.[24] Most recently, $PI(4,5)P_2$ has been reported to stimulate the activation of the EGFR.[87] The data suggest, in contrast to what has been previously proposed, that the interactions of the JMD with $PI(4,5)P_2$ should increase the formation of active dimers as pharmacological or genetic downregulation of $PI(4,5)P_2$ levels decreases EGF-induced receptor phosphorylation, whereas upregulation of $PI(4,5)P_2$ levels augments it.

The signaling cascades initiated upon ligand binding by EGFR are not restricted to changes of the cellular phosphoproteome but in fact also alter the lipid content in the membrane. EGFR activity is modulated by $PI(4,5)P_2$ and at the same time the receptor's activation leads to the turnover of $PI(4,5)P_2$, which might serve as a mechanism of self-desensitization. EGFR not only stimulates PLC, which hydrolyzes $PI(4,5)P_2$ into DAG and IP3, but also activates the phosphoinositide 3-kinase (PI3K), which turns $PI(4,5)P_2$ into $PI(3,4,5)P_3$ and which would presumably interact with the same region of the EGFR. Apart from phosphoinositide turnover, EGFR activation induces hydrolysis of plasma membrane phosphatidylcholine by phospholipase D2 producing PA and choline. This creates a local microdomain rich in PA, which also contains an elevated number of EGFRs.[88] This is not surprising since the EGFR can bind to acidic lipids in the plasma membrane.[49,85,86] It is likely that the receptor interacts with newly synthesized PA to form this protein–lipid complex. By regulating the production of critical second messenger lipids and modifying the local membrane lipid environment, enriched in PA or $PI(3,4,5)P_3$, EGFR activation drives the formation of a membrane lipid signaling hub, where adaptor proteins are recruited and the transduced signal is further amplified. The rearrangement of inner leaflet lipids around activated EGFR is reflected also in changes on the extracellular leaflet. Stimulation with EGF results in the colocalization of EGFR and GPI–GFP, which does not occur under resting conditions.[69]

These examples raise the important question whether lipids can—through either direct interaction or active control of adaptor protein recruitment, or both—modulate EGFR's function and therefore take an active role in ligand binding and EGFR receptor activation. The grand challenge in analyzing and understanding the underlying regulatory mechanisms lies within the compositional diversity and dynamic nature of the plasma membrane. A major issue is that lipids are not genetically accessible and fluorescent modification leads to major physicochemical changes. Silencing or knocking down enzymes involved in lipid synthesis pathways result in several alterations among various lipids as lipid synthesis occurs sequentially. Furthermore, lipids are not only synthetized de novo but a substantial part is recycled or synthetized through the salvage pathway.

Modulation of EGFR Activity by Lipids

Lipid	Effect on EGFR	Other Effects
Cholesterol ↑	Increases number of monomeric receptors and inhibits EGFR activity[29]	Changes membrane thickness and fluidity[65]
Cholesterol ↓	Increases EGFR dimerization/oligomerization and increases ligand binding and activity[29] Induces ligand-independent activation[74,78]	Inhibits non-clathrin-mediated endocytosis[7] Induces a wide range of cellular responses[75–77]
GM3 ↑	Inhibits activity[54,78,80]	Non-glycosylated EGFR is insensitive to GM3 inhibition[83]
GD1a ↑	Increases the number of high-affinity receptors[79]	
GD3 ↓	Reduces expression levels of EGFR and accelerates degradation of activated receptor[84]	
PA ↑	Induces dimerization/oligomerization and induces ligand-independent endocytosis and recycling[88,97]	
PI(4,5)P$_2$ ↑	Stimulates activation of EGFR[87]	
PI(3,4,5)P$_3$ ↑	Induces dimerization/oligomerization and induces ligand-independent endocytosis and recycling[101]	

3.5   EGFR ENDOCYTOSIS AND REGULATION

Upon ligand stimulation, the EGFR is rapidly internalized, permitting removal of activated receptors from the cell surface. The major mechanism of EGFR internalization occurs via clathrin-mediated endocytosis, whereby the receptor is removed from the surface in clathrin-coated pits and then routed to early endosomes from where it is destined to lysosomal degradation or recycling. Activation-induced endocytosis and subsequent degradation in lysosomes constitute an important negative feedback control for EGFR signaling.[89–92] Nevertheless, EGFR internalization is not necessarily equivalent to immediate signal attenuation, as specific signals also arise from the endosomal compartment.[93,94] Depending on its subcellular localization, activated EGFR associates with different signaling complexes, modulating the signaling output.[90,93–95] Cell fate decisions initiated by EGF are controlled by the recruitment of adaptor proteins activating distinct pathways. The Shc adaptor protein associates with EGFR located at the plasma membrane or within endosomes. In contrast, target proteins such as Grb2 and Eps8 are primarily found to bind to activated plasma membrane EGFR and to endosomal receptors, respectively.[90] Hence, receptor trafficking substantially affects the overall outcome of receptor signaling.

Clathrin-coated vesicles are generally accepted to be the main entry portal for the EGFR at low EGF concentrations, which is believed to result in signal abrogation owing to degradation but is apparently also followed by recycling of a major pool of the receptors, leading to prolonged signaling.[96] High ligand concentrations additionally activate internalization via ubiquitin-dependent, non-clathrin-mediated endocytosis, which subjects the receptor to lysosomal degradation, eventually resulting in signal termination.[7] Non-clathrin-mediated endocytosis is greatly decreased upon perturbation of cholesterol homeostasis by filipin, which leads to cholesterol sequestration. Furthermore, interference with cholesterol results in an increased recycling of the activated and internalized EGFR back to the plasma membrane rather than to lysosomal degradation.[96]

Endocytosis seems to be mediated by clathrin-dependent and -independent pathways, both leading to receptor accumulation in juxtanuclear recycling endosomes, where the internalized EGFR can remain without degradation for several hours or return rapidly to the cell surface upon discontinuation of the stimulus.[97] Similarly, diacylglycerol mimicking phorbol esters have been shown to induce ligand-independent EGFR internalization, which involves the activation of protein kinase C that directly phosphorylates threonine 654 of the EGFR. Threonine 654 phosphorylated receptors have been shown to undergo normal internalization, but instead of being sorted for lysosomal degradation, they recycle back to the cell surface. Moreover, T654 phosphorylation is also known to decrease the number of high-affinity EGFRs, though the exact molecular mechanism remains unclear.[23,98,99]

EGFR activation is not a prerequisite for receptor internalization. Apparently, other cellular mechanisms exist, which lead to the desensitization of the cell by removing unliganded and non-activated surface receptors. Interestingly, the pharmacological or mutational inhibition of the EGFR kinase activation does not block EGF-induced EGFR internalization, whereas the deletion of the extracellular dimerization loop of EGFR is sufficient to impede it. EGFR kinase inhibition results in enhanced recycling of the receptor instead of lysosomal degradation.[100] In summary, receptor internalization might depend on the ligand-induced dimerization step, rather than on the activation of the kinase domain. The EGFR also undergoes ligand-independent endocytosis invoked for instance by the accumulation of PI(3,4,5)P_3 or PA.[97,101]

The generation of PI(3,4,5)P_3 or PA occurs in the immediate vicinity of the activated EGFR as a result of activation of PI3K or PLD2, respectively, leading to local remodeling of the lipid bilayer.[88] Both of these lipids have been demonstrated to cluster EGFR and sequester (non-activated and non-ubiquitinated) it in the recycling endosome compartment.[97,101] Therefore, the interaction of the JMD or the tyrosine kinase domain with negatively charged lipids could be a general mechanism involved in receptor sequestration to recycling endocytic compartments, which results in temporal desensitization of the cell. It remains an open question how these different lipids, PS, PA, and PIPs crosstalk and what their actual contribution to regulation of EGFR activation and signaling is.

3.6   CONCLUSION AND PERSPECTIVES

For a comprehensive analysis of EGFR activation, the spatiotemporal distribution of the receptor and specific lipid–protein interaction needs to be considered. Increasing the concentration of EGFRs at the plasma membrane results in the formation of preformed dimers, which have been shown to be primed for ligand binding and receptor activation.[28,30,31] These receptors are mostly located at the cell periphery or at the leading edge of migrating cells. Interestingly, receptor dimerization has been shown to be sufficient for inducing receptor internalization as even kinase-dead EGFR mutants undergo endocytosis.[100] Whether preformed dimers in EGFR-overexpressing cells also follow rapid endocytosis and recycling remains to be shown. In summary, preformed dimers might reflect the high-affinity receptors at the nucleation sites of endocytic pits or just about to undergo ligand-independent internalization. Dimer formation might, however, directly depend on the local membrane properties guiding receptor dimerization and thus the formation and the spatiotemporal distribution of the high-affinity receptors. It should be noted that the cell periphery is highly enriched in actin cytoskeleton that forms numerous attachment sites with the membrane through adaptor proteins and therefore greatly reduces diffusion within the membrane. The attachment of the cortical meshwork to the membrane is predominantly based on the interactions with negatively charged phosphoinositides. Among these lipids, the predominant $PI(4,5)P_2$ has been shown to be actively involved in the nucleation of clathrin-coated pits.[102,103] A possible mechanism for the formation of high-affinity receptors would involve the interactions of the EGFR JMD with phosphoinositides; such interactions might even be necessary to compete with the interactions of the entire kinase domain with phosphatidylserine for the activation process.[44,49,86] In fact, EGFR reconstituted in liposomes containing phosphoinositides shows increased affinity for its ligand and the activity of EGFR correlates with the level of $PI(4,5)P_2$.[52,87] Most probably, other phosphoinositides $(PI(3,4,5)P3, PI(3,4)P2, PI(5)P$ and $PI(3)P)$, which change in concentration along the endocytic route, and PA, which is reported to influence EGFR endocytosis,[88,97,104] might also directly regulate receptor signaling fate decisions through adaptor protein recruitment. Importantly, outer leaflet lipids, especially gangliosides, contribute to the activation process, as well.[4,72,78,79] In migrating T cells, a distinct segregation of GM1 and GM3 is observed in the tailing and leading edge, respectively,[105] implying an additional level of complexity in receptor regulation and signaling response. Understanding precisely how the various membrane components influence lateral EGFR distribution, its membrane domain association/partitioning and activation, and how this connects to receptor endocytosis and signaling remains a challenge.

ACKNOWLEDGMENTS

The authors acknowledge Dr. Cornelia Schroeder for critical reading of the manuscript. This work was supported by Deutsche Forschungsgemeinschaft "Transregio 83" Grant TRR83 TP18 and by the German Federal Ministry of Education and Research grant to the German Center for Diabetes Research (DZD e.V.).

REFERENCES

1. Lemmon, M. A., and J. Schlessinger. "Cell Signaling by Receptor Tyrosine Kinases." *Cell* 141, no. 7 (2010): 1117–34.
2. Citri, A., and Y. Yarden. "EGF-ERBB Signalling: Towards the Systems Level." *Nat Rev Mol Cell Biol* 7, no. 7 (2006): 505–16.

3. Coskun, U., and K. Simons. "Cell Membranes: The Lipid Perspective." *Structure* 19, no. 11 (2011): 1543–8.

4. Miljan, E. A., and E. G. Bremer. "Regulation of Growth Factor Receptors by Gangliosides." *Sci STKE* 2002, no. 160 (2002): re15.

5. Lopez, P. H., and R. L. Schnaar. "Gangliosides in Cell Recognition and Membrane Protein Regulation." *Curr Opin Struct Biol* 19, no. 5 (2009): 549–57.

6. Yarden, Y., and M. X. Sliwkowski. "Untangling the ErbB Signalling Network." *Nat Rev Mol Cell Biol* 2, no. 2 (2001): 127–37.

7. Sigismund, S., T. Woelk, C. Puri et al. "Clathrin-Independent Endocytosis of Ubiquitinated Cargos." *Proc Natl Acad Sci U S A* 102, no. 8 (2005): 2760–5.

8. Avraham, R., and Y. Yarden. "Feedback Regulation of EGFR Signalling: Decision Making by Early and Delayed Loops." *Nat Rev Mol Cell Biol* 12, no. 2 (2011): 104–17.

9. Higashiyama, S., J. A. Abraham, J. Miller, J. C. Fiddes, and M. Klagsbrun. "A Heparin-Binding Growth Factor Secreted by Macrophage-Like Cells That Is Related to EGF." *Science* 251, no. 4996 (1991): 936–9.

10. Shing, Y., G. Christofori, D. Hanahan et al. "Betacellulin: A Mitogen from Pancreatic Beta Cell Tumors." *Science* 259, no. 5101 (1993): 1604–7.

11. Plowman, G. D., J. M. Green, V. L. McDonald et al. "The Amphiregulin Gene Encodes a Novel Epidermal Growth Factor-Related Protein with Tumor-Inhibitory Activity." *Mol Cell Biol* 10, no. 5 (1990): 1969–81.

12. Toyoda, H., T. Komurasaki, D. Uchida et al. "Epiregulin. A Novel Epidermal Growth Factor with Mitogenic Activity for Rat Primary Hepatocytes." *J Biol Chem* 270, no. 13 (1995): 7495–500.

13. Moriki, T., H. Maruyama, and I. N. Maruyama. "Activation of Preformed EGF Receptor Dimers by Ligand-Induced Rotation of the Transmembrane Domain." *J Mol Biol* 311, no. 5 (2001): 1011–26.

14. Nagy, P., J. Claus, T. M. Jovin, and D. J. Arndt-Jovin. "Distribution of Resting and Ligand-Bound ErbB1 and ErbB2 Receptor Tyrosine Kinases in Living Cells Using Number and Brightness Analysis." *Proc Natl Acad Sci U S A* 107, no. 38 (2010): 16524–9.

15. Livneh, E., R. Prywes, O. Kashles et al. "Reconstitution of Human Epidermal Growth Factor Receptors and Its Deletion Mutants in Cultured Hamster Cells." *J Biol Chem* 261, no. 27 (1986): 12490–7.

16. King, A. C., and P. Cuatrecasas. "Resolution of High and Low Affinity Epidermal Growth Factor Receptors. Inhibition of High Affinity Component by Low Temperature, Cycloheximide, and Phorbol Esters." *J Biol Chem* 257, no. 6 (1982): 3053–60.

17. Felder, S., J. LaVin, A. Ullrich, and J. Schlessinger. "Kinetics of Binding, Endocytosis, and Recycling of EGF Receptor Mutants." *J Cell Biol* 117, no. 1 (1992): 203–12.

18. Livneh, E., M. Benveniste, R. Prywes et al. "Large Deletions in the Cytoplasmic Kinase Domain of the Epidermal Growth Factor Receptor Do Not Affect Its Laternal Mobility." *J Cell Biol* 103, no. 2 (1986): 327–31.

19. Garrett, T. P., N. M. McKern, M. Lou et al. "Crystal Structure of a Truncated Epidermal Growth Factor Receptor Extracellular Domain Bound to Transforming Growth Factor Alpha." *Cell* 110, no. 6 (2002): 763–73.

20. Ogiso, H., R. Ishitani, O. Nureki et al. "Crystal Structure of the Complex of Human Epidermal Growth Factor and Receptor Extracellular Domains." *Cell* 110, no. 6 (2002): 775–87.

21. Defize, L. H. K., J. Boonstra, J. Meisenhelder et al. "Signal Transduction by Epidermal Growth Factor Occurs through the Subclass of High Affinity Receptors." *J Cell Biol* 109, no. 5 (1989): 2495–507.

22. Bellot, F., W. Moolenaar, R. Kris et al. "High-Affinity Epidermal Growth Factor Binding Is Specifically Reduced by a Monoclonal Antibody, and Appears Necessary for Early Responses." *J Cell Biol* 110, no. 2 (1990): 491–502.

23. Livneh, E., T. J. Dull, E. Berent et al. "Release of a Phorbol Ester-Induced Mitogenic Block by Mutation at Thr-654 of the Epidermal Growth Factor Receptor." *Mol Cell Biol* 8, no. 6 (1988): 2302–8.

24. Uyemura, T., H. Takagi, T. Yanagida, and Y. Sako. "Single-Molecule Analysis of Epidermal Growth Factor Signaling That Leads to Ultrasensitive Calcium Response." *Biophys J* 88, no. 5 (2005): 3720–30.

25. Krall, J. A., E. M. Beyer, and G. MacBeath. "High- and Low-Affinity Epidermal Growth Factor Receptor-Ligand Interactions Activate Distinct Signaling Pathways." *PLoS One* 6, no. 1 (2011): e15945.

26. Gadella Jr., T. W., and T. M. Jovin. "Oligomerization of Epidermal Growth Factor Receptors on A431 Cells Studied by Time-Resolved Fluorescence Imaging Microscopy. A Stereochemical Model for Tyrosine Kinase Receptor Activation." *J Cell Biol* 129, no. 6 (1995): 1543–58.

27. Sako, Y., S. Minoghchi, and T. Yanagida. "Single-Molecule Imaging of EGFR Signalling on the Surface of Living Cells." *Nat Cell Biol* 2, no. 3 (2000): 168–72.

28. Teramura, Y., J. Ichinose, H. Takagi et al. "Single-Molecule Analysis of Epidermal Growth Factor Binding on the Surface of Living Cells." *EMBO J* 25, no. 18 (2006): 4215–22.

29. Saffarian, S., Y. Li, E. L. Elson, and L. J. Pike. "Oligomerization of the EGF Receptor Investigated by Live Cell Fluorescence Intensity Distribution Analysis." *Biophys J* 93, no. 3 (2007): 1021–31.

30. Chung, I., R. Akita, R. Vandlen et al. "Spatial Control of EGF Receptor Activation by Reversible Dimerization on Living Cells." *Nature* 464, no. 7289 (2010): 783–7.

31. Macdonald, J. L., and L. J. Pike. "Heterogeneity in EGF-Binding Affinities Arises from Negative Cooperativity in an Aggregating System." *Proc Natl Acad Sci U S A* 105, no. 1 (2008): 112–7.

32. Pike, L. J. "Negative Co-Operativity in the EGF Receptor." *Biochem Soc Trans* 40, no. 1 (2012): 15–9.

33. Ferguson, K. M. "Structure-Based View of Epidermal Growth Factor Receptor Regulation." *Annu Rev Biophys* 37 (2008): 353–73.

34. Lemmon, M. A., Z. Bu, J. E. Ladbury et al. "Two EGF Molecules Contribute Additively to Stabilization of the EGFR Dimer." *EMBO J* 16, no. 2 (1997): 281–94.

35. Ferguson, K. M., M. B. Berger, J. M. Mendrola et al. "EGF Activates Its Receptor by Removing Interactions That Autoinhibit Ectodomain Dimerization." *Mol Cell* 11, no. 2 (2003): 507–17.

36. Dawson, J. P., Z. Bu, and M. A. Lemmon. "Ligand-Induced Structural Transitions in ErbB Receptor Extracellular Domains." *Structure* 15, no. 8 (2007): 942–54.

37. Burgess, A. W., H. S. Cho, C. Eigenbrot et al. "An Open-and-Shut Case? Recent Insights into the Activation of EGF/ErbB Receptors." *Mol Cell* 12, no. 3 (2003): 541–52.

38. Dawson, J. P., M. B. Berger, C. C. Lin et al. "Epidermal Growth Factor Receptor Dimerization and Activation Require Ligand-Induced Conformational Changes in the Dimer Interface." *Mol Cell Biol* 25, no. 17 (2005): 7734–42.

39. Cho, H. S., K. Mason, K. X. Ramyar et al. "Structure of the Extracellular Region of HER2 Alone and in Complex with the Herceptin Fab." *Nature* 421, no. 6924 (2003): 756–60.

40. Alvarado, D., D. E. Klein, and M. A. Lemmon. "Structural Basis for Negative Cooperativity in Growth Factor Binding to an EGF Receptor." *Cell* 142, no. 4 (2010): 568–79.

41. Jura, N., N. F. Endres, K. Engel et al. "Mechanism for Activation of the EGF Receptor Catalytic Domain by the Juxtamembrane Segment." *Cell* 137, no. 7 (2009): 1293–307.

42. Red Brewer, M., S. H. Choi, D. Alvarado et al. "The Juxtamembrane Region of the EGF Receptor Functions as an Activation Domain." *Mol Cell* 34, no. 6 (2009): 641–51.

43. Jura, N., X. Zhang, N. F. Endres et al. "Catalytic Control in the EGF Receptor and Its Connection to General Kinase Regulatory Mechanisms." *Mol Cell* 42, no. 1 (2011): 9–22.

44. Endres, N. F., R. Das, A. W. Smith et al. "Conformational Coupling across the Plasma Membrane in Activation of the EGF Receptor." *Cell* 152, no. 3 (2013): 543–56.

45. Yu, X. C., K. D. Sharma, T. Takahashi, R. Iwamoto, and E. Mekada. "Ligand-Independent Dimer Formation of Epidermal Growth Factor Receptor (EGFR) Is a Step Separable from Ligand-Induced EGFR Signaling." *Mol Biol Cell* 13, no. 7 (2002): 2547–57.

46. Siddle, K. "Signalling by Insulin and IGF Receptors: Supporting Acts and New Players." *J Mol Endocrinol* 47, no. 1 (2011): R1–10.

47. Mi, L. Z., C. Lu, Z. Li et al. "Simultaneous Visualization of the Extracellular and Cytoplasmic Domains of the Epidermal Growth Factor Receptor." *Nat Struct Mol Biol* 18, no. 9 (2011): 984–9.

48. Mi, L. Z., M. J. Grey, N. Nishida et al. "Functional and Structural Stability of the Epidermal Growth Factor Receptor in Detergent Micelles and Phospholipid Nanodiscs." *Biochemistry* 47, no. 39 (2008): 10314–23.

49. Arkhipov, A., Y. Shan, R. Das et al. "Architecture and Membrane Interactions of the EGF Receptor." *Cell* 152, no. 3 (2013): 557–69.

50. Kozer, N., C. Henderson, J. T. Jackson et al. "Evidence for Extended YFP-EGFR Dimers in the Absence of Ligand on the Surface of Living Cells." *Phys Biol* 8, no. 6 (2011): 066002.

51. Ziomkiewicz, I., A. Loman, R. Klement et al. "Dynamic Conformational Transitions of the EGF Receptor in Living Mammalian Cells Determined by FRET and Fluorescence Lifetime Imaging Microscopy." *Cytometry A* 83, no. 9 (2013): 794–805.

52. den Hartigh, J. C., P. M. van Bergen en Henegouwen, J. Boonstra, and A. J. Verkleij. "Cholesterol and Phosphoinositides Increase Affinity of the Epidermal Growth Factor Receptor." *Biochim Biophys Acta* 1148, no. 2 (1993): 249–56.

53. Lewis, R. E., and M. P. Czech. "Phospholipid Environment Alters Hormone-Sensitivity of the Purified Insulin Receptor Kinase." *Biochem J* 248, no. 3 (1987): 829–36.

54. Bremer, E. G., J. Schlessinger, and S. Hakomori. "Ganglioside-Mediated Modulation of Cell Growth. Specific Effects of GM3 on Tyrosine Phosphorylation of the Epidermal Growth Factor Receptor." *J Biol Chem* 261, no. 5 (1986): 2434–40.

55. Ernst, A. M., F. X. Contreras, B. Brugger, and F. Wieland. "Determinants of Specificity at the Protein–Lipid Interface in Membranes." *FEBS Lett* 584, no. 9 (2010): 1713–20.

56. Simons, K., and E. Ikonen. "Functional Rafts in Cell Membranes." *Nature* 387, no. 6633 (1997): 569–72.

57. Lingwood, D., and K. Simons. "Lipid Rafts as a Membrane-Organizing Principle." *Science* 327, no. 5961 (2010): 46–50.

58. Shevchenko, A., and K. Simons. "Lipidomics: Coming to Grips with Lipid Diversity." *Nat Rev Mol Cell Biol* 11, no. 8 (2010): 593–8.

59. Cherezov, V., D. M. Rosenbaum, M. A. Hanson et al. "High-Resolution Crystal Structure of an Engineered Human Beta(2)-Adrenergic G Protein-Coupled Receptor." *Science* 318, no. 5854 (2007): 1258–65.

60. Zhou, M., N. Morgner, N. P. Barrera et al. "Mass Spectrometry of Intact V-Type ATPases Reveals Bound Lipids and the Effects of Nucleotide Binding." *Science* 334, no. 6054 (2011): 380–5.

61. Gerl, M. J., J. L. Sampaio, S. Urban et al. "Quantitative Analysis of the Lipidomes of the Influenza Virus Envelope and MDCK Cell Apical Membrane." *J Cell Biol* 196, no. 2 (2012): 213–21.

62. Kalvodova, L., J. L. Sampaio, S. Cordo et al. "The Lipidomes of Vesicular Stomatitis Virus, Semliki Forest Virus, and the Host Plasma Membrane Analyzed by Quantitative Shotgun Mass Spectrometry." *J Virol* 83, no. 16 (2009): 7996–8003.

63. Burger, K., G. Gimpl, and F. Fahrenholz. "Regulation of Receptor Function by Cholesterol." *Cell Mol Life Sci* 57, no. 11 (2000): 1577–92.

64. Lingwood, D., H. J. Kaiser, I. Levental, and K. Simons. "Lipid Rafts as Functional Heterogeneity in Cell Membranes." *Biochem Soc Trans* 37, Pt 5 (2009): 955–60.

65. Maxfield, F. R., and G. van Meer. "Cholesterol, the Central Lipid of Mammalian Cells." *Curr Opin Cell Biol* 22, no. 4 (2010): 422–9.

66. Ringerike, T., F. D. Blystad, F. O. Levy, I. H. Madshus, and E. Stang. "Cholesterol Is Important in Control of EGF Receptor Kinase Activity but EGF Receptors Are Not Concentrated in Caveolae." *J Cell Sci* 115, Pt 6 (2002): 1331–40.

67. Pike, L. J., and L. Casey. "Cholesterol Levels Modulate EGF Receptor-Mediated Signaling by Altering Receptor Function and Trafficking." *Biochemistry* 41, no. 32 (2002): 10315–22.

68. Pike, L. J. "Growth Factor Receptors, Lipid Rafts and Caveolae: An Evolving Story." *Biochim Biophys Acta* 1746, no. 3 (2005): 260–73.

69. Hofman, E. G., M. O. Ruonala, A. N. Bader et al. "EGF Induces Coalescence of Different Lipid Rafts." *J Cell Sci* 121, Pt 15 (2008): 2519–28.

70. Nagy, P., G. Vereb, Z. Sebestyen et al. "Lipid Rafts and the Local Density of ErbB Proteins Influence the Biological Role of Homo- and Heteroassociations of ErbB2." *J Cell Sci* 115, Pt 22 (2002): 4251–62.

71. Yamabhai, M., and R. G. Anderson. "Second Cysteine-Rich Region of Epidermal Growth Factor Receptor Contains Targeting Information for Caveolae/Rafts." *J Biol Chem* 277, no. 28 (2002): 24843–6.

72. Miljan, E. A., E. J. Meuillet, B. Mania-Farnell et al. "Interaction of the Extracellular Domain of the Epidermal Growth Factor Receptor with Gangliosides." *J Biol Chem* 277, no. 12 (2002): 10108–13.

73. Anderson, R. G., and K. Jacobson. "A Role for Lipid Shells in Targeting Proteins to Caveolae, Rafts, and Other Lipid Domains." *Science* 296, no. 5574 (2002): 1821–5.

74. Chen, X., and M. D. Resh. "Cholesterol Depletion from the Plasma Membrane Triggers Ligand-Independent Activation of the Epidermal Growth Factor Receptor." *J Biol Chem* 277, no. 51 (2002): 49631–7.

75. Kwik, J., S. Boyle, D. Fooksman et al. "Membrane Cholesterol, Lateral Mobility, and the Phosphatidylinositol 4,5-Bisphosphate-Dependent Organization of Cell Actin." *Proc Natl Acad Sci U S A* 100, no. 24 (2003): 13964–9.

76. Doherty, G. J., and H. T. McMahon. "Mediation, Modulation, and Consequences of Membrane-Cytoskeleton Interactions." *Annu Rev Biophys* 37 (2008): 65–95.

77. Peres, C., A. Yart, B. Perret, J. P. Salles, and P. Raynal. "Modulation of Phosphoinositide 3-Kinase Activation by Cholesterol Level Suggests a Novel Positive Role for Lipid Rafts in Lysophosphatidic Acid Signalling." *FEBS Lett* 534, no. 1–3 (2003): 164–8.

78. Coskun, U., M. Grzybek, D. Drechsel, and K. Simons. "Regulation of Human EGF Receptor by Lipids." *Proc Natl Acad Sci U S A* 108, no. 22 (2011): 9044–8.

79. Liu, Y., R. Li, and S. Ladisch. "Exogenous Ganglioside GD1a Enhances Epidermal Growth Factor Receptor Binding and Dimerization." *J Biol Chem* 279, no. 35 (2004): 36481–9.

80. Yoon, S. J., K. I. Nakayama, T. Hikita, K. Handa, and S. I. Hakomori. "Epidermal Growth Factor Receptor Tyrosine Kinase Is Modulated by GM3 Interaction with N-Linked GlcNAc Termini of the Receptor." *Proc Natl Acad Sci U S A* 103, no. 50 (2006): 18987–91.

81. Nishio, M., O. Tajima, K. Furukawa, T. Urano, and K. Furukawa. "Over-Expression of GM1 Enhances Cell Proliferation with Epidermal Growth Factor without Affecting the Receptor Localization in the Microdomain in PC12 Cells." *Int J Oncol* 26, no. 1 (2005): 191–9.

82. Zurita, A. R., H. J. Maccioni, and J. L. Daniotti. "Modulation of Epidermal Growth Factor Receptor Phosphorylation by Endogenously Expressed Gangliosides." *Biochem J* 355, Pt 2 (2001): 465–72.

83. Wang, X. Q., P. Sun, M. O'Gorman, T. Tai, and A. S. Paller. "Epidermal Growth Factor Receptor Glycosylation Is Required for Ganglioside GM3 Binding and GM3-Mediated Suppression [Correction of Suppresion] of Activation." *Glycobiology* 11, no. 7 (2001): 515–22.

84. Wang, J., and R. K. Yu. "Interaction of Ganglioside GD3 with an EGF Receptor Sustains the Self-Renewal Ability of Mouse Neural Stem Cells In Vitro." *Proc Natl Acad Sci U S A* 110, no. 47 (2013): 19137–42.

85. Sengupta, P., E. Bosis, E. Nachliel et al. "EGFR Juxtamembrane Domain, Membranes, and Calmodulin: Kinetics of Their Interaction." *Biophys J* 96, no. 12 (2009): 4887–95.

86. McLaughlin, S., S. O. Smith, M. J. Hayman, and D. Murray. "An Electrostatic Engine Model for Autoinhibition and Activation of the Epidermal Growth Factor Receptor (EGFR/ErbB) Family." *J Gen Physiol* 126, no. 1 (2005): 41–53.

87. Michailidis, I. E., R. Rusinova, A. Georgakopoulos et al. "Phosphatidylinositol-4,5-Bisphosphate Regulates Epidermal Growth Factor Receptor Activation." *Pflugers Arch* 461, no. 3 (2011): 387–97.

88. Ariotti, N., H. Liang, Y. Xu et al. "Epidermal Growth Factor Receptor Activation Remodels the Plasma Membrane Lipid Environment to Induce Nanocluster Formation." *Mol Cell Biol* 30, no. 15 (2010): 3795–804.

89. Baulida, J., M. H. Kraus, M. Alimandi, P. P. Di Fiore, and G. Carpenter. "All ErbB Receptors Other Than the Epidermal Growth Factor Receptor Are Endocytosis Impaired." *J Biol Chem* 271, no. 9 (1996): 5251–7.

90. Burke, P., K. Schooler, and H. S. Wiley. "Regulation of Epidermal Growth Factor Receptor Signaling by Endocytosis and Intracellular Trafficking." *Mol Biol Cell* 12, no. 6 (2001): 1897–910.

91. Alwan, H. A., E. J. van Zoelen, and J. E. van Leeuwen. "Ligand-Induced Lysosomal Epidermal Growth Factor Receptor (EGFR) Degradation Is Preceded by Proteasome-Dependent EGFR De-Ubiquitination." *J Biol Chem* 278, no. 37 (2003): 35781–90.

92. Renfrew, C. A., and A. L. Hubbard. "Degradation of Epidermal Growth Factor Receptor in Rat Liver. Membrane Topology through the Lysosomal Pathway." *J Biol Chem* 266, no. 31 (1991): 21265–73.

93. Platta, H. W., and H. Stenmark. "Endocytosis and Signaling." *Curr Opin Cell Biol* 23, no. 4 (2011): 393–403.

94. Sadowski, L., I. Pilecka, and M. Miaczynska. "Signaling from Endosomes: Location Makes a Difference." *Exp Cell Res* 315, no. 9 (2009): 1601–9.

95. Sousa, L. P., I. Lax, H. Shen et al. "Suppression of EGFR Endocytosis by Dynamin Depletion Reveals That EGFR Signaling Occurs Primarily at the Plasma Membrane." *Proc Natl Acad Sci U S A* 109, no. 12 (2012): 4419–24.

96. Sigismund, S., E. Argenzio, D. Tosoni et al. "Clathrin-Mediated Internalization Is Essential for Sustained EGFR Signaling but Dispensable for Degradation." *Dev Cell* 15, no. 2 (2008): 209–19.

97. Norambuena, A., C. Metz, J. E. Jung et al. "Phosphatidic Acid Induces Ligand-Independent Epidermal Growth Factor Receptor Endocytic Traffic through PDE4 Activation." *Mol Biol Cell* 21, no. 16 (2010): 2916–29.

98. Downward, J., M. D. Waterfield, and P. J. Parker. "Autophosphorylation and Protein Kinase C Phosphorylation of the Epidermal Growth Factor Receptor. Effect on Tyrosine Kinase Activity and Ligand Binding Affinity." *J Biol Chem* 260, no. 27 (1985): 14538–46.

99. Bao, J., I. Alroy, H. Waterman et al. "Threonine Phosphorylation Diverts Internalized Epidermal Growth Factor Receptors from a Degradative Pathway to the Recycling Endosome." *J Biol Chem* 275, no. 34 (2000): 26178–86.

100. Wang, Q., G. Villeneuve, and Z. X. Wang. "Control of Epidermal Growth Factor Receptor Endocytosis by Receptor Dimerization, Rather Than Receptor Kinase Activation." *EMBO Rep* 6, no. 10 (2005): 942–8.

101. Laketa, V., S. Zarbakhsh, A. Traynor-Kaplan et al. "PIP_3 Induces the Recycling of Receptor Tyrosine Kinases." *Sci Signal* 7, no. 308 (2014): ra5.

102. McMahon, H. T., and E. Boucrot. "Molecular Mechanism and Physiological Functions of Clathrin-Mediated Endocytosis." *Nat Rev Mol Cell Biol* 12, no. 8 (2011): 517–33.

103. Di Paolo, G., and P. De Camilli. "Phosphoinositides in Cell Regulation and Membrane Dynamics." *Nature* 443, no. 7112 (2006): 651–7.

104. Ramel, D., F. Lagarrigue, V. Pons et al. "Shigella Flexneri Infection Generates the Lipid PI5P to Alter Endocytosis and Prevent Termination of EGFR Signaling." *Sci Signal* 4, no. 191 (2011): ra61.

105. Gomez-Mouton, C., J. L. Abad, E. Mira et al. "Segregation of Leading-Edge and Uropod Components into Specific Lipid Rafts during T Cell Polarization." *Proc Natl Acad Sci U S A* 98, no. 17 (2001): 9642–7.

4 Tetraspanins as Master Organizers of the Plasma Membrane

Cindy K. Miranti, Alexis Bergsma,
and Annemiek B. van Spriel

CONTENTS

4.1 INTRODUCTION—THE PRINCIPLE OF MEMBRANE COMPARTMENTALIZATION

Inspired by the fluid mosaic cell membrane model of Singer and Nicolson,[1] cell biologists have extensively investigated the biochemical and biophysical properties of the plasma membrane in the last decades. The identification of separate compartments in the cell membrane that are enriched in specific proteins and lipids has been a major advance in membrane science.[2,3] This principle, referred to as *membrane compartmentalization*, is essential for efficient transmission of extracellular stimuli into intracellular signals. Different types of membrane compartments (also called microdomains or nanodomains) have been characterized on the basis of their different protein–lipid composition, size, and biophysical behavior. Classical lipid nanodomains (rafts) are dependent on strong interactions between cholesterol and sphingolipids, which can sequester specific signaling proteins, allowing for the formation of large signaling assemblies.[4] In the "picket fence" model, transmembrane proteins and phospholipids can undergo hop diffusion between membrane compartments, whereas they can move freely within a compartment formed by the actin-based membrane skeleton.[5] This chapter focuses on the biological functions and molecular mechanisms of tetraspanin-enriched microdomains (TEMs), with the goal of presenting a unifying concept for tetraspanin function in the plasma membrane.

4.2   TETRASPANIN-ENRICHED MICRODOMAINS

Tetraspanins belong to a subset of the transmembrane 4 superfamily (TM4SF) that consists of small (20–50 kDa) transmembrane proteins that are expressed at the cell surface and in intracellular membranes. Tetraspanins are highly conserved between species and have been identified in multicellular eukaryotic organisms as diverse as plants, fungi, and mammals. Key structural features that tetraspanins share include the presence of conserved cysteines and a CCG motif in the large extracellular domain, four transmembrane domains, and palmitoylation sites at intracellular juxtamembrane regions[6] (http://www.ebi.ac.uk/interpro/entry/IPR000301?q=tetraspanin). To date, 33 different tetraspanins have been identified in humans. Whereas multiple tetraspanins (CD9, CD63, CD81, CD82, and CD151 among others) have a broad tissue distribution, restricted expression is documented for CD37 and CD53 (immune system), Tssc6 and Tspan33 (hematopoietic), Rom-1 and RDS (ocular), and uroplakins (bladder epithelium).

Tetraspanins are important in several fundamental cellular processes including migration, proliferation, differentiation, and immune surveillance and in malignant and infectious disease[7–10] (Table 4.1). The major functional characteristic of tetraspanins is that they control the lateral organization (*in cis*) of membrane proteins at the plasma membrane. Tetraspanins interact with each other (as homo- or heterodimers) and with transmembrane receptors, enzymes, and signaling proteins, whereby they form functional complexes in the membrane that are called *tetraspanin-enriched microdomains* (TEMs).[11] TEMs are variable in composition and size in different cell types, but they can cover up to 400 nm^2 of the plasma membrane. The composition and localization of TEMs are dynamic, thereby building up an interacting network or "tetraspanin web" in the plasma membrane.[12] At the inner leaflet of the plasma membrane, TEMs can be connected to the underlying actin cytoskeleton by tetraspanin interactions with cytoskeleton-associating receptors (integrins, receptor tyrosine kinases [RTKs]). For example, the C-terminal domain of tetraspanin CD81 has been demonstrated to interact directly with ezrin–radixin–moesin (ERM) actin linkers.[13] TEMs are discrete units that are clearly distinct from "classical" lipid rafts as evidenced by biochemical, proteomic, and imaging studies.[14–16] First, partitioning of tetraspanins into low-density fractions of sucrose gradients is preserved at 37°C

TABLE 4.1
Tetraspanins, Tissue-Specific Functions, and Their Targets

Function	Signaling/Partners
Migration/invasion	Integrins/RTKs/RhoGTPases/SrcK/PKC/PI4K/GPCRs/cadherins/MMPs
Tumor cells	CD151, CD82, CD9, Tspan8
Trophoblasts	CD82
Oligodendrocytes	CD82, CD9, Tspan2, CD81
Immune cells	CD82, CD37, CD81
Pathogen entry/exit/trans	Coreceptors/cytoskeleton/fusion/claudin/EWI
HCV	CD81
HIV	CD81, CD9, CD82, CD63
HTLV	CD81
Plasmodium	CD81
Immune surveillance	TCR/BCR/integrins/MHC/PKC/ERM/TLR/Dectin-1/CD19
T-cells	CD82, CD9, CD81, CD37, Tssc6, CD151
B-cells	CD37, CD81, CD53
APC	CD82, CD37, Tssc6, CD53, CD151
Platelets	CD9, CD151, CD82, Tssc6
Development/differentiation	Notch/ADAM10/fusion/cadherins
Caenorhabditis elegans	Tspan15
Drosophila	TspanC8s, sunglasses, late bloomer
Eye	ROM/RDS/Tspan12
Osteoclasts	CD82, CD9, Tspan13, Tspan5
Platelet/RBC/EC	TspanC8s, CD151, CD82
Skin	CD151
Muscle	CD9, CD81
Brain	CD81, Tspan7
Fertility	Integrins/Ca+
Egg/sperm	CD9, CD81
Membrane structure	
Eye	RDS
Bladder	Uroplakin
Intracellular trafficking	RTKs/integrins/ADAM10/E-cad/MHC/CD19/syntenin
Immune cells	CD63, CD82, CD81
Tumor cells	CD82
Platelet/RBC/EC	TspanC8s

using mild detergents, whereas rafts are disrupted under these conditions. Second, TEMs are more difficult to disrupt with cholesterol-depleting agents, such as methyl-β-cyclodextrin, in contrast to lipid rafts.[17] Third, proteomic analysis of TEMs has identified no raft-like proteins (glycosylphosphatidylinositol [GPI]-anchored proteins, caveolin).[15] Finally, single-molecule tracking of the raft GPI-anchored protein CD55 and tetraspanin CD9 demonstrates that they have different dynamic behavior in living cells.[16]

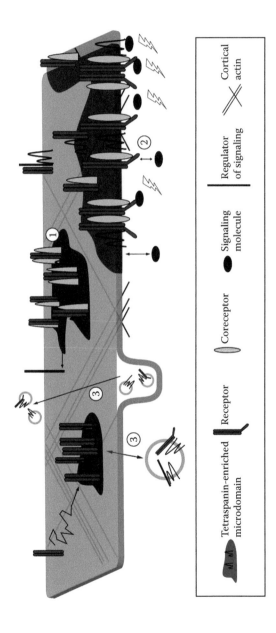

FIGURE 4.1 Unifying model illustrating TEMs in the plasma membrane that can facilitate receptor clustering, signal transduction, and membrane trafficking and exchange. (1) Complex assembly. Receptors can be clustered within TEMs leading to an increase of receptor avidity. TEMs provide a local environment that facilitates cross talk between different receptors, their coreceptors, and regulators, resulting in enhancement (or dampening) of their function. (2) Signaling. Signaling molecules are specifically recruited toward membrane domains, where stable signaling complexes are being created. (3) Membrane trafficking and exchange. Tetraspanins regulate the trafficking of specific membrane proteins to the plasma membrane and are involved in cell fusion, internalization, and transport to intracellular and extracellular compartments. (Modified from Zuidscherwoude, M. et al., *J Leukoc Biol*, 95, 251–63, 2014.)

4.3 THE UNIFYING CONCEPT OF TETRASPANINS

Tetraspanins are implicated in a wide variety of different cell functions, ranging from migration, immune surveillance, development, and protein trafficking to membrane fusion. This can be explained by the large number of tetraspanin interactions with different partner molecules that have been identified in diverse tissues and cell types (Table 4.1). Still, the molecular mechanism underlying the formation of TEMs is the same: that is, the lateral organization of specific membrane proteins and signaling molecules into dynamic units. This provides cells with a high level of plasticity to modulate the transduction of extracellular and intracellular signals essential for cell function. On the basis of the evidence presented in numerous biochemical and molecular tetraspanin studies, we present three major molecular mechanisms underlying tetraspanin function in the membrane, namely, (1) complex assembly, (2) modulation of signal transduction, and (3) membrane trafficking and exchange (Figure 4.1).[18]

4.4 TETRASPANIN FUNCTION IN MEMBRANE BIOLOGY

4.4.1 COMPLEX ASSEMBLY

Tetraspanins interact with one another (as homo- or heterodimers) and with a wide variety of transmembrane receptors, enzymes, and signaling proteins, whereby they form multimolecular complexes at the cell surface (reviewed in Refs. 7, 12, and 19). This complex assembly induces local clustering of receptors that leads to an increase of receptor avidity. Moreover, TEMs provide a local environment that facilitates cross talk between different receptors and their coreceptors resulting in enhancement (or dampening) of their function. Research on TEMs was, as most membrane research, initially based on biochemical approaches (isolation of detergent-resistant membranes, coimmunoprecipitation, proteomics). This provided insight into the biochemical principles underlying tetraspanin–partner interactions resulting in their classification into three different categories on the basis of their strength of interaction. Level 1 (primary) interactions represent direct interactions, whereas levels 2 and 3 (secondary and tertiary) represent indirect interactions.[7,14] In this chapter, we use the word *partner* only when referring to a level 1 (direct) tetraspanin interaction. Complex assembly at different levels may provide the cell with a mechanism to continually adapt to its environment and explain why many tetraspanin–protein interactions are transient and thus dynamic. The recent development of advanced microscopy techniques now provides the tools to investigate TEM dynamics in living cells. Pioneering imaging studies of tetraspanin CD9 in living cells revealed that CD9 mostly exhibits Brownian diffusion at the plasma membrane but is transiently confined to platforms that are enriched in CD9 and its interacting proteins, demonstrating the existence of different complexes that are diverse in their size, localization, and composition.[16] In addition, the recruitment of adhesion receptors (VCAM-1, ICAM-1) into TEMs of endothelial cells occurs independently of receptor–ligand engagement, actin cytoskeleton anchorage, and heterodimer formation.[20] We anticipate that the recent advances in the microscopy field will make important contributions to further unravel the biology of TEMs in the plasma membrane of living cells. In particular, super-resolution microscopy techniques (stochastic optical reconstruction microscopy, near-field scanning optical microscopy, and stimulated emission depletion microscopy) can directly map the nanoscale landscape of the cell surface, whereas single-molecule imaging, such as Förster resonance energy transfer and fluorescence lifetime imaging microscopy (FRET–FLIM) and multicolor single particle tracking, can provide insight into the dynamic behavior of membrane proteins at the molecular level.[21]

4.4.1.1   Complex Assembly of Integrins and Immune Receptors

Instead of attempting to list all tetraspanin–protein interactions, we will now discuss typical examples of complex assembly by tetraspanins that have functional consequences in different cell types and tissues (epithelium, immune system, and tumor cells).

One of the best characterized complex assemblies is the clustering of integrins into TEMs, which is important for downstream integrin signaling, adhesion strengthening, and cell migration. The interaction of tetraspanin CD151 with laminin-binding integrin α3β1 as a direct partner maps within the large extracellular domain (EC2) of CD151.[22] The integrin α7 subunit also binds directly to the same CD151 domain,[23] whereas CD151 interacts indirectly with α6β1 and α6β4 integrins.[24] Palmitoylation of the cytoplasmic tails of CD151 and the integrin α3, α6, and β4 subunits is required for the assembly of CD151/integrin complexes into TEMs (level 3 interaction) and their association with other tetraspanins.[25,26] In the immune system, we recently demonstrated that tetraspanin CD37 is essential for B-cell survival, antibody (immunoglobulin G) production, and long-lived protective immunity.[27] CD37-deficient B-cells show impaired Akt signaling mediated through α4β1 integrin molecules. At the molecular level, CD37 is required for the mobility and clustering of α4β1 integrins in the plasma membrane, thus regulating the membrane distribution of α4β1 integrin that is necessary for activation of the Akt survival pathway in the immune system.[27] Although the interaction of CD37 with α4β1 integrin is a level 2 or 3 interaction, this study demonstrates that indirect interactions do have important physiological relevance. The other reported tetraspanin that is essential for B-cell function and humoral immunity is CD81.[10,28] CD81 facilitates α4β1 integrin-mediated rolling and arrest under shear flow in line with CD37 function.[29] Moreover, CD81 is a direct partner of CD19 in the BCR coreceptor complex, and CD81 is essential for CD19 complex formation in the plasma membrane.[30,31] The large extracellular loop of CD81 associates physically with CD19 early during biosynthesis and CD81 facilitates the exit of CD19 from the endoplasmic reticulum (ER).[32] The importance of CD81 in BCR activation was elegantly demonstrated in super-resolution microscopy studies showing that CD81 assembles CD19 molecules in TEMs to facilitate interaction with mobile BCR nanoclusters that are released after cytoskeleton disruption.[33] The importance of tetraspanins in the immune system is underlined by the impaired humoral and cellular immune responses in tetraspanin-deficient mice and humans (discussed in Section 4.5).

4.4.1.2   Complex Assembly in Tumor Cells

Tetraspanins play a major role in tumor cell migration and invasion through their ability to cluster integrins, metalloproteases, or growth factor receptors (reviewed in Refs. 34–36). An intriguing correlation between the expression of tetraspanins

(Tspan7, Tspan8, Tspan31, CD9, CD63, CD82, and CD151) and tumor development has been reported. Tetraspanins do not appear to be involved in primary tumor growth; instead, they are important in tumor metastasis. However, we recently observed that CD37-deficient mice spontaneously develop B-cell lymphomas upon aging (unpublished data, AvS). Both tumor-suppressing (e.g., CD9 and CD82) and tumor-promoting (e.g., CD151 and Tspan8) effects have been reported in a number of different cancers (reviewed in Refs. 35 and 37). Tetraspanin CD82 is a well-known tumor suppressor protein that inhibits cancer cell motility, invasiveness, and survival (reviewed in Refs. 38 and 39). Different mechanisms have been attributed to CD82 function, including regulation of growth factor receptor signaling (epidermal growth factor receptor [EGFR], Met), β1 integrin function, stabilization of E-cadherin/β-catenin complex formation at the cell surface, and coupling to different signaling pathways (protein kinase C [PKC], Src, discussed in Section 4.4.2.1). Studies using CD82 mutants that are unable to inhibit tumor cell migration and invasion revealed that the membrane-proximal palmitoylation cysteine residues are essential for the tumor suppressor function of CD82.[40] CD151 strengthens tumor cell laminin adhesion and metastasis.[41,42] In addition, CD151 stimulates HGF (hepatocyte growth factor)/Met signaling in breast cancer cells and TGF (transforming growth factor) β1-induced activation and is associated with reduced survival in breast cancer patients.[43–45]

4.4.1.3 Complex Assembly of Membrane Enzymes

Tetraspanins interact with different proteases (and their substrates), which are critically important in cell migration, adhesion, and proliferation (reviewed in Ref. 46). Tetraspanins interact with membrane proteases belonging to the matrix metalloproteinase (MMP), a disintegrin and metalloprotease (ADAM), and γ-secretase families. The assembly of these proteases and their specific substrates into TEMs has been shown to affect their enzymatic activity. For example, the collagenolytic activity of MT1-MMP is regulated by tetraspanin CD151 in endothelial cells. Biochemical and FRET analyses showed that CD151 associates tightly with the hemopexin domain in MT1-MMP, thereby inducing the formation of ternary membrane complexes of α3β1 integrin/CD151/MT1-MMP.[47] Complex assembly of CD151 with MT1-MMP and α3β1 integrin induces cross talk and thereby spatiotemporally controls pericellular proteolysis during endothelial cell migration and angiogenesis. CD151 knockdown inhibits MT1-MMP inclusion into TEMs, prevents its biochemical association with α3β1 integrins, and results in enhanced MT1-MMP-mediated activation of MMP2. In tumor cells, MT1-MMP was found to interact with tetraspanins CD81, CD9, and Tspan12. Tetraspanin deletion decreased MT1-MMP expression levels at the plasma membrane resulting in impaired matrix degradation in these cells and decreased invasive capacity.[48] The underlying mechanism involved tetraspanin-induced MT1-MMP protein protection from lysosomal degradation and support of MT1-MMP delivery to the cell surface. Recently, another functional interaction between tetraspanins of the TspanC8 members (Tspan5, Tspan10, Tspan14, Tspan15, Tspan17, and Tspan33) with the metalloprotease ADAM10 has been reported.[49,50] ADAM10 is a ubiquitous transmembrane metalloprotease that cleaves the extracellular regions from multiple transmembrane proteins and is crucial in development, immunity, and cancer. TspanC8 tetraspanins were found to be crucial for the trafficking (discussed in Section 4.4.3), maturation, and stabilization of ADAM10 in the plasma membrane. The finding that certain tetraspanins inhibit the proteolytic capacity of membrane enzymes (CD151-MT1-MMP) whereas others (CD81/CD9/Tspan12-MT1-MMP and TspanC8-ADAM10) stimulate their activity by recruitment into TEMs highlights that tetraspanins can have opposing functions. Although the different cell types used in these studies may have contributed to these different results, we also envisage that TEMs of different composition and localization in the membrane exist within the same cell. In particular, evidence is now accumulating that tetraspanins interact dynamically with many different molecules at the cell surface. Thus, the dynamic regulation of compartmentalization of enzymes and their substrates into TEMs would enable rapid regulation of their enzymatic activity and accessibility to substrates in the plasma membrane.

Taken together, there is a plethora of literature demonstrating that tetraspanins induce complex assembly of their partner molecules in TEMs, and mapping the precise domains in tetraspanin proteins that are responsible for this molecular organization and function is still an active area of research. The importance of intracellular palmitoylation on juxtamembrane cysteine residues of tetraspanins for the stabilization of tetraspanin–tetraspanin interactions is well established (reviewed in Ref. 51). This contributes directly to the stability of TEMs and facilitates level 2 and level 3 (indirect) tetraspanin interactions. In addition, a role for the tetraspanin EC2 domain in the direct interaction with specific partners has been shown (reviewed in Refs. 6, 32, and 52). Recently, studies on the intracellular tails of CD9 revealed that the short C-terminus contains a well-conserved domain of three amino acids (Glu–Met–Val) that is involved in CD9-mediated cell adhesion and molecular organization of CD9 in the plasma membrane.[53] It will be interesting to investigate whether homologous regions in the C-terminal tails of other tetraspanins are required for TEM assembly and function. Moreover, the complete crystal structure of a tetraspanin protein interacting with a specific partner protein has not been resolved to date.

4.4.2 MODULATION OF SIGNAL TRANSDUCTION

Because of their lack of intrinsic enzymatic motifs, tetraspanins are frequently thought to facilitate signaling events rather than acting directly in a given pathway. While this is generally the case, it should not discount their significance in influencing major signal transduction pathways. In fact, tetraspanins interact with a surfeit of kinases, phosphatases, and signaling receptors that each serve an important role in inhibiting or promoting cell motility and invasiveness. This section will emphasize a handful of examples of tetraspanins, their associated signaling molecules, and the subsequent consequences on cell motility, invasion, and survival. How tetraspanins link these processes with the underlying cytoskeleton will also be discussed.

4.4.2.1 RTK Signaling

RTKs are the high-affinity cell surface receptors for many polypeptide growth factors, cytokines, and hormones. EGFR and its related ErbB family members typically respond to growth factors such as EGF, amphiregulin, and neuregulin by inducing the intrinsic tyrosine kinase activity to autophosphorylate its cytoplasmic domain. In this chapter, we will also discuss Met, which is the receptor for hepatocyte growth factor or scatter factor (HGF/SF), and the immune-specific RTKs, B-cell and T-cell receptors (BCR/TCR), which interact with antigen/major histocompatibility complex (MHC) complexes on antigen-presenting cells (APCs) to activate a similar tyrosine phosphorylation cascade.

Tetraspanins CD82 and CD151 are well known for their interactions with various components of the RTK signaling pathways. For example, CD82 positively regulates TCR signaling in T-cells but negatively regulates Met and EGFR in epithelial cells.[54–56] Conversely, CD151 stimulates Met activity in epithelial cells. Met is known to promote prostate cancer metastasis,[57] while CD82 is best known for its metastasis suppressing abilities where its expression is lost in almost all metastatic cancers. CD151 on the other hand is associated with more aggressive cancers. These opposing biological activities are likely a direct reflection of their effects on RTK signaling.

CD151 not only interacts with Met but also is required for functional Met–β4 integrin complexes in the plasma membrane of cancer cells.[58,59] Although the interaction between CD151 and Met is indirect, CD151 stimulates Met-induced phosphorylation of integrin β4 in tumor cells, thereby stimulating tumor growth by propagating MAPK proliferative signals.[60] In CD151-deficient cells, FAK phosphorylation by HGF at Src sites is impaired and this trend is exacerbated in CD151-null breast cancer cells where total HGF/Met signaling is lost.[44,59] In addition, CD151 and Met expression correlate with poor prognosis in pancreatic ductal adenocarcinoma patients, demonstrating the significant translational value of CD151–RTK interactions.[61]

As will be discussed in Section 4.4.3, the primary mechanism by which CD82 suppresses RTKs is through regulation of their internalization. In addition, CD82 prevents ligand-induced dimerization of EGFR and subsequent propagation of downstream signaling events to survival and proliferation pathways MAPK, STAT, and mTOR[62,63] as well as regulating EGFR ubiquitylation.[64]

One of the downstream signaling targets of RTKs is PKC, which is a family of serine/threonine kinases whose activation is highly membrane associated and dependent on lipid binding. Both CD82 and CD151 associate with PKC.[65,66] Through its interaction with PKC along with caveolin-1 and ganglioside GM3, CD82 associates with and desensitizes EGFR-induced signaling.[67] Integrins that interact with CD82 and CD151 are another target of PKC signaling.[65,66] In the case of CD151, this target is Ser1424 in the cytoplasmic tail of integrin β4. CD151 association with PKC and integrin β4 was shown to be necessary to promote skin carcinogenesis.[66] In the case of CD82 stimulation of PKC, integrin α3 cytoplasmic tail phosphorylation was the target.[65] The direct effect of these phosphorylation events on integrin signaling was not assessed in these studies, but the downstream biological effects on integrin β4 are consistent with a positive action on integrin function toward migration. The basis for the association between tetraspanins and PKC has not been fully explored, except for the cytoplasmic loop between the two tails, and for CD151, the cysteine residues therein are important. Interestingly, PKC is known to be palmitoylated,[68] a lipid modification that also occurs at the membrane-proximal cysteines on the cytoplasmic domains of tetraspanins.[40,69] As discussed in Section 4.4.1, palmitoylation is critical for the assembly of tetraspanins into TEMs.[51] Thus, PKC is likely to associate with the TEM via its palmitoylation, which enhances its ability to target palmitoylated integrins also present within the TEM.

Src kinases, downstream targets of both RTKs and integrins, are potent activators of migratory and invasive characteristics.[70] CD82 is a powerful suppressor of Src kinases, resulting in subsequent deactivation of several Src substrates, including p130CAS, FAK, and CDCP1.[55,71] The mechanism by which Src kinases are inhibited by CD82 has not been clearly elucidated. In one study, the effect was not caused by inhibition of the upstream RTK Met.[55] In another study, gangliosides were shown to inhibit Src, suggesting the possible recruitment of Src into TEMs.[56] Src itself is not palmitoylated, although other members such as Yes, Fyn, and Lyn are, but it is associated with the membrane through myristylation. Src activity and its ability to transform cells are suppressed through its association with cholesterol-enriched microdomains.[72] The extent to which CD82 might shuttle between TEMs and cholesterol-containing microdomains[73] may play an important role in how Src is regulated.

Alternatively, a more recent report demonstrated that CDCP1 (aka gp140/Trask), a CUB domain-containing protein, was responsible for suppressing Src activity via CD82. This is particularly striking given the association of CDCP1 with aggressive cancer, RTK and integrin signaling, and extracellular matrix proteases. It is also palmitoylated and reportedly associates with TEMs.[74,75] In addition, it serves as a scaffold to facilitate PKC activation.[76] Thus, CDCP1 seems to be poised to act as an interface between several different signaling pathways affected by tetraspanins. A better understanding of CDCP1 and other molecules that might control signaling between different membrane microdomains will be essential for fully understanding how tetraspanins regulate cellular signaling processes.

E-cadherin and claudins are transmembrane proteins that constitute adherens and tight junctions, respectively, to mediate cell–cell adhesion and recognition. Tetraspanins can influence cell–cell junctions. CD82 strongly promotes E-cadherin-induced adhesion by stabilizing E-cadherin's association with β-catenin, a complex required for E-cadherin function and stability.[77] On the other hand, while junction stability in CD151-deficient cells is normal when α3β1 integrin is present, localization of E-cadherin is impaired.[78] Tetraspanins (CD9, Tspan3, CO-029, CD81, and CD151) have been reported to associate with claudins.[79,80] For example, oligodendrocyte migration is stimulated under the association of claudin-11, Tspan3, and β1 integrin[81] and may be critical for normal myelination and repair. Furthermore, cross-linking studies in nonpolarized cells demonstrate a direct association between CD9 and claudin-1 in TEMs, yet this complex is not detectable at tight junctions in polarized cells.[79] Similarly, the association between claudin-7 and another adhesion molecule, EpCAM, which occurs within the TEM, enhanced tumorigenic properties including proliferation, Erk signaling, increased cell survival, drug resistance, and motility, but had no effect on EpCAM-mediated cell–cell adhesion.[82] Thus, the picture emerging for tetraspanins and claudins is for their association outside of tight junctions.

RTKs, such as Met or EGFR, in combination with Src, signal to dissociate cell–cell junctions in epithelial cells to promote migration during wound healing and similarly promote invasion during metastasis (Figure 4.2, right-hand cell). Upon signaling initiated by wounding, Src directly phosphorylates substrates within the

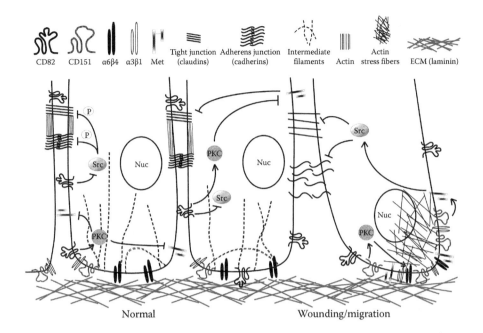

CD82 CD151 α6β4 α3β1 Met   Tight junction   Adherens junction   Intermediate   Actin   ECM (laminin)
                     (claudins)   (cadherins)   filaments   Actin   stress fibers

Normal   Wounding/migration

FIGURE 4.2 Reciprocal signaling by tetraspanins CD82 and CD151 and their control of intercellular adhesion and migration in epithelial cells. (left) In normal epithelial cells, CD82 localization at the lateral cell junction prevents migration by inhibiting Src and Met through PKC stimulation, strengthening adherens and tight junctions. CD82 and CD151 are also situated on the basal/lateral surface where they associate with integrin α3β1 and α6β4. (right) During migration induced by events such as wound healing or growth factor signaling through RTKs such as Met, CD151 relocalizes with integrins and RTKs to the leading edge of the migrating cells, where it stimulates PKC and subsequent integrin β4 activation, which dissolves α6β4–hemidesmosome and intermediate filaments. In addition, CD151 activates Met signaling. Met activation subsequently transmits signaling to stimulate Src, resulting in loose junctional arrangements and decreased cell–cell adhesion. Organized actin fibers at the tight and adherens junctions dissociate and actin reassembles at the leading edge, along with CD151 and integrin complexes, in a coordinated effort to promote cell migration. In the absence of CD82, this migratory capacity is perpetuated. When CD82 is present, it suppresses RTK and Src signaling to reestablish hemidesmosomes, cell–cell junctions, and cell polarity.

tight and adherens junctions that promote their dissociation. Moreover, Src phosphorylates molecules that disrupt the underlying actin cytoskeleton at the junctions. The same signaling pathway also disrupts the integrin α6β4–hemidesmosome complex at the basement membrane disrupting intermediate filaments. This wholesale change in cell cytoskeleton is accompanied by assembly of integrin/actin/RTK complexes at the leading edge. Tetraspanins can be found within the leading edge assembly where they are poised to regulate the resulting signaling and biological events. The presence of specific tetraspanins may dictate the ultimate outcome of continued migration and invasion as seen in cancer cells or an eventual regression and reestablishment of tissue integrity seen in normal cells. For instance, positive PKC activation by CD151 would promote the actin rearrangements and integrin activation and further stimulate RTK signaling (Figure 4.2, right-hand cell), whereas CD82 would balance the signal by directing PKC toward suppressing RTK and Src to limit the response (Figure 4.2, left-hand cells). This would ultimately permit restoration of cell–cell junctions, α6β4–hemidesmosomal structures, and cell polarity (Figure 4.2, left-hand cells). Thus, it is possible to envision how loss of either tetraspanin might disrupt this delicate balance. As is seen in metastatic cancers, loss of CD82 would remove the negative feedback loop and keep cells perpetually in a migratory state.

This model further serves to demonstrate how different pairings of tetraspanins, at times working toward the same purpose, and at times working to balance each other's response, are poised to tightly regulate biological responses in complex multicellular organisms. Given that the same opposing activities between CD82 and CD37 are seen in migrating APCs in vivo strongly suggests the potential for reciprocal signaling paradigms that may exist between other tetraspanin pairs as well. It also points to the importance of taking into consideration the whole tetraspanin repertoire expressed within a cell to fully understand the biological outcome when manipulating individual components. The underlying mechanism for how different tetraspanins within the TEM work together or work in opposition still needs to be determined, whether the outcome is dictated by specific partner proteins or is intrinsic to the tetraspanin.

4.4.2.2 Tetraspanin Effects on the Cytoskeleton

The net effect of much of the signaling controlled by tetraspanins is to have a downstream impact on actin-based events. However, tetraspanins themselves also directly contribute to actin reorganization through controlling signals via the Rho small GTPases, Rho, Rac, and Cdc42. Under adherent conditions where CD151-associated integrins engage the cytoskeleton, CD151 recruits Rac1, and Cdc42, as well as Ras, but not RhoA, into a complex and subsequently activates cytoskeletal remodeling as well as Ras signaling events.[83] The ability to activate Ras is dependent on adhesion; when these integrins are dissociated from the matrix, CD151 is unable to assemble the Ras complex, resulting in Ras inactivation.[84] Conversely, in the absence of CD151, there is a dramatic increase in RhoA signaling causing disruption of cell–cell adhesion at the lateral surface and the assembly of actin stress fibers at the basal surface,[78] that is, a switch in membrane localization for actin assembly. Additionally, preliminary evidence suggests that CD151 may need to associate with integrin α3β1 to suppress RhoA activity.[78] Together, these data indicate that there is a functional integration of tetraspanins and integrins in order to signal normally. While proteomic analysis can be used to identify protein–protein interactions, advanced immunofluorescence microscopy techniques have been important in verifying these signaling interactions in living cells. Such methods have been used to identify the Rac–CD81 complex and its localization at the leading edges of migrating cells and to demonstrate negative regulation of Rac1 by CD82.[85,86] The CD81–Rac complex is also necessary for normal dendritic cell migration, as shown in CD81-deficient dendritic cells that are incapable of forming adequate actin-based membrane protrusions owing to impaired CD81–Rac complex assembly.[87] Moreover, integrin clustering at the leading edge of the migrating cell appears to be regulated by CD81, as CD81-deficient cells and wild-type cells demonstrated similar cluster size and distribution around the cell surface. These examples demonstrate how tetraspanins play a significant role in regulating GTPase signaling and consequently affect cellular cytoskeletal arrangements in events such as migration and metastasis.

Single-pass Ig-like EWI proteins have been shown to partner with tetraspanins CD9, CD81, and CD82.[13,88] EWI proteins, through their direct interaction with ERM proteins, act as linkers to connect TEMs to the actin cytoskeleton to regulate cell motility and polarity.[13] EWI-2 and EWI-F colocalized with ERM proteins at microspikes and microvilli of adherent cells and at the cellular uropod in polarized migrating leukocytes. Biochemical studies using the cytoplasmic domains of EWI proteins corroborated the strong and direct interaction between ERMs and the tetraspanin-binding EWI-2 and EWI-F proteins. In addition, direct association of EWI partner CD81 C-terminal domain with ERMs was also demonstrated. Functionally, silencing of endogenous EWI-2 expression in lymphoid cells augmented cell migration and cellular polarity and increased phosphorylation of ERMs. Thus, EWI acting through tetraspanins may act to limit the extent of actin polymerization and control migration. This is further supported by the demonstration that EWI-2 is necessary for CD82 inhibition of cell migration in prostate cancer cells.[88] Additional support for the involvement of CD81 in actin rearrangements was demonstrated in B-cells, where engagement of CD81 induced Syk tyrosine kinase activation. Syk was responsible for inducing the tyrosine phosphorylation of ezrin and inducing a complex between ezrin and F-actin.[89] Moreover, CD81 has been shown to mediate B-cell survival in the event of actin rearrangement.[33] Cytoskeletal reorganization induces the release of BCR nanoclusters that can subsequently reassemble with CD81-stabilized CD19. Tetraspanin CD81 thus holds coreceptor CD19 in place to interact with mobile BCR nanoclusters released after cytoskeleton disruption.

4.4.2.3 hemITAM Signaling

That tetraspanins themselves may act as signaling proteins had not been appreciated until a recent report demonstrated the presence of functional ITIM (immunoreceptor tyrosine-based inhibition motif)-like and ITAM (immunoreceptor tyrosine-based activation motif)-like motifs on tetraspanin CD37.[90] ITIMs and ITAMs are motifs on immune cell receptors that, when engaged by ligand, are phosphorylated and transformed into docking sites for proteins that negatively or positively regulate signaling events, respectively. Akt signaling was shown to be regulated by p85-PI3Kδ recruitment to the ITAM-like motif in the C-terminal cytoplasmic tail of CD37 after phosphorylation by Syk kinase. Conversely, tyrosine phosphorylation of the N-terminal cytoplasmic domain in an ITIM-like motif by the Src kinase Lyn recruited the SHP1 phosphatase, which in turn upregulated the pro-apoptotic protein Bim, leading to apoptosis. Thus, CD37 acts as a binary switch to regulate survival in B-cells, which is confirmed in the defective humoral immune responses in mice lacking CD37. Impaired α4β1 integrin-dependent Akt signaling via CD37 was shown to be responsible for the decreased survival of plasma cells in CD37-deficient mice.[27] Whether this signaling is dependent on CD37 association with the TEM and whether the association with other partners determines the net effect on cell survival remain to be investigated.

4.4.3 TETRASPANINS IN MEMBRANE TRAFFICKING AND EXCHANGE

In addition to modulating signaling molecules and complex assembly through localized lateral interactions within the plasma membrane, tetraspanins affect larger membrane interactions such as intracellular trafficking of membrane proteins, exosome biogenesis, and membrane fusion. Nonetheless, the principles of lateral diffusion, complex assembly, and control of signaling through microdomains still likely apply. In this section, we will provide a few examples of how tetraspanins modulate larger membrane processes, including intracellular trafficking, exosomes, and membrane fusion.

4.4.3.1 Intracellular Trafficking

Many tetraspanins reside both on the cell surface and within intracellular membranes. One exception is CD63, which is predominately found on intracellular vesicles. CD63 harbors at its C-terminal cytoplasmic tail a classical YXXΦ sorting motif, GYEVM, which is required for directing it to the late endosomal compartment.[91] Several tetraspanins, including CD151, CD82, CD37, and Tspan1, 3, 6, 7, and 8, also contain similar motifs in their C-terminal tails.[6] The importance of this motif has been reported for CD151, where specific mutation of the YRSL sequence markedly attenuates CD151 internalization.[92] Support for this motif being important for CD82 function is provided by a C-terminal deletion mutant, which inhibits its own endocytic trafficking.[64] Additionally, specific mutation of the lysine in the CD82 YSKV motif similarly reduced CD82 internalization (unpublished data, CKM).

Both CD63 and CD82, localized on endosomal vesicles, are involved in innate immune responses to pathogens.[93] The mechanisms involved are not well defined, but preliminary studies in CD82-null mice demonstrate defects in endosomal-specific Toll-like receptor-mediated signaling (unpublished data, CKM). However, the best characterized role of tetraspanins on internal membranes is the turnover of cell surface proteins, such as integrins and RTKs. The internalization, trafficking, and recycling of integrins are postulated to regulate cell migration. Internalized CD151 was found to colocalize with several integrins, and mutation of the CD151 internalization motif impaired integrin internalization and reduced cell migration.[92] This was not limited to only integrin α3β1, which is tightly associated with CD151, but included α6 and α5 integrin subunits. The CD151 mutant had no effect on CD9 internalization, indicating that integrin internalization was not being mediated globally through TEMs. Therefore, some aspects of specificity are involved, but it cannot wholly be explained by the direct association between CD151 and integrin α3β1 since other less strongly associated integrins were similarly affected. This suggests the presence of additional proteins within the internalizing complex. Similarly, CD82 expression was shown to cause internalization of integrin α6 and reduce cell adhesion.[94]

As noted in Section 4.4.2, CD82 is a suppressor of EGFR and Met RTK signaling. Based on several studies, EGFR suppression is mediated through recruitment of PKCα and direct phosphorylation of EGFR at Thr654 triggering its internalization.[62,67] This response is dependent upon cholesterol and enhanced by gangliosides, indicating that the events are dependent on cholesterol-enriched membrane microdomains such as rafts or TEMs. In parallel studies, CD82 was shown to suppress

EGFR ubiquitylation, enhance its internalization, and promote phosphorylation of both EGFR and Cbl (the EGFR E3 ligase) by PKC. Deletion of the C-terminal cytoplasmic domain inhibited the ability of CD82 to suppress EGFR signaling.[64] The mechanism by which CD82 suppresses Met is less well characterized, but there is evidence for the involvement of gangliosides in assisting CD82 in Met suppression,[95] analogous to what was reported for EGFR. Given that Met internalization is regulated by a similar PKC- and Cbl-dependent mechanism as EGFR suggests that a shared mechanism is likely to be involved generally in suppressing RTK signaling by CD82. As noted in Section 4.4.2, CD151 has the opposite effect on Met from CD82, enhancing its activity. It is unknown whether this involves altered internalization of Met by CD151. The ability of CD82 to control membrane protein internalization is not limited to RTKs. CD82 has been shown to promote enhanced cell–cell adhesion through E-cadherin in epithelial cells.[77] E-cadherin internalization induced by Ca^{2+} depletion was attenuated in cells expressing the CD82 internalization YSKV motif mutant (unpublished data, CKM).

Thus, dynamic control of the recycling and internalization of cell surface molecules is controlled by tetraspanins. These studies also clearly demonstrate that tetraspanins have the capacity to dictate the signal response of RTKs and do so through interactions with the RTK internalization machinery. Although complexes can be detected between tetraspanins and RTKs, to date these have not been shown to be direct. Thus, as in the examples above, the mechanisms that target tetraspanins to control the responses of specific partners still need further investigation but are likely to involve the assembly of microdomains based on their enhancement by gangliosides.

Recent studies suggest that the role of tetraspanins in controlling surface expression of partner molecules is much more universal than originally realized. Furthermore, this is not limited to those tetraspanins with classic internalization motifs. A subclass of tetraspanins, termed TspanC8, because of the presence of four cysteine–cysteine disulfide bonds in the EC2 domain, was recently shown by two independent studies to control the surface expression of the extracellular metalloprotease ADAM10[49,50] by enhancing its departure from the ER. Tspan5, 10, 14, 15, 17, and 33 (aka Penumbra) were shown to directly interact with ADAM10, and loss of one or more tetraspanin reduced ADAM10 surface expression and activity.[49] In some cell types of knock-out mice, loss of one TspanC8 member was compensated by the presence of another. Furthermore, three TspanC8 genes in *Drosophila* were able to activate Notch1 signaling in vivo and human Tspan5 and Tspan14 promoted ADAM10-dependent Notch1 signaling in cells in vitro,[50] demonstrating the importance of tetraspanin proteins throughout evolution. The stability of claudin-1 expression, which associates with CD9 and CD151 in TEMs but not at tight junctions, was reduced when either tetraspanin was deleted,[79] just as is the CD81 partner protein CD19, which is destabilized when CD81 is lost.[31,96] Stabilization of CD19, like ADAM10, occurs during ER trafficking.

Based on the number of examples studied thus far, tetraspanins appear to regulate partner membrane protein expression by three distinct mechanisms. The first is to facilitate partner protein stabilization, appearance, and clustering at the cell surface. The second is to facilitate partner protein internalization. The third is to promote trafficking from the ER–Golgi system to the plasma membrane (CD81–CD19, Tspans–ADAM10). However, the mechanisms of these processes appear to be somewhat different. Molecules whose surface expression is enhanced by tetraspanins appear to be through direct interactions with the partner protein, while those that control internalization do so by an indirect mechanism carrying not only partner molecules but also other associated complexes.

Most studies have focused on the role of tetraspanins in partner protein internalization, but the processes that control the expression and subcellular localization of tetraspanins themselves also warrant some consideration. CD82 is very sensitive to changes in protein folding and undergoes extensive glycosylation and processing before appearing at the cell surface.[97] Whether CD82, like the TspanC8 family members or CD81, has a direct partner that it helps to traffic to the cell surface is unknown as no direct interacting partner has been identified to date. Interestingly, Tspan10, CD231, and Tssc6 contain potential dileucine sorting motifs in their cytoplasmic N-terminal domains that may facilitate exit from the ER.[98] The finding that some tetraspanins facilitate internalization and others only facilitate surface expression of their partners may be explained by the presence of specific subclasses of tetraspanins. Whether they work together in some way to coordinate responses is yet to be determined.

4.4.3.2 Exosomes

Tetraspanins are not only involved in intracellular trafficking of membrane proteins but also intimately associated with the export or exocytosis of membrane vesicles, more specifically those described as exosomes. In fact, tetraspanin proteins are the markers by which exosomes are defined. Despite the known association between tetraspanins and exosomes, the absolute requirement for tetraspanins in the formation or functioning of exosomes has not been investigated until very recently.

Many tetraspanins regulate the expression and functioning of MHC class II receptors on APCs during adaptive immunity. The effect is observed at several different stages, including control of MHC II trafficking on endosomes, assembly of the peptide complexes, clustering at the cell surface, and T-cell costimulation.[99] MHC II is crucial to the proper assembly of the synaptic junction between APCs and T-cells. Recently, exosomes were demonstrated to contribute to the adaptive immune response. CD63-positive exosomes were released from T-cells, which transferred miRNAs to the APCs upon synaptic junction formation. In a study designed to test the reverse process, that is, transfer from APCs to T-cells, it was found that knockdown of CD63 in the APC resulted in enhanced exosome production with a resulting enhancement of CD4+ T-cell stimulation.[99] Thus, not only are tetraspanins associated with exosomes, in this context, CD63 is important for regulating their biogenesis.

It is interesting to note that exosomes are also released at synaptic clefts by neurons, suggesting that they might have the ability to influence synaptic transmission analogous to the synaptic signaling in immune cells. The role of tetraspanins in neurotransmission has not yet been investigated. Given the known association of at least one tetraspanin gene mutation in humans that causes mental retardation (Tpsan7) and the reported expression of several others in the brain, it would not be surprising if some of them also regulate synaptic functions in the brain through exosomes.

A role for tetraspanins in regulating exosome recognition and uptake by receiving cells was demonstrated for Tspan8 (aka CO-029), where exosomes expressing Tspan8 displayed a distinct preference for uptake by endothelial cells. Furthermore, coexpression of integrin β4 changed the specificity. The ability of endothelial cells to specifically take up Tspan8-containing exosomes was correlated with enhanced angiogenesis and metastatic niche remodeling.[100]

Finally, a role for CD81 in controlling the exocytosis and secretion of wnt proteins was recently described.[101] In this study, a breast cancer model was characterized where enhanced tumor cell migration is mediated by factors secreted from fibroblasts. They demonstrated that the fibroblasts secreted factors that were involved in enhancing a wnt autocrine signaling pathway in the tumor cells. This was found to involve the release of CD81-containing exosomes from the fibroblasts, which were then taken up by the tumor cells via the endocytic pathway. Within this pathway, they encountered wnt11. Wnt11 was then secreted out of the cell through CD81-positive exosomes to interact with the tumor cells and promote their migration. This process was completely dependent on CD81. Knockdown of CD81 in the fibroblasts did not prevent exosome formation but prevented the exosomes received by the tumor cell from secreting wnt11. Knockdown of CD82 or CD63 had no effect on the wnt11 pathway or on cell migration.[101] These data suggest that it is the presence of CD81 specifically in the exosomes that is responsible for the packaging and secretion of wnt11 in exosomes.

Now that there is evidence supporting active involvement of tetraspanins in exosome biogenesis and function, the mechanisms by which this happens need to be studied further. No doubt a role for establishing specific membrane microdomains is required for both the production and functioning of exosomes. Furthermore, identifying the factors on the receiving cells that the exosomes interact with will be important as well as determining how that fusion is mediated. As discussed in Section 4.4.3.3, membrane fusion is another important function of tetraspanins; thus, their appearance on exosomes may be essential for dictating the proper target for fusion.

4.4.3.3 Membrane Fusion

Tetraspanins enter the evolutionary tree at the point of multicellular organisms, being absent in yeast. The switch from a single cell to a multicellular organism requires compartmentalization of cells causing distinct physical and physiological differences to arise between the cell types. Tetraspanins may have evolved to help in the processing of signals that ensure proper organization and correct signaling. To date, we have focused primarily on what is happening at the cell surface in isolated cells and have not wholly addressed how tetraspanins coordinate signaling throughout a tissue to control its development and maintain homeostasis. The ability of tetraspanins to control larger membrane interactions may be a vital part of being multicellular.

This point may be exceedingly important when it comes to controlling cell fusion. Making sure the right cells fuse at the right time, to the proper extent, and with the right partner is fundamental to normal development. Primary examples include myoblast fusion in muscle, osteoclast fusion in bone development, and syncytiotrophoblasts in the embryo. A crucial role for tetraspanins in controlling cell fusion is most exemplified by two tetraspanins, CD9 and CD81, which mediate the fusion reaction between sperm and egg.

Both CD9 and CD81 knock-out female mice are less fertile than wild-type mice[102–105] owing to failed egg–sperm fusion. Loss of both CD9 and CD81 creates completely infertile mice. Microinjection of CD9 mRNA into oocytes can rescue fusion deficiency in both CD9-null and CD81-null oocytes, but CD81 mRNA cannot rescue CD9-null oocytes, indicating both unique and overlapping functions for each tetraspanin. Neither integrins nor ADAM proteases are required for egg–sperm fusion, indicating that these are not the partner molecules being targeted by tetraspanins in gamete production.[106] The EC2 domain of CD9 is required for fusion,[107] and loss of an Ig domain-containing protein, Izumo, on sperm also blocks fusion, suggesting that CD9 is directly involved in binding a partner on an adjoining cell. It was later discovered that CD9 released in exosomes by the egg is responsible for interacting with sperm via Izumo and promoting the fusion reaction.[108] The role of CD81 in this process is currently less clear but may be involved in assisting CD9 localization.

This primary ability of cells to control cell–cell fusion is usurped by membrane-encased viruses to gain entry into cells. The mechanism for viral entry in liver cells is best characterized for hepatitis C virus (HCV). HCV entry is mediated through a direct extracellular interaction of the viral E1E2 protein with CD81 in complex with its partner protein EWI-2. It is EWI-2, in its truncated version (2wint) found specifically in liver cells, which is responsible for the liver-specific infectivity of HCV.[109] EWI-2 requires its transmembrane glycine zipper motif and palmitoylation on two juxtamembranous cysteines in its cytosolic tail to interact with CD81.[110] Once assembled, this complex then interacts with claudin-1 via its first extracellular loop with residues T149, E152, and T153 in the EC2 domain of CD81.[111] Fusion is mediated through a low-pH conformational change in E1E2 that makes it competent to interact with the cell fusion machinery. The role of CD81 appears to be one of presentation or priming of E1E2 to facilitate its proper conformational change. Recently, it was demonstrated that RTKs, specifically EGFR or Ephrin A2, serve as cofactors for assembly of the CD81/claudin-1 complex.[112] This highlights the potential importance of how signaling may help establish the correct microdomain distribution to facilitate assembly of complexes. The requirement for RTK signaling is likely a mechanism for release of claudin-1 from its normal association with tight junctions to make it available to the virus. The added benefit is the cells are then primed for proliferation to assist in virus production. Thus, the virus, through coevolution, has adapted to take full advantage of tightly controlled tetraspanin membrane assemblies.

Just as in signaling and other membrane interactions, tetraspanins exert their effects on cell fusion by regulating the assembly of complexes necessary to facilitate the fusion reaction in a controlled fashion. That these cell–cell or membrane–membrane interactions are mediated through specific microdomains controlled by tetraspanins has not been formally demonstrated, but is highly likely given what is known about how tetraspanins work on single membranes. This would be accomplished specifically through microdomains in cell–cell contacts and interactions.

4.5 TETRASPANIN DEFICIENCIES AND DISEASE

The importance of tetraspanins in human biology is further supported by human genetic mutations known to be associated with specific human syndromes. At least six human tetraspanin gene mutations are directly associated with disease.

Tspan7 (A15) deletions and mutations are causative for a nonspecific X-linked form of mental retardation.[113] Tspan7 mRNA is highly expressed in the cerebral cortex and hippocampus. A recent study found that Tspan7 is critical for AMPA receptor trafficking in neurons.[114] This is mediated through the C-terminal tail interaction with PDZ-containing protein PICK1 to limit its association with AMPA receptors and likely accounts for the intellectual disability when Tspan7 is nonfunctional.

Familial exudative vitreoretinopathy is an inherited blinding disorder of the retinal vascular system, and two independent studies have demonstrated that dominant autosomal mutations in Tspan12 are a relatively frequent cause of this retinal disease.[115] Although the precise underlying mechanisms have not been defined, the ability of Tspan12 to regulate retinal vascular development by promoting Norrin/β-catenin signaling may underlie these findings.[116]

Tspan22, also known as RDS (peripherin), is a component of the photoreceptor outer segments (OSs) in rods and cones of the eye. The proper functioning of OSs is highly dependent on the precise stacking of hundreds of membranous disks. RDS directly generates the membrane curvature required for membrane stacking through the amphipathic helix within its C-terminal domain.[117] Numerous heterozygous point mutations within the RDS gene, including Arg172Trp, Gly208Asp, Pro210Arg, and Cys213Ty, lead to structural abnormalities in the cones and cause a broad variety of progressive retinal degenerations in humans.[118] These phenotypes are mimicked in murine and *Xenopus* models.

Tspan23, also known as ROM1 (peripherin2), is expressed in rods of the eye and is a partner of RDS. Mutations within ROM1 itself are rarely associated with eye pathology, but a form of retinitis pigmentosa occurs in patients with double heterozygous mutations in both ROM1 and RDS, but not with single mutations in either.[119] RDS/ROM1 appear to function as a tetramer in photoreceptor biology; thus, mutations that disrupt oligomerization are predicted to affect photoreceptor health. During night/sleep phase, the membranes of photoreceptor cells are degraded and turned over through a fusogenic process. ROM1, in cooperation with RDS, is critical for mediating membrane fusion during photoreceptor renewal.[120] In mouse models, full loss of ROM1 results in photoreceptor degeneration, indicating that ROM1 may also function independently to promote cell survival.[121]

The CD151 (Tspan24) gene encodes the MER2 blood group antigen. MER2-negative patients have a single nucleotide insertion in exon 5 that creates a frameshift and premature stop, creating a product, which, if made, would lack the integrin-binding domain. These patients present with hereditary nephritis, deafness, epidermolysis bullosa, and beta-thalassemia minor bleeding disorder,[122] which resembles the phenotypes present in CD151 knock-out mice.

Patients homozygous for a single point mutation at a splice acceptor site in exon 6 (exon6+1 G>A) of the CD81 (Tspan28) gene generate a 13-nucleotide insertion leading to a frameshift and premature stop upstream of the fourth transmembrane domain.[31] These patients present with severe nephropathy and profound hypogam-maglobulinemia. The latter syndrome is attributable to an absence of CD19 expression on B-cells in these patients. The same immune deficiency and lack of CD19 partner expression is observed in CD81-null mice.

Lack of CD53 expression on neutrophils was found to be the cause of an immune deficiency syndrome in a family that suffered from opportunistic infections and reactivation of chronic silent mutations.[123] Although the mechanism underlying this defect in immune cell function was not studied, a role for CD53 in negatively regulating the immune response was postulated. The importance of tetraspanins in the immune system has been validated in studies with tetraspanin-deficient mice. Central processes during cellular immunity (antigen presentation, T-cell activation, and dendritic cell migration) and humoral immunity (antibody production) are controlled by tetraspanins CD37, CD81, CD151, Tssc6 (reviewed in Refs. 8 and 28), CD82, and CD53 (unpublished data, Wright and van Spriel). The underlying mechanisms involve modulation of the molecular interactions between tetraspanins and important immune cell surface molecules including antigen-presenting MHC proteins, T-cell coreceptors CD4 and CD8, pattern-recognition receptors, and signaling molecules such as Lck and PKC (reviewed in Refs. 8, 10, and 124).

What is most striking about the human pathologies associated with inherited tetraspanin mutations is how well they fit into the three basic functional paradigms of complex assembly, signal transduction, and membrane trafficking/exchange arrived at through in vitro cell models. Tspan7 and Tspan12 are controlling receptor signaling by regulating complex assembly, ROM/RDS are controlling membrane structure and fusion as a complex, CD151 is controlling integrin functions through complex assembly and signaling, and CD81 is stabilizing its partner. Also very satisfying is how well the tetraspanin mouse models effectively recapitulate human syndromes, providing a very strong rationale for continuing to pursue the genetic approach to link tetraspanins with human diseases.

4.6   CONCLUDING REMARKS

Efficient inter- and intracellular communication is dependent on the spatial and temporal organization of proteins and lipids in the plasma membrane. Tetraspanins control the lateral organization of specific membrane proteins and signaling molecules into TEMs. The diversity in fundamental cell functions (migration, immune surveillance, development, protein trafficking, and membrane fusion) modulated by tetraspanins can be explained by the multiple tetraspanin interactions with different receptors and signaling molecules that have been identified in diverse tissues and cell types. Still, the molecular mechanism underlying the formation of TEMs is the same: that is, the lateral organization of specific membrane proteins and signaling molecules into dynamic units. Accordingly, TEMs are hotspots for (1) complex assembly and cross talk, (2) modulation of signal transduction, and (3) membrane trafficking and exchange in the 3D plasma membrane environment (Figure 4.1). We propose that the high level of molecular organization within TEMs defined by hierarchical interactions between tetraspanins and their interacting molecules defines the specificity of their function. Recent studies demonstrate that tetraspanins can have equivalent or opposing functions, which strongly suggests the potential for reciprocal signaling paradigms that exist between tetraspanin pairs. Disrupting the balance in tetraspanin pairing by loss of one or overexpression of another would be expected to have a major impact on the signaling pathways involved. It also emphasizes the importance of taking into consideration the whole tetraspanin repertoire expressed within a cell to fully understand their role in the final biological outcome. Although we are only at the beginning of understanding the complex biology of TEMs in the plasma membrane, pioneering studies at the single-molecule level in living cells revealed that the dynamic behavior of tetraspanins is heterogeneous, ranging from rapid diffusion to confinement. This may provide cells with the capacity to delicately regulate the formation of receptor signaling complexes in the plasma membrane that is essential for the biological responses in complex multicellular organisms. Indeed, recent studies have shown that tetraspanin proteins regulate the mobility of their interacting receptors in the plasma membrane. The identification of different human pathologies that are caused by specific tetraspanin deficiencies warrants further comprehensive investigation of these intriguing four-transmembrane proteins. Excitingly, targeting TEMs as a novel therapeutic approach for the treatment of infectious and malignant diseases is currently under investigation in (pre-)clinical studies.[36,125,126]

ACKNOWLEDGMENTS

Annemiek van Spriel is supported by the Netherlands Organization for Scientific Research (NWO-ALW VIDI Grant 864.11.006). Cindy Miranti is supported by the Van Andel Research Institute. Alexis Bergsma is supported by the Van Andel Institute Graduate School program.

REFERENCES

1. Singer, S. J., and G. L. Nicolson. "The Fluid Mosaic Model of the Structure of Cell Membranes." *Science* 175, no. 4023 (1972): 720–31.
2. Laude, A. J., and I. A. Prior. "Plasma Membrane Microdomains: Organization, Function and Trafficking." *Mol Membr Biol* 21, no. 3 (2004): 193–205.
3. Lingwood, D., and K. Simons. "Lipid Rafts as a Membrane-Organizing Principle." *Science* 327, no. 5961 (2010): 46–50.
4. Simons, K., and J. L. Sampaio. "Membrane Organization and Lipid Rafts." *Cold Spring Harb Perspect Biol* 3, no. 10 (2011): a004697.
5. Kusumi, A., T. K. Fujiwara, R. Chadda et al. "Dynamic Organizing Principles of the Plasma Membrane That Regulate Signal Transduction: Commemorating the Fortieth Anniversary of Singer and Nicolson's Fluid-Mosaic Model." *Annu Rev Cell Dev Biol* 28 (2012): 215–50.
6. Stipp, C. S., T. V. Kolesnikova, and M. E. Hemler. "Functional Domains in Tetraspanin Proteins." *Trends Biochem Sci* 28, no. 2 (2003): 106–12.
7. Boucheix, C., and E. Rubinstein. "Tetraspanins." *Cell Mol Life Sci* 58, no. 9 (2001): 1189–205.
8. Tarrant, J. M., L. Robb, A. B. van Spriel, and M. D. Wright. "Tetraspanins: Molecular Organisers of the Leukocyte Surface." *Trends Immunol* 24, no. 11 (2003): 610–7.
9. Hemler, M. E. "Tetraspanin Functions and Associated Microdomains." *Nat Rev Mol Cell Biol* 6, no. 10 (2005): 801–11.

10. Levy, S., and T. Shoham. "The Tetraspanin Web Modulates Immune-Signalling Complexes." *Nat Rev Immunol* 5, no. 2 (2005): 136–48.
11. Hemler, M. E. "Tetraspanin Proteins Mediate Cellular Penetration, Invasion, and Fusion Events and Define a Novel Type of Membrane Microdomain." *Annu Rev Cell Dev Biol* 19 (2003): 397–422.
12. Charrin, S., F. le Naour, O. Silvie et al. "Lateral Organization of Membrane Proteins: Tetraspanins Spin Their Web." *Biochem J* 420, no. 2 (2009): 133–54.
13. Sala-Valdes, M., A. Ursa, S. Charrin et al. "EWI-2 and EWI-F Link the Tetraspanin Web to the Actin Cytoskeleton through Their Direct Association with Ezrin–Radixin–Moesin Proteins." *J Biol Chem* 281, no. 28 (2006): 19665–75.
14. Claas, C., C. S. Stipp, and M. E. Hemler. "Evaluation of Prototype Transmembrane 4 Superfamily Protein Complexes and Their Relation to Lipid Rafts." *J Biol Chem* 276, no. 11 (2001): 7974–84.
15. Le Naour, F., M. Andre, C. Boucheix, and E. Rubinstein. "Membrane Microdomains and Proteomics: Lessons from Tetraspanin Microdomains and Comparison with Lipid Rafts." *Proteomics* 6, no. 24 (2006): 6447–54.
16. Espenel, C., E. Margeat, P. Dosset et al. "Single-Molecule Analysis of CD9 Dynamics and Partitioning Reveals Multiple Modes of Interaction in the Tetraspanin Web." *J Cell Biol* 182, no. 4 (2008): 765–76.
17. Charrin, S., S. Manie, C. Thiele et al. "A Physical and Functional Link between Cholesterol and Tetraspanins." *Eur J Immunol* 33, no. 9 (2003): 2479–89.
18. Zuidscherwoude, M., C. M. de Winde, A. Cambi, and A. B. van Spriel. "Microdomains in the membrane landscape shape antigen-presenting cell function." *J Leukoc Biol* 95, no. 2 (2014): 251–63.
19. Yanez-Mo, M., O. Barreiro, M. Gordon-Alonso, M. Sala-Valdes, and F. Sanchez-Madrid. "Tetraspanin-Enriched Microdomains: A Functional Unit in Cell Plasma Membranes." *Trends Cell Biol* 19, no. 9 (2009): 434–46.
20. Barreiro, O., M. Zamai, M. Yanez-Mo et al. "Endothelial Adhesion Receptors Are Recruited to Adherent Leukocytes by Inclusion in Preformed Tetraspanin Nanoplatforms." *J Cell Biol* 183, no. 3 (2008): 527–42.
21. Lidke, D. S., and B. S. Wilson. "Caught in the Act: Quantifying Protein Behaviour in Living Cells." *Trends Cell Biol* 19, no. 11 (2009): 566–74.
22. Berditchevski, F., E. Gilbert, M. R. Griffiths et al. "Analysis of the CD151-Alpha3beta1 Integrin and CD151-Tetraspanin Interactions by Mutagenesis." *J Biol Chem* 276, no. 44 (2001): 41165–74.
23. Sterk, L. M., C. A. Geuijen, J. G. van den Berg et al. "Association of the Tetraspanin CD151 with the Laminin-Binding Integrins Alpha3beta1, Alpha6beta1, Alpha6beta4 and Alpha7beta1 in Cells in Culture and In Vivo." *J Cell Sci* 115, Pt 6 (2002): 1161–73.
24. Sterk, L. M., C. A. Geuijen, L. C. Oomen et al. "The Tetraspan Molecule CD151, a Novel Constituent of Hemidesmosomes, Associates with the Integrin Alpha6beta4 and May Regulate the Spatial Organization of Hemidesmosomes." *J Cell Biol* 149, no. 4 (2000): 969–82.
25. Yang, X., O. V. Kovalenko, W. Tang et al. "Palmitoylation Supports Assembly and Function of Integrin-Tetraspanin Complexes." *J Cell Biol* 167, no. 6 (2004): 1231–40.
26. Berditchevski, F., E. Odintsova, S. Sawada, and E. Gilbert. "Expression of the Palmitoylation-Deficient CD151 Weakens the Association of Alpha 3 Beta 1 Integrin with the Tetraspanin-Enriched Microdomains and Affects Integrin-Dependent Signaling." *J Biol Chem* 277, no. 40 (2002): 36991–7000.
27. van Spriel, A. B., S. de Keijzer, A. van der Schaaf et al. "The Tetraspanin CD37 Orchestrates the Alpha(4)Beta(1) Integrin-Akt Signaling Axis and Supports Long-Lived Plasma Cell Survival." *Sci Signal* 5, no. 250 (2012): ra82.

28. van Spriel, A. B. "Tetraspanins in the Humoral Immune Response." *Biochem Soc Trans* 39, no. 2 (2011): 512–7.
29. Feigelson, S. W., V. Grabovsky, R. Shamri, S. Levy, and R. Alon. "The CD81 Tetraspanin Facilitates Instantaneous Leukocyte VLA-4 Adhesion Strengthening to Vascular Cell Adhesion Molecule 1 (VCAM-1) under Shear Flow." *J Biol Chem* 278, no. 51 (2003): 51203–12.
30. Bradbury, L. E., G. S. Kansas, S. Levy, R. L. Evans, and T. F. Tedder. "The CD19/CD21 Signal Transducing Complex of Human B Lymphocytes Includes the Target of Antiproliferative Antibody-1 and Leu-13 Molecules." *J Immunol* 149, no. 9 (1992): 2841–50.
31. van Zelm, M. C., J. Smet, B. Adams et al. "CD81 Gene Defect in Humans Disrupts CD19 Complex Formation and Leads to Antibody Deficiency." *J Clin Invest* 120, no. 4 (2010): 1265–74.
32. Shoham, T., R. Rajapaksa, C. C. Kuo, J. Haimovich, and S. Levy. "Building of the Tetraspanin Web: Distinct Structural Domains of CD81 Function in Different Cellular Compartments." *Mol Cell Biol* 26, no. 4 (2006): 1373–85.
33. Mattila, P. K., C. Feest, D. Depoil et al. "The Actin and Tetraspanin Networks Organize Receptor Nanoclusters to Regulate B Cell Receptor-Mediated Signaling." *Immunity* 38, no. 3 (2013): 461–74.
34. Wright, M. D., G. W. Moseley, and A. B. van Spriel. "Tetraspanin Microdomains in Immune Cell Signalling and Malignant Disease." *Tissue Antigens* 64, no. 5 (2004): 533–42.
35. Zoller, M. "Tetraspanins: Push and Pull in Suppressing and Promoting Metastasis." *Nat Rev Cancer* 9, no. 1 (2009): 40–55.
36. Sala-Valdes, M., N. Ailane, C. Greco, E. Rubinstein, and C. Boucheix. "Targeting Tetraspanins in Cancer." *Expert Opin Ther Targets* 16, no. 10 (2012): 985–97.
37. Richardson, M. M., L. K. Jennings, and X. A. Zhang. "Tetraspanins and Tumor Progression." *Clin Exp Metastasis* 28, no. 3 (2011): 261–70.
38. Liu, W. M., and X. A. Zhang. "KAI1/CD82, a Tumor Metastasis Suppressor." *Cancer Lett* 240, no. 2 (2006): 183–94.
39. Miranti, C. K. "Controlling Cell Surface Dynamics and Signaling: How CD82/KAI1 Suppresses Metastasis." *Cell Signal* 21, no. 2 (2009): 196–211.
40. Zhou, B., L. Liu, M. Reddivari, and X. A. Zhang. "The Palmitoylation of Metastasis Suppressor KAI1/CD82 Is Important for Its Motility- and Invasiveness-Inhibitory Activity." *Cancer Res* 64, no. 20 (2004): 7455–63.
41. Zijlstra, A., J. Lewis, B. Degryse, H. Stuhlmann, and J. P. Quigley. "The Inhibition of Tumor Cell Intravasation and Subsequent Metastasis via Regulation of In Vivo Tumor Cell Motility by the Tetraspanin CD151." *Cancer Cell* 13, no. 3 (2008): 221–34.
42. Stipp, C. S. "Laminin-Binding Integrins and Their Tetraspanin Partners as Potential Antimetastatic Targets." *Expert Rev Mol Med* 12 (2010): e3.
43. Sadej, R., H. Romanska, G. Baldwin et al. "CD151 Regulates Tumorigenesis by Modulating the Communication between Tumor Cells and Endothelium." *Mol Cancer Res* 7, no. 6 (2009): 787–98.
44. Klosek, S. K., K. Nakashiro, S. Hara et al. "CD151 Regulates HGF-Stimulated Morphogenesis of Human Breast Cancer Cells." *Biochem Biophys Res Commun* 379, no. 4 (2009): 1097–100.
45. Sadej, R., H. Romanska, D. Kavanagh et al. "Tetraspanin CD151 Regulates Transforming Growth Factor Beta Signaling: Implication in Tumor Metastasis." *Cancer Res* 70, no. 14 (2010): 6059–70.
46. Yanez-Mo, M., F. Sanchez-Madrid, and C. Cabanas. "Membrane Proteases and Tetraspanins." *Biochem Soc Trans* 39, no. 2 (2011): 541–6.

47. Yanez-Mo, M., O. Barreiro, P. Gonzalo et al. "MT1-MMP Collagenolytic Activity Is Regulated through Association with Tetraspanin CD151 in Primary Endothelial Cells." *Blood* 112, no. 8 (2008): 3217–26.

48. Lafleur, M. A., D. Xu, and M. E. Hemler. "Tetraspanin Proteins Regulate Membrane Type-1 Matrix Metalloproteinase-Dependent Pericellular Proteolysis." *Mol Biol Cell* 20, no. 7 (2009): 2030–40.

49. Haining, E. J., J. Yang, R. L. Bailey et al. "The TspanC8 Subgroup of Tetraspanins Interacts with a Disintegrin and Metalloprotease 10 (ADAM10) and Regulates Its Maturation and Cell Surface Expression." *J Biol Chem* 287, no. 47 (2012): 39753–65.

50. Dornier, E., F. Coumailleau, J. F. Ottavi et al. "TspanC8 Tetraspanins Regulate ADAM10/ Kuzbanian Trafficking and Promote Notch Activation in Flies and Mammals." *J Cell Biol* 199, no. 3 (2012): 481–96.

51. Charrin, S., S. Manie, M. Oualid et al. "Differential Stability of Tetraspanin/Tetraspanin Interactions: Role of Palmitoylation." *FEBS Lett* 516, no. 1–3 (2002): 139–44.

52. Zevian, S., N. E. Winterwood, and C. S. Stipp. "Structure-Function Analysis of Tetraspanin CD151 Reveals Distinct Requirements for Tumor Cell Behaviors Mediated by Alpha3beta1 Versus Alpha6beta4 Integrin." *J Biol Chem* 286, no. 9 (2011): 7496–506.

53. Wang, H. X., T. V. Kolesnikova, C. Denison, S. P. Gygi, and M. E. Hemler. "The C-Terminal Tail of Tetraspanin Protein CD9 Contributes to Its Function and Molecular Organization." *J Cell Sci* 124, Pt 16 (2011): 2702–10.

54. Delaguillaumie, A., C. Lagaudriere-Gesbert, M. R. Popoff, and H. Conjeaud. "Rho GTPases Link Cytoskeletal Rearrangements and Activation Processes Induced via the Tetraspanin CD82 in T Lymphocytes." *J Cell Sci* 115, Pt 2 (2002): 433–43.

55. Sridhar, S. C., and C. K. Miranti. "Tetraspanin KAI1/CD82 Suppresses Invasion by Inhibiting Integrin-Dependent Crosstalk with c-Met Receptor and Src Kinases." *Oncogene* 25, no. 16 (2006): 2367–78.

56. Todeschini, A. R., J. N. Dos Santos, K. Handa, and S. I. Hakomori. "Ganglioside GM2/ GM3 Complex Affixed on Silica Nanospheres Strongly Inhibits Cell Motility through CD82/cMet-Mediated Pathway." *Proc Natl Acad Sci U S A* 105, no. 6 (2008): 1925–30.

57. Knudsen, B. S., and M. Edlund. "Prostate Cancer and the Met Hepatocyte Growth Factor Receptor." *Adv Cancer Res* 91 (2004): 31–67.

58. Klosek, S. K., K. Nakashiro, S. Hara et al. "CD151 Forms a Functional Complex with c-Met in Human Salivary Gland Cancer Cells." *Biochem Biophys Res Commun* 336, no. 2 (2005): 408–16.

59. Franco, M., C. Muratori, S. Corso et al. "The Tetraspanin CD151 Is Required for Met-Dependent Signaling and Tumor Cell Growth." *J Biol Chem* 285, no. 50 (2010): 38756–64.

60. Michieli, P., M. Mazzone, C. Basilico et al. "Targeting the Tumor and Its Microenvironment by a Dual-Function Decoy Met Receptor." *Cancer Cell* 6, no. 1 (2004): 61–73.

61. Zhu, G. H., C. Huang, Z. J. Qiu et al. "Expression and Prognostic Significance of CD151, c-Met, and Integrin Alpha3/Alpha6 in Pancreatic Ductal Adenocarcinoma." *Dig Dis Sci* 56, no. 4 (2011): 1090–8.

62. Odintsova, E., T. Sugiura, and F. Berditchevski. "Attenuation of EGF Receptor Signaling by a Metastasis Suppressor, the Tetraspanin CD82/KAI-1." *Curr Biol* 10, no. 16 (2000): 1009–12.

63. Odintsova, E., J. Voortman, E. Gilbert, and F. Berditchevski. "Tetraspanin CD82 Regulates Compartmentalisation and Ligand-Induced Dimerization of EGFR." *J Cell Sci* 116, Pt 22 (2003): 4557–66.

64. Odintsova, E., G. van Niel, H. Conjeaud et al. "Metastasis Suppressor Tetraspanin CD82/KAI1 Regulates Ubiquitylation of Epidermal Growth Factor Receptor." *J Biol Chem* 288, no. 36 (2013): 26323–34.

65. Zhang, X. A., A. L. Bontrager, and M. E. Hemler. "Transmembrane-4 Superfamily Proteins Associate with Activated Protein Kinase C (PKC) and Link PKC to Specific Beta(1) Integrins." *J Biol Chem* 276, no. 27 (2001): 25005–13.

66. Li, Q., X. H. Yang, F. Xu et al. "Tetraspanin CD151 Plays a Key Role in Skin Squamous Cell Carcinoma." *Oncogene* 32, no. 14 (2013): 1772–83.

67. Wang, X. Q., Q. Yan, P. Sun et al. "Suppression of Epidermal Growth Factor Receptor Signaling by Protein Kinase C-Alpha Activation Requires CD82, Caveolin-1, and Ganglioside." *Cancer Res* 67, no. 20 (2007): 9986–95.

68. Ford, D. A., C. C. Horner, and R. W. Gross. "Protein Kinase C Acylation by Palmitoyl Coenzyme a Facilitates Its Translocation to Membranes." *Biochemistry* 37, no. 34 (1998): 11953–61.

69. Sharma, C., X. H. Yang, and M. E. Hemler. "DHHC2 Affects Palmitoylation, Stability, and Functions of Tetraspanins CD9 and CD151." *Mol Biol Cell* 19, no. 8 (2008): 3415–25.

70. Rahimi, N., W. Hung, E. Tremblay, R. Saulnier, and B. Elliott. "C-Src Kinase Activity Is Required for Hepatocyte Growth Factor-Induced Motility and Anchorage-Independent Growth of Mammary Carcinoma Cells." *J Biol Chem* 273, no. 50 (1998): 33714–21.

71. Zhang, X. A., B. He, B. Zhou, and L. Liu. "Requirement of the p130CAS-Crk Coupling for Metastasis Suppressor KAI1/CD82-Mediated Inhibition of Cell Migration." *J Biol Chem* 278, no. 29 (2003): 27319–28.

72. Oneyama, C., T. Iino, K. Saito et al. "Transforming Potential of Src Family Kinases Is Limited by the Cholesterol-Enriched Membrane Microdomain." *Mol Cell Biol* 29, no. 24 (2009): 6462–72.

73. Xu, C., Y. H. Zhang, M. Thangavel et al. "CD82 Endocytosis and Cholesterol-Dependent Reorganization of Tetraspanin Webs and Lipid Rafts." *FASEB J* 23, no. 10 (2009): 3273–88.

74. Park, J. J., Y. B. Jin, Y. J. Lee et al. "KAI1 Suppresses HIF-1alpha and VEGF Expression by Blocking CDCP1-Enhanced Src Activation in Prostate Cancer." *BMC Cancer* 12 (2012): 81.

75. Alvares, S. M., C. A. Dunn, T. A. Brown, E. E. Wayner, and W. G. Carter. "The Role of Membrane Microdomains in Transmembrane Signaling through the Epithelial Glycoprotein Gp140/CDCP1." *Biochim Biophys Acta* 1780, no. 3 (2008): 486–96.

76. Stahelin, R. V., K. F. Kong, S. Raha et al. "Protein Kinase Ctheta C2 Domain Is a Phosphotyrosine Binding Module That Plays a Key Role in Its Activation." *J Biol Chem* 287, no. 36 (2012): 30518–28.

77. Abe, M., T. Sugiura, M. Takahashi et al. "A Novel Function of CD82/KAI-1 on E-Cadherin-Mediated Homophilic Cellular Adhesion of Cancer Cells." *Cancer Lett* 266, no. 2 (2008): 163–70.

78. Johnson, J. L., N. Winterwood, K. A. DeMali, and C. S. Stipp. "Tetraspanin CD151 Regulates Rhoa Activation and the Dynamic Stability of Carcinoma Cell-Cell Contacts." *J Cell Sci* 122, Pt 13 (2009): 2263–73.

79. Kovalenko, O. V., X. H. Yang, and M. E. Hemler. "A Novel Cysteine Cross-Linking Method Reveals a Direct Association between Claudin-1 and Tetraspanin CD9." *Mol Cell Proteomics* 6, no. 11 (2007): 1855–67.

80. Harris, H. J., M. J. Farquhar, C. J. Mee et al. "CD81 and Claudin 1 Coreceptor Association: Role in Hepatitis C Virus Entry." *J Virol* 82, no. 10 (2008): 5007–20.

81. Tiwari-Woodruff, S. K., A. G. Buznikov, T. Q. Vu et al. "Osp/Claudin-11 Forms a Complex with a Novel Member of the Tetraspanin Super Family and Beta1 Integrin and Regulates Proliferation and Migration of Oligodendrocytes." *J Cell Biol* 153, no. 2 (2001): 295–305.

82. Nubel, T., J. Preobraschenski, H. Tuncay et al. "Claudin-7 Regulates EpCAM-Mediated Functions in Tumor Progression." *Mol Cancer Res* 7, no. 3 (2009): 285–99.

83. Hong, I. K., D. I. Jeoung, K. S. Ha, Y. M. Kim, and H. Lee. "Tetraspanin CD151 Stimulates Adhesion-Dependent Activation of Ras, Rac, and Cdc42 by Facilitating Molecular Association between Beta1 Integrins and Small GTPases." *J Biol Chem* 287, no. 38 (2012): 32027–39.

84. Sawada, S., M. Yoshimoto, E. Odintsova, N. A. Hotchin, and F. Berditchevski. "The Tetraspanin CD151 Functions as a Negative Regulator in the Adhesion-Dependent Activation of Ras." *J Biol Chem* 278, no. 29 (2003): 26323–6.

85. Tejera, E., V. Rocha-Perugini, S. Lopez-Martin et al. "CD81 Regulates Cell Migration through Its Association with Rac GTPase." *Mol Biol Cell* 24, no. 3 (2013): 261–73.

86. Choi, U. J., B. K. Jee, Y. Lim, and K. H. Lee. "KAI1/CD82 Decreases Rac1 Expression and Cell Proliferation through PI3K/Akt/mTOR Pathway in H1299 Lung Carcinoma Cells." *Cell Biochem Funct* 27, no. 1 (2009): 40–7.

87. Quast, T., F. Eppler, V. Semmling et al. "CD81 Is Essential for the Formation of Membrane Protrusions and Regulates Rac1-Activation in Adhesion-Dependent Immune Cell Migration." *Blood* 118, no. 7 (2011): 1818–27.

88. Zhang, X. A., W. S. Lane, S. Charrin, E. Rubinstein, and L. Liu. "EWI2/PGRL Associates with the Metastasis Suppressor KAI1/CD82 and Inhibits the Migration of Prostate Cancer Cells." *Cancer Res* 63, no. 10 (2003): 2665–74.

89. Coffey, G. P., R. Rajapaksa, R. Liu et al. "Engagement of CD81 Induces Ezrin Tyrosine Phosphorylation and Its Cellular Redistribution with Filamentous Actin." *J Cell Sci* 122, Pt 17 (2009): 3137–44.

90. Lapalombella, R., Y. Y. Yeh, L. Wang et al. "Tetraspanin CD37 Directly Mediates Transduction of Survival and Apoptotic Signals." *Cancer Cell* 21, no. 5 (2012): 694–708.

91. Rous, B. A., B. J. Reaves, G. Ihrke et al. "Role of Adaptor Complex AP-3 in Targeting Wild-Type and Mutated CD63 to Lysosomes." *Mol Biol Cell* 13, no. 3 (2002): 1071–82.

92. Liu, L., B. He, W. M. Liu et al. "Tetraspanin CD151 Promotes Cell Migration by Regulating Integrin Trafficking." *J Biol Chem* 282, no. 43 (2007): 31631–42.

93. Artavanis-Tsakonas, K., P. V. Kasperkovitz, E. Papa et al. "The Tetraspanin CD82 Is Specifically Recruited to Fungal and Bacterial Phagosomes Prior to Acidification." *Infect Immun* 79, no. 3 (2011): 1098–106.

94. He, B., L. Liu, G. A. Cook et al. "Tetraspanin CD82 Attenuates Cellular Morphogenesis through Down-Regulating Integrin Alpha6-Mediated Cell Adhesion." *J Biol Chem* 280, no. 5 (2005): 3346–54.

95. Todeschini, A. R., J. N. Dos Santos, K. Handa, and S. I. Hakomori. "Ganglioside GM2-Tetraspanin CD82 Complex Inhibits Met and Its Cross-Talk with Integrins, Providing a Basis for Control of Cell Motility through Glycosynapse." *J Biol Chem* 282, no. 11 (2007): 8123–33.

96. Shoham, T., R. Rajapaksa, C. Boucheix et al. "The Tetraspanin CD81 Regulates the Expression of CD19 during B Cell Development in a Postendoplasmic Reticulum Compartment." *J Immunol* 171, no. 8 (2003): 4062–72.

97. Cannon, K. S., and P. Cresswell. "Quality Control of Transmembrane Domain Assembly in the Tetraspanin CD82." *EMBO J* 20, no. 10 (2001): 2443–53.

98. Berditchevski, F., and E. Odintsova. "Tetraspanins as Regulators of Protein Trafficking." *Traffic* 8, no. 2 (2007): 89–96.

99. Petersen, S. H., E. Odintsova, T. A. Haigh et al. "The Role of Tetraspanin CD63 in Antigen Presentation via MHC Class II." *Eur J Immunol* 41, no. 9 (2011): 2556–61.

100. Nazarenko, I., S. Rana, A. Baumann et al. "Cell Surface Tetraspanin Tspan8 Contributes to Molecular Pathways of Exosome-Induced Endothelial Cell Activation." *Cancer Res* 70, no. 4 (2010): 1668–78.

101. Luga, V., L. Zhang, A. M. Viloria-Petit et al. "Exosomes Mediate Stromal Mobilization of Autocrine Wnt-PCP Signaling in Breast Cancer Cell Migration." *Cell* 151, no. 7 (2012): 1542–56.

102. Le Naour, F., E. Rubinstein, C. Jasmin, M. Prenant, and C. Boucheix. "Severely Reduced Female Fertility in CD9-Deficient Mice." *Science* 287, no. 5451 (2000): 319–21.
103. Miyado, K., G. Yamada, S. Yamada et al. "Requirement of CD9 on the Egg Plasma Membrane for Fertilization." *Science* 287, no. 5451 (2000): 321–4.
104. Kaji, K., S. Oda, T. Shikano et al. "The Gamete Fusion Process Is Defective in Eggs of CD9-Deficient Mice." *Nat Genet* 24, no. 3 (2000): 279–82.
105. Rubinstein, E., A. Ziyyat, M. Prenant et al. "Reduced Fertility of Female Mice Lacking CD81." *Dev Biol* 290, no. 2 (2006): 351–8.
106. Rubinstein, E., A. Ziyyat, J. P. Wolf, F. Le Naour, and C. Boucheix. "The Molecular Players of Sperm-Egg Fusion in Mammals." *Semin Cell Dev Biol* 17, no. 2 (2006): 254–63.
107. Zhu, G. Z., B. J. Miller, C. Boucheix et al. "Residues SFQ (173–175) in the Large Extracellular Loop of CD9 Are Required for Gamete Fusion." *Development* 129, no. 8 (2002): 1995–2002.
108. Miyado, K., K. Yoshida, K. Yamagata et al. "The Fusing Ability of Sperm Is Bestowed by CD9-Containing Vesicles Released from Eggs in Mice." *Proc Natl Acad Sci U S A* 105, no. 35 (2008): 12921–6.
109. Potel, J., P. Rassam, C. Montpellier et al. "EWI-2wint Promotes CD81 Clustering That Abrogates Hepatitis C Virus Entry." *Cell Microbiol* 15, no. 7 (2013): 1234–52.
110. Montpellier, C., B. A. Tews, J. Poitrimole et al. "Interacting Regions of CD81 and Two of Its Partners, EWI-2 and EWI-2wint, and Their Effect on Hepatitis C Virus Infection." *J Biol Chem* 286, no. 16 (2011): 13954–65.
111. Davis, C., H. J. Harris, K. Hu et al. "In Silico Directed Mutagenesis Identifies the CD81/Claudin-1 Hepatitis C Virus Receptor Interface." *Cell Microbiol* 14, no. 12 (2012): 1892–903.
112. Lupberger, J., M. B. Zeisel, F. Xiao et al. "EGFR and EphA2 Are Host Factors for Hepatitis C Virus Entry and Possible Targets for Antiviral Therapy." *Nat Med* 17, no. 5 (2011): 589–95.
113. Zemni, R., T. Bienvenu, M. C. Vinet et al. "A New Gene Involved in X-Linked Mental Retardation Identified by Analysis of an X;2 Balanced Translocation." *Nat Genet* 24, no. 2 (2000): 167–70.
114. Bassani, S., and M. Passafaro. "Tspan7: A New Player in Excitatory Synapse Maturation and Function." *Bioarchitecture* 2, no. 3 (2012): 95–7.
115. Nikopoulos, K., C. Gilissen, A. Hoischen et al. "Next-Generation Sequencing of a 40 Mb Linkage Interval Reveals Tspan12 Mutations in Patients with Familial Exudative Vitreoretinopathy." *Am J Hum Genet* 86, no. 2 (2010): 240–7.
116. Junge, H. J., S. Yang, J. B. Burton et al. "Tspan12 Regulates Retinal Vascular Development by Promoting Norrin- but Not Wnt-Induced FZD4/Beta-Catenin Signaling." *Cell* 139, no. 2 (2009): 299–311.
117. Khattree, N., L. M. Ritter, and A. F. Goldberg. "Membrane Curvature Generation by a C-Terminal Amphipathic Helix in Peripherin-2/rds, a Tetraspanin Required for Photoreceptor Sensory Cilium Morphogenesis." *J Cell Sci* 126, no. 20 (2013): 659–70.
118. Duncan, J. L., K. E. Talcott, K. Ratnam et al. "Cone Structure in Retinal Degeneration Associated with Mutations in the Peripherin/RDS Gene." *Invest Ophthalmol Vis Sci* 52, no. 3 (2011): 1557–66.
119. Goldberg, A. F., and R. S. Molday. "Defective Subunit Assembly Underlies a Digenic Form of Retinitis Pigmentosa Linked to Mutations in Peripherin/RDS and ROM-1." *Proc Natl Acad Sci U S A* 93, no. 24 (1996): 13726–30.
120. Boesze-Battaglia, K., F. P. Stefano, C. Fitzgerald, and S. Muller-Weeks. "ROM-1 Potentiates Photoreceptor Specific Membrane Fusion Processes." *Exp Eye Res* 84, no. 1 (2007): 22–31.
121. Clarke, G., A. F. Goldberg, D. Vidgen et al. "ROM-1 Is Required for Rod Photoreceptor Viability and the Regulation of Disk Morphogenesis." *Nat Genet* 25, no. 1 (2000): 67–73.

122. Karamatic Crew, V., N. Burton, A. Kagan et al. "CD151, the First Member of the Tetraspanin (TM4) Superfamily Detected on Erythrocytes, Is Essential for the Correct Assembly of Human Basement Membranes in Kidney and Skin." *Blood* 104, no. 8 (2004): 2217–23.
123. Mollinedo, F., G. Fontan, I. Barasoain, and P. A. Lazo. "Recurrent Infectious Diseases in Human CD53 Deficiency." *Clin Diagn Lab Immunol* 4, no. 2 (1997): 229–31.
124. Figdor, C. G., and A. B. van Spriel. "Fungal Pattern-Recognition Receptors and Tetraspanins: Partners on Antigen-Presenting Cells." *Trends Immunol* 31, no. 3 (2010): 91–6.
125. Hemler, M. E. "Targeting of Tetraspanin Proteins—Potential Benefits and Strategies." *Nat Rev Drug Discov* 7, no. 9 (2008): 747–58.
126. Hassuna, N., P. N. Monk, G. W. Moseley, and L. J. Partridge. "Strategies for Targeting Tetraspanin Proteins: Potential Therapeutic Applications in Microbial Infections." *BioDrugs* 23, no. 6 (2009): 341–59.

5 B Cell Receptor Signaling

Christoph Feest, Andreas Bruckbauer,
and Facundo D. Batista

CONTENTS

5.1   INTRODUCTION

5.1.1   B Cells in the Immune System

Immunity is the capability to detect, resist, and overcome a challenge that is posed by any foreign substance. This is carried out by a set of organs and tissues that are collectively referred to as the immune system. Its adaptive branch is able to respond to virtually any feature on a pathogen by the generation of highly specific receptors that recognize this so-called antigen—it adapts to the challenge and also ensures highly specific and long-lasting protection.[1]

The main groups of cells in the adaptive immune system are B and T lymphocytes; B cells get activated when a pathogenic challenge is detected. B cells carry a special surface receptor, the B cell receptor (BCR; Figure 5.1a), which evolves during a challenge to better bind the antigen. After activation, B cells secrete a soluble form of BCR as antibodies (Figure 5.1b, Ref. 2) that bind to, and thus highlight, a pathogen for other players in the immune system.

The tremendous flexibility and potency of the adaptive immune system require that the activation of lymphocytes must be tightly regulated to prevent aberrant activity that could provoke autoimmune diseases or cancer. That is why a detailed cellular and molecular description of the events underlying lymphocyte activation will be of immense value—not only to achieve a more complete understanding of the function of the immune system but also to design novel therapeutics that allow tailored control of lymphocyte activity.

5.1.2   The BCR and B Cell Activation

The BCR is an immunoglobulin (Ig) structure that can bind proteins, lipids, and sugars. Structurally, the BCR is a very flexible tetrameric structure composed of Ig domains (Figure 5.1a). As the BCR main body has no significant cytoplasmic tail, the associated Igα/β heterodimer carries immunotyrosine activation motifs (ITAMs) that mediate intracellular signaling.[3] Full B cell activation leads to proliferation and differentiation and is achieved when B cells receive two signals that are separated in space and time: First, binding of antigen to the BCR initiates rapid phosphorylation of ITAMs within the Igα/β sheath by Src family kinases and leads to the recruitment of numerous intracellular signaling molecules and adaptors in an assembly known as the signalosome.[4–6] Such activation leads to the BCR-mediated internalization of antigen into intracellular endosomes. Internalized antigen is broken down into smaller polypeptides that are loaded onto major histocompatibility complex II (MHCII). Hours after the first signal, peptide-loaded MHCII is displayed on the B cell surface and attracts a type of helping T cells with specificity for the same antigen.[7] These T helper cells provide the second signal in the form of secreted messengers and through binding of coreceptors, without which a B cell would not be fully activated.

After the successful reception of signals 1 and 2, B cells either differentiate to form extrafollicular plasma cells that are capable of the rapid secretion of low-affinity antibodies[8] or undergo affinity maturation to generate extremely high-affinity antibodies and long-lasting memory cells.[9]

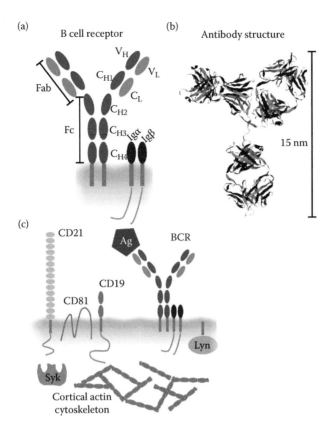

FIGURE 5.1 Secreted antibodies and the BCR are Igs. (a) The BCR, here the IgM isotype, consists of two heavy chains (with the variable domain V_H and constant domains C_{H1-4}) and two light chains (one variable, V_L, and one constant, C_L, domain). The BCR main body has no significant cytoplasmic tail and thus the associated Igα/β heterodimer carries ITAMs that mediate signaling. (b) The crystal structure of the human antibody IgG1 b12 against HIV-1. (Adapted from Saphire et al., *Science* [2001] 293: 1155–1159.) (c) The first steps in the canonical BCR signaling pathway are as follows: Antigen binding through the BCR is followed by the activation of Lyn, which phosphorylates the ITAMs on the Igα/β heterodimer. These activated ITAMs can then recruit cytoplasmic effectors such as Syk. The CD19 complex with CD81 and CD21 can bring in further activatory molecules.

5.1.3 IMAGING THE MOLECULAR EVENTS OF EARLY B CELL ACTIVATION

Historically, B cell activation has been characterized using global biochemical analysis after stimulation with soluble antigen. Then, early imaging investigations found that after engagement with multivalent soluble antigen, BCRs were redistributed to form a "cap" structure on the B cell membrane.[10–12] While these strategies provided a critical foundation for the understanding of B cell activation, there was also evidence that B cells receive antigen through cell–cell contacts with antigen-presenting cells (APC).[13,14] Recent multiphoton microscopy investigations in lymph nodes in vivo have underpinned the notion that B cells can recognize antigen on the surface of a number of APCs, including macrophages and dendritic cells, and it is now accepted that membrane-bound antigen is the predominant form of antigen that initiates B cell activation in vivo.[15,16] This cellular response leads to the formation of an immunological synapse,[17] a feature also associated with the activation of T cells and natural killer cells.[18–21] Consequently, B cell activation cannot simply be viewed as a result of ligand engagement of the BCR but must rather be considered in the context of the complex morphological changes that occur within B cells: A host of intracellular, membrane-proximal, and extracellular cues have to be integrated.

Studies of the early events during B cell activation with optical microscopy rely on experimental setups that mimic some but never truly all features of a cell–cell contact. Many approaches have been adapted from seminal, analogous investigations in T cells.[19,21–23] The most common modes for imaging-centered B cell activation studies are summarized in Figure 5.2.

Useful model systems to mimic APCs are planar lipid bilayers and antigen-coated glass coverslips. Antigen on a supported lipid bilayer is the experimental setup closest to a cell–cell contact as it allows a B cell to perform its characteristic spreading-and-contraction response.[24] On a bilayer, antigen is mobile: It can be aggregated into signaling microclusters, concentrated in one larger central cluster (reminiscent of an antigen cap), and can also be extracted from the bilayer for internalization. Bilayers also allow for the tethering of additional ligands that can, for example, bind to integrins.[25] However, the mobility of antigen on a supported lipid bilayer is higher than what is to be expected on an APC. Also, it is difficult to engineer nonstimulatory bilayers and the still high substrate stiffness might interfere with mechanosensing of

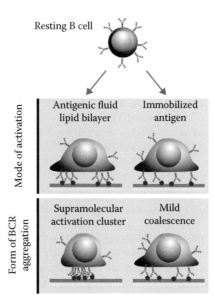

FIGURE 5.2 Experimental setups to study molecular events of B cell activation with TIRFM: Antigen can be presented immobilized on coverslips or mobile on supported lipid bilayers. Especially on lipid bilayers, antigen is actively aggregated into microclusters.

B cells.[26] In contrast, immobilized antigen on a glass substrate allows the B cell to spread but frustrates microcluster formation and cell contraction.

Planar lipid bilayers and antigen-coated glass coverslips are especially insightful model systems when they are imaged with total internal reflection fluorescence microscopy (TIRFM).[27] A TIRFM setup allows the highly selective imaging of an approximately 100-nm-thin slice just above the coverslip—putting both the antigen and the B cell membrane into the same focal plane. This technique greatly enhances signal-to-noise ratio, which enables the detection of single fluorescent molecules, and can be combined with fast image acquisition to study the dynamics of several molecular players simultaneously at video rate.

Using the technologies described above, it has been shown that upon recognition of cognate antigen on the surface of a presenting cell, B cells undergo a rapid spreading-and-contraction response to maximize the antigen uptake.[24] The molecular events underlying this spreading-and-contraction response after antigenic stimulation on lipid bilayers have been first dissected with sequential three-color TIRFM.[28,29] There, the formation of BCR and antigen microclusters (containing between 100 and 500 antigen molecules) is regarded as the earliest observable molecular event. Subsequent effector recruitment to these microclusters is concomitant with the initiation of calcium signaling, which led us to redefine these microclusters as microsignalosomes and to suggest that they are common units of signaling in lymphocytes.[28,30] Signaling through several small, mobile microclusters that recruit positive and negative regulators provides a means to actively shape BCR-mediated signaling. However, this highly dynamic nature of BCR signaling and the mere number of cues that need to be integrated into the signaling process add complexity when characterizing the events underlying B cell activation.

5.2 NANOSCALE ORGANIZATION OF BCR

5.2.1 Receptor Counting on B Cells

To establish the copy numbers of receptors and coreceptors, we performed a counting assay (Simply Cellular, Bangs Laboratories) that is based on bead standards with a known number of binding sites that bind the FC region of a rat-raised antibody. Beads were stained with saturating amounts of antibody to cover all binding sites. The beads with increasing number of binding sites allow the construction of a linear calibration curve that is obtained after linear regression. From this calibration curve, the number of target sites, that is, receptors, on the cell surface can be calculated. To this end, primary B cells (PBCs) were purified, labeled with monoclonal antibodies against IgM, IgD, and CD19 that were conjugated to APC, PE, AF488, or AF647, and then analyzed by flow cytometry (Table 5.1).

On wild-type (wt) PBCs, we find that IgD is highly expressed—up to 260,000 copies—while IgM and CD19 are expressed in the same, lower range—55,000–80,000. On PBCs that are specific for the hen egg lysozyme (HEL) antigen, that is, PBCs from MD4 transgenic mice, IgM expression is higher. Having quantified the expression level of receptors, we went on to estimate the surface density of receptors on the membrane. First, we determined the average total surface area of a PBC by

TABLE 5.1
Copy Number of Receptors and Surface Density

Receptor, Cell Type	Mean	Standard Deviation	Density (1/μm²)	Coverage (%)
IgD, wt	260,000	50,000	1300–1700	6.5–8.5
IgD, MD4	225,000	55,000	1100–1500	5.5–7.5
IgM, wt	60,000	25,000	280–380	1.4–1.9
IgM, MD4	155,000	60,000	800–1000	4.0–5.0
CD19, wt	75,000	5000	380–500	1.0–1.3
CD19, MD4	80,000	10,000	400–520	1.0–1.3

Note: The copy number of receptors as determined by a counting assay allowed us to estimate their surface density. We find that, in PBCs, more than 10% of the surface is occupied by both isotypes of BCR (IgM and IgD) and the positive coreceptor CD19 combined.

multiplying the surface area of a sphere with radius $r = 2.5$ μm ($A = 4\pi r^2 = 78$ μm²) with a "ruffle factor" of 2. From several sources, for example, electron microscopy images,[24] we know that the B cell membrane is strongly ruffled, and with data from Thaunat et al.,[31] we estimated this factor to be approximately 2. Finally, we calculated what proportion of the plasma membrane is covered by the respective receptors. We estimated that the BCR (two Ig domains fused, where the spatial extension of an Ig domain is 4–7 nm) occupies an area of 50 nm² and that CD19 (one Ig domain) occupies an area of 25 nm². This leads us to gauge that more than 10% of the surface of PBCs is occupied by both isotypes of BCR and CD19 combined.

5.2.2 Fast Multicolor TIRFM and Single-Particle Tracking

Existing imaging methods such as sequential three-color TIRFM with a typical imaging speed of 2 frames/s have proved useful in the definition and characterization of the signalosome, but they are inadequately slow to investigate highly dynamic changes at the molecular level prior to and during B cell activation. Interactions between the molecular players happen on a millisecond timescale, necessitating a high temporal resolution of at least 20 frames/s. Multiplexed acquisition can be achieved through either hyperspectral setups[32,33] or optical splitters. We use optical splitters, which allows the simultaneous observation of up to four colors, but comes at the expense of a smaller field of view. The TIRF microscopes we use in our studies are based on 2- and 3-laser line Olympus cell^R TIRF systems, which are equipped with a two- and four-color optical splitter and additional air-coupled laser lines to extend our excitation options.

Single-particle tracking (SPT) combined with TIRFM is well suited to study dynamic processes in lymphocytes. Here, we use the term *SPT* specifically to signify the tracking of fluorescently labeled molecules on a B cell membrane. The general assumption behind SPT is that a molecule on the surface of the plasma membrane is subject to many forces that determine its mobility. These influences can impossibly be taken individually into account, so a simple value that condenses all this information offers a handle to describe particles' behavior; this number is the diffusion coefficient D. In our case of SPT, D describes the lateral motion of molecules on the membrane. This gives an idea how explorative a molecule is—how far does it travel in a set time? From the mobility, we can broadly conclude how strongly it interacts with other molecules. Then, by tweaking parameters in our system, for example, removing a specific interaction partner, one can study the strength of an interaction. To conduct an SPT experiment, the number of labeled receptors must be low. Yet, all of the receptors of interest on a B cell are expressed at high copy number. In order to follow individual receptors, labeling strategies are employed to achieve staining that labels only a tiny proportion of the receptors but in turn allows their tracking as their fluorescence no longer overlaps. Competitive staining uses Fab fragments that are conjugated and unconjugated at ratios of 1:100–1:1000 to label individual molecules. In effect, only a few out of many receptors are stained with a fluorescent dye.

We prepared Fab fragments from purified antibodies through digestion with papain. After antibody digestion, the Fab fragments are separated from the remaining undigested antibody and Fc region in a two-step process: First, gel filtration to narrow down the size of the protein, followed by the second step, an anion exchange column to separate Fab and Fc. Eventually, the Fab fragment is conjugated to an organic dye at a degree of labeling less than one dye molecule per Fab fragment. Our preferred choice of dyes for labeling are manufactured by ATTO-TEC, as these are very photostable and allow acquisition times of up to 1 min.

Our typical SPT acquisition time is 50–80 ms/frame, with 200–300 frames/movie recorded. Analysis of SPT movies is done with custom MATLAB® scripts based on established algorithms:[34,35] In every frame, particle candidates are identified by intensity and shape criteria; then, their positions are determined via a centroid calculation and linked over several frames to give particle tracks in time. Criteria for this linking are kept stringent; tracks needed to link particles over a minimum of 10 frames[36] and the maximum allowed jumping distance between frames was kept at 4 pixels (430 nm).

Employing simultaneous two-color SPT to investigate the dynamics of the BCR in resting PBCs,[37] we observed that the median diffusion coefficient of IgD was 10-fold lower than that of IgM (0.032 μm^2/s), suggesting that an isotype-specific feature determines BCR mobility. The influence of the cytoskeleton on BCR mobility will be discussed later.

5.2.3 LOCALIZATION MICROSCOPY

SPT is an excellent tool to study the dynamics of receptors at high temporal resolution and high position accuracy. However, to resolve the organization—the landscape—of receptors, a larger proportion has to be labeled and imaged at super-resolution in every cell. Today, several fluorescence techniques are available that provide resolution beyond the diffraction limit. They have sprung from the realization that both the properties of the excitation light and the properties of the fluorescent molecules could be exploited. This led first to the nonlinear method of stimulated emission depletion (STED)[38] and later to the linear methods structured illumination microscopy,[39,40] and localization microscopy (LM).[41–43] LM largely comprises the seminal techniques of fluorescence photoactivation localization microscopy (fPALM),[42] photoactivated localization microscopy (PALM),[41] and stochastic optical reconstruction microscopy (STORM).[43] From a conceptual perspective, all of these techniques are equal as they break the diffraction barrier in a similar way: The position of a single, isolated fluorescent molecule can be determined with accuracy beyond the diffraction limit.[44] The challenge is to separate the fluorescence of the molecules in a densely labeled sample. These seminal LM approaches are based on the temporal isolation of fluorescence emitting molecules, which was achieved using photoactivatable dyes (as in fPALM, the first available was PA-GFP[45]), photoswitchable dyes (as in PALM, the first set of dyes was Eos and Kaede), and organic dye pairs (as in STORM, demonstrated with the pair Cy5–Cy3). To study structures in PBCs, the application of organic labels is often preferable to genetically expressed proteins, because PBCs usually become plasmablasts after any such transduction. That is why we have used the cyanine dyes Cy5 and Alexa647, which have a desirable switching behavior that depends on the buffer conditions.[46] This approach is similar to STORM but does not require a second dye in the proximity of the first one; consequently, it has been termed directSTORM or dSTORM.[47,48] In dSTORM, the initially fluorescent dye molecules are transferred into a metastable dark state with high-intensity illumination. The longevity of that metastable dark state is determined by the buffer conditions. Also, additional illumination with light of the appropriate wavelength (usually somewhere between 300 and 500 nm) encourages a return to the ground state. This return process is stochastic, meaning that an unpredictable set of fluorophores is returned to their ground state. From there, they will get excited again and either reenter the dark state or fluoresce. The buffer conditions make a fluorescence event much less likely than a transfer to the dark state, which eventually leads to only sparse fluorescence events. If their fluorescence does not overlap, their individual positions can be determined with high accuracy. dSTORM data were recorded in TIRF mode with acquisition times of 150–300 ms/frame at a laser power density of 0.1–0.3 kW/cm^2. Usually, 3000–6000 frames were recorded, leading to acquisition times of approximately 15–30 min per sample. We found that the mean photon count consistently lies around 2000–3000 and that this results in a localization precision of 10–15 nm. This gave further confidence in the utility of dSTORM as a tool to resolve receptor distributions in super-resolution. Over the time of acquisition, up to 30 min, the microscope stage inevitably moves owing to thermal drift and alternating airflows. This stage movement was recorded by monitoring the position of gold fiducial particles (of 40–100 nm diameter) in the sample. Their positions were tracked and used to calculate and correct the sample drift over time in postprocessing. To analyze dSTORM data, we basically followed the protocol laid out in the study by Betzig et al.[41] Switched molecules are detected as peaks in differential images $I_D = I_{k+1} - I_k$. A field of 7 × 7 pixels around these was then used to fit a single-mode 2D Gaussian to the peak position. Fits closer than 400 nm to a molecule localized in any of the two preceding frames were discarded. Similarly, fits that did not fulfill criteria in terms of intensity and shape or width of the fitted PSF were discarded.

Several papers have addressed the question whether LM can be regarded as a quantitative tool.[49–52] All LM techniques rely on the blinking/switching behavior of the fluorescent probe, which makes it difficult to reliably count how often each individual molecule has been recorded. We followed the strategies described in the aforementioned papers to account for overcounting in our system: Through a combination of pair-correlation and blinking analysis, it was determined that we localize every molecule approximately twice.[53] This is less than the roughly 10 expected switching cycles for Cy5,[54] but our usual acquisition time per frame is longer (150–300 ms) than what most groups use; thus, our acquisition time covers several short blinks of Cy5. Between these bursts of short blinks lie many minutes before the molecule fluoresces again. Apart from the rather mathematical analysis, dilute labeling gave further confidence that we can actually count molecules reliably. In a dilute labeling regime, only 20–50 molecules on a single cell were labeled and most of these molecules were recorded only once over the acquisition period.

5.2.4 SPATIAL STATISTICS TO DESCRIBE CLUSTERING BEHAVIOR

A dSTORM image is basically a table that contains the x and y coordinates of the registered molecules. This point pattern can be further analyzed to derive parameters that describe the organization more quantitatively.

Originally derived in the field of botany,[55] the Hopkins index has become a popular and effective measure. In short, it declares how strongly the probed data set deviates from a random distribution. This means that the null hypothesis is that points are distributed randomly. The three major pros of the Hopkins index are as follows: it is an effective indicator of structure, it is dimensionless, and it is straightforward to implement. A fully random distribution does achieve a Hopkins index of 0.5 while a completely nonrandom distribution would achieve 1.

Our second tool to describe spatial distributions is Ripley's K statistic, which was also first applied in an ecological context—redwood seedlings.[56] The goal is, similar to the Hopkins index, to quantify the extent to which a given distribution of points deviates from a random distribution. The original Ripley's K statistic is usually modified to give visually more interpretable graphics[57] and can be easily extended to 3D.[58] The most common modification leads to the distance-dependent so-called H function, which is a valuable source of information: First, at any given distance, the H function is hovering around 0 for a random distribution, is greater than 0 for a nonrandom distribution, and is below 0 for a dispersed distribution. Second, for distributions of roundish clusters, the H function's peak position is a good proxy for the radius of strongest aggregation and the peak's height for the compactness of clusters. In short, the H function is a valuable descriptive measure that compliments the Hopkins index.

5.2.5 ON THE NANOSCALE, BOTH ISOTYPES OF BCR
EXIST AS PREFORMED NANOCLUSTERS

Controversy surrounds the organization of BCR on the nanoscale. A better understanding of the precise state of the BCR in the resting state has strong implications for how signaling is prohibited, initiated, and amplified. Mono- and oligomeric BCR organization has been proposed: There is evidence for monomeric organization from a lack of fluorescence resonance energy transfer (FRET) between BCRs in a reconstituted system,[59] as well as for oligomeric complexes from early biochemical methods[60] and a FRET-based assay in a reconstituted system.[61] It is significant to clarify this organization to improve models of B cell activation with respect to explaining the wide range of affinities of antigens that can be recognized by the BCR,[62,63] tonic survival signaling,[64] and BCR signal amplification via coreceptors.

To visualize the organization of BCR, we used the super-resolution microscopy method dSTORM as outlined in Section 5.2.3.[47] PBCs were purified and labeled with Fab fragments against IgD or IgM that were conjugated to the dSTORM-compatible dye Cy5. After washing, the cells were resuspended in imaging buffer and settled onto coverslips that were coated with antibody against MHCII, which provides a nonstimulatory protein coating. Cells were left to adhere at 37°C for 4 min and then fixed with a mixture of 4% paraformaldehyde and 0.1% glutaraldehyde for 45 min to sufficiently immobilize receptors. After washing, samples were imaged in TIRF mode to selectively visualize those receptors that are in proximity to the coverslip. Data were recorded at 150 ms exposure time for up to 45 min. We routinely achieve a localization precision of approximately 10 nm, and as we use small fluorescently tagged Fab fragments, the recorded localization should be less than 5 nm from the labeled receptor. We do not need a secondary antibody, which would further decrease the true localization precision for the BCR. Based on the receptor counting, we estimate that we are visualizing 5–15% of all receptors. The collected localizations are corrected for sample drift, overlaid, and built into a single pseudocolor image in postprocessing.

To highlight the contrast between TIRFM and super-resolution dSTORM, Figure 5.3a juxtaposes images for IgD and IgM in these respective imaging modes. The dSTORM images are rendered in a way that they represent a 10-fold increase in resolution compared to TIRFM. It is apparent that both isotypes of BCR exist in a clustered organization, with IgD being more clustered (Figure 5.3b). Given that we are able to visualize approximately 10% of molecules, we extrapolate that IgD clusters contain 30–120 IgD molecules while IgM clusters contain 20–50 IgM molecules. With regard to the quantification on nonstimulatory coating, both IgD and IgM demonstrate a nonrandom distribution with Hopkins indices of 0.83 and 0.66, respectively (Figure 5.3c). From the H function, we can conclude that for IgD and IgM, the radius of aggregation was similar at approximately 60–80 nm, while IgD was clustered move heavily (Figure 5.3d). A very straightforward way of quantifying clustering is to take the obtained radius of aggregation from the H function and then group molecules according to them having more (clustered) or less (not clustered) neighbors within a circular area of that radius compared to what is predicted for a random distribution (Figure 5.3b). Using this criterion, we found 70% of IgD molecules and 38% of IgM molecules to reside in clusters (Figure 5.3e, clustered molecules are dark, unclustered ones are gray). It is also noteworthy that even a random distribution displays some degree of clustering, usually 2–5%, when using this criterion. This simple clustering index reproduces the results of the Hopkins index qualitatively. Underpinned by the spatial statistics, the important conclusion from our dSTORM experiments is that both isotypes of BCR exist as preformed nanoclusters.

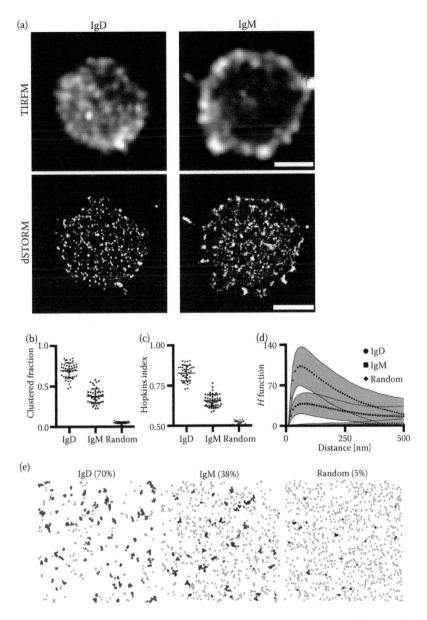

FIGURE 5.3 The organization of both isotypes of BCR on the nanoscale is revealed by dSTORM. (a) The improvement on conventional TIRFM is clearly visible in the dSTORM images; the scale bar represents 2 μm. (b–d) Spatial statistics reveal that BCR is nonrandomly distributed in the steady state and that IgD clusters more strongly than IgM. BCR nanoclusters have a radius of aggregation of approximately 60–80 nm. Bars are mean ± SD; error bands are 95% confidence intervals. (e) In a 9 μm² area, 900 individual localizations of IgD, IgM, and a random distribution are plotted and the localizations classed as clustered are shown in darker tones.

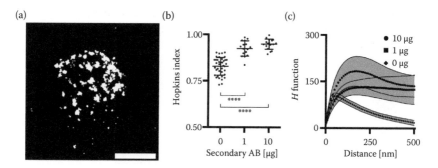

FIGURE 5.4 BCR cross-linking can be sensitively induced and detected with dSTORM. (a) IgD on PBCs is heavily cross-linked by anti-rat antibody against IgD-labeling Fab; the scale bar represents 2 µm. (b and c) Spatial statistics reveal that IgD clusters grow dependent on the amount of cross-linking reagent. Bars are mean ± SD; error bands are 95% confidence intervals.

5.2.6 CROSS-LINKED BCR FORMS LARGER CLUSTERS

B cells are activated when the BCR binds its ligand, the antigen. Many antigens, especially those that are capable of eliciting T-independent responses, are assumed to be multivalent and thus to heavily cross-link BCRs[65]—providing a simple mechanism for signal amplification. We wanted to see if dSTORM is able to detect cross-linked BCR on the nanoscale. PBCs were labeled on ice with increasing amounts of F(ab)$_2$ and imaged with dSTORM. We observed clearly visible cross-linking of IgM.[53] We were keen to show similar cross-linking for IgD that already exhibits a stronger preclustering. To find such increased clustering, PBCs were first labeled with Fab fragments against IgD (raised in rat), washed and resuspended, and then labeled with increasing amounts of anti-rat antibody before being settled, fixed, and imaged in dSTORM. As expected, we found cross-linking of Fab-labeled IgD to induce clearly visible stronger clustering (Figure 5.4a).

The quantification shows the Hopkins index to further increase from 0.83 over 0.92 to 0.95, depending on the amount of cross-linking antibody (Figure 5.4b). The H function shifts its peak position to larger sizes and rises dramatically in amplitude (Figure 5.4c). Taken together, these cross-linking experiments demonstrated that we could sensitively induce and detect changes in the nanoscale organization of BCR on PBCs. It should also be noted that cells with cross-linked BCRs spread more reluctantly, which is an indication of ongoing signaling that makes resources less available for spreading.

5.2.7 BCR NANOCLUSTER INTEGRITY DOES NOT DEPEND ON CORTICAL ACTIN

We wanted to establish if the reorganization of the cytoskeleton affects the observed clustering of BCR. To investigate the effect of cytoskeleton reorganization, PBCs were settled onto nonstimulatory coverslips. Then, the buffer was quickly exchanged against prewarmed imaging buffer containing 1 µM Latrunculin A (LatA), a drug that inhibits polymerization of actin by sequestering G-actin in a 1:1 stoichiometry. After 4 min of incubation, cells were fixed and imaged in dSTORM. Surprisingly, cytoskeleton reorganization did not change the extent of either IgM or IgD clustering at this early stage of activation;[53] neither Hopkins index nor H function was altered significantly. Similar results were obtained when cells were treated with 10–50 µM Cytochalasin D (CytoD), which disrupts actin polymerization by end-capping of existing actin filaments. Our dSTORM data indicate that both isotypes of BCR exist as preformed nanoclusters that are not significantly altered during cytoskeleton reorganization, which suggests that their integrity is maintained through a cytoskeleton-independent mechanism. Even when cells were incubated with LatA or CytoD for up to 60 min, there was again no detectable change in BCR organization, but after such prolonged treatment, the cells' morphology became strongly affected. With the results obtained after cross-linking BCR, we feel confident that we would have detected any such changes, although we cannot rule out changes on the scale of a few nanometers that were reported with FRET.[59]

5.2.8 BCR Nanocluster Organization Is Unperturbed upon Antigen Stimulation on Glass

Until now, we focused on the steady-state organization of BCR. How does this organization relate to the more physiological scenario in which B cell activation is triggered through antigen engagement on the surface of a presenting cell? To investigate PBCs under specific antigenic stimulation, we took advantage of the MD4 transgenic system: B cells from these mice carry a BCR that is highly specific for HEL. MD4 PBCs were labeled with Fab fragments against IgM or IgD and settled onto coverslips that were coated with either nonstimulatory antibody or HEL to provide a specific stimulatory protein coating for MD4 PBCs. To our surprise, we again observed no visual difference in IgM or IgD organization between nonstimulatory and stimulatory coating. Quantification with Hopkins index and H function did not yield any differences either.[53] We confirmed that under these experimental conditions, strong stimulation occurred by fluorescence staining of activation markers.

The organization of BCR in the plasma membrane has been and still is controversial. In summary, we provide evidence that both isotypes of BCR exist as preformed nanoclusters in PBCs—a fact that is reminiscent of T cell receptor (TCR) organization in protein islands.[66,67] In particular, IgD clusters more strongly than IgM, which is in line with the low lateral mobility of IgD and the higher mobility of IgM.[68] At early times after activation, through either antigen or cytoskeleton disruption, the nanoscale organization of BCR appeared largely unchanged, which means that robust BCR-mediated signaling can occur without a global reorganization of receptors.

This raises the question of how activation is accomplished. One road to explore is the contribution of coreceptors. Physiologically, there is evidence that the impact of coreceptors is not only important but rather fundamental in bringing about successful BCR signaling. In B cells, the prime example is the coreceptor CD19, which is absolutely required to achieve a BCR signaling response to membrane-bound ligands.[28] Section 5.3 will therefore be dedicated to CD19.

5.3 CD19 IS REGULATED BY THE TETRASPANIN NETWORK

We have established an oligomeric organization of the BCR that remains unchanged upon cytoskeleton reorganization and antigen stimulation. It is therefore sound to assume that the BCR cooperates with another molecule to bring about the trans-membrane signaling that leads to full B cell activation. Indeed, it has been known for some time that B cell signaling is positively and negatively regulated by coreceptors.[69–73] Our laboratory has previously shown that the positive coreceptor CD19 is required for B cell activation with membrane-bound antigen and a requirement to form antigen-containing microclusters during B cell activation.[28] CD19 is a 95 kDa glycoprotein that serves as a B cell lineage marker[74] and has been implicated in immune disease.[75] It has no known ligand but was shown to cocap with the BCR during soluble stimulation[76] and to massively lower the threshold for BCR signaling.[77] CD19 exists in a complex with CD21/CD35[78] and the tetraspanin CD81.[79] While CD81 is important for correct trafficking of CD19 to the plasma membrane,[80] CD21 is assumed to function as a bridge between innate and adaptive immunity[78] but unimportant for the actual BCR signaling.[28]

5.3.1 CD19 EXISTS IN PREFORMED NANOCLUSTERS

As a first step, we set out to image the distribution of CD19 in the plasma membrane with dSTORM. To probe the distribution of CD19 in steady state and under antigenic stimulation, PBCs from MD4 transgenic mice were settled onto coverslips that were coated with either anti-MHCII or HEL. The first finding was that CD19 is nonrandomly distributed into preformed nanoclusters,[53] which are reminiscent of what we found for BCR before. CD19 nanoclusters also do not change during antigenic stimulation. In comparison to BCR, the quantification yields a slightly smaller cluster radius (50–60 nm compared to 60–70 nm). Also, it was noticeable in the statistics that we observed a broader range of behavior than was observed for BCR. Whether or not this hints at subpopulations of differentially organized CD19 clusters, for example, different tetraspanin content or interactions, could not be deduced from this experiment.

5.3.2 CD19 NANOCLUSTER INTEGRITY DOES NOT DEPEND ON CORTICAL ACTIN

CD19 was found to be of paramount importance in B cell stimulation when antigen was presented in a membrane-bound way on a lipid bilayer.[28] This confirmed that CD19 has an indispensable role when B cells are activated in response to membrane-bound antigen and suggested that there is a connection between CD19 and the cytoskeleton. To study how cytoskeleton reorganization affects the distribution and clustering of CD19, PBCs were settled onto nonstimulatory coverslips before treatment with LatA through buffer exchange. Astoundingly, cytoskeleton reorganization did not bring about any detectable difference in CD19 nanoclustering, indicating that CD19 is similarly structured during cytoskeleton rearrangement and thus suggesting that the cytoskeleton is no direct regulator of CD19. We also reported SPT experiments in which CD19 is largely immobile with a median diffusion coefficient of 0.005 µm²/s, which is as slow as IgD and does not change upon LatA treatment.[53] When viewed in light of this unaffected dynamics during cytoskeleton reorganization, it is less surprising to find no influence of the cytoskeleton on the nanoclustering of CD19.

5.3.3 THE TETRASPANIN CD81 REGULATES CD19 NANOCLUSTERS

In order to understand the molecular mechanism that restrains CD19 mobility and maintains its nanocluster integrity, we turned to the tetraspanin CD81. Tetraspanins are capable of organizing membrane proteins in a static and dynamic way[81] and are expressed widely in the immune system.[82,83] Therefore, we studied the distribution of CD19 in the plasma membrane of PBCs that lacked CD81 or were double heterozygous in CD81 and CD19. These 2xHET mice serve as a control, because CD19 expression is reduced in the absence of CD81,[84] but the 2xHET cells show a similar reduction in CD19 expression level[53] while all the components remain present. The staining efficiency of anti-CD19 Fab fragments in CD81 was too low to achieve sufficient labeling density for dSTORM. For that reason, we used the full anti-CD19 antibody, which, importantly, did not alter the detected clustering in wt controls. On nonstimulatory coating, we observed a marked increase in the clustering of CD19 in the CD81-deficient cells, which also manifested in higher Hopkins index and rising H function amplitude. Interestingly, in CD81-deficient cells, the number of CD19 molecules per nanocluster increased by more than 80%. These data show that the tetraspanin network, mediated through CD81, plays an important role in organizing CD19 nanoclusters. It is tempting to speculate that CD81 works as a spacer in CD19 nanoclusters and might thus bring about an optimal density of those clusters. However, it is also possible that CD81 mediates an interaction with another component of that cluster or other molecules in the plasma membrane.

Having established a role for CD81 in maintaining a physiologically important organization of CD19 nanoclusters, the question arose in how far does it affect the dynamics of CD19. We performed SPT on PBCs from wt and CD81KO mice and also disrupted the cytoskeleton to check for differential interactions with the cytoskeleton. While CD19 is largely immobile in wt cells (0.005 µm²/s), it is threefold faster in CD81KO cells (0.015 µm²/s). This means that the absence of CD81 affects both the nanoclustering and the mobility of CD19. Interestingly, when cells were treated with LatA, there was no effect on CD19 mobility in wt cells, but in CD81KO cells, there was a further doubling of the median diffusion coefficient from 0.015 to 0.29 µm²/s.

Finding such a marked increase in the mobility of CD19 nanoclusters when one component of these nanoclusters is missing raised the question whether all clusters or just a fraction are affected. That is why we performed a two-population analysis of the diffusion coefficients—as the existence of two distinct subpopulations had been reported for other receptors before.[85] For this analysis, the diffusion coefficients were imported into MATLAB (immobile particles were excluded with a cutoff at either 0.001 or 0.0001 µm²/s) and fitted to a bimodal model curve that simply adds up two lognormal distributions. Such lognormal distributions are the best current model to describe a population of diffusion coefficients.[86] In our calculation, the center of the slow diffusion component in CD81-deficient cells was capped at the wt value. The

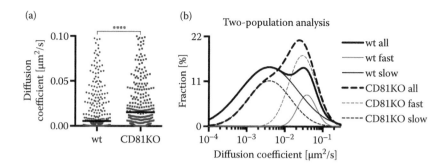

FIGURE 5.5 Mobility of the coreceptor CD19 is restrained by the tetraspanin CD81. (a) SPT of CD19 in wt and CD81KO PBCs shows a significant increase in the median diffusion coefficient. Bars are median. (b) A refined two-population analysis reveals a bimodal distribution of CD19 diffusion coefficients in wt PBCs. In the absence of CD81, a swap from the slower to the faster subpopulation takes place, which indicates that the tetraspanin network is responsible for restraining CD19 mobility.

analysis shows that there is not simply a shift of the whole population but rather a swap from slower to faster diffusion (Figure 5.5). In numbers, this manifests as a drop from 85% to 52% in the slow component and a corresponding rise from 15% to 48% in the faster diffusing component, from wt to CD81-deficient cells. This is the first time that we see a distinct swap in the diffusing populations; a similar analysis for BCR revealed a uniform shift of the whole population toward faster diffusion during cytoskeleton reorganization. These studies of CD19 dynamics provide evidence that a considerable part of CD19 nanoclusters is restrained in mobility by CD81. Bearing in mind the dSTORM results, it thus appears likely that the tetraspanin CD81 acts as a spacer and restrainer, thereby organizing CD19 nanoclusters in an optimal way to support BCR signaling.

5.3.4 CD19 Nanoclusters Coalesce with IgM in Areas of Signaling

How could synergy between BCR and CD19 be brought about dynamically? To answer that question, the SPT experiments lack an important piece of information: Where does signaling happen? It is clear that BCR signaling does not happen homogeneously on the whole surface area that is engaged by an APC. Rather small entities termed *signalosomes* are hotspots of signaling, as evidenced by the rapid recruitment of effector kinases.[28,29] We therefore highlighted areas of ongoing signaling by using GFP-tagged Syk as an indicator for early BCR-mediated signaling in a B cell line that also expressed a HEL-specific IgM-BCR. First, the distribution of IgM in these cells was checked with dSTORM. IgM behaved largely similar to what was observed for PBCs, with the exception of a larger radius of aggregation on stimulatory coverslips. This pointed to a slightly more ordered distribution of IgM during stimulation. The distribution of CD19 in these cells appeared consistently nonrandom but slightly more clustered than in PBCs. A most interesting observation was that Syk indeed formed microcluster-like structures during antigenic stimulation on glass.

The induction of these structures worked robustly and they colocalized with higher IgM intensity when we stained cells for IgM. This meant that we could locate signaling hotspots and that they overlapped with higher local IgM intensity.

We compared the nanoscale distribution of IgM and CD19 inside and outside of Syk clusters by dSTORM imaging. To perform such correlative dSTORM in fixed cells, first an image of the GFP channel was taken to capture the distribution of Syk microclusters. This image was thresholded to give a mask of high Syk. Then, dSTORM of IgM or CD19 was performed to elucidate their nanoscale distribution. The resulting dSTORM images were then overlaid with the Syk mask, and the extent to which either IgM or CD19 would be different inside or outside Syk clusters was quantified. Individual molecule localizations were counted as being inside or outside of these Syk clusters and the density of these so-classed molecules was divided by their overall density. This analysis revealed that inside Syk clusters, the number of IgM and CD19 molecules is 50% higher than the overall density.[53] Surprisingly, we could not detect any changes in the molecular densities of individual CD19 or IgM nanoclusters. That means that the nanoclusters themselves are unchanged in the different conditions and that their abundance in Syk microclusters is a significant local divergence from the global mean for both molecules. Together with the unchanged density of IgM and CD19, it indicates that in areas of ongoing signaling through the BCR, there is a coalescence of BCR and the costimulatory molecule CD19 without any alteration to their individual nanocluster makeup.

In conclusion, we showed that CD19 exists in preformed nanoclusters that are on a similar length scale as those of BCR. We found that the tetraspanin CD81 regulates the size and mobility of CD19 nanoclusters, although the mechanism through which that is achieved is not entirely clear, but palmitoylation of CD81 has been reported[87,88] which could provide the linkage to the plasma membrane that restricts mobility of the CD19 nanoclusters. As tetraspanins tend to interact with each other dynamically, there may be further interactions involved in this compartmentalization mechanism.

During antigenic stimulation, it was shown that while the individual nanoclusters of CD19 and BCR remained unchanged, their number in Syk-rich areas was increased. This local divergence from the mean concentration could explain the synergy of CD19 and BCR, but this static observation offers no clue as to how it is brought about.

With SPT, we did not find any evidence of correlated motion or dynamic interaction between BCR and CD19 (Christoph Feest, unpublished data). This attempt could have been hampered by the weakness and transience of the interaction—it may be only of short duration and thus lie well below what we can expect to detect. Indeed, determining such correlations from SPT experiments is far from effortless[89] and the slow diffusion of CD19 makes it rather difficult to put forward a model, in which a highly dynamic process leads to recruitment. However, the density of CD19 and BCR on the membrane is very high and we are labeling only a tiny fraction of the nanoclusters in SPT experiments. This is probably the major obstacle in such a single-molecule approach. It is simply very unlikely to find any coincidences when we are following so few particles. Alternative ways to probe the coincidence and coconfinement of molecules in the plasma membrane are fluorescence correlation spectroscopy (FCS)[90] and STED-FCS.[91] Both methods could provide additional experimental insight into the nanoscale organization and interaction of BCR and CD19.

5.4 COMPARTMENTALIZATION EMERGES AS A CONCEPT FROM IMAGING STUDIES

5.4.1 COMPARTMENTALIZATION OF THE PLASMA MEMBRANE BY THE ACTIN-BASED MEMBRANE SKELETON

In the description of the membrane by the fluid-mosaic model, proteins diffuse freely and are randomly distributed at long range.[92] This view has since been overhauled.[93] The discrepancy between protein mobility in artificial systems[94,95] as well as membrane blebs, which show high mobility, and biological systems[96] with 20 times lower mobility suggested that the membrane cortex hinders lateral mobility. The principal current proposition is the picket-fence model by the Kusumi laboratory.[97,98] In this model, actin filaments function as membrane skeleton fences to which transmembrane proteins are anchored. This arrangement leads to the creation of compartments of sizes between 40 and 400 nm,[99] which hinder the lateral mobility of transmembrane proteins and lipids. They can be trapped in these compartments for some milliseconds before they are able to "hop" to another compartment.[97] The complexities of interactions between several parts of the cytoskeleton are today of wide interest in understanding receptor-mediated cell signaling.[100–103]

5.4.2 REGULATION OF BCR MOBILITY AND B CELL SIGNALING THROUGH THE ACTIN CYTOSKELETON

Regulation of receptor diffusion through the membrane cortex was soon associated with signaling and activation of lymphocytes.[104] Specifically in B cells, association between BCR, BCR caps, and cytoskeletal components such as actin,[105–107] myosin,[10] and tubulin[108] was found.

Simultaneous two-color TIRFM SPT was used to investigate the dynamic distribution of the BCR in relation to the cytoskeleton. By visualizing F-actin and BCR in a B cell line through LifeAct-GFP at 20 frames/s, we observed that actin forms a dense meshwork and that the density of that actin meshwork is inversely correlated with BCR mobility: BCR diffusion was lower in regions of higher actin density and higher in regions of actin paucity,[37] demonstrating that the cortical actin cytoskeleton forms barriers that hinder BCR diffusion, most likely in interaction with the Igβ sheath.

A further factor mediating BCR diffusion is proteins from the highly conserved family of ezrin–radixin–moesin (ERM) proteins:[109] ERM proteins provide a linkage between the plasma membrane and the underlying actin cytoskeleton when they cycle between an open, actin-binding and a closed state.[110] In a B cell line, we found that both networks did not fully overlap and the ezrin network underwent more dynamic remodeling.[68] Similarly to actin density, steady-state BCR mobility correlated inversely with ezrin density. During B cell activation, ERM proteins were quickly dephosphorylated, suggesting an important role in mediating activation and microcluster integrity depended on the proper functionality of ERM proteins.[111]

Consequently, we examined the effect of drug-induced cytoskeleton reorganization on the mobility of BCR in PBCs. With SPT, we observed that during cytoskeleton reorganization, both isotypes of BCR exhibited a marked increase of diffusion. Moreover, this cytoskeleton reorganization led to the phosphorylation of specific kinases downstream of BCR,[68] while the release of intracellular calcium under this treatment had been reported before.[112] Finding that the removal of diffusion barriers triggers ligand-independent B cell signaling that is concomitant with increased BCR diffusion was a direct indication that compartmentalization of the plasma membrane plays a role in B cell signaling.

At this stage, it was unknown whether such ligand-independent signaling would require the BCR. We then directly demonstrated that BCR expression is a requirement for such signaling[53] via a transgenic mouse model in which the expression of BCR was genetically abolished in mature B cells.[113] This link between BCR, actin cytoskeleton, and B cell signaling suggests that restriction of BCR diffusion is a mechanism of signaling inhibition. However, CD19 is still required for signaling initiated by cytoskeleton disruption. When CD19-deficient PBCs were stimulated with LatA or CytoD, we found a dramatic diminution of an intracellular calcium flux response and an absence of phosphorylation of Akt and ERK[53]—while heavily cross-linking with anti-IgM F(ab)$_2$ elicited a normal signaling response.

5.4.3 BCR and CD19 Exist as Cytoskeleton-Independent Nanoclusters

Through the application of dSTORM, we showed that both isotypes of BCR and CD19 exist in preformed nanoclusters, whose diameter varies between 100 and 200 nm.[53] For the regulation of the organization and dynamics of receptors and co-receptors in B cells, different layers have emerged. While the cytoskeleton influences the lateral mobility of BCR nanoclusters, their integrity seems to be dependent on isotype-intrinsic interactions of BCR. Nanoclusters of the activatory coreceptor CD19 remain unaffected during drug-induced cytoskeleton rearrangements. Instead, the tetraspanin molecule CD81 is indispensable for CD19 organization.

Such a nanocluster organization appears to be an overarching principle for surface receptors in many cell types. In the T cell field, TCR signaling-related molecules and the TCR itself were found to exist in protein islands[66,67,114,115]—BCR nanoclusters resemble that form of organization. It is noticeable that in various fields, the length and time scales seem to converge on similar values for size and mobility, further supporting the notion that nanoclusters are a pervasive organizing principle.

During stimulation, CD19 and BCR coalesce into signaling areas—creating areas of enrichment in both. This local divergence from the mean concentration could explain the synergy of CD19 and BCR. Here, the kinetic segregation model[116] could explain how it is achieved: In areas where BCR binds tightly to antigen, inhibitory molecules with larger ectodomains are pushed away from the contact site, which allows a higher concentration of molecules with smaller ectodomains, such as CD19. Taken together, through a series of genetic dissections and high-resolution imaging, we have collected data that suggest a molecular mechanism for B cell activation, in which BCR gains better access to the positive regulator CD19 through the breakdown of cytoskeleton-imposed diffusion barriers.

Successful B cell activation integrates several intracellular, membrane-proximal, and extracellular cues. It appears certain that this web of interactions will be further untangled through advances in high-resolution imaging techniques.

ACKNOWLEDGMENT

We would like to thank Francesca Gasparrini from the Lymphocyte Interaction Lab for critical reading of the manuscript. This work was supported by Cancer Research UK and a Royal Society Wolfson Research Merit Award (FDB).

REFERENCES

1. Rajewsky, K., Clonal selection and learning in the antibody system. *Nature*, 1996; Vol. 381, pp. 751–758.
2. Saphire, E. O.; Parren, P. W.; Pantophlet, R. et al., Crystal structure of a neutralizing human IGG against HIV-1: A template for vaccine design. *Science*, 2001; Vol. 293, pp. 1155–1159.
3. Reth, M., Antigen receptor tail clue. *Nature*, 1989; Vol. 338, pp. 383–384.
4. Dal Porto, J. M.; Gauld, S. B.; Merrell, K. T. et al., B cell antigen receptor signaling 101. *Mol Immunol*, 2004; Vol. 41, pp. 599–613.
5. Kurosaki, T., Genetic analysis of B cell antigen receptor signaling. *Annu Rev Immunol*, 1999; Vol. 17, pp. 555–592.
6. DeFranco, A. L., The complexity of signaling pathways activated by the BCR. *Curr Opin Immunol*, 1997; Vol. 9, pp. 296–308.
7. Lanzavecchia, A., Antigen-specific interaction between T and B cells. *Nature*, 1985; Vol. 314, pp. 537–539.
8. MacLennan, I. C. M.; Toellner, K.-M.; Cunningham, A. F. et al., Extrafollicular antibody responses. *Immunol Rev*, 2003; Vol. 194, pp. 8–18.
9. MacLennan, I. C., Germinal centers. *Annu Rev Immunol*, 1994; Vol. 12, pp. 117–139.
10. Schreiner, G. F.; Unanue, E. R., Calcium-sensitive modulation of Ig capping: Evidence supporting a cytoplasmic control of ligand-receptor complexes. *J Exp Med*, 1976; Vol. 143, pp. 15–31.
11. Stackpole, C. W.; Jacobson, J. B.; Lardis, M. P., Two distinct types of capping of surface receptors on mouse lymphoid cells. *Nature*, 1974; Vol. 248, pp. 232–234.
12. Unanue, E. R.; Perkins, W. D.; Karnovsky, M. J., Ligand-induced movement of lymphocyte membrane macromolecules. I. Analysis by immunofluorescence and ultrastructural radioautography. *J Exp Med*, 1972; Vol. 136, pp. 885–906.
13. Szakal, A. K.; Kosco, M. H.; Tew, J. G., A novel in vivo follicular dendritic cell-dependent iccosome-mediated mechanism for delivery of antigen to antigen-processing cells. *J Immunol*, 1988; Vol. 140, pp. 341–353.
14. Wykes, M.; Pombo, A.; Jenkins, C.; MacPherson, G. G., Dendritic cells interact directly with naive B lymphocytes to transfer antigen and initiate class switching in a primary T-dependent response. *J Immunol*, 1998; Vol. 161, pp. 1313–1319.
15. Batista, F. D.; Harwood, N. E., The who, how and where of antigen presentation to B cells. *Nat Rev Immunol*, 2009; Vol. 9, pp. 15–27.
16. Yuseff, M.-I.; Pierobon, P.; Reversat, A.; Lennon-Duménil, A.-M., How B cells capture, process and present antigens: A crucial role for cell polarity. *Nat Rev Immunol*, 2013; Vol. 13, pp. 475–486.

17. Batista, F. D.; Iber, D.; Neuberger, M. S., B cells acquire antigen from target cells after synapse formation. *Nature*, 2001; Vol. 411, pp. 489–494.
18. Monks, C. R.; Freiberg, B. A.; Kupfer, H.; Sciaky, N.; Kupfer, A., Three-dimensional segregation of supramolecular activation clusters in T cells. *Nature*, 1998; Vol. 395, pp. 82–86.
19. Grakoui, A.; Bromley, S. K.; Sumen, C. et al., The immunological synapse: A molecular machine controlling T cell activation. *Science*, 1999; Vol. 285, pp. 221–227.
20. Davis, D. M.; Chiu, I.; Fassett, M. et al., The human natural killer cell immune synapse. *Proc Natl Acad Sci USA*, 1999; Vol. 96, pp. 15062–15067.
21. Krummel, M. F.; Sjaastad, M. D.; Wülfing, C.; Davis, M. M., Differential clustering of CD4 and CD3zeta during T cell recognition. *Science*, 2000; Vol. 289, pp. 1349–1352.
22. Dustin, M. L.; Olszowy, M. W.; Holdorf, A. D. et al., A novel adaptor protein orchestrates receptor patterning and cytoskeletal polarity in T-cell contacts. *Cell*, 1998; Vol. 94, pp. 667–677.
23. Bunnell, S. C.; Hong, D. I.; Kardon, J. R. et al., T cell receptor ligation induces the formation of dynamically regulated signaling assemblies. *J Cell Biol*, 2002; Vol. 158, pp. 1263–1275.
24. Fleire, S. J.; Goldman, J. P.; Carrasco, Y. R. et al., B cell ligand discrimination through a spreading and contraction response. *Science*, 2006; Vol. 312, pp. 738–741.
25. Carrasco, Y. R.; Batista, F. D., B-cell activation by membrane-bound antigens is facilitated by the interaction of VLA-4 with VCAM-1. *EMBO J*, 2006; Vol. 25, pp. 889–899.
26. Wan, Z.; Zhang, S.; Fan, Y. et al., B cell activation is regulated by the stiffness properties of the substrate presenting the antigens. *J Immunol*, 2013; Vol. 190, pp. 4661–4675.
27. Axelrod, D., Total internal reflection fluorescence microscopy in cell biology. *Traffic*, 2001; Vol. 2, pp. 764–774.
28. Depoil, D.; Fleire, S.; Treanor, B. L. et al., CD19 is essential for B cell activation by promoting B cell receptor-antigen microcluster formation in response to membrane-bound ligand. *Nat Immunol*, 2008; Vol. 9, pp. 63–72.
29. Weber, M.; Treanor, B.; Depoil, D. et al., Phospholipase C-gamma2 and Vav cooperate within signaling microclusters to propagate B cell spreading in response to membrane-bound antigen. *J Exp Med*, 2008; Vol. 205, pp. 853–868.
30. Harwood, N. E.; Batista, F. D., New insights into the early molecular events underlying B cell activation. *Immunity*, 2008; Vol. 28, pp. 609–619.
31. Thaunat, O.; Granja, A. G.; Barral, P. et al., Asymmetric segregation of polarized antigen on B cell division shapes presentation capacity. *Science*, 2012; Vol. 335, pp. 475–479.
32. Andrews, N. L.; Pfeiffer, J. R.; Martinez, A. M. et al., Small, mobile FcepsilonRI receptor aggregates are signaling competent. *Immunity*, 2009; Vol. 31, pp. 469–479.
33. Cutler, P. J.; Malik, M. D.; Liu, S. et al., Multi-color quantum dot tracking using a high-speed hyperspectral line-scanning microscope. *PLoS ONE*, 2013; Vol. 8, p. e64320.
34. Crocker, J. C.; Grier, D. G., Methods of digital video microscopy for colloidal studies. *J Colloid Interface Sci*, 1996; Vol. 179, pp. 298–310.
35. Gao, Y.; Kilfoil, M. L., Accurate detection and complete tracking of large populations of features in three dimensions. *Opt Express*, 2009; Vol. 17, pp. 4685–4704.
36. Ritchie, K.; Shan, X.-Y.; Kondo, J. et al., Detection of non-Brownian diffusion in the cell membrane in single molecule tracking. *Biophys J*, 2005; Vol. 88, pp. 2266–2277.
37. Treanor, B.; Batista, F. D., Organisation and dynamics of antigen receptors: Implications for lymphocyte signalling. *Curr Opin Immunol*, 2010; Vol. 22, pp. 299–307.
38. Klar, T. A.; Jakobs, S.; Dyba, M.; Egner, A.; Hell, S. W., Fluorescence microscopy with diffraction resolution barrier broken by stimulated emission. *Proc Natl Acad Sci USA*, 2000; Vol. 97, pp. 8206–8210.
39. Gustafsson, M. G., Surpassing the lateral resolution limit by a factor of two using structured illumination microscopy. *J Microsc*, 2000; Vol. 198, pp. 82–87.

40. Heintzmann, R.; Cremer, C. G., Laterally modulated excitation microscopy: Improvement of resolution by using a diffraction grating. *Proc SPIE 3568*, 1999; Vol. 185, pp. 185–196. International Society for Optics and Photonics.

41. Betzig, E.; Patterson, G. H.; Sougrat, R. et al., Imaging intracellular fluorescent proteins at nanometer resolution. *Science*, 2006; Vol. 313, pp. 1642–1645.

42. Hess, S. T.; Girirajan, T. P. K.; Mason, M. D., Ultra-high resolution imaging by fluorescence photoactivation localization microscopy. *Biophys J*, 2006; Vol. 91, pp. 4258–4272.

43. Rust, M. J.; Bates, M.; Zhuang, X., Sub-diffraction-limit imaging by stochastic optical reconstruction microscopy (STORM). *Nat Methods*, 2006; Vol. 3, pp. 793–795.

44. Thompson, R. E.; Larson, D. R.; Webb, W. W., Precise nanometer localization analysis for individual fluorescent probes. *Biophys J*, 2002; Vol. 82, pp. 2775–2783.

45. Patterson, G. H.; Lippincott-Schwartz, J., A photoactivatable GFP for selective photolabeling of proteins and cells. *Science*, 2002; Vol. 297, pp. 1873–1877.

46. Heilemann, M.; Margeat, E.; Kasper, R.; Sauer, M.; Tinnefeld, P., Carbocyanine dyes as efficient reversible single-molecule optical switch. *J Am Chem Soc*, 2005; Vol. 127, pp. 3801–3806.

47. Heilemann, M.; van de Linde, S.; Schüttpelz, M. et al., Subdiffraction-resolution fluorescence imaging with conventional fluorescent probes. *Angew Chem (Int Ed in English)*, 2008; Vol. 47, pp. 6172–6176.

48. van de Linde, S.; Sauer, M.; Heilemann, M., Subdiffraction-resolution fluorescence imaging of proteins in the mitochondrial inner membrane with photoswitchable fluorophores. *J Struct Biol*, 2008; Vol. 164, pp. 250–254.

49. Annibale, P.; Vanni, S.; Scarselli, M.; Rothlisberger, U.; Radenovic, A., Quantitative photo activated localization microscopy: Unraveling the effects of photoblinking. *PLoS ONE*, 2011; Vol. 6, p. e22678.

50. Lee, S.-H.; Shin, J. Y.; Lee, A.; Bustamante, C., Counting single photoactivatable fluorescent molecules by photoactivated localization microscopy (PALM). *Proc Natl Acad Sci USA*, 2012; Vol. 109, pp. 17436–17441.

51. Sengupta, P.; Jovanovic-Talisman, T.; Lippincott-Schwartz, J., Quantifying spatial organization in point-localization superresolution images using pair correlation analysis. *Nat Protoc*, 2013; Vol. 8, pp. 345–354.

52. Sengupta, P.; Jovanovic-Talisman, T.; Skoko, D. et al., Probing protein heterogeneity in the plasma membrane using PALM and pair correlation analysis. *Nat Methods*, 2011; Vol. 8, pp. 969–975.

53. Mattila, P. K.; Feest, C.; Depoil, D. et al., The actin and tetraspanin networks organize receptor nanoclusters to regulate B cell receptor-mediated signaling. *Immunity*, 2013; Vol. 38, pp. 461–474.

54. Dempsey, G. T.; Vaughan, J. C.; Chen, K. H.; Bates, M.; Zhuang, X., Evaluation of fluorophores for optimal performance in localization-based super-resolution imaging. *Nat Methods*, 2011; Vol. 8, pp. 1027–1036.

55. Hopkins, B.; Skellam, J., A new method for determining the type of distribution of plant individuals. *Ann Bot*, 1954; Vol. 18, pp. 213–227.

56. Ripley, B. D., The second-order analysis of stationary point processes. *J Appl Probab*, 1976; Vol. 13, pp. 255–266.

57. Kiskowski, M. A.; Hancock, J. F.; Kenworthy, A. K., On the use of Ripley's K-function and its derivatives to analyze domain size. *Biophys J*, 2009; Vol. 97, pp. 1095–1103.

58. Owen, D. M.; Williamson, D. J.; Boelen, L. et al., Quantitative analysis of three-dimensional fluorescence localization microscopy data. *Biophys J*, 2013; Vol. 105, pp. L05–L07.

59. Tolar, P.; Sohn, H. W.; Pierce, S. K., The initiation of antigen-induced B cell antigen receptor signaling viewed in living cells by fluorescence resonance energy transfer. *Nat Immunol*, 2005; Vol. 6, pp. 1168–1176.

60. Schamel, W. W.; Reth, M., Monomeric and oligomeric complexes of the B cell antigen receptor. *Immunity*, 2000; Vol. 13, pp. 5–14.
61. Yang, J.; Reth, M., Oligomeric organization of the B-cell antigen receptor on resting cells. *Nature*, 2010; Vol. 467, pp. 465–469.
62. Batista, F. D.; Neuberger, M. S., Affinity dependence of the B cell response to antigen: A threshold, a ceiling, and the importance of off-rate. *Immunity*, 1998; Vol. 8, pp. 751–759.
63. Carrasco, Y. R.; Fleire, S. J.; Cameron, T.; Dustin, M. L.; Batista, F. D., LFA-1/ICAM-1 interaction lowers the threshold of B cell activation by facilitating B cell adhesion and synapse formation. *Immunity*, 2004; Vol. 20, pp. 589–599.
64. Lam, K. P.; Kühn, R.; Rajewsky, K., In vivo ablation of surface immunoglobulin on mature B cells by inducible gene targeting results in rapid cell death. *Cell*, 1997; Vol. 90, pp. 1073–1083.
65. Vinuesa, C. G.; Chang, P.-P., Innate B cell helpers reveal novel types of antibody responses. *Nat Immunol*, 2013; Vol. 14, pp. 119–126.
66. Lillemeier, B. F.; Pfeiffer, J. R.; Surviladze, Z.; Wilson, B. S.; Davis, M. M., Plasma membrane-associated proteins are clustered into islands attached to the cytoskeleton. *Proc Natl Acad Sci USA*, 2006; Vol. 103, pp. 18992–18997.
67. Lillemeier, B. F.; Mörtelmaier, M. A.; Forstner, M. B. et al., TCR and Lat are expressed on separate protein islands on T cell membranes and concatenate during activation. *Nat Immunol*, 2010; Vol. 11, pp. 90–96.
68. Treanor, B.; Depoil, D.; Gonzalez-Granja, A. et al., The membrane skeleton controls diffusion dynamics and signaling through the B cell receptor. *Immunity*, 2010; Vol. 32, pp. 187–199.
69. Cambier, J. C.; Pleiman, C. M.; Clark, M. R., Signal transduction by the B cell antigen receptor and its coreceptors. *Annu Rev Immunol*, 1994; Vol. 12, pp. 457–486.
70. O'Rourke, L.; Tooze, R.; Fearon, D. T., Co-receptors of B lymphocytes. *Curr Opin Immunol*, 1997; Vol. 9, pp. 324–329.
71. Peaker, C. J., Transmembrane signalling by the B-cell antigen receptor. *Curr Opin Immunol*, 1994; Vol. 6, pp. 359–363.
72. Tooze, R. M.; Doody, G. M.; Fearon, D. T., Counterregulation by the coreceptors CD19 and CD22 of MAP kinase activation by membrane immunoglobulin. *Immunity*, 1997; Vol. 7, pp. 59–67.
73. Weiss, A.; Littman, D. R., Signal transduction by lymphocyte antigen receptors. *Cell*, 1994; Vol. 76, pp. 263–274.
74. Nadler, L. M.; Anderson, K. C.; Marti, G. et al., B4, a human B lymphocyte-associated antigen expressed on normal, mitogen-activated, and malignant B lymphocytes. *J Immunol*, 1983; Vol. 131, pp. 244–250.
75. Engel, P.; Zhou, L. J.; Ord, D. C. et al., Abnormal B lymphocyte development, activation, and differentiation in mice that lack or overexpress the CD19 signal transduction molecule. *Immunity*, 1995; Vol. 3, pp. 39–50.
76. Pesando, J. M.; Bouchard, L. S.; McMaster, B. E., CD19 is functionally and physically associated with surface immunoglobulin. *J Exp Med*, 1989; Vol. 170, pp. 2159–2164.
77. Carter, R. H.; Fearon, D. T., CD19: Lowering the threshold for antigen receptor stimulation of B lymphocytes. *Science*, 1992; Vol. 256, pp. 105–107.
78. Matsumoto, A. K.; Kopicky-Burd, J.; Carter, R. H. et al., Intersection of the complement and immune systems: A signal transduction complex of the B lymphocyte-containing complement receptor type 2 and CD19. *J Exp Med*, 1991; Vol. 173, pp. 55–64.
79. Bradbury, L. E.; Kansas, G. S.; Levy, S.; Evans, R. L.; Tedder, T. F., The CD19/CD21 signal transducing complex of human B lymphocytes includes the target of antiproliferative antibody-1 and Leu-13 molecules. *J Immunol*, 1992; Vol. 149, pp. 2841–2850.

80. Shoham, T.; Rajapaksa, R.; Kuo, C.-C.; Haimovich, J.; Levy, S., Building of the tetraspanin web: Distinct structural domains of CD81 function in different cellular compartments. *Mol Cell Biol*, 2006; Vol. 26, pp. 1373–1385.
81. Charrin, S.; Le Naour, F.; Silvie, O. et al., Lateral organization of membrane proteins: Tetraspanins spin their web. *Biochem J*, 2009; Vol. 420, pp. 133–154.
82. Jones, E. L.; Demaria, M. C.; Wright, M. D., Tetraspanins in cellular immunity. *Biochem Soc Trans*, 2011; Vol. 39, pp. 506–511.
83. Levy, S.; Shoham, T., The tetraspanin web modulates immune-signalling complexes. *Nat Rev Immunol*, 2005; Vol. 5, pp. 136–148.
84. Maecker, H. T.; Levy, S., Normal lymphocyte development but delayed humoral immune response in CD81-null mice. *J Exp Med*, 1997; Vol. 185, pp. 1505–1510.
85. Cairo, C. W.; Mirchev, R.; Golan, D. E., Cytoskeletal regulation couples LFA-1 conformational changes to receptor lateral mobility and clustering. *Immunity*, 2006; Vol. 25, pp. 297–308.
86. Saxton, M. J., Single-particle tracking: Models of directed transport. *Biophys J*, 1994; Vol. 67, pp. 2110–2119.
87. Cherukuri, A.; Carter, R. H.; Brooks, S. et al., B cell signaling is regulated by induced palmitoylation of CD81. *J Biol Chem*, 2004; Vol. 279, pp. 31973–31982.
88. Cherukuri, A.; Shoham, T.; Sohn, H. W. et al., The tetraspanin CD81 is necessary for partitioning of coligated CD19/CD21-B cell antigen receptor complexes into signaling-active lipid rafts. *J Immunol*, 2004; Vol. 172, pp. 370–380.
89. Radhakrishnan, K.; Halász, Á.; McCabe, M. M.; Edwards, J. S.; Wilson, B. S., Mathematical simulation of membrane protein clustering for efficient signal transduction. *Ann Biomed Eng*, 2012; Vol. 40, pp. 2307–2318.
90. He, H.-T.; Marguet, D., Detecting nanodomains in living cell membrane by fluorescence correlation spectroscopy. *Annu Rev Phys Chem*, 2011; Vol. 62, pp. 417–436.
91. Eggeling, C.; Ringemann, C.; Medda, R. et al., Direct observation of the nanoscale dynamics of membrane lipids in a living cell. *Nature*, 2009; Vol. 457, pp. 1159–1162.
92. Singer, S. J.; Nicolson, G. L., The fluid mosaic model of the structure of cell membranes. *Science*, 1972; Vol. 175, pp. 720–731.
93. Kusumi, A.; Fujiwara, T. K.; Chadda, R. et al., Dynamic organizing principles of the plasma membrane that regulate signal transduction: Commemorating the fortieth anniversary of Singer and Nicolson's fluid-mosaic model. *Annu Rev Cell Dev Biol*, 2012; Vol. 28, pp. 215–250.
94. Poo, M.; Cone, R. A., Lateral diffusion of rhodopsin in the photoreceptor membrane. *Nature*, 1974; Vol. 247, pp. 438–441.
95. Saffman, P. G.; Delbrück, M., Brownian motion in biological membranes. *Proc Natl Acad Sci USA*, 1975; Vol. 72, pp. 3111–3113.
96. Sheetz, M. P.; Schindler, M.; Koppel, D. E., Lateral mobility of integral membrane proteins is increased in spherocytic erythrocytes. *Nature*, 1980; Vol. 285, pp. 510–511.
97. Fujiwara, T.; Ritchie, K.; Murakoshi, H.; Jacobson, K.; Kusumi, A., Phospholipids undergo hop diffusion in compartmentalized cell membrane. *J Cell Biol*, 2002; Vol. 157, pp. 1071–1081.
98. Kusumi, A.; Nakada, C.; Ritchie, K. et al., Paradigm shift of the plasma membrane concept from the two-dimensional continuum fluid to the partitioned fluid: High-speed single-molecule tracking of membrane molecules. *Annu Rev Biophys Biomol Struct*, 2005; Vol. 34, pp. 351–378.
99. Kusumi, A.; Fujiwara, T. K.; Morone, N. et al., Membrane mechanisms for signal transduction: The coupling of the meso-scale raft domains to membrane-skeleton-induced compartments and dynamic protein complexes. *Semin Cell Dev Biol*, 2012; Vol. 23, pp. 126–144.
100. Grecco, H. E.; Schmick, M.; Bastiaens, P. I. H., Signaling from the living plasma membrane. *Cell*, 2011; Vol. 144, pp. 897–909.

101. Jaqaman, K.; Grinstein, S., Regulation from within: The cytoskeleton in transmembrane signaling. *Trends Cell Biol*, 2012; Vol. 22, pp. 515–526.

102. Kusumi, A.; Shirai, Y. M.; Koyama-Honda, I.; Suzuki, K. G. N.; Fujiwara, T. K., Hierarchical organization of the plasma membrane: Investigations by single-molecule tracking vs. fluorescence correlation spectroscopy. *FEBS Lett*, 2010; Vol. 584, pp. 1814–1823.

103. Mostowy, S.; Cossart, P., Septins: The fourth component of the cytoskeleton. *Nat Rev Mol Cell Biol*, 2012; Vol. 13, pp. 183–194.

104. Braun, J.; Hochman, P. S.; Unanue, E. R., Ligand-induced association of surface immunoglobulin with the detergent-insoluble cytoskeletal matrix of the B lymphocyte. *J Immunol*, 1982; Vol. 128, pp. 1198–1204.

105. Flanagan, J.; Koch, G. L., Cross-linked surface Ig attaches to actin. *Nature*, 1978; Vol. 273, pp. 278–281.

106. Sundqvist, K. G.; Ehrnst, A., Cytoskeletal control of surface membrane mobility. *Nature*, 1976; Vol. 264, pp. 226–231.

107. Toh, B. H.; Hard, C. C., Actin co-caps with concanavalin A receptors. *Nature*, 1977; Vol. 269, pp. 695–697.

108. Gabbiani, G.; Chaponnier, C.; Zumbe, A.; Vassalli, P., Actin and tubulin co-cap with surface immunoglobulins in mouse B lymphocytes. *Nature*, 1977; Vol. 269, pp. 697–698.

109. Gupta, N.; Wollscheid, B.; Watts, J. D. et al., Quantitative proteomic analysis of B cell lipid rafts reveals that ezrin regulates antigen receptor-mediated lipid raft dynamics. *Nat Immunol*, 2006; Vol. 7, pp. 625–633.

110. Bretscher, A.; Edwards, K.; Fehon, R. G., ERM proteins and merlin: Integrators at the cell cortex. *Nat Rev Mol Cell Biol*, 2002; Vol. 3, pp. 586–599.

111. Treanor, B.; Depoil, D.; Bruckbauer, A.; Batista, F. D., Dynamic cortical actin remodeling by ERM proteins controls BCR microcluster organization and integrity. *J Exp Med*, 2011; Vol. 208, pp. 1055–1068.

112. Baeker, T. R.; Simons, E. R.; Rothstein, T. L., Cytochalasin induces an increase in cytosolic free calcium in murine B lymphocytes. *J Immunol*, 1987; Vol. 138, pp. 2691–2697.

113. Srinivasan, L.; Sasaki, Y.; Calado, D. P. et al., PI3 kinase signals BCR-dependent mature B cell survival. *Cell*, 2009; Vol. 139, pp. 573–586.

114. Sherman, E.; Barr, V.; Manley, S.; Patterson, G.; Balagopalan, L.; Akpan, I.; Regan, C. K.; Merrill, R. K.; Sommers, C. L.; Lippincott-Schwartz, J.; Samelson, L. E., Functional nanoscale organization of signaling molecules downstream of the T cell antigen receptor. *Immunity*, 2011; Vol. 35, pp. 705–720.

115. Williamson, D. J.; Owen, D. M.; Rossy, J.; Magenau, A.; Wehrmann, M.; Gooding, J. J.; Gaus, K., Pre-existing clusters of the adaptor Lat do not participate in early T cell signaling events. *Nat Immunol*, 2011; Vol. 12, pp. 655–662.

116. Davis, S. J.; van der Merwe, P. A., The kinetic-segregation model: TCR triggering and beyond. *Nat Immunol*, 2006; Vol. 7, pp. 803–809.

6 Imaging the Complexity, Plasticity, and Dynamics of Caveolae

Asier Echarri and Miguel A. Del Pozo

CONTENTS

6.1 INTRODUCTION

Communication between a cell and its environment is mostly mediated through the signals received and processed at the plasma membrane. The plasma membrane therefore needs to be able to sense and sort these signals, and in order to achieve this, it is organized into domains that accommodate specific populations of resident membrane molecules. Plasma membrane domains can be composed of specific lipids, such as lipid rafts,[1] proteins,[2,3] or a combination of both. Caveolae are plasma membrane domains with a specific lipid and protein composition[4] that confers them with a characteristic membrane curvature, defining them as flask-shaped inward plasma membrane invaginations with a diameter of 60–80 nm (Figure 6.1). These membrane microdomains were first noticed in 1953 by Nobel laureate microscopist G.E. Palade and were described and named "caveola intracellularis" by E. Yamada in 1955. It took approximately 40 years to identify caveolin-1 (Cav1), the main

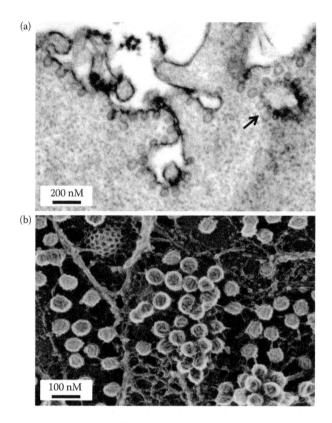

FIGURE 6.1 Electron microscopy (EM) images showing different organizations of caveolae. (a) Mouse embryo fibroblasts were detached from the substratum and held in suspension for 20 min. Glutaraldehyde-fixed cells in the presence of ruthenium red, to label surface-connected structures, were embedded in epon and imaged by EM. Caveolae and a surface-connected rosette (arrow) are observed. (b) Deep-etch replicas imaged by EM of differentiated 3T3-L1 adipocytes, revealing individual and clustered caveolae. A clathrin-coated pit is visible in the upper left corner. (Produced in the Heuser laboratory by N. Morone and obtained from Krijnse Locker, J., and S. L. Schmid, *PLoS Biology*, 11, e1001639, doi:10.1371/journal.-pbio.1001639, 2013.)

structural component of caveolae,[5] followed a decade later by the discovery of a second family of proteins, the cavins, which have emerged as key regulators of caveolae formation and stability.[6–8] Now, after 60 years of research, we are just beginning to understand the physiology of caveolae, and the advent of new imaging tools is revealing the secrets of these enigmatic membrane invaginations.

6.2   CAVEOLAE AND THEIR FORMATION REQUIREMENTS

6.2.1   Caveolins, The Main Component of Caveolae

The main constituent proteins of caveolae are proteins of the caveolin family. There are three mammalian caveolin genes: Cav1, caveolin-2 (Cav2), and caveolin-3 (Cav3). Cav1 and Cav2 are expressed in most cell types except skeletal muscle, whereas

Cav3 is restricted to muscle. Cells of mice lacking Cav1 or Cav3 in their respective tissues do not have caveolae,[9–11] strongly suggesting that Cav1 and Cav3 are the main essential caveolae components. Cav2 contributes to caveolae formation in some cell types but is not needed in vivo.[4] The abundance of caveolins in mammalian cells is highly variable, with some cell types, such as lymphocytes, neurons, and hepatocytes, expressing Cav1 at low level, while cells in mechanically stressed tissues express Cav1 (adipocytes, fibroblasts, and endothelial cells) or Cav3 (muscle) at high abundance.[4] Caveolins are restricted to metazoans and are thus absent from fungi, plants, and nonmetazoan parasites.[12] Some organisms, such as *Caenorhabditis elegans*, express caveolin but do not contain caveolae.[12] While expression of honeybee caveolin in mouse cells devoid of caveolae is able to form caveolae, no caveolin gene has been identified in the fruit fly.[12] Expression of Cav1 in bacteria was recently shown to induce formation of caveolae-like invaginations, suggesting that Cav1 is able by itself to bend the membrane to some extent.[13]

Cav1 is an integral membrane protein that is posttranslationally modified by the addition of palmitic acid on three cysteine residues.[14] Cav1 is inserted in the membrane through a central region with a putative hairpin structure, leaving both ends of the protein in the cytosol.[4] Cav1 oligomerizes, and an estimated 144 Cav1 molecules can incorporate into a single caveolae.[15] The ability of Cav1 to bind cholesterol[16] and fatty acids[17] indicates a role in lipid biology. Many proteins have been shown to interact with Cav1, many of them through the scaffolding domain,[18] although this view has been challenged.[19,20] Cav1 binding proteins include membrane receptors, ion channels, adaptors, kinases, and other signaling molecules, although many of these interactions may be indirect. Cav1 also interacts with proteins such as filamin A that link it to the actin cytoskeleton.[21] Some protein interactions are dependent on phosphorylation of Cav1 on tyrosine 14.[4]

6.2.2 Caveolae Regulatory Molecules

In the early phase of caveolae research, attention focused exclusively on Cav1, mainly because of the absence of caveolae in Cav1 knockout mice. But subsequent studies provided a richer view of the players involved in the formation and regulation of caveolae. A proteomics screen for molecules abundant in caveolae identified PTRF (polymerase I and transcription release factor), SDPR (serum deprivation response, also known as sdr), and SRBC (sdr-related gene product that binds to C-kinase).[7] These proteins were later renamed cavin1, cavin2, and cavin3,[8,22] and a fourth cavin, cavin4 (also called Murc), was identified in muscle cells.[23,24] These molecules form the cavin complex that is important for the stability of caveolae.[25] The functions of caveolins and cavins are highly interdependent. Cavin1 is required for the stability and expression of all the other cavins and of caveolins, while Cav1 is required for the stability and expression of all cavins except for cavin4.[26] In contrast, cavin2 and cavin3 do not contribute to the stability of other known caveolar residents.[26] Cavin1 stabilizes Cav1 at the plasma membrane by facilitating its oligomerization and preventing its degradation.[26,27] Cavin1 reaches the plasma membrane after Cav1[28] and can be released from this location upon osmotic swelling,[29] suggesting that cavin1 has roles unrelated to its participation in caveolae; indeed, cavin1 was originally isolated as a direct transcriptional regulator in the nucleus.[30] Analysis of cavin2 knockout mice showed that cavin2 is required for caveolae formation in lung endothelium and adipose tissue but is dispensable in the endothelium of the heart. In contrast, caveolae in cavin3 knockout appear to be normal, at least structurally;[26] however, analysis of cavin3 silenced cells revealed a role in the trafficking of Cav1-positive spots.[31]

Although the biochemical details of the interactions between the cavin complex and caveolins or other caveolar residents are still unknown, cavin1 appears to interact with Cav1 and directly with cavin2[32] and therefore seems to be more important for caveolae formation than the other members of the complex. Furthermore, cavin1 is the only cavin to induce caveolae biogenesis in PC3 prostate cancer cells, which express Cav1 but not cavins, and recruits the other members to caveolae.[23] Protein cross-linking before cell lysis allowed the immunopurification of a larger complex containing Cav1, Cav2, and cavin1, cavin2, and cavin3 in a constant proportion independent of the immunotargeted protein. The most abundant protein in this complex is Cav1/2, followed by cavin1—four times less—and cavin2 and cavin3, which compete with each other for binding to the complex.[25] This complex has been proposed to form the core that determines the shape of caveolae.[25] Cavins may also be important for the recruitment of signaling molecules to caveolae. Purified cavin2 in the presence of phophatidylserine binds PKCα, a regulator of caveolae endocytosis, and cavin2 is required for the caveolar localization of this enzyme, suggesting that cavin2 may recruit proteins to caveolae.[6] Together, these studies suggest that cavin1 is essential, together with Cav1, for the formation of caveolae and the stability of key caveolae regulators,[27] while the other cavins appear to play regulatory roles.

Other proteins that localize to caveolae or regulate its organization and trafficking properties include some that are able to shape membranes and tubulate them under specific conditions. For example, pacsin2, an F-BAR protein involved in clathrin-mediated endocytosis,[33] localizes to a pool of caveolae and plays a role in shaping them.[34,35] Other studies provide evidence suggesting that the mobility of caveolae is dependent on EHD2, an ATPase that binds and tubulates the plasma membrane by oligomerization.[36,37] This ATPase localizes to a pool of caveolae and prevents the mobility of Cav1 by favoring its anchorage to stress fibers by an unknown mechanism.[38,39] In endothelium and some other tissues, the neck of caveolae is capped by the stomatal diaphragm, a structure formed by plasmalemmal vesicle–associated protein.[40,41]

Caveolar membrane domains are highly complex, and caveolae can be present as single units or groups, depending on the cell type and conditions. When several caveolae are interconnected, they are referred to as racesome invaginations, caveolar rosettes, or simply rosettes (Figures 6.1a [arrow] and b and 6.3 later in the chapter). The molecules responsible for this plasticity are not known, but Abl kinases and mDia1-regulated actin fibers have been shown to impinge on this organization.[42]

6.3   CAVEOLAE TRAFFICKING

6.3.1   EXOCYTOSIS AND RECYCLING OF CAVEOLAE

Caveolae are formed exclusively at the plasma membrane and are not observed in endomembranes. However, newly synthesized Cav1 forms a complex in the Golgi, where it associates with cholesterol and forms a precursor of caveolae.[28,43] After reaching the plasma membrane, cavins and possibly other factors are recruited and contribute to the formation of caveolae.[28] Exocytosis of caveolae is dependent on SNAP23 and syntaxin4,[44] and other factors required for membrane fusion have been identified in caveolae.[45] Upon loss of cell adhesion, Cav1 accumulates in the Rab11 positive recycling endosomes and, upon readhesion, recycles back to the plasma membrane in a process tightly regulated by integrins.[46–48] In this pathway, integrin-linked kinase, mDia1, and IQGAP regulate the transport of Cav1 vesicles to the plasma membrane in a microtubule-dependent manner.[49] The recycling of Cav1 upon cycles of de-adhesion and adhesion has also been shown to be regulated by the exocyst component Exo70, actin, and microtubules.[50]

6.3.2 ENDOCYTOSIS OF CAVEOLAE

The endocytosis of caveolae is difficult to analyze for various reasons. First, under basal conditions, endocytosis of caveolae is infrequent.[51] Second, there is no known specific cargo of caveolae to facilitate tracking, since cargoes assigned to caveolae, such as cholera toxin B subunit or SV40, can enter Cav1-deficient cells because of their ability to enter through other routes.[51,52] Finally, surface-connected caveolae can be observed deep in the cytosol, frequently in groups referred to as rosettes, making it difficult to distinguish endocytosed caveolae from membrane folds containing caveolae (Figures 6.1a [arrow] and 6.3).[53] For these reasons, many studies have tracked the inward trafficking of membrane receptors or Cav1 itself and have characterized the involvement of Cav1 in the trafficking of particular receptor or the involvement of factors in the regulation of Cav1 inward trafficking. Several membrane residents have been shown to traffic in a Cav1-dependent manner, suggesting that they are endocytosed through caveolae. Multiple studies link Cav1 with TGFβ signaling,[54,55] and TGFβ receptor itself has been shown to traffic through caveolae under certain conditions, which negatively regulates its stability.[56] Similarly, Wnt signaling uses caveolae as a regulatory platform in the trafficking of LRP6, a subfamily of low-density lipoprotein receptor–related proteins. Stimulation of LRP6 with Dkk1 induces its endocytosis through clathrin-mediated endocytosis, while stimulation with Wnt3a redirects it to caveolae, resulting in different signaling outputs,[57] such that Wnt3a induced β-catenin translocation to the nucleus is dependent on Cav1.[58] Caveolae are highly abundant in the endothelium and various studies show a role of caveolae trafficking in this tissue. Endothelin, a potent vasoconstrictor, induces endocytosis of the endothelin receptor type B through caveolae.[59] The role of caveolae in transcytosis in the endothelium has been debated for many years,[60–62] but the presence of caveolae in tubulovesicular structures penetrating deep into the cytosol might favor this type of specialized transport. A role for caveolae in tissue permeability has been linked to its ability to endocytose membrane proteins such as occludin[63] and E-cadherins.[64]

The trafficking properties of caveolae are highly dependent on integrins. Integrins not only regulate the recycling of Cav1[48] but also, under specific conditions, regulate caveolae endocytosis.[65] β1 integrins and fibronectin are themselves endocytosed in a Cav1-dependent manner in some cell types[66–68] but not in others.[69] A recent paper showed that syndecan-4-stimulated cells induce α5β1 integrin endocytosis in a Cav1- and RhoG-dependent manner.[70] Interestingly, RhoG was previously implicated in caveolae endocytosis.[71] The trafficking of Cav1 to the perinuclear area upon loss of cell adhesion is highly dependent on actin filaments and microtubules,[42] as is Cav1 endocytosis induced by other stimuli.[72,73] Regulators of stress fibers, including Abl tyrosine kinases, mDia1, and filamin A, regulate this process.[42,47,74] Caveolae entry is also regulated by the tyrosine kinase Src.[75,76] The Abl and Src kinases phosphorylate Cav1 on tyrosine 14, a residue involved in trafficking.[48,77] Integrin signaling and the stress fiber regulatory machinery thus appear to play a key role in controlling the plasma membrane Cav1 pool. Similar to clathrin-mediated endocytosis, caveolae endocytosis requires dynamin2.[42,47,75,76,78,79] Shortly after the identification of Cav1, a role was identified for PKCα in caveolae endocytosis, and this has since been corroborated.[47,80] PKCα phosphorylates filamin A and c-Abl, key regulators of caveolae trafficking.[47,81] Caveolae endocytosis is also triggered by other stimuli, including hyperosmotic medium and okadaic acid,[73] mitosis,[82] and certain viruses.[83–85] Furthermore, the stability of caveolae at the plasma membrane is also strongly influenced by the membrane lipid composition.[75,76]

6.4   VISUALIZATION OF CAVEOLAE

6.4.1   ELECTRON MICROSCOPY-BASED TECHNOLOGY TO STUDY CAVEOLAE MORPHOLOGY

The most obvious characteristic of caveolae is their shape, and since this can only be identified unambiguously by electron microscopy (EM), caveolae can only be unequivocally identified using EM techniques (Figure 6.1). Even though this morphological criterion is generally accepted, given the relatively constant and unique diameter and shape of caveolae, in some cases, additional immunolabeling with caveolin antibodies may be required. The precise shape of caveolae differs depending on the EM technique used, ranging from flask-shaped in glutaraldehyde-fixed samples to open cups, without a clear constricted neck, in cryofixed samples.[86] It is important to take these differences into account for visualization and analysis.

Circular vesicles with a caveolar diameter can frequently be observed in the cytosol (Figures 6.1a and 6.3), and immunolabeling with Cav1 may be needed to assign a caveolar origin if a caveolar shape is not clear. Tomography, the three-dimensional (3D) reconstruction from thin serial sections, has been successfully employed to define the surface connection of these internal caveolae-like vesicles and the complexity in the organization of caveolar domains.[87–89] The surface connection of these internal caveolar structures can be established by the use of cell nonpermeable labels such as ruthenium red during fixation[42,53] or by using membrane-impermeable quenching agents, such as ascorbic acid, targeted against HRP bound to cholera toxin.[51] This last approach, using anti-Cav1 specific immunogold labeling, detected the budding of a small fraction of clustered and what appear to be individual caveolae.[51] However, individual caveolae were not detected by tomography, so it is possible that the apparently individual caveolae detected by immunogold labeling are part of clusters centered outside the section plane.

Freeze-fracture immunolabeling of plasma membrane Cav1 in unfixed cells shows that Cav1 concentrates toward the neck of the caveolae,[90] a finding supported by scanning EM in combination with tungsten labeling.[91] These findings suggest that the neck region might be a functionally distinct subdomain within caveolae.[92] However, analysis of carbon-platinum fast-freeze, deep-etch replicas by immuno-EM showed Cav1 staining in the caveolar bulb,[5] and a recent study using nanogold-conjugated secondary antibodies revealed a caveolar bulb distribution of Cav1, cavin1, cavin2, and cavin3.[25] The coating of the caveolar bulb appears striated or spiked depending on the EM protocol used (Figure 6.1b).[93,94] Although the exact protein composition of this structure is not fully determined, it appears to include Cav1.[5,88,89,95] A recent study used a mini singlet oxygen generator (mini-SOG) approach to study the distribution of caveolar components. This technique is based on the ability of an engineered fluorescent flavoprotein from *Arabidopsis* to generate reactive oxygen upon illumination; the oxygen radicals catalyze the polymerization of diaminobenzidine, producing a dark, electrodense precipitate used to localize the protein by EM.[96] Fusion constructs of the mini-SOG with the protein of interest allow its identification with better spatial resolution than classical immunogold techniques because of the small size of the flavoprotein compared with the antibodies used in immuno-EM techniques. Using this approach, Nichols and coworkers showed that caveolae are coated by a structure, the caveolar coat complex, likely consisting of Cav1, Cav2, and cavin1, cavin2, and cavin3.[25] Dual-tilt tomograms and mini-SOG EM reveal that this structure is repeated with a constant spacing over the surface of the caveolar bulb.[25]

The link between caveolae and the actin cytoskeleton was suggested by the first antiserum raised against caveolin, which revealed caveolae decorating actin cables.[5] This was also observed by quick-freeze, deep-etch studies on rat aortic endothelium.[97] Similarly, electron tomography of the cytoplasmic surface using rapidly frozen, deeply etched, platinum-replicated plasma membranes showed that 93% of caveolae are associated with the actin filaments of the membrane skeleton, similar to the proportion of actin-associated clathrin-coated pits.[93] A tight link between the caveolar system and the cytoskeleton was confirmed by studies of fast-frozen/freeze-substituted cells and immunolabeled plasma membrane lawns, together with analysis by 3D electron tomography, and these studies also revealed a heterogeneous organization of caveolae.[89]

The potential of CLEM (correlative light and electron microscopy) has yet to be fully exploited in the caveolae field. To the best of our knowledge, three studies have used this approach. A study of exocytosis measured SNAP23- and syntaxin4-mediated fusion of caveolar vesicles with the plasma membrane and showed that the presence of SNAP23 correlates with different vesicle fusion states.[44] A recent study used immunofluorescence techniques to show that cavin3 is enriched together with Cav1 at the rear of migrating cells, and EM analysis of this pattern revealed multiple caveolae, rosettes, and caveolae-like vesicles at the plasma membrane and penetrating relatively deep into the cell body,[25] once again demonstrating the ability of caveolae to form complex structures. Immunostaining has also showed an association of Cav1 with curved caveolae in human placenta samples.[98] The resolution of caveolae structures observed by light microscopy at the EM level will be highly informative.

6.4.2 ANALYSIS OF CAVEOLAE BY EPIFLUORESCENCE, CONFOCAL, AND TOTAL INTERNAL REFLECTION FLUORESCENCE MICROSCOPY

The Z-resolution in epifluoresence and confocal microscopy does not differentiate caveolae at the plasma membrane from internal vesicles, but these techniques have nonetheless provided valuable information about the motility and organization of caveolae and Cav1. Confocal fluorescence microscopy has been universally applied to study caveolin localization in cells, showing that Cav1 staining is concentrated in retracting areas of the cell (Figure 6.2b), early or recycling endosomes, and coaligned with stress fibers (Figure 6.2c).[5,42,47,85] In epithelial cells, Cav1 accumulates at cell–cell junctions,[99] whereas in transmigrating endothelial cells, Tyr 14-phosphorylated Cav1 accumulates in the forward extensions.[100] In muscle cells, Cav3 localizes to T-tubules.[101] The dynamics of caveolae have been studied indirectly by intravital fluorescence microscopy to investigate the role of caveolae in endothelial cells.[102,103]

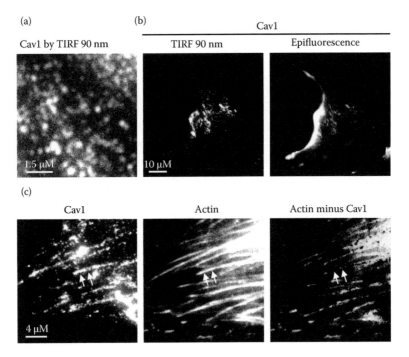

FIGURE 6.2 Images of different patterns of endogenous Cav1 distribution. (a) NIH3T3 cells were stained for endogenous Cav1 and imaged by TIRF-m with a penetration of 90 nm. Spots of differing sizes and intensities are visible. (b) Mouse adult fibroblasts were plated on fibronectin-coated dishes and imaged 24 h later. The same polarized cell was imaged by TIRF-m at 90 nm penetration or by epifluorescence (right image). The pool of Cav1 in the retracting area is only visible in the epifluorescence image, indicating that it is located in the upper part of the cell. (c) Cav1 coaligns with stress fibers. NIH3T3 cells were fixed and stained for Cav1 and actin with phalloidin Alexa-rhodamine. In the right image, the Cav1 image was subtracted from the actin staining, revealing the empty spaces on stress fibers corresponding to the alignment of Cav1 spots with stress fibers (arrows).

Confocal microscopy, alone or in combination with FRAP (fluorescence recovery after photobleaching), has been used to study the dynamics of GFP-tagged Cav1 or other caveolar components, such as cavins or EHD2.[31,39,104] Gervásio and colleagues used fluorescence resonance energy transfer (FRET) to indirectly study the flattening of caveolae upon membrane stretching. Exploiting the relative enrichment of caveolae with the sphingolipid GM1,[105] they used cholera toxin B subunit (which binds GM1) tagged with Alexa Fluor 555 or 647 as FRET donor and acceptor, respectively. FRET efficiency increased upon Cav3 expression, suggesting that Cav3 reduces the distance between GM1 molecules. This was reversed by stretching, indicating increased separation, probably caused by flattening of caveolae.[106] A similar approach using FLIM (fluorescence lifetime imaging microscopy)/FRET showed that the cavin complex is formed in the cytosol and associates with caveolae at the plasma membrane.[23] Image cross-correlation spectroscopy has been used to study the colocalization of BMP receptors with Cav1-positive structures and their dynamic behavior after stimulation.[107]

The complexity of caveolae is clearly revealed by the EM techniques described in Section 6.4.1 and by total internal reflection fluorescence microscopy (TIRF-m) (Figures 6.1a, b and 6.2a). TIRF-m analysis of immunostained endogenous Cav1 or Cav1-GFP allows identification of the different Cav1-positive populations on the basis of their fluorescence intensity in diffraction-limited fixed spots.[15,42] Although this analysis only quantifies the "amount" of fluorescence in a defined region that correlates with the number of molecules, it allows comparison of the effects of a given treatment on the organization of caveolar domains. This analysis reveals a quite large diversity in caveolar structures, correlating with the diversity observed by EM techniques (Figures 6.1a and 6.2a). However, TIRF-m cannot be used to define or count the number of caveolae since flattened Cav1-positive domains—flattened caveolae—coexist with invaginated caveolae[5] and many caveolae can fit into a diffraction-limited spot. In addition, the dimmer spots detected by this technique could represent internal Cav1 spots that are further from the TIRF plane and are not necessarily caveolae. Despite these limitations, TIRF-m is a powerful tool for studying caveolae organization and dynamics. Using TIRF-m, the dynamic behavior of plasma membrane-proximal Cav1 spots can be precisely followed in the xy and z axes.[15,42,47] The so-called kiss-and-run movement of Cav1-GFP observed by TIRF-m is not sensitive to dynamin2, Abl kinases, or mDia1, all regulators of Cav1 inward trafficking;[42] however, this movement is slightly sensitive to cytochalasin D (Echarri A and Del Pozo MA, unpublished observations), suggesting that different caveolar pools exist. Flattening of caveolae was suggested by TIRF-m, although this required confirmation by EM and immuno-EM analysis.[29]

6.4.3 SUPER-RESOLUTION MICROSCOPY APPLIED TO CAVEOLAE

The use of super-resolution microscopy has begun to be applied in the caveolae field and has been used to describe other plasma membrane invaginations, such as clathrin-coated pits.[108] A study using FPALM (fluorescence photoactivation localization microscopy) showed that CRFB1, a subunit of the zebrafish IFN-R (type I interferon receptor) complex, colocalized with caveolin in clusters at the plasma membrane.

Caveolin silencing reduced the numbers of these CRFB1 clusters,[109] suggesting that caveolin forms clusters that condition the organization of other molecules. A super-resolution optical imaging approach using STORM (stochastic optical reconstruction microscopy) showed that Cav3 in mouse cardiac myocytes is present in different-sized clusters colocalized with ryanodine receptors.[110] Diffraction-limited resolution indicated 28.6% colocalization between these molecules, whereas super-resolution showed a colocalization of just 4.9%, suggesting that optical blurring was responsible for the higher colocalization observed by diffraction-limited resolution.[111] Dual-color super-resolution was also used to observe different-sized Cav1 spots labeled with anti-GFP camelid nanobodies.[112]

Stimulated emission depletion (STED) gives a significantly better resolution of Cav1 spots than confocal microscopy,[113] reaching around 128 nm in cells express-ing low levels of Cav1. These spots are probably Cav1 scaffolds, since they were significantly smaller than the average diameter of spots in cells expressing normal levels of Cav1.[114] STED has also been used to study the response of Cav3-positive domains in transverse tubules after myocardial infarction. Myocardial infarction sig-nificantly alters the distribution of Cav3, and STED revealed an increase in the num-ber of Cav3-positive longitudinal structures between striations, concomitant with an increase in other longitudinal transverse tubule components.[115] However, the shape of caveolae in these structures could not be resolved.[113,115]

The further application of super-resolution microscopy will undoubtedly reveal new information about the structure of caveolae and the spatial relationship between caveolins and other caveolar components such as cavins, EHD2, pacsin2, and dyna-min2. Super-resolution microscopy also has the potential to provide valuable infor-mation about the interplay between caveolae and filamin A, stress fibers, and other cytoskeleton-related molecules. It is unclear how this technology will visualize the different levels of caveolar curvature—flattened, curved, or in a fission/fusion pro-cess—but if dynamic behavior is included, it will certainly increase our understand-ing of caveolae biology.

6.5 CAVEOLAR FUNCTIONS AND HUMAN DISEASE

Although mice lacking caveolae are viable and fertile, the presence of caveolae in cells provides certain advantages that facilitate optimal cell function.[116] The exact function of caveolae is still debated. The phenotypes of mice lacking Cav1, Cav3, or cavin1–cavin3 and of human patients with natural mutations provide important clues. The most marked effects of the absence of caveolae are observed in adipose and muscle tissue, where caveolae are highly abundant. The numerous other minor abnormalities of caveolin-deficient mice have been reviewed previously.[116] Patients with Cav1, Cav3, or cavin1 mutations have lipodystrophy, muscular dystrophies, and, to a lesser extent, cardiac alterations. The first human mutations in Cav3 were described in muscular dystrophy patients,[117,118] and various Cav1 mutations have been found in patients with lipodystrophy.[119,120] Cav1 deficiency leads to less body fat and smaller and more fragile adipocytes.[121–123] The identification of cavin1 as a key caveolae protein[124] was followed by reports of mutations in cavin1 in patients with lipodystrophy and muscular dystrophies.[125–130] Human cardiac syndromes associated with cavin1 mutations have also been reported,[125,131] and lack of cavin1 in humans and mice is linked to metabolic alterations.[124,128]

The role of Cav1 in regulating signaling pathways involved in proliferation, migration, and adhesion indicated that Cav1 would be important in some stages of cancer progression.[132–134] Several studies showed that Cav1 acts as a tumor suppressor through its ability to block cell proliferation and metastasis.[133–137] In addition, several potent oncogenes induce the downregulation of Cav1, suggesting that Cav1 counteracts the action of these oncogenes.[138] Other studies, however, appear to show a role for Cav1 in tumor progression in melanoma and prostate and breast cancers.[139–142] The absence of cavin1, cavin2, and cavin3 from some tumor samples also links the cavin family to cancer progression.[143–146] The complex involvement of caveolae components in tumor progression reflects the involvement of caveolae in multiple signaling cascades and the complexity of cancer in terms of altered signaling, types, and tumor stages and the interplay between stroma and tumor cells.

The general function of caveolae as platforms that regulate the emanation of signals from the plasma membrane is detailed above (Figure 6.3). The shape of caveolae might be explained by its ability to endocytose, although endocytosis is uncommon and most caveolae retain a constant invaginated shape. The fact that caveolae can flatten in response to increased tension[29,42,147] suggests that caveolae could serve as

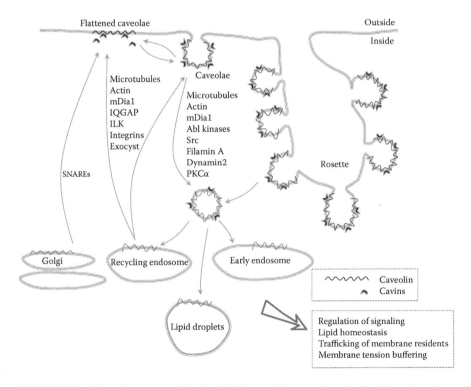

FIGURE 6.3 Caveolae: organization, trafficking regulators, and major Cav1/caveolae functions. Flattened caveolae, isolated caveolae, and caveolae in rosettes are depicted. Known proteins involved in endocytosis and exocytosis/recycling are indicated.

membrane reservoirs that buffer the cellular adaptation to mechanical stress. This change in curvature would simultaneously modulate signaling for an appropriate response to this stress.[147] In this context, the pathologies associated with caveolae and the abundance of caveolae in mechanically stressed tissues and the diseases with which they are associated suggest that the regulation of mechanotransduction may be the principal function of caveolae.[148]

Caveolae and Cav1 also appear to be important in lipid homeostasis. In Cav1-deficient cells, free cholesterol accumulates in mitochondria, resulting in susceptibility to apoptosis.[149] Cav1 localizes to lipid droplets, and lipid droplet trafficking is disrupted by a dominant-negative form of Cav1.[150] Furthermore, the trafficking properties of Cav1 are regulated by the levels of cholesterol and fatty acids[76,151] and the curvature of caveolae is dependent on cholesterol.[5] Caveolae are thus tightly linked to lipid biology. This, together with a mechanoprotective role of caveolae,[121] could explain the lipodystrophy phenotypes of humans and mice lacking functional Cav1 genes. Imaging the structure, organization, and movement of caveolae in vivo is still a challenge, but this approach could contribute to the understanding of the function of this important membrane curvature domain.

ACKNOWLEDGMENTS

This work was supported by grants from the MINECO (Spanish Ministry of Economy and Competitiveness) to MADP (SAF2011-25047 and CSD2009-00016). Simon Bartlett (CNIC) provided English editing. The CNIC is supported by the MINECO and the Pro-CNIC Foundation.

REFERENCES

1. Simons, K., and M. J. Gerl. "Revitalizing Membrane Rafts: New Tools and Insights." *Nature Reviews. Molecular Cell Biology* 11, no. 10 (2010): 688–99.
2. Yanez-Mo, M., O. Barreiro, M. Gordon-Alonso, M. Sala-Valdes, and F. Sanchez-Madrid. "Tetraspanin-Enriched Microdomains: A Functional Unit in Cell Plasma Membranes." *Trends in Cell Biology* 19, no. 9 (2009): 434–46.
3. Frick, M., N. A. Bright, K. Riento et al. "Coassembly of Flotillins Induces Formation of Membrane Microdomains, Membrane Curvature, and Vesicle Budding." *Current Biology: CB* 17, no. 13 (2007): 1151–6.
4. Parton, R. G., and M. A. del Pozo. "Caveolae as Plasma Membrane Sensors, Protectors and Organizers." *Nature Reviews. Molecular Cell Biology* 14, no. 2 (2013): 98–112.
5. Rothberg, K. G., J. E. Heuser, W. C. Donzell et al. "Caveolin, a Protein Component of Caveolae Membrane Coats." *Cell* 68, no. 4 (1992): 673–82.
6. Mineo, C., Y. S. Ying, C. Chapline, S. Jaken, and R. G. Anderson. "Targeting of Protein Kinase Calpha to Caveolae." *The Journal of Cell Biology* 141, no. 3 (1998): 601–10.
7. Aboulaich, N., J. P. Vainonen, P. Stralfors, and A. V. Vener. "Vectorial Proteomics Reveal Targeting, Phosphorylation and Specific Fragmentation of Polymerase I and Transcript Release Factor (PTRF) at the Surface of Caveolae in Human Adipocytes." *Biochemical Journal* 383, Pt 2 (2004): 237–48.
8. Vinten, J., A. H. Johnsen, P. Roepstorff, J. Harpoth, and J. Tranum-Jensen. "Identification of a Major Protein on the Cytosolic Face of Caveolae." *Biochimica et Biophysica Acta* 1717, no. 1 (2005): 34–40.

9. Razani, B., J. A. Engelman, X. B. Wang et al. "Caveolin-1 Null Mice Are Viable but Show Evidence of Hyperproliferative and Vascular Abnormalities." *The Journal of Biological Chemistry* 276, no. 41 (2001): 38121–38.

10. Drab, M., P. Verkade, M. Elger et al. "Loss of Caveolae, Vascular Dysfunction, and Pulmonary Defects in Caveolin-1 Gene-Disrupted Mice." *Science* 293, no. 5539 (2001): 2449–52.

11. Galbiati, F., D. Volonte, C. Minetti, D. B. Bregman, and M. P. Lisanti. "Limb-Girdle Muscular Dystrophy (LGMD-1C) Mutants of Caveolin-3 Undergo Ubiquitination and Proteasomal Degradation. Treatment with Proteasomal Inhibitors Blocks the Dominant Negative Effect of LGMD-1C Mutanta and Rescues Wild-Type Caveolin-3." *The Journal of Biological Chemistry* 275, no. 48 (2000): 37702–11.

12. Kirkham, M., S. J. Nixon, M. T. Howes et al. "Evolutionary Analysis and Molecular Dissection of Caveola Biogenesis." *Journal of Cell Science* 121, Pt 12 (2008): 2075–86.

13. Walser, P. J., N. Ariotti, M. Howes et al. "Constitutive Formation of Caveolae in a Bacterium." *Cell* 150, no. 4 (2012): 752–63.

14. Dietzen, D. J., W. R. Hastings, and D. M. Lublin. "Caveolin Is Palmitoylated on Multiple Cysteine Residues. Palmitoylation Is Not Necessary for Localization of Caveolin to Caveolae." *The Journal of Biological Chemistry* 270, no. 12 (1995): 6838–42.

15. Pelkmans, L., and M. Zerial. "Kinase-Regulated Quantal Assemblies and Kiss-and-Run Recycling of Caveolae." *Nature* 436, no. 7047 (2005): 128–33.

16. Murata, M., J. Peranen, R. Schreiner et al. "VIP21/Caveolin Is a Cholesterol-Binding Protein." *Proceedings of the National Academy of Sciences of the United States of America* 92, no. 22 (1995): 10339–43.

17. Trigatti, B. L., R. G. Anderson, and G. E. Gerber. "Identification of Caveolin-1 as a Fatty Acid Binding Protein." *Biochemical and Biophysical Research Communications* 255, no. 1 (1999): 34–9.

18. Couet, J., S. Li, T. Okamoto, T. Ikezu, and M. P. Lisanti. "Identification of Peptide and Protein Ligands for the Caveolin-Scaffolding Domain. Implications for the Interaction of Caveolin with Caveolae-Associated Proteins." *The Journal of Biological Chemistry* 272, no. 10 (1997): 6525–33.

19. Byrne, D. P., C. Dart, and D. J. Rigden. "Evaluating Caveolin Interactions: Do Proteins Interact with the Caveolin Scaffolding Domain through a Widespread Aromatic Residue-Rich Motif?" *PLoS One* 7, no. 9 (2012): e44879.

20. Collins, B. M., M. J. Davis, J. F. Hancock, and R. G. Parton. "Structure-Based Reassessment of the Caveolin Signaling Model: Do Caveolae Regulate Signaling through Caveolin-Protein Interactions?" *Developmental Cell* 23, no. 1 (2012): 11–20.

21. Stahlhut, M., and B. van Deurs. "Identification of Filamin as a Novel Ligand for Caveolin-1: Evidence for the Organization of Caveolin-1-Associated Membrane Domains by the Actin Cytoskeleton." *Molecular Biology of the Cell* 11, no. 1 (2000): 325–37.

22. Hansen, C. G., and B. J. Nichols. "Exploring the Caves: Cavins, Caveolins and Caveolae." *Trends in Cell Biology* 20, no. 4 (2010): 177–86.

23. Bastiani, M., L. Liu, M. M. Hill et al. "MURC/Cavin-4 and Cavin Family Members Form Tissue-Specific Caveolar Complexes." *The Journal of Cell Biology* 185, no. 7 (2009): 1259–73.

24. Ogata, T., T. Ueyama, K. Isodono et al. "MURC, a Muscle-Restricted Coiled-Coil Protein That Modulates the Rho/Rock Pathway, Induces Cardiac Dysfunction and Conduction Disturbance." *Molecular and Cellular Biology* 28, no. 10 (2008): 3424–36.

25. Ludwig, A., G. Howard, C. Mendoza-Topaz et al. "Molecular Composition and Ultrastructure of the Caveolar Coat Complex." *PLoS Biology* 11, no. 8 (2013): e1001640.

26. Hansen, C. G., E. Shvets, G. Howard, K. Riento, and B. J. Nichols. "Deletion of Cavin Genes Reveals Tissue-Specific Mechanisms for Morphogenesis of Endothelial Caveolae." *Nature Communications* 4 (2013): 1831.

27. Hill, M. M., M. Bastiani, R. Luetterforst et al. "PTRF-Cavin, a Conserved Cytoplasmic Protein Required for Caveola Formation and Function." *Cell* 132, no. 1 (2008): 113–24.

28. Hayer, A., M. Stoeber, C. Bissig, and A. Helenius. "Biogenesis of Caveolae: Stepwise Assembly of Large Caveolin and Cavin Complexes." *Traffic* 11, no. 3 (2010): 361–82.

29. Sinha, B., D. Koster, R. Ruez et al. "Cells Respond to Mechanical Stress by Rapid Disassembly of Caveolae." *Cell* 144, no. 3 (2011): 402–13.

30. Jansa, P., S. W. Mason, U. Hoffmann-Rohrer, and I. Grummt. "Cloning and Functional Characterization of PTRF, a Novel Protein Which Induces Dissociation of Paused Ternary Transcription Complexes." *The EMBO Journal* 17, no. 10 (1998): 2855–64.

31. McMahon, K. A., H. Zajicek, W. P. Li et al. "SRBC/Cavin-3 Is a Caveolin Adapter Protein That Regulates Caveolae Function." *The EMBO Journal* 28, no. 8 (2009): 1001–15.

32. Hansen, C. G., N. A. Bright, G. Howard, and B. J. Nichols. "SDPR Induces Membrane Curvature and Functions in the Formation of Caveolae." *Nature Cell Biology* 11, no. 7 (2009): 807–14.

33. Suetsugu, S., and A. Gautreau. "Synergistic BAR-NPF Interactions in Actin-Driven Membrane Remodeling." *Trends in Cell Biology* 22, no. 3 (2012): 141–50.

34. Senju, Y., Y. Itoh, K. Takano, S. Hamada, and S. Suetsugu. "Essential Role of PACSIN2/ Syndapin-II in Caveolae Membrane Sculpting." *Journal of Cell Science* 124, Pt 12 (2011): 2032–40.

35. Hansen, C. G., G. Howard, and B. J. Nichols. "Pacsin 2 Is Recruited to Caveolae and Functions in Caveolar Biogenesis." *Journal of Cell Science* 124, Pt 16 (2011): 2777–85.

36. Daumke, O., R. Lundmark, Y. Vallis et al. "Architectural and Mechanistic Insights into an EHD ATPase Involved in Membrane Remodelling." *Nature* 449, no. 7164 (2007): 923–7.

37. Lee, D. W., X. Zhao, S. Scarselletta et al. "ATP Binding Regulates Oligomerization and Endosome Association of RME-1 Family Proteins." *The Journal of Biological Chemistry* 280, no. 17 (2005): 17213–20.

38. Moren, B., C. Shah, M. T. Howes et al. "EHD2 Regulates Caveolar Dynamics Via ATP-Driven Targeting and Oligomerization." *Molecular Biology of the Cell* 23, no. 7 (2012): 1316–29.

39. Stoeber, M., I. K. Stoeck, C. Hanni et al. "Oligomers of the ATPase EHD2 Confine Caveolae to the Plasma Membrane through Association with Actin." *The EMBO Journal* 31, no. 10 (2012): 2350–64.

40. Stan, R. V., E. Tkachenko, and I. R. Niesman. "PV1 Is a Key Structural Component for the Formation of the Stomatal and Fenestral Diaphragms." *Molecular Biology of the Cell* 15, no. 8 (2004): 3615–30.

41. Herrnberger, L., K. Ebner, B. Junglas, and E. R. Tamm. "The Role of Plasmalemma Vesicle-Associated Protein (PLVAP) in Endothelial Cells of Schlemm's Canal and Ocular Capillaries." *Experimental Eye Research* 105 (2012): 27–33.

42. Echarri, A., O. Muriel, D. M. Pavon et al. "Caveolar Domain Organization and Trafficking Is Regulated by Abl Kinases and mDia1." *Journal of Cell Science* 125, Pt 13 (2012): 3097–113.

43. Tagawa, A., A. Mezzacasa, A. Hayer et al. "Assembly and Trafficking of Caveolar Domains in the Cell: Caveolae as Stable, Cargo-Triggered, Vesicular Transporters." *The Journal of Cell Biology* 170, no. 5 (2005): 769–79.

44. Predescu, S. A., D. N. Predescu, K. Shimizu, I. K. Klein, and A. B. Malik. "Cholesterol-Dependent Syntaxin-4 and SNAP-23 Clustering Regulates Caveolar Fusion with the Endothelial Plasma Membrane." *The Journal of Biological Chemistry* 280, no. 44 (2005): 37130–8.

45. Schnitzer, J. E., J. Liu, and P. Oh. "Endothelial Caveolae Have the Molecular Transport Machinery for Vesicle Budding, Docking, and Fusion Including VAMP, NSF, SNAP, Annexins, and GTPases." *The Journal of Biological Chemistry* 270, no. 24 (1995): 14399–404.

46. Lapierre, L. A., N. A. Ducharme, K. R. Drake, J. R. Goldenring, and A. K. Kenworthy. "Coordinated Regulation of Caveolin-1 and Rab11a in Apical Recycling Compartments of Polarized Epithelial Cells." *Experimental Cell Research* 318, no. 2 (2012): 103–13.

47. Muriel, O., A. Echarri, C. Hellriegel et al. "Phosphorylated Filamin A Regulates Actin-Linked Caveolae Dynamics." *Journal of Cell Science* 124, Pt 16 (2011): 2763–76.

48. del Pozo, M. A., N. Balasubramanian, N. B. Alderson et al. "Phospho-Caveolin-1 Mediates Integrin-Regulated Membrane Domain Internalization." *Nature Cell Biology* 7, no. 9 (2005): 901–8.

49. Wickstrom, S. A., A. Lange, M. W. Hess et al. "Integrin-Linked Kinase Controls Microtubule Dynamics Required for Plasma Membrane Targeting of Caveolae." *Developmental Cell* 19, no. 4 (2010): 574–88.

50. Hertzog, M., P. Monteiro, G. Le Dez, and P. Chavrier. "Exo70 Subunit of the Exocyst Complex Is Involved in Adhesion-Dependent Trafficking of Caveolin-1." *PLoS One* 7, no. 12 (2012): e52627.

51. Kirkham, M., A. Fujita, R. Chadda et al. "Ultrastructural Identification of Uncoated Caveolin-Independent Early Endocytic Vehicles." *The Journal of Cell Biology* 168, no. 3 (2005): 465–76.

52. Damm, E. M., L. Pelkmans, J. Kartenbeck et al. "Clathrin- and Caveolin-1-Independent Endocytosis: Entry of Simian Virus 40 into Cells Devoid of Caveolae." *The Journal of Cell Biology* 168, no. 3 (2005): 477–88.

53. Parton, R. G., J. C. Molero, M. Floetenmeyer, K. M. Green, and D. E. James. "Characterization of a Distinct Plasma Membrane Macrodomain in Differentiated Adipocytes." *The Journal of Biological Chemistry* 277, no. 48 (2002): 46769–78.

54. Del Galdo, F., M. P. Lisanti, and S. A. Jimenez. "Caveolin-1, Transforming Growth Factor-Beta Receptor Internalization, and the Pathogenesis of Systemic Sclerosis." *Current Opinion in Rheumatology* 20, no. 6 (2008): 713–9.

55. Meyer, C., Y. Liu, A. Kaul, I. Peipe, and S. Dooley. "Caveolin-1 Abrogates TGF-Beta Mediated Hepatocyte Apoptosis." *Cell Death & Disease* 4 (2013): e466.

56. Di Guglielmo, G. M., C. Le Roy, A. F. Goodfellow, and J. L. Wrana. "Distinct Endocytic Pathways Regulate TGF-Beta Receptor Signalling and Turnover." *Nature Cell Biology* 5, no. 5 (2003): 410–21.

57. Yamamoto, H., H. Komekado, and A. Kikuchi. "Caveolin Is Necessary for Wnt-3a-Dependent Internalization of LRP6 and Accumulation of Beta-Catenin." *Developmental Cell* 11, no. 2 (2006): 213–23.

58. Glinka, A., C. Dolde, N. Kirsch et al. "LGR4 and LGR5 Are R-Spondin Receptors Mediating Wnt/Beta-Catenin and Wnt/PCP Signalling." *EMBO Reports* 12, no. 10 (2011): 1055–61.

59. Oh, P., T. Horner, H. Witkiewicz, and J. E. Schnitzer. "Endothelin Induces Rapid, Dynamin-Mediated Budding of Endothelial Caveolae Rich in ET-B." *The Journal of Biological Chemistry* 287, no. 21 (2012): 17353–62.

60. Gumbleton, M. "Caveolae as Potential Macromolecule Trafficking Compartments within Alveolar Epithelium." *Advanced Drug Delivery Reviews* 49, no. 3 (2001): 281–300.

61. Palade, G. E., M. Simionescu, and N. Simionescu. "Structural Aspects of the Permeability of the Microvascular Endothelium." *Acta Physiologica Scandinavica. Supplementum* 463 (1979): 11–32.

62. Komarova, Y., and A. B. Malik. "Regulation of Endothelial Permeability Via Paracellular and Transcellular Transport Pathways." *Annual Review of Physiology* 72 (2010): 463–93.

63. Marchiando, A. M., L. Shen, W. V. Graham et al. "Caveolin-1-Dependent Occludin Endocytosis Is Required for TNF-Induced Tight Junction Regulation In Vivo." *The Journal of Cell Biology* 189, no. 1 (2010): 111–26.

64. Orlichenko, L., S. G. Weller, H. Cao et al. "Caveolae Mediate Growth Factor-Induced Disassembly of Adherens Junctions to Support Tumor Cell Dissociation." *Molecular Biology of the Cell* 20, no. 19 (2009): 4140–52.

65. Singh, R. D., E. L. Holicky, Z. J. Cheng et al. "Inhibition of Caveolar Uptake, SV40 Infection, and Beta1-Integrin Signaling by a Nonnatural Glycosphingolipid Stereoisomer." *The Journal of Cell Biology* 176, no. 7 (2007): 895–901.

66. Shi, F., and J. Sottile. "Caveolin-1-Dependent Beta1 Integrin Endocytosis Is a Critical Regulator of Fibronectin Turnover." *Journal of Cell Science* 121, Pt 14 (2008): 2360–71.

67. Du, J., X. Chen, X. Liang et al. "Integrin Activation and Internalization on Soft ECM as a Mechanism of Induction of Stem Cell Differentiation by ECM Elasticity." *Proceedings of the National Academy of Sciences of the United States of America* 108, no. 23 (2011): 9466–71.

68. Upla, P., V. Marjomaki, P. Kankaanpaa et al. "Clustering Induces a Lateral Redistribution of Alpha 2 Beta 1 Integrin from Membrane Rafts to Caveolae and Subsequent Protein Kinase C-Dependent Internalization." *Molecular Biology of the Cell* 15, no. 2 (2004): 625–36.

69. Arjonen, A., J. Alanko, S. Veltel, and J. Ivaska. "Distinct Recycling of Active and Inactive Beta1 Integrins." *Traffic* 13, no. 4 (2012): 610–25.

70. Bass, M. D., R. C. Williamson, R. D. Nunan et al. "A Syndecan-4 Hair Trigger Initiates Wound Healing through Caveolin- and RhoG-Regulated Integrin Endocytosis." *Developmental Cell* 21, no. 4 (2011): 681–93.

71. Prieto-Sanchez, R. M., I. M. Berenjeno, and X. R. Bustelo. "Involvement of the Rho/Rac Family Member RhoG in Caveolar Endocytosis." *Oncogene* 25, no. 21 (2006): 2961–73.

72. Mundy, D. I., T. Machleidt, Y. S. Ying, R. G. Anderson, and G. S. Bloom. "Dual Control of Caveolar Membrane Traffic by Microtubules and the Actin Cytoskeleton." *Journal of Cell Science* 115, Pt 22 (2002): 4327–39.

73. Parton, R. G., B. Joggerst, and K. Simons. "Regulated Internalization of Caveolae." *The Journal of Cell Biology* 127, no. 5 (1994): 1199–215.

74. Sverdlov, M., V. Shinin, A. T. Place, M. Castellon, and R. D. Minshall. "Filamin A Regulates Caveolae Internalization and Trafficking in Endothelial Cells." *Molecular Biology of the Cell* 20, no. 21 (2009): 4531–40.

75. Sharma, D. K., J. C. Brown, A. Choudhury et al. "Selective Stimulation of Caveolar Endocytosis by Glycosphingolipids and Cholesterol." *Molecular Biology of the Cell* 15, no. 7 (2004): 3114–22.

76. Le Lay, S., E. Hajduch, M. R. Lindsay et al. "Cholesterol-Induced Caveolin Targeting to Lipid Droplets in Adipocytes: A Role for Caveolar Endocytosis." *Traffic* 7, no. 5 (2006): 549–61.

77. Salani, B., M. Passalacqua, S. Maffioli et al. "IGF-IR Internalizes with Caveolin-1 and PTRF/Cavin in HaCat Cells." *PLoS One* 5, no. 11 (2010): e14157.

78. Henley, J. R., E. W. Krueger, B. J. Oswald, and M. A. McNiven. "Dynamin-Mediated Internalization of Caveolae." *The Journal of Cell Biology* 141, no. 1 (1998): 85–99.

79. Oh, P., D. P. McIntosh, and J. E. Schnitzer. "Dynamin at the Neck of Caveolae Mediates Their Budding to Form Transport Vesicles by GTP-Driven Fission from the Plasma Membrane of Endothelium." *The Journal of Cell Biology* 141, no. 1 (1998): 101–14.

80. Smart, E. J., Y. S. Ying, and R. G. Anderson. "Hormonal Regulation of Caveolae Internalization." *The Journal of Cell Biology* 131, no. 4 (1995): 929–38.

81. Pendergast, A. M., J. A. Traugh, and O. N. Witte. "Normal Cellular and Transformation-Associated Abl Proteins Share Common Sites for Protein Kinase C Phosphorylation." *Molecular and Cellular Biology* 7, no. 12 (1987): 4280–9.

82. Boucrot, E., M. T. Howes, T. Kirchhausen, and R. G. Parton. "Redistribution of Caveolae During Mitosis." *Journal of Cell Science* 124, Pt 12 (2011): 1965–72.

83. Pelkmans, L., D. Puntener, and A. Helenius. "Local Actin Polymerization and Dynamin Recruitment in SV40-Induced Internalization of Caveolae." *Science* 296, no. 5567 (2002): 535–9.

84. Moriyama, T., J. P. Marquez, T. Wakatsuki, and A. Sorokin. "Caveolar Endocytosis Is Critical for BK Virus Infection of Human Renal Proximal Tubular Epithelial Cells." *Journal of Virology* 81, no. 16 (2007): 8552–62.

85. Richterova, Z., D. Liebl, M. Horak et al. "Caveolae Are Involved in the Trafficking of Mouse Polyomavirus Virions and Artificial VP1 Pseudocapsids toward Cell Nuclei." *Journal of Virology* 75, no. 22 (2001): 10880–91.

86. Schlormann, W., F. Steiniger, W. Richter et al. "The Shape of Caveolae Is Omega-Like after Glutaraldehyde Fixation and Cup-Like after Cryofixation." *Histochemistry and Cell Biology* 133, no. 2 (2010): 223–8.

87. Bundgaard, M., P. Hagman, and C. Crone. "The Three-Dimensional Organization of Plasmalemmal Vesicular Profiles in the Endothelium of Rat Heart Capillaries." *Microvascular Research* 25, no. 3 (1983): 358–68.

88. Lebbink, M. N., N. Jimenez, K. Vocking et al. "Spiral Coating of the Endothelial Caveolar Membranes as Revealed by Electron Tomography and Template Matching." *Traffic* 11, no. 1 (2010): 138–50.

89. Richter, T., M. Floetenmeyer, C. Ferguson et al. "High-Resolution 3D Quantitative Analysis of Caveolar Ultrastructure and Caveola-Cytoskeleton Interactions." *Traffic* 9, no. 6 (2008): 893–909.

90. Westermann, M., F. Steiniger, and W. Richter. "Belt-Like Localisation of Caveolin in Deep Caveolae and Its Re-Distribution after Cholesterol Depletion." *Histochemistry and Cell Biology* 123, no. 6 (2005): 613–20.

91. Thorn, H., K. G. Stenkula, M. Karlsson et al. "Cell Surface Orifices of Caveolae and Localization of Caveolin to the Necks of Caveolae in Adipocytes." *Molecular Biology of the Cell* 14, no. 10 (2003): 3967–76.

92. Foti, M., G. Porcheron, M. Fournier, C. Maeder, and J. L. Carpentier. "The Neck of Caveolae Is a Distinct Plasma Membrane Subdomain That Concentrates Insulin Receptors in 3T3-L1 Adipocytes." *Proceedings of the National Academy of Sciences of the United States of America* 104, no. 4 (2007): 1242–7.

93. Morone, N., T. Fujiwara, K. Murase et al. "Three-Dimensional Reconstruction of the Membrane Skeleton at the Plasma Membrane Interface by Electron Tomography." *The Journal of Cell Biology* 174, no. 6 (2006): 851–62.

94. Peters, K. R., W. W. Carley, and G. E. Palade. "Endothelial Plasmalemmal Vesicles Have a Characteristic Striped Bipolar Surface Structure." *The Journal of Cell Biology* 101, no. 6 (1985): 2233–8.

95. Izumi, T., Y. Shibata, and T. Yamamoto. "Striped Structures on the Cytoplasmic Surface Membranes of the Endothelial Vesicles of the Rat Aorta Revealed by Quick-Freeze, Deep-Etching Replicas." *The Anatomical Record* 220, no. 3 (1988): 225–32.

96. Shu, X., V. Lev-Ram, T. J. Deerinck et al. "A Genetically Encoded Tag for Correlated Light and Electron Microscopy of Intact Cells, Tissues, and Organisms." *PLoS Biology* 9, no. 4 (2011): e1001041.

97. Izumi, T., Y. Shibata, and T. Yamamoto. "Quick-Freeze, Deep-Etch Studies of Endothelial Components, with Special Reference to Cytoskeletons and Vesicle Structures." *Journal of Electron Microscopy Technique* 19, no. 3 (1991): 316–26.

98. Takizawa, T., and J. M. Robinson. "Correlative Microscopy of Ultrathin Cryosections Is a Powerful Tool for Placental Research." *Placenta* 24, no. 5 (2003): 557–65.

99. Kronstein, R., J. Seebach, S. Grossklaus et al. "Caveolin-1 Opens Endothelial Cell Junctions by Targeting Catenins." *Cardiovascular Research* 93, no. 1 (2012): 130–40.

100. Parat, M. O., B. Anand-Apte, and P. L. Fox. "Differential Caveolin-1 Polarization in Endothelial Cells During Migration in Two and Three Dimensions." *Molecular Biology of the Cell* 14, no. 8 (2003): 3156–68.

101. Parton, R. G., M. Way, N. Zorzi, and E. Stang. "Caveolin-3 Associates with Developing T-Tubules During Muscle Differentiation." *The Journal of Cell Biology* 136, no. 1 (1997): 137–54.

102. Oh, P., P. Borgstrom, H. Witkiewicz et al. "Live Dynamic Imaging of Caveolae Pumping Targeted Antibody Rapidly and Specifically across Endothelium in the Lung." *Nature Biotechnology* 25, no. 3 (2007): 327–37.

103. Chen, J., F. Braet, S. Brodsky et al. "VEGF-Induced Mobilization of Caveolae and Increase in Permeability of Endothelial Cells." *American Journal of Physiology. Cell Physiology* 282, no. 5 (2002): C1053–63.

104. Thomsen, P., K. Roepstorff, M. Stahlhut, and B. van Deurs. "Caveolae Are Highly Immobile Plasma Membrane Microdomains, Which Are Not Involved in Constitutive Endocytic Trafficking." *Molecular Biology of the Cell* 13, no. 1 (2002): 238–50.

105. Parton, R. G. "Ultrastructural Localization of Gangliosides; GM1 Is Concentrated in Caveolae." *The Journal of Histochemistry and Cytochemistry* 42, no. 2 (1994): 155–66.

106. Gervasio, O. L., W. D. Phillips, L. Cole, and D. G. Allen. "Caveolae Respond to Cell Stretch and Contribute to Stretch-Induced Signaling." *Journal of Cell Science* 124, Pt 21 (2011): 3581–90.

107. Nohe, A., E. Keating, T. M. Underhill, P. Knaus, and N. O. Petersen. "Dynamics and Interaction of Caveolin-1 Isoforms with BMP-Receptors." *Journal of Cell Science* 118, Pt 3 (2005): 643–50.

108. Jones, S. A., S. H. Shim, J. He, and X. Zhuang. "Fast, Three-Dimensional Super-Resolution Imaging of Live Cells." *Nature Methods* 8, no. 6 (2011): 499–508.

109. Gabor, K. A., C. R. Stevens, M. J. Pietraszewski et al. "Super Resolution Microscopy Reveals That Caveolin-1 Is Required for Spatial Organization of CRFB1 and Subsequent Antiviral Signaling in Zebrafish." *PLoS One* 8, no. 7 (2013): e68759.

110. Wong, J., D. Baddeley, E. A. Bushong et al. "Nanoscale Distribution of Ryanodine Receptors and Caveolin-3 in Mouse Ventricular Myocytes: Dilation of T-Tubules near Junctions." *Biophysical Journal* 104, no. 11 (2013): L22–4.

111. Baddeley, D., D. Crossman, S. Rossberger et al. "4D Super-Resolution Microscopy with Conventional Fluorophores and Single Wavelength Excitation in Optically Thick Cells and Tissues." *PLoS One* 6, no. 5 (2011): e20645.

112. Ries, J., C. Kaplan, E. Platonova, H. Eghlidi, and H. Ewers. "A Simple, Versatile Method for GFP-Based Super-Resolution Microscopy Via Nanobodies." *Nature Methods* 9, no. 6 (2012): 582–4.

113. Hein, B., K. I. Willig, C. A. Wurm et al. "Stimulated Emission Depletion Nanoscopy of Living Cells Using Snap-Tag Fusion Proteins." *Biophysical Journal* 98, no. 1 (2010): 158–63.

114. Zheng, Y. Z., C. Boscher, K. L. Inder et al. "Differential Impact of Caveolae and Caveolin-1 Scaffolds on the Membrane Raft Proteome." *Molecular & Cellular Proteomics: MCP* 10, no. 10 (2011): M110.007146.

115. Wagner, E., M. A. Lauterbach, T. Kohl et al. "Stimulated Emission Depletion Live-Cell Super-Resolution Imaging Shows Proliferative Remodeling of T-Tubule Membrane Structures after Myocardial Infarction." *Circulation Research* 111, no. 4 (2012): 402–14.

116. Le Lay, S., and T. V. Kurzchalia. "Getting Rid of Caveolins: Phenotypes of Caveolin-Deficient Animals." *Biochimica et Biophysica Acta* 1746, no. 3 (2005): 322–33.

117. Minetti, C., F. Sotgia, C. Bruno et al. "Mutations in the Caveolin-3 Gene Cause Autosomal Dominant Limb-Girdle Muscular Dystrophy." *Nature Genetics* 18, no. 4 (1998): 365–8.

118. McNally, E. M., E. de Sa Moreira, D. J. Duggan et al. "Caveolin-3 in Muscular Dystrophy." *Human Molecular Genetics* 7, no. 5 (1998): 871–7.
119. Cao, H., L. Alston, J. Ruschman, and R. A. Hegele. "Heterozygous CAV1 Frameshift Mutations (MIM 601047) in Patients with Atypical Partial Lipodystrophy and Hypertriglyceridemia." *Lipids in Health and Disease* 7 (2008): 3.
120. Kim, C. A., M. Delepine, E. Boutet et al. "Association of a Homozygous Nonsense Caveolin-1 Mutation with Berardinelli-Seip Congenital Lipodystrophy." *The Journal of Clinical Endocrinology and Metabolism* 93, no. 4 (2008): 1129–34.
121. Martin, S., M. A. Fernandez-Rojo, A. C. Stanley et al. "Caveolin-1 Deficiency Leads to Increased Susceptibility to Cell Death and Fibrosis in White Adipose Tissue: Characterization of a Lipodystrophic Model." *PLoS One* 7, no. 9 (2012): e46242.
122. Cohen, A. W., B. Razani, X. B. Wang et al. "Caveolin-1-Deficient Mice Show Insulin Resistance and Defective Insulin Receptor Protein Expression in Adipose Tissue." *American Journal of Physiology. Cell Physiology* 285, no. 1 (2003): C222–35.
123. Razani, B., T. P. Combs, X. B. Wang et al. "Caveolin-1 Deficient Mice Are Lean, Resistant to Diet-Induced Obesity, and Show Hyper-Triglyceridemia with Adipocyte Abnormalities." *The Journal of Biological Chemistry* 5 (2001): 5.
124. Liu, L., D. Brown, M. McKee et al. "Deletion of Cavin/PTRF Causes Global Loss of Caveolae, Dyslipidemia, and Glucose Intolerance." *Cell Metabolism* 8, no. 4 (2008): 310–7.
125. Rajab, A., V. Straub, L. J. McCann et al. "Fatal Cardiac Arrhythmia and Long-QT Syndrome in a New Form of Congenital Generalized Lipodystrophy with Muscle Rippling (CGL4) Due to PTRF-Cavin Mutations." *PLoS Genetics* 6, no. 3 (2010): e1000874.
126. Hayashi, Y. K., C. Matsuda, M. Ogawa et al. "Human PTRF Mutations Cause Secondary Deficiency of Caveolins Resulting in Muscular Dystrophy with Generalized Lipodystrophy." *The Journal of Clinical Investigation* 119, no. 9 (2009): 2623–33.
127. Dwianingsih, E. K., Y. Takeshima, K. Itoh et al. "A Japanese Child with Asymptomatic Elevation of Serum Creatine Kinase Shows PTRF-Cavin Mutation Matching with Congenital Generalized Lipodystrophy Type 4." *Molecular Genetics and Metabolism* 101, no. 2–3 (2010): 233–7.
128. Murakami, N., Y. K. Hayashi, Y. Oto et al. "Congenital Generalized Lipodystrophy Type 4 with Muscular Dystrophy: Clinical and Pathological Manifestations in Early Childhood." *Neuromuscular Disorders* 23, no. 5 (2013): 441–4.
129. Shastry, S., M. R. Delgado, E. Dirik et al. "Congenital Generalized Lipodystrophy, Type 4 (CGL4) Associated with Myopathy Due to Novel PTRF Mutations." *American Journal of Medical Genetics* Part A 152A, no. 9 (2010): 2245–53.
130. Ardissone, A., C. Bragato, L. Caffi et al. "Novel PTRF Mutation in a Child with Mild Myopathy and Very Mild Congenital Lipodystrophy." *BMC Medical Genetics* 14, no. 1 (2013): 89.
131. Rodriguez, G., T. Ueyama, T. Ogata et al. "Molecular Genetic and Functional Characterization Implicate Muscle-Restricted Coiled-Coil Gene (MURC) as a Causal Gene for Familial Dilated Cardiomyopathy." *Circulation. Cardiovascular Genetics* 4, no. 4 (2011): 349–58.
132. Grande-Garcia, A., A. Echarri, J. de Rooij et al. "Caveolin-1 Regulates Cell Polarization and Directional Migration through Src Kinase and Rho GTPases." *The Journal of Cell Biology* 177, no. 4 (2007): 683–94.
133. Cerezo, A., M. C. Guadamillas, J. G. Goetz et al. "The Absence of Caveolin-1 Increases Proliferation and Anchorage-Independent Growth by a Rac-Dependent, Erk-Independent Mechanism." *Molecular and Cellular Biology* 29, no. 18 (2009): 5046–59.
134. Williams, T. M., and M. P. Lisanti. "Caveolin-1 in Oncogenic Transformation, Cancer, and Metastasis." *American Journal of Physiology. Cell Physiology* 288, no. 3 (2005): C494–506.

135. Capozza, F., T. M. Williams, W. Schubert et al. "Absence of Caveolin-1 Sensitizes Mouse Skin to Carcinogen-Induced Epidermal Hyperplasia and Tumor Formation." *The American Journal of Pathology* 162, no. 6 (2003): 2029–39.

136. Witkiewicz, A. K., A. Dasgupta, F. Sotgia et al. "An Absence of Stromal Caveolin-1 Expression Predicts Early Tumor Recurrence and Poor Clinical Outcome in Human Breast Cancers." *The American Journal of Pathology* 174, no. 6 (2009): 2023–34.

137. Quann, K., D. M. Gonzales, I. Mercier et al. "Caveolin-1 Is a Negative Regulator of Tumor Growth in Glioblastoma and Modulates Chemosensitivity to Temozolomide." *Cell Cycle* 12, no. 10 (2013): 1510–20.

138. Koleske, A. J., D. Baltimore, and M. P. Lisanti. "Reduction of Caveolin and Caveolae in Oncogenically Transformed Cells." *Proceedings of the National Academy of Sciences of the United States of America* 92, no. 5 (1995): 1381–5.

139. Hayashi, K., S. Matsuda, K. Machida et al. "Invasion Activating Caveolin-1 Mutation in Human Scirrhous Breast Cancers." *Cancer Research* 61, no. 6 (2001): 2361–4.

140. Felicetti, F., I. Parolini, L. Bottero et al. "Caveolin-1 Tumor-Promoting Role in Human Melanoma." *International Journal of Cancer* 125, no. 7 (2009): 1514–22.

141. Yang, G., T. L. Timme, A. Frolov, T. M. Wheeler, and T. C. Thompson. "Combined C-Myc and Caveolin-1 Expression in Human Prostate Carcinoma Predicts Prostate Carcinoma Progression." *Cancer* 103, no. 6 (2005): 1186–94.

142. Goetz, J. G., S. Minguet, I. Navarro-Lerida et al. "Biomechanical Remodeling of the Microenvironment by Stromal Caveolin-1 Favors Tumor Invasion and Metastasis." *Cell* 146, no. 1 (2011): 148–63.

143. Xu, X. L., L. C. Wu, F. Du et al. "Inactivation of Human SRBC, Located within the 11p15.5-p15.4 Tumor Suppressor Region, in Breast and Lung Cancers." *Cancer Research* 61, no. 21 (2001): 7943–9.

144. Zochbauer-Muller, S., K. M. Fong, J. Geradts et al. "Expression of the Candidate Tumor Suppressor Gene hSRBC Is Frequently Lost in Primary Lung Cancers with and without DNA Methylation." *Oncogene* 24, no. 41 (2005): 6249–55.

145. Bai, L., X. Deng, Q. Li et al. "Down-Regulation of the Cavin Family Proteins in Breast Cancer." *Journal of Cellular Biochemistry* 113, no. 1 (2012): 322–8.

146. Nassar, Z. D., M. M. Hill, R. G. Parton, and M. O. Parat. "Caveola-Forming Proteins Caveolin-1 and PTRF in Prostate Cancer." *Nature Reviews. Urology* 10, no. 9 (2013): 529–36.

147. Kozera, L., E. White, and S. Calaghan. "Caveolae Act as Membrane Reserves Which Limit Mechanosensitive I(Cl,Swell) Channel Activation During Swelling in the Rat Ventricular Myocyte." *PLoS One* 4, no. 12 (2009): e8312.

148. Nassoy, P., and C. Lamaze. "Stressing Caveolae New Role in Cell Mechanics." *Trends in Cell Biology* 22, no. 7 (2012): 381–9.

149. Bosch, M., M. Mari, A. Herms et al. "Caveolin-1 Deficiency Causes Cholesterol-Dependent Mitochondrial Dysfunction and Apoptotic Susceptibility." *Current Biology: CB* 21, no. 8 (2011): 681–6.

150. Pol, A., S. Martin, M. A. Fernandez et al. "Dynamic and Regulated Association of Caveolin with Lipid Bodies: Modulation of Lipid Body Motility and Function by a Dominant Negative Mutant." *Molecular Biology of the Cell* 15, no. 1 (2004): 99–110.

151. Pol, A., S. Martin, M. A. Fernandez et al. "Cholesterol and Fatty Acids Regulate Dynamic Caveolin Trafficking through the Golgi Complex and between the Cell Surface and Lipid Bodies." *Molecular Biology of the Cell* 16, no. 4 (2005): 2091–105.

7 Membrane Microdomains Enriched in Ceramides
From Generation to Function

Sibylle Schneider-Schaulies,
Nora Müller, and Erich Gulbins

CONTENTS

7.1 INTRODUCTION

Regardless as to whether they accumulate owing to de novo synthesis or subsequent to sphingomyelin (SM) breakdown, ceramides are membrane constituents that (1) biochemically, (2) biophysically, and (3) functionally strongly affect membrane activity. They do so (1) in serving as central hubs in the sphingolipid (SL) metabolism as they represent central building blocks for complex glycosylated SL (glycosphingolipids, or GSLs), as well as precursors for biologically active metabolites; (2) in altering membrane fluidity and rigidity, thereby promoting dynamics of inward/outward curvature and vesiculation; and (3) by compartmentalizing and segregating membrane proteins and lipids, thereby acting as organizers of signal perception and propagation. Their activity is confined to membranes. Therefore, they are no classical second messengers. Because of their multifunctional properties, their biological activities range from conveying apoptotic stimuli to affecting cell differentiation, adhesion, migration, cell–cell communication, and endo/phagocytosis, as well as pathogen interactions especially in uptake and release. Ceramide derivatives, which are permanently generated along with ceramide accumulation under rheostat and activated conditions, are bioactive lipids as well and do influence or exert biological processes. This has been documented in numerous studies describing biological activities of ceramide metabolites that are not dealt with within this chapter. As a recent example, the neutral sphingomyelinase (NSM) activity associated with a mitochondrial proximal compartment has been found required for lowering the threshold for BAX and BAK activation in mitochondrial apoptosis. However, cooperation between these proteins relied on the ceramide metabolites sphingosine-1-phosphate (S1P) and hexadecenal rather than ceramide itself.[1] For the sake of clarity and to meet the topic, we will focus on effects directly associated with the activity of sphingomyelinases and ceramides. What should, however, also be made initially clear is that ceramide-enriched domains may not be considered as nanodomains. This is because, when generated in response to SM breakdown, they fuse into large domains that range between a few hundred nanometers to micrometers and are easily visible by standard confocal microscopy.

7.2 NANODOMAINS, LIPID RAFTS, AND CERAMIDE-ENRICHED PLATFORMS

Molecular organization of the membrane landscape as achieved by dynamic clustering of lipid and protein components essentially regulates key processes including endo/exocytosis and signal initiation and termination.[1] Consequently, alterations of membrane patterning in response to external stimuli such as receptor ligation result in lateral reorganization of membrane building blocks, thereby strongly affecting these cellular processes.

Lipids partition into discrete membrane subdomains, and it was only with the advent of suitable tools and methodology that the heterogeneity of lipid membrane microdomains could be established, which differ with regard to size, lipid content, and driving forces for condensation or maintenance (Ref. 2, and reviewed in detail in Chapters 10 through 13). This also applies to microdomains enriched in SLs and cholesterol, commonly referred to as "lipid rafts."[1,3] These are defined as nanometric membrane domains with saturated acyl chains, which confers them a high degree of lipid order (l_o domains). For obvious reasons, saturation and length of the acyl side chains critically influence the degree of membrane order of and fluidity within these microdomains.

They share similarities to domains revealed in model membranes where the requirement of SLs (in this case, SM) and cholesterol for large-scale phase separation into l_o domains was demonstrated. Within these domains, the hydrophilic phosphoryl headgroups of SM tightly interact with each other, the hydroxygroups of GSLs, and the hydrophilic parts of cholesterol.[3–5] There, hydrophobic interactions tightly link cholesterol with the ceramide moiety of SLs and both hydrophilic and hydrophobic interactions mediate lateral segregation of these lipids into distinct domains. Cholesterol depletion results in loss of separation and increases membrane fluidity, while turnover of SM into ceramide results in transition from the l_o into gel-like domains.[6,7] A recent study employing fluorescent SM with a conjugated pentaene system in its fatty acids suggests that at least at low cholesterol concentrations, certain SM species preferentially interact with cholesterol, while others prefer their kin.[8]

Lipophilic dyes reporting the polarity of local environment (and changes thereof) such as ANEP or Laurdan (eventually in combination with fluorescence correlation spectroscopy, FCS) have been widely used to reveal coexistence of differentially ordered phases in biomembranes but do not distinguish between lipids.[9–13] Mass spectroscopy has been established as a powerful analytical method to define and quantify SLs at the level of whole cells or compartments.[14] The existence of SL-enriched microdomains in natural membranes has been documented by a number of techniques. CTxB (cholera toxin B subunit) is often used to detect a subspecies of membrane microdomains (containing GM1 or GM3) in both fixed and living cells where, as a pentameric ligand, however, it actually induced GM1 clustering itself.[15,16] This ability has been used for single-particle tracking experiments to monitor inclusion of quantum dot-labeled glycophosphatidylinositol (GPI)-anchored proteins into CTxB-induced GM1 clusters.[16,17] Fluorescence-based live cell detection in the absence of cross-linking has long been hampered by the lack of suitable reagents that do not affect lateral organization. Thus, lipid fluorophores such as NBD- or BODIPY-labeled fatty acids have an enormous impact on the chemical structure of the resulting lipid, in particular, in conferring a lysophospholipid character, and not only can alter lateral aggregation but also can lead to mislocalization of the labeled lipid.[18–20] Moreover, conventional fluorescence imaging methods are restricted in their spatial resolution and cannot resolve the distribution of SLs in nanodomains or clusters with a size of 2–300 nm.[21]

SL-enriched microdomains substantially differ in size, and in addition to those at nanometric scale, SL-containing membrane domains of micrometer size have also been revealed by using incorporation of ^{15}N-labeled SLs and direct imaging by nanoSIMS as well as fluorophore-tagged SM analogs.[22–24] Micrometer-sized SL patches consisting of numerous microclusters were found continuously present in discrete areas of the plasma membrane of fibroblasts with nonrandom SL clustering being much more sensitive to disruption of cortical actin rather than to that of cholesterol.[24] This mode of compartmentalization resembles the fencing concept described for lipid and GPI-anchored protein clusters where loss of integrity has been linked to perturbation of cholesterol subsequent to that of actin organization.[25,26] These patches are clearly different from classical lipid rafts and were suggested to represent membrane compartments that are confined by a protein scaffold consisting of the actin cytoskeleton and associated proteins.[24]

7.3 BIOSYNTHESIS AND METABOLIZATION OF SLs

There are excellent reviews describing the biosynthesis and turnover of SLs.[27–29] We will therefore just give a simplified view on this pathway to introduce the complexity of this class of lipids and key enzymes involved in generating ceramides referred to later in this chapter (Figure 7.1).

During their de novo synthesis in the endoplasmic reticulum (ER), ceramides differing in acyl chain length are generated owing to the activity of six different ceramide synthases. Because ceramides (and their complex derivatives) affect membrane order and fluidity depending on length and saturation of the acyl side chains,[30] differing acyl chain lengths should attribute specific biophysical properties or unique biological functions. As they are membrane-associated molecules with no solubility in aequous environment, transfer of ceramides from the ER involves either vesicular or protein-bound (ceramide transfer protein [CERT]) transport to the Golgi compartment where they are used as building blocks for generation of GSLs or SMs. The latter requires activity of SM synthases (SMSs), which transfer a phosphocholine headgroup from phosphatidycholine to ceramides either at the luminal membrane of the trans-Golgi (SMS1) or at the plasma membrane to directly regulate the SM pool there (SMS2). Also within the trans-Golgi, ceramides can be converted into ceramide-1-phosphates (C1P) by the resident ceramide kinase.

Reversing their biosynthesis pathway, complex SLs are catalyzed into their building blocks due to the activity of enzymes resident at compartments where they accumulate. Thus, ceramide can be generated from C1P by a plasma membrane–associated C1P phosphatase,[31,32] by reverse activities of acid ceramidase acting on sphingosine,[33] or by endoglycoceramidase on complex GSLs.[34]

As a complex SL containing a bulky headgroup, SM very inefficiently flips between membrane leaflets in the absence of flippase activity, thereby explaining why it is most abundant in leaflets where it has been generated, that is, the luminal Golgi leaflet or the extrafacial layer of the plasma membrane. There, it serves as substrate for the lysosomal acid sphingomyelinase (ASM [*SMPD1*]) for the human,

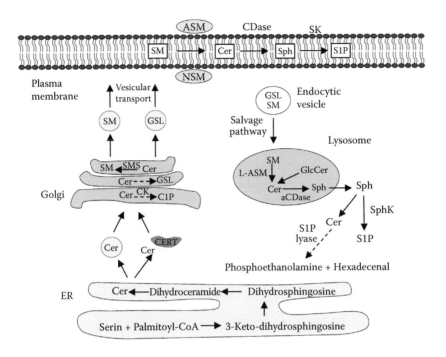

FIGURE 7.1 Schematic illustration of the SL metabolic cycle. After synthesis from its precursors in the endoplasmic reticulum (ER), ceramide (cer) is tranlocated to Golgi membranes in a process involving vesicular or CERT-mediated transport. At Golgi membranes, ceramide is converted into ceramide 1 phosphate (C1P), GSLs, or SM by the activity of the ceramide kinase (CK), glycosyltransferases (not indicated herein), or sphingomyelin synthases (SMS), respectively, which subsequently undergo anterograde vesicular plasma membrane transport. At the plasma membrane, SM is converted into cer by the activity of acid or neutral sphingomyelinase (ASM or NSM, respectively) and further to sphingosine (Sph) and sphingosine-1-phosphate (S1P) due to the activity of ceramidases (CD) and sphingosine kinases (SK). In the salvage pathway, GSL and SM are degraded in an analogous manner into their metabolites in the lysosomal compartment. Finally, the S1P lyase catalyzes breakdown of S1P into phosphoethanolamine and hexadecenal.

Asm [*Smpd1*] for the murine enzyme) residing in a lysosomal compartment, which fuses with substrate-containing vesicles or the plasma membrane to generate phosphocholin and ceramide. The best characterized NSM (NSM2 [*SMPD3*] in humans, Nsm2 [*Smpd3*] in mice) hydrolyzes SM at the cytosolic leaflets where it is much less abundant. Once generated, ceramides, if not reused as building blocks in the salvage pathway, are deacetylated to generate sphingosine by the activity of lysosomal acid and plasma membrane-associated neutral or alkaline ceramidases, the isoforms of which locate in the ER, the Golgi, or both compartments. Sphingosine is sufficiently amphipatic to diffuse between membranes and is modified further to S1P by the activity of sphingosine-1- or -2-kinase (SK1 and SK2), respectively. In response to growth factor and survival signals, SK1 translocates to the plasma membrane where it generates S1P, which has a prosurvival function there. In contrast, perinuclear SK2 activity enhances or even induces apoptosis (excellent reviews on the activities of S1P and SKs are available, also including Refs. 35 and 36). The final step in SL breakdown is exerted by the S1P lyase, an ER transmembrane protein exposing its catalytic site into the cytosol, which hydrolyzes sphingoid bases into hexadecenal and phosphoethanolamine.

The crucial importance of homeostasis and tightly regulated activation of SL generation and turnover is highlighted by severe pathophysiology and disease associated with its deregulation (recent reviews on this issue are summarized in Ref. 37). These not surprisingly include lipid storage diseases (sphingolipidoses) such as Farber and Niemann Pick type A and B (which are genetically deficient for acid ceramidase or ASM, respectively),[38–40] as well as infectious diseases, cystic fibrosis, chronic obstructive pulmonary disorder, diabetes, metabolic disorders, immune disorders, cancer, and others.[41]

7.4 SPHINGOMYELINASES: ENZYMES PROMOTING HOMEOSTATIC AND ACTIVATION-INDUCED SM BREAKDOWN AND CERAMIDE GENERATION

Three sphingomyelinase species mediate SM breakdown, which are named by their pH optimum: the alkaline sphingomyelinase is an intestine- and liver-specific enzmye involved in dietary SM digestion (not further considered herein), and the ASM/Asm (*SMPD1/Smpd1*), NSM2/Nsm2 (*SMPD3/Smpd3*), and the more recently discovered NSM3 (*SMPD4*), which are ubiquitously expressed and are major regulators of SM breakdown in cellular membranes.

7.4.1 ACID SPHINGOMYELINASE

The ASM localizes in conventional or specialized lysosomal compartments as an inactive precursor protein, which is N-glycosylated on at least six positions and mannnose-6-phosphorylated as important for acquisition of a stable secondary structure (L-ASM) (Figure 7.2a and b).

A secretory isoform ASM (S-ASM) produced from the same gene differs from the lysosomal isoform with regard to N-glycosylation and N-terminal processing.[42] The lysosomal ASM is the major enzyme catalyzing membrane SM breakdown and its complete or partial genetic ablation causes the progressive neurodegenerative Niemann–Pick disease type A or B, respectively, in humans (first described in Ref. 43) and Asm knockout mice, which is characterized by massive SM deposition in various tissues, especially the brain.[44,45] Depending on the experimental system analyzed, oxidation, proteolytic cleavage, phosphorylation, or acidification of the environment have been implicated in the biochemical activation of the enzyme.[42,46,47] It is activated in response to a variety of stimuli including UV, oxidative stress, or drugs such as cisplatin,[48–52] ligation of death receptors,[53–57] CD40,[58] CD28,[59] CD5,[60] and receptors involved in pathogen interaction or uptake, also including phagocytosis of IgG-coated beads.[12,61–70]

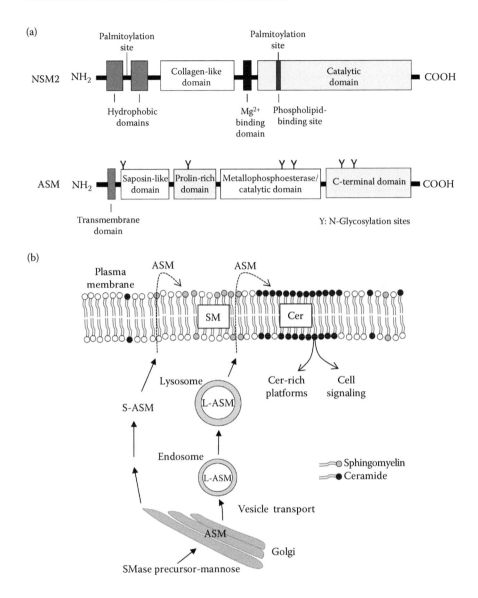

FIGURE 7.2 (a) Domain organization of human ASM and NSM2; the ASM C-terminal domain is not known to harbor an active site; however, it is indicated as a boxed region because it contains two glycosylation sites that are functionally important. (b) Trafficking and activity of ASM. Secretory ASM (S-ASM) and lysosomal ASM (L-ASM) originated from a common precursor that enters the Golgi as mannosylated precursor. The L-ASM undergoes vesicular transport and is stored within a lysosomal compartment. When activated, L-ASM is displayed at the extrafacial layer of the plasma membrane (or, not shown in this figure, the anticytoplasmic layer of vesicular compartments) where it acts to catalyze ceramide release from SM. Cer-enriched membrane microdomains fuse into large ceramide-enriched platforms that regulate cell apoptosis, receptor and signalosome recruitment, and, biophysically, membrane fluidity, fusogenicity, and vesicle formation.

The ASM catalyzes SM breakdown within the anticytosolic leaflets of lysosomal compartments or the plasma and requires translocation of the enzyme involving a fusion process with the target compartment. This can be the plasma membrane where ASM translocation is followed by its surface display and extrafacial ceramide generation. This NEM-sensitive exocytic process may involve actin remodeling and can occur Ca^{2+} dependently and independently (eventually involving PKCδ) and depends on syntaxin 4 for fusion.[46,49,56,71-73] Examples for this particular transport studied mechanistically in more detail have been provided after ligation of CD95 on glioma cells,[73] DC-SIGN on dendritic cells,[61] peroxide exposure of Jurkat cells,[49] or cisplatin treatment of MCF-7 cells.[48] Interestingly, fusion during exocytosis does not apparently rely on the activity of the ASM itself. In Jurkat cells, for instance, ASM translocation and surface codisplay with LAMP-1 upon oxidative stress was unaffected by ASM deficiency.[49] Similarly, IFN-γ discharge of cytolytic granules from CD8+ T cells was sensitive to Asm abrogation, but their trafficking toward and fusion with the plasma membrane at the IS was not.[71] In contrast, Asm activity and ceramide release may be critical for fusion of intracellular compartments as revealed by substantially impaired phagosomal/lysosomal fusion in Asm-deficient macrophages.[74,75]

Consequences of ASM-generated ceramides at the plasma membrane are numerous. In TNFR1 signaling, the receptor is internalized by a clathrin-dependent mechanism followed by recruitment of the DISC complex containing the initiator caspase 8 to the TNFR1, a process that finally results in the formation of the TNF receptosome. The receptosome accesses a multivesicular compartment to which the lysosomal compartment harboring the ASM also fuses. There, the enzyme is proteolytically activated presumably by a compartment resident, caspase-7 (the activation of which occurs with caspase-8 dependently), followed by ceramide release, cathepsin D activation, Bid cleavage, tBid generation, and activation of executor caspase-9 and caspase-3 too.[47,53,76] Thus, caspase-7-dependent ASM activation is of crucial importance to transmission of death signals from an endosomal compartment after TNFR1 ligation while TNFR1 signaling from the plasma membrane activates NSM and is proinflammatory. Similar to that of TNFR1, compartmentalization of CD95 on the cell surface regulates its biological activities.[77-79] CD95 proapoptotic signaling also involves caspase-8-dependent surface translocation and thereby activation of ASM. Surface display of ASM within minutes was clearly documented and was found to be required for CD95 clustering, caspase-3 and -9 cleavage, and decrease of mitochondrial membrane potential.

Finally, there is evidence for cross-regulation of sphingomyelinases. In addition to its specific siRNA and pharmacological ablation, ASM surface display and subsequent ceramide production were largely ablated upon NSM interference after measles virus (MV) interaction with T cells,[66] suggesting that NSM acts as an upstream activator of ASM. In contrast, Asm was elevated at the level of both mRNA and enzyme activity in fibroblasts derived from mice homologous for the fragilis ossium allele (*fro/fro*) that causes Nsm deficiency. Strikingly, under homeostatic conditions, loss of Nsm in this system was associated with a more marked loss of total ceramides than Asm deficiency.[80] Reasons for these seemingly discordant observations are unknown as yet but may include cell type or induction/compartment-specific effects.

7.4.2 NEUTRAL SPHINGOMYELINASE

The NSM family consists of three members: NSM1 does not metabolize SM and will not be further considered here. NSM2/Nsm2 (*SMPD3/Smpd3*) is associated via its two hydrophobic domains flanking a cysteine-rich palmitoylation site with the cytosolic membrane leaflet of the plasma membrane, the Golgi, the endo/lyosomal compartment, and a mitochondrial-associated compartment. The NSM3 (*SMPD4*) contains a transmembrane domain and is anchored to the ER and possibly the Golgi[81–88] (Figure 7.2a). NSM2 can be activated by glutathione, proteases, heat shock protein 60, and phospholipids; is phosphorylated at serine residues; and appears to be a p38 and protein kinase C effector. Phosphorylation and activity of the enzyme can be enhanced upon stimulation and counteracted by calcineurin (PP2B).[89] TNFR1 ligation increases NSM2 activity at the plasma membrane, and this is in line with enrichment of phosphatidylserine there, which, as other anionic phospholipids, stimulates NSM2 activity.[82,90] NSM2 can be activated by a variety of drugs and inflammatory (TNF, IL-1, LPS) and stress signals (cigarette smoke, oxidative and heat stress) with outcomes ranging from supporting inflammatory responses to apoptosis. Interestingly, nonapoptotic signaling conveyed by TNFR1 relies on NSM2 activation rather than that of the internalized ASM. NSM2 activation is initiated by recruitment of FAN (factor associated with NSM activation) to the NSD (NSM activating domain) within the TNFR1 cytosolic tail. FAN recruits RACK1, which couples to and activates NSM after plasma membrane translocation of EED from the nucleus.[53,57,91–93] Because both NSM2 and NSM3 hydrolyze SM in vitro and localize to or have their catalytic site exposed to the cytosolic layers of membranes, it is as yet unclear whether they are also able to give rise to larger ceramide-enriched domains. This is because their substrate is much less abundant there than in the extrafacial layers/luminal vesicle layer, as for instance revealed by lysenin binding experiments.[94] The physiological importance of the NSM2, however, has been impressively documented in mice deficient for the Nsm2 (Nsm2KO)[95] or harboring a mutant Nsm2 allele lacking the catalytic domain (*fro/fro* mice).[96] Both mouse lines suffer from severe chondroplasia and dwarfism, indicating that Nsm2 has a central role in regulating bone development and formation. Pointing to the importance of this NSM family member, abrogation of Nsm in both models was associated with an up to 90% loss of NSM activity in all tissues analyzed.

7.5 CHARACTERISTICS OF CERAMIDE-ENRICHED DOMAINS AND FUNCTIONAL CONSEQUENCES

This part focuses on what has been established with regard to biophysical properties of ceramide-enriched membrane domains and, later on, on their interaction with proteins and lipids. It should be noted that it summarizes data generated in both model membranes and tissue culture cells where especially dynamic changes of ceramide generation and protein association have been difficult to monitor for the time being owing to lack of suitable reagents (see also Section 7.2). Availability of pharmacological inhibitors, knockdown strategies in tissue culture, and mice genetically deficient for sphingomyelinases, however, has been instrumental to evaluate the biological relevance of SM breakdown in functional terms.

7.5.1 Consequences of Biophysical Alterations Relating to Ceramide Accumulation

In model membranes, ceramide addition induced phase separation and catalyzed formation of small ceramide-enriched microdomains, from which cholesterol is displaced and thereby excluded.[97–100] Whether this also applies to rafts in cellular membranes has not been formally proven. As revealed in both model systems and living cells, ceramide-enriched membrane microdomains tend to fuse into macrodomains, referred to as ceramide-enriched membrane platforms that range between a few hundred nanometers to micrometers.[58,101–103] These can be detected using antibodies[61,66,101,104,105] or, indirectly, by loss of lysenin binding owing to SM depletion.[48,94] Because these acquire a lipid-ordered (l_o) state, membrane dyes reporting domains of low polarity and high order such as Laurdan or ANEP by standard and confocal fluorescence microscopy can be used.[10,12,106,107] Magnetic resonance spectroscopy and atomic force microscopy have been used to reveal laminar phase separation in model membranes and confirmed biophysical studies, indicating that increase in ceramide content supported transition of fluid into gel-like phases, thereby supporting the role of ceramide to establish stabilized l_o domains.[102,108,109]

7.5.1.1 Ceramides in Regulating Membrane Curvature, Vesiculation, and Phagocytosis

While lipid-disordered domains are more prone to accomodate curved regions, l_o domains are rather flat shaped but project from the surface. Upon enrichment of l_o domains with cone-shaped lipids (such as ceramides), these can promote curvature on the opposite side of the leaflet in model membranes. Because SM-enriched domains are converted into those enriched in ceramides within one leaflet of the bilayer only, the higher degree of condensation and altered biophysical properties of the latter translated into alterations of membrane curvature and asymmetrical budding of vesicles in giant liposomes.[97,110] Thus, sphingomyelinase-catalyzed SM breakdown within the outer layer caused inward budding and vesicle shedding while outward vesicle shedding was observed when the enzyme acted on the inner leaflet. Similarly, inward vesiculation was observed after exposure of DOPC/SM/cholesterol containing giant unilamellar vesicles to exogenous sphingomyelinase.[88]

Whether these studies on synthetic membranes that lack proteins and cytoskeletal components reflect properties of sphingomyelinase-dependent ceramide, platform formation in vivo is not established. It has, however, been shown that inward budding of intralumenal vesicles into multivesicular bodies that are subsequently shed as exosomes depended on ceramide generation by NSM2 in oligodendroglial cells.[88] There is increasing evidence for the prominent role of NSM2 in exosome generation and, thereby, intercellular transfer. For instance, NSM2 was found required for production and transfer of miRNAs from HEK293 cells or cancer cells where this was crucial for angiogenesis in the tumor milieu[111,112] or from T to dendritic cells in the immune synapse.[113] NSM2-driven transfer of viral RNA from infected cells to plasmacytoid dendritic cells revealed to be crucial for the production of type I IFN from these cells.[114] A most recent study provides in vitro and in vivo evidence for transfer of type I interferon-induced effector proteins and mRNAs by exosomes that depended on NSM/Nsm activity and was essential for controlling hepatitis B virus replication in vitro and in vivo. NSM-dependent transfer of antiviral activity extended to control of other viruses as well and thereby for the first time revealed the prominent role of NSM activity in infection control.[115]

Blebbing and release of plasma membrane-derived microparticles (MPs) have been related to ASM activation.[116,117] In astrocytes, stimulation of the P2X7 receptor by ATP caused surface display and activation of ASM in an src and p38 MAP kinase-dependent manner. Shedded plasma membrane-derived MPs were enriched in ASM in the inner leaflet and phosphatidylserine in the outer leaflet and carried IL-1β as a cargo. MP release was monitored by prelabeling cells with NBD C_6-HPC (fluorophore-conjugated phosphocholin) and was sensitive to inhibitors of ASM, actin polymerization (cytoD), and Ca^{2+} homeostasis. Because exposure to recombinant sphingomyelinase was sufficient to promote MP and thereby IL-1β release, ceramide generation appeared to be crucial for this particular system where IL-1β release is MP dependent. It appears, however, that IL-1β release may not be generally dependent on ASM. While levels of this proinflammatory cytokine were lower after intracerebral Sindbis virus infection in Asm-deficient mice than in wild-type mice, massive IL-1β release was seen in *Pseudomonas*-infected Asm-deficient mice.[118,119] Probably also relating to SM/ceramide-related biophysical properties of vesicular membranes, discharge of IFN-γ containing granulae from CD8+ T cells at the cytolytic synapse was impaired in LCMV-infected Asm-deficient mice. Interestingly, discharge of RANTES containing granulae was not affected,[71] indicating that Asm has the propensity to affect vesicle production and/or discharge differentially and this may vary depending on the cell type, compartment, and type of vesicle.

Membrane blebbing followed by MP release was also observed in HEK293 cells after SLO-mediated plasma membrane damaging and subsequent Ca^{2+} influx and ASM activation. In this context, ceramide accumulation likely served as an important component in the removal of plasma membrane regions by outward vesiculation and subsequent shedding of microvesicles or, alternatively, endocytosis followed by degradation.[120,121] A role of ASM in membrane healing after SLO exposure by rapid endocytosis or injured regions was confirmed in another study that, however, did not support a role of ASM in lysosomal exocytosis for plasma repair.[122]

The role of sphingomyelinase activation/ceramide generation in phagocytosis has been clearly documented in bacterial uptake (see Section 7.7.1). In macrophages measuring dynamic membrane order during phagocytic bead uptake in macrophages, lipid condensation (and thereby increase in general membrane order) occured prior to phagocytic cup formation.[12] Phagosomal membranes were largely devoid of cholesterol, but selectively enriched for SM and ceramide, and both formation of these structures and phagocytosis were largely abolished upon ASM inhibition. Formation of ordered phagosomal membranes was required for coordination of F-actin remodeling. In contrast to rapid F-actin polymerization at the cup followed by fast dissociation (after cup closure), lowering of membrane order and enhancement fluidity by 7-ketocholesterol (7KC) prefeeding resulted in structures resembling frustrated early phagosomes: F-actin slowly accumulated but did not dissociate from the cup structure. Though abrogating cup formation and F-actin remodeling, 7KC feeding did not affect overall accumulation of SM and ceramide, indicating that local membrane condensation into areas of high lipid order was crucial for initiation of phagocytosis rather than lipid composition.

7.5.1.2   Ceramides in Membrane Fusion

In addition to promoting/supporting membrane curvature, ceramide-enriched membrane domains were implicated in membrane fusogenicity.[74] This property has been assigned to the conversion of the cylindrical SM into the cone-shaped ceramide lacking the polar headgroup. When accumulating locally to high levels, ceramide was suggested to promote formation of hexagonal phase II structures that increase asymmetrical membrane tension leading to vesicular fusion, or alternatively, when affecting both membrane layers, ceramide was thought to stimulate flexibility, which may support plasma membrane fusion and thereby, giant cell formation. This hypothesis has been supported by the observation that lysosomal hydrolases and fluid phase markers were inefficiently transferred to phagosomes in Asm-deficient macrophages infected with *Listeria monocytogenes*.[75] Supporting a role of ceramide-enriched platforms in fusion, these domains have also been suggested in endo/exocyosis-dependent plasma membrane repair (see Section 7.5.1.1 and Refs. 120, 121, and 123). Whether ceramides in addition to mediating receptor segregation directly act to support fusion of enveloped viruses with their target cells during entry has not yet been addressed.

7.5.2   Proteins Associating with SM- or Ceramide-Enriched Membrane Domains

Proteins embedded into lipid membrane microdomains have been difficult to analyze and were mostly studied after extraction from detergent micelles and, more recently, mass spectrometry.[124] Methods to directly reveal intramembrane protein–lipid interactions specifically included feeding of cells with modified lipids (labeled with isotopes or, more recently, inclusion of azide moieties for click reactions) through which target proteins can be studied after photoactivated cross-linking followed by immunoprecipitation.[125,126]

Proteins partitioning into SL-enriched domains do so because they harbor specific lipid anchors (that preferentially insert into l_o domains such as myristoylated or palmitoylated proteins) or protein signatures. This was for instance documented in a Forster resonance energy transfer-based approach for the p24 COPI unit, which directly and specifically interacted with SM.[127] First, both the acyl chains and the polar headgroup were involved in binding, and second, a signature sequence within p24 was required for both SM binding and SM-induced dimerization. Supporting the general importance of these findings, SM interaction could also be confirmed for signature sequence containing proteins other than p24 and, interestingly, might be also dependent on interaction with exogenous ligands as revealed for the IFN-γ receptor.[127] The requirement to interact with both the acyl chains and the headgroup for p24 would predict that this (and other proteins bearing this particular signature sequence) would not firmly interact with ceramides and, therefore, likely be excluded from membrane microdomains where ceramide has been generated at the expense of SM.

Ceramide-enriched domains were shown to concentrate receptors by increasing their local density and lateral confinement and amplifying their biological function in signal transmission. There are many receptors promoting sphingomyelinase activation, but trapping of those into ceramide-enriched platforms has only been investigated for a few. The best studied examples are CD40 and CD95. CD95 activates ASM upon ligation to generate ceramide-enriched membrane microdomains where it subsequently clusters.[101,128,129] ASM-dependent clustering is functionally important because CD95 signaling with regard to FADD recruitment and caspase-8 activation was almost entirely abrogated in Asm-deficient lymphocytes, however, could be restored upon exogenous supply of ceramides,[56] supporting a direct role of those in CD95 clustering and signal initiation. CD40 signals from SL-enriched membrane domains in B and dendritic cells and, similar to CD95, causes outer membrane display of ASM and ceramide within enlarged clusters on ligation to which it also localizes for signaling.[58,130,131] Exchange of the CD40 transmembrane domain by that of CD45 did not abolish generation of ceramide platforms, but rather partitioning of the recombinant molecule therein and, to a major extent, CD40 signaling. The latter was partially restored upon forced cross-linking of the recombinant protein, indicating that clustering is required for CD40 signaling.[132] Recruitment into ceramide-enriched domains is, however, not always supporting the biological activity of membrane proteins. For instance, the potassium channel Kv1.3 is active nanodomains enriched in SL, but tyrosine phosphorylated and inactive in exogenously generated ceramide-enriched platforms.[133,134] Differential outcomes of ceramide generation and receptor sorting have also been reported for pathogen uptake into cells (see Section 7.7).

A number of plasma membrane resident or proximal proteins including c-Raf,[61,135] PKCζ,[136] PP2A and PP1,[137,138] RhoA,[139] or CRAC channels[140,141] were identified as ceramide effectors. Direct interaction with ceramides has so far, however, only been revealed for some proteins such as phospholipase A2,[142] KSR1 (kinase suppressor of Ras), c-Raf, and PKCζ.[135,143–145] Recent studies indicated that ceramide also binds to LC3B, implying an important function of ceramide in autophagy.[146]

Ceramide binds the C1 domains of and activates KSR1 most likely by targeting the enzyme to GSL-enriched plasma membrane platforms.[143] KSR1, formerly referred to as CAP (ceramide-activated protein) kinase, is a positive regulator of the Ras–Raf–MAPK pathway by activating Raf-1 because of its kinase and scaffolding function.[147–149] For TNFR1 signaling, generation of KSR1-activating ceramides has been placed downstream of FAN-dependent activation of NSM.[150] Physical interaction and codistribution of PKCζ with ceramide relied on both its atypical C1 domain and a C-terminal 20 kDa protein fragment, which has been found essential for regulating formation of junctional complexes in epithelial cells.[144,151]

Bcl-2 family members are crucial effectors in ceramide-mediated apoptosis. As highly relevant for mitochondrial outer membrane permeabilization (MOMP)-mediated apoptosis, the channel-forming activity of ceramides in the outer membrane of mitochondria in the absence of proteins was revealed in vitro. There, ceramides might be acquired by transfer from the ER.[152,153] Binding of antiapoptotic Bcl-2 proteins Bcl-xL and Ced-9 antagonized channel formation and disassembled ceramide channels, while these were enhanced upon binding of the proapoptotic Bax protein, which, by itself, was capable to synergize in channel formation.[152,154,155] Ceramides were, however, also placed upstream of Bax activation in MOMP, and it has been shown that Bax integrates into mitochondrial membranes via ceramide-enriched domains.[156–158] This also refers to TNFR1 signaling, where activated ASM is a downstream effector of caspases-8 and -7 to promote ceramides and cause activation of Bid into tBid, Bad/Bax-mediated MOMP, and that of executor caspases-9 and -3.[47,76] A ceramide-mediated additional mechanism promoting MOMP apoptosis was recently suggested in tumor cells where drug-induced activation of the proapoptotic Bak caused activation of ceramide synthase and subsequent ceramide accumulation, thereby placing a Bcl-2 protein upstream of ceramide release.[159] Mechanistically, support of MOMP apoptosis by this mechanism was proposed to follow regulation of outer membrane channel formation as detailed above, though it remained unclear which SL acted upstream to Bak in response to drug exposure. Studies by Kolesnick et al. demonstrated that irradiation induces the formation of ceramide in mitochondria and presumably the formation of ceramide-enriched membrane domains in mitochondria.[158] These domains serve to trap and integrate Bax into the outer mitochondrial membrane to execute death. Indpendently of apoptosis, ceramide can mediate lethal autophagy by promoting mitophagy.[146] There, it acts as a receptor for the lipidated LC3B (LCB3-II), thereby targeting autophagolysosomes to mitochondrial membranes.

7.5.3 THE CERAMIDE-ENRICHED POLARITY COMPLEX

A ceramide–protein complex consisting of ceramide, PKCζ, the Rho GTPase Cdc42, and polarity protein 3 (Par3) (also referred to as ceramide aPKC polarity complex [CAP-PC]) forms a functional key element in cell polarity. This has as yet been evidenced by the initial observation that ceramide-activated PKCζ formed complexes with polarity proteins (Par6) and Cdc42 both in vitro and in living cells, thereby establishing that ceramide can organize cell polarity on the molecular level.[144,145,160] This view was supported by codetection of ceramide with PKCζ, Cdc42, F-actin, and β-catenin in the apical membrane of primitive ectoderm cells of embryoid bodies.[160] More recently, an "apical ceramide-enriched compartment" (ACEC) was defined as a novel cis-Golgi compartment at the base of primary cilia in polarized epithelial cells. Its formation relied on endocytosed ceramides generated by ASM at the plasma membrane of epithelial cells. It consists of the CAP-PC, which recruited fusion (exocyst proteins Sec10, Sec8, and Sec15), vesicular transport (Rab11a, Rabin8, Rab8), and Bardet–Biedl syndrome 1 (BBS1) proteins to anchor the nascent cilium and protect tubulin strands by preventing HDAC6-mediated deacetylation.[104,105,151] It therefore appears that the CAP-CA is a basic module in defining cell polarity, which can be further modified by recruitment of proteins (to form the sphingolipid-induced protein scaffold [SLIPS]) that determine functional specificity.[151]

7.5.4 TRANSBILAYER COMMUNICATION PROMOTES INTERACTION OF CYTOSOLIC PROTEINS WITH SL-ENRICHED MEMBRANE DOMAINS

In addition to the eventual direct binding to interacting proteins, SM/ceramide can also regulate binding of proteins to the inner leaflet of the plasma membrane as a result of transbilayer communication. This has, for instance, been evidenced for annexins, which have been identified as sensors for lipid microdomain dynamics, and especially for annexin A1, which reports (and was therefore used for visualization of) formation and subsequent internalization of ceramide-enriched membrane platforms in fixed and living cells.[161] Interaction of the unique N-terminal domain of annexin A1 with these domains is strictly dependent on Ca^{2+}. This is, however, most likely based on ceramide-mediated increase in annexin A1 affinity to negatively charged phospholipids and l_o domains of the inner membrane leaflet rather than on direct interaction with ceramides. Inhibitor-based experiments evidenced that ceramide platform formation as reported by annexin A1 recruitment was dependent on Ca^{2+}-mediated ASM activation, while platform dissociation was prevented upon SMS inhibition, which would expectedly catalyze ceramide consumption by conversion to SM.

In T lymphocytes, formation and integrity of SL/cholesterol domains were required for stimulated plasma membrane recruitment and partitioning of the Akt kinase and other PH domain-containing proteins into raft nanodomains. SM generation was important in this process, because loss of Akt activation upon pharmacologic inhibition of SM generation was reversed when nanodomains were restored by addition of exogenous SM.[162] While the impact of sphingomyelinases was not addressed in this study, another study revealed the ability of the enzyme to strongly affect transbilayer communication when exogenously provided. Using a nontoxic version of lysenin to monitor concentration of SM in the outer leaflet of the cleavage furrow in HeLa cells, the authors showed that SM was required for localization of phosphatidylinositol-4,5-phosphate (PIP$_2$) to this site and formation of PIP$_2$-enriched domains there. As a result of SM depletion, recruitment of phosphatidyl-inositol-4-phosphate 5-kinase β (producing phosphatidyl-inositol-4-phosphate) and RhoA to the furrow was largely ablated and aberrant cytokinesis occurred.[94] In this study, external supplementation with SM but not with ceramide restored PIP$_2$ accumulation and cleavage furrow formation, indicating that transbilayer communication relied on integrity of SM and not on ceramide release upon SM breakdown.

7.6 SM/CERAMIDE-ENRICHED PLATFORMS AS SITES OF DOWNSTREAM EFFECTOR REGULATION

As they segregate and concentrate certain receptors, ceramide-enriched membrane domains can serve to amplify and thereby transform weak into strong signals. This has particularly been revealed in the context of death receptor signaling as referred to already in Section 7.5.2. Radiation or UV light-induced apoptosis particularly in certain cell types also relied on ASM activity, but there, downstream effectors have not been defined.[51,163,164] This also applies to cell death induced upon chemotherapeutical drugs such as doxorubicin, cisplatin, and gemcitabine or anti-CD20 (ritumximab) exposure of leukemic cells. As clustering of TNFR1, CD95, and DR5 into lipid rafts after radiation or drug treatment in a variety of cell lines has been observed, cell death induced by these compounds shares downstream effectors with those exerted in ceramide-enriched domains.[165,166]

7.6.1 Regulation of Akt Kinase Activity

Activation of Akt by various stimuli has revealed one of the major targets of ceramide induction in a variety of cells. When exogenously added, ceramides were directly implicated in preventing Akt activation by recruitment or stimulation of lipid and protein phosphatases or by targeting and retaining Akt in caveolin-enriched membrane microdomains where phosphorylation at Ser34 interferes with binding to phosphatidylinositol-3 lipids.[167–171] PKCζ-mediated inhibitory Akt phosphorylation was identified as a major mechanism in vascular smooth muscle cells[169] and in adipocytes or muscle cells, where the Akt kinase was retained in caveolin-enriched microdomains to which both PTEN and PKCζ cosegregated.[171] As revealed in a follow-up study, exogenously added ceramide exerted its inhibitory activity on the Akt kinase predominantly via activation of PP2A in cells that were less abundant in caveolin-enriched domains.[170] These experiments relied on exogenous supply of short-chain ceramides, and therefore, formal proof is lacking that ceramides generated de novo or in response to sphingomyelinase activity counteract Akt activation and if so, by which mechanism. The same holds true for the ability of ceramide to activate autophagy in this system, which was partially attributed to inhibition of Akt, and, thereby, its downstream effector, mTOR, where ceramides had been elevated by exogenous C_2 or C_6 supplementation.[172,173]

7.6.2 ERM Proteins and Actin Cytoskeleton

Ezrin–radixin–moesin (ERM) proteins were found to be ceramide effectors in MCF-7 breast cancer cells.[48] Because the pan-pERM antibody only detected a single ezrin specific band, these cells may lack moesin and radixin, and thus, it is unclear whether phosphorylation and thereby activity of these proteins are also subject to ceramide-mediated control. In T cells induced to activate ASM and NSM in response to MV, moesin was found to be much less sensitive to ceramide-induced dephosphorylation than ezrin.[66] Interestingly, ceramide and its metabolite S1P exert opposing activities on the ezrin phosphorylation status in HeLa cells: while accumulation of ceramide induced by exogenous bacterial sphingomyelinase caused ezrin dephosphorylation, addition of S1P or exogenous ceramidase rescued loss of pERM.[138,174] ERM proteins serve to link certain plasma membrane receptors to the actin cytoskeleton and, as such, contain domains binding to PIP_2 and to actin. These domains are unfolded and available for their respective interactions after phosphorylation at residues located at their very C-termini.[175] In addition to phosphorylation/dephosphorylation, the ERM protein activity is sensitive to PIP_2 depletion as seen after phospholipase C activation.[138] ERM proteins locate to actin-dependent membrane extension such as ruffles, lamellopodia, and microvilli. Processes involving rapid reorganization of cortical actin, including migration and adhesion, as well as formation of tight interaction platforms such as immunological synapses, usually involve rapid cycling of ERM protein activity.[175–177] In HeLa cells, ceramide-mediated ezrin dephosphorylation was not due to loss of SM or PIP_2 but rather to activation of PP1α (and not PP2A), thereby identifying this phosphatase as a direct ceramide effector at the plasma membrane.[138] In line with earlier studies where ERM proteins were genetically depleted,[178,179] ceramide-mediated dephosphorylation went along with loss of cell polarity, actin-based protrusions, and motility in MCF-7 cells and T cells exposed to MV, bacterial sphingomyelinase, or ceramide[48,66,138,174] (Figure 7.3).

This does, however, by no means indicate that ERM protein deactivation and actin cytoskeletal collapse are general consequences of ceramide release at the plasma membrane. First, ERM proteins are only associated with certain membrane receptors that may or may not be included into ceramide-enriched platforms; second, their distribution is cell type specific; and finally, they may be differentially sensitive to ceramide-mediated effects, which, in other cell types or other stimulation conditions, may also target PIP_2 nanodomain integrity owing to SM depletion.[94,162] Interestingly, ERM proteins were also found associated with CD95-enriched lipid rafts in drug-treated cells, yet there, the phosphorylation status of these proteins was

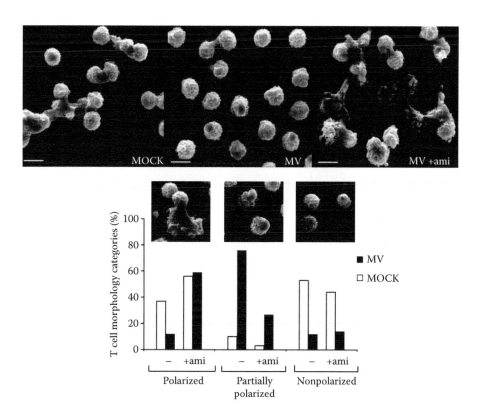

FIGURE 7.3 ASM activation accounts for MV-induced loss of T cell polarization. In human T cells seeded onto fibronectin, exposure to MV but not a control cell preparation (MOCK) results in loss of polarization. This is completely rescued if ASM activation is inhibited by amitriptyline (MV +ami). A quantative assessement of this experiment is shown in the bottom graph where phenotypes of cells in each category are also indicated as insets (Schneider-Schaulies et al., unpublished data). Rescue of MV-induced loss of actin-based protrusions has been similarly observed in Asm-deficient murine spleen cells.

not analyzed.[180] The outcome of sphingomyelinase activation/ceramide generation on actin dynamics may also be entirely different. Actin polymerization accompanies phagocytic cup formation that relies on SM activity,[12] and attachment, invasion, and phagocytosis of certain bacteria involve acid sphingomyelinase activation and definitely actin remodeling.[67,119,181] Similarly, increase in filamentous actin, Cdc42-dependent pseudopodia formation, and cell motility occur after ligation of the TNF-R1, which, however, involved PIP_2-dependent FAN recruitment followed by NSM2 activation.[182–184]

7.6.3 DOWNSTREAM EFFECTORS: TRANSCRIPTION FACTORS

There are several candidates for membrane distal pathways and effectors involved in ceramide-dependent signaling. In death signaling, these include activation of p53, which preceeds increase in Bax/Bcl-2 ratio and caspase activity in neuroblastoma cells exposed to exogenous ceramides. Irradiation-induced cell death requiring ASM can, however, occur in both p53-proficient and -deficient cells.[185,186] In Asm- and p53-deficient mice, the dependence of Asm-induced cell death from p53 may be cell type specific.[187] The SAP/JNK pathway has been shown to be activated in cell death in response to CD95 ligation or exposure to exogenous ceramide, and its targets may vary in a cell type-specific manner.[188,189] In lymphoid and myeloid cells, c-jun appears to be an essential JNK target in ceramide-induced apoptosis because this is prevented by dominant-negative c-Jun.[190] The SAPK/JNK pathway is also activated in a ceramide-dependent manner by PKCζ, which is a direct ceramide effector (see Section 7.5.2).[136,191]

Ceramide-activated PKCζ can, however, also relay a proliferative/survival signal. This was shown in PC12 cells where exposure to low dose of C_2 ceramides activated NF-κB along with JNK to promote cell survival rather than cell death.[192] In addition to promoting apoptosis by ASM activation, TNFR1 ASM-independently relays proinflammatory signals from the plasma membrane and these involve NF-κB activation.[193] Apparently, NF-κB activation rather involves NSM2, as shown for iNOS transcription in vascular smooth muscle cells.[194] NF-κB activation was also placed downstream of NSM2 in regulation of cyclooxygenase-2 expression in human alveolar epithelial cells in response to TNF-α and peptidoglycan in macrophages.[195,196] NSM2 activity promoted activation of RelA/p52 and RelA/p50 heterodimers in TNF-α-treated human colon carcinoma cells, where, interestingly, ASM-dependent formation of inactive p50/p50 homodimers was also observed.[197] Finally, the ability of recombinant sphingomyelinase to promote degradation of IκB in a cell-free system has also been documented.[198] Sphingomyelinase activation and ceramide release can thus promote but also impair NF-κB activation. In dendritic cells, ligation of the DC-SIGN by mannan, antibodies, or MV activated ASM, and this was required for activation of Raf-1 and ERK through DC-SIGN, yet interfered with LPS-dependent activation of NF-κB.[61] Similarly, inhibition of NF-κB activation was also reported in MCF-7 and Jurkat cells exposed to exogeous ceramides or sphingomyelinase.[199,200] Not surprisingly, the impact of ceramide release on NF-κB activation apparently depends on the sphingomyelinase activated, dose, compartment, mode of induction, and cell type.

7.7   BIOLOGICAL CONSEQUENCES OF SM BREAKDOWN AND CERAMIDE ACCUMULATION: ROLE IN PATHOGEN UPTAKE, RELEASE, AND HOST DEFENSES

Genetic or pharmacologic ablation of sphingomyelinase has provided valuable insights into the requirement of ceramides and its derivatives for the biological processes to be discussed in the following. Technically, it is still challenging to perform "gain of function" experiments where ceramide levels are raised and specifically investigated in physiological concentrations and conditions. Thus, exogenous sphingomyelinase is often used, which efficiently depletes SM from the outer membrane layer, and thereby, positional effects (i.e., generation of ceramides at defined areas on nonpolarized cells) are lost. Addition of exogenous ceramides has also been widely employed, which is mainly confined to short-chain ceramides because of the low water solubility of natural C_{16}–C_{24} ceramides. Short-chain ceramides can but do not have to be converted into long-chain ceramides or derivatives, and thus, various ceramide species may be present within the same experiment, again questioning the physiological relevance in the absence of control experiments involving complementary strategies. We and others have recently shown that mice lacking the acid ceramidase or being heterozygous for this enzyme accumulate ceramide and may serve to study cellular effects of increased ceramide levels.[201–202]

7.7.1   Pathogen Uptake

In line with their particular biophysical structure and ability to organize membrane domains with regard to segregation of transmembrane proteins and their signalosomes, membrane domains enriched in ceramide principally regulate pathogen uptake at the level of surface interaction (with ceramides or metabolites directly or segregation of [protein] receptors) or endo-phagosomal uptake into phagocytic or nonphagocytic cells.

7.7.1.1   Bacterial/Parasite Internalization and Induction of Host Cell Death

In vivo, the importance of ASM for endo/phagocytosis has been studied in a number of systems. The enzyme was found to be required for mannose-6-phosphate receptor-mediated endocytosis as revealed in Asm-deficient macrophages.[203] Studies with pathogens revealed that the ASM/Asm is required for internalization of *Neisseria gonorrhoeae* and *Pseudomonas aeruginosa* into human and murine epithelial and airway epithelial cells, respectively,[67,119] while uptake of *L. monocytogenes* and *Escherichia coli* into Asm macrophages does not appear to be impaired by deficiency of the enzyme.[74,75] Internalization of pathogens into epithelial cells by the ASM is mediated by the formation of ceramide-enriched membrane domains that colocalize with the pathogens. However, whether these domains serve to cluster specific receptors that mediate internalization is unknown. Ceramide-enriched membrane platforms formed by *P. aeruginosa*-triggered activation of the ASM are also required for the induction of apoptosis of infected epithelial cells and the controlled release of cytokines from infected cells.[119] A similar role applies to the infection of endothelial cells with *Staphylococcus aureus*.[204] Infection of endothelial cells with

S. aureus results in ASM activation and a subsequent release of ceramide, stimulation of caspases and Jun-N-terminal kinases, a release of cytochrome *c* from mitochondria, and finally apoptosis.

The role of sphingomyelinases and ceramide is even more complex for the infection of mammalian cells with parasites: *Plasmodium falciparum* expresses an endogenous sphingomyelinase that serves to generate ceramide in mammalian host cells and to mediate uptake of the parasite by erythrocytes.[205] On the other hand, pharmacological inhibition or genetic deficiency of the host acid sphingomyelinase is involved in the regulation of death of *P. falciparum*-infected human erythrocytes and thereby in vivo parasitemia and survival of *Plasmodium berghei*-infected mice.[206] Finally, *Leishmania donovani* promastigotes were shown to trigger an activation of the acid sphingomyelinase, which is required for internalization of the parasite.[207] While the acid sphingomyelinase mediates early release of ceramide upon infection with *L. donovani*, the parasite induces de novo synthesis of ceramide in a later phase, which is required for antigen presentation to T lymphocytes.

7.7.1.2   Viral Uptake

7.7.1.2.1   *HIV: The Role of Complex Glycosylated Ceramides*

GSLs have been implicated in modulating uptake of HIV into target cells, which per se relies on interaction of HIV env protein gp120 with its attachment and fusion receptors, CD4 and CCR5 or CXCR4, respectively.[208] A motif within the gp120 V3 loop also interacts with the carbohydrate moieties of Gb3 (Galα1-4Gal1β1-4 glucosyl ceramide or globotriasyl-ceramide), while galactosyl-ceramide (Gal-Cer) can bind both the gp120 and the gp41 subunit of the HIV env protein. Unlike chemokine receptor binding, gp120 interaction with Gb3 does not require that with CD4, and because of the proximity of the Gb3 binding and the chemokine receptor binding site within the V3 loop, Gb3 binding was suggested to regulate HIV fusion and uptake.[209,210] The importance of GSLs in HIV entry was revealed by the sensitivity of HIV entry to compounds affecting conversion of ceramide into glucosylceramide or by variations of the cellular GSL content.[211,212] In model membranes, gp120 efficiently bound to C_{16}, C_{22}, and C_{24} Gb3 isoforms while C_{18} and C_{20} were not recognized and rather acted dominant negatively in lipid mixtures.[210,213] Whether these in vitro observations translate into in vivo conditions, where binding affinities may further differ between monomeric and biologically active trimeric gp120, is, however, still unclear.[214]

Gb3 and Ga-Cer support HIV uptake into CD4+ as well as into CD4− cells such as mucosal epithelial cells, during transcytosis, and support HIV transmission to T cells or DCs.[215,216] A soluble Gb3-mimic, where the ceramide moiety is replaced by a rigid adamantane hydrocarbon frame, efficiently prevented HIV infection of primary lymphoid cells.[217] Gb3 levels can, however, also inversely correlate with susceptibility and thereby confer resistance to HIV infection as revealed for PBMCs of Fabry disease patients[218] and in cell lines where levels of Gb3 were constitutively high.[219]

Gal-Cer was proposed to act as mucosal epithelial cell apical receptor for both HIV gp120 and gp41 to promote internalization followed by transcytosis and release from the basolateral membrane.[220,221] Gal-Cer trapping by mammary epithelial cells efficiently enhanced HIV transmission to T cells where raft-dependent endocytosis was proposed to act as an alternative route to the clathrin-mediated uptake after CD4 interaction.[222] Because gp41 also attaches to Gal-Cer expressed on DCs isolated from human blood and mucosal tissue and in situ on mucosal tissues, this mode of transmission to T cells appears to be pathogenically relevant.[223]

7.7.1.2.2 Ceramides in Segregating Viral Protein Receptors and Viral Endocytosis

Membrane domains enriched in ceramides were suggested to support vesicular fusion,[74] and therefore, conditions favoring generation of these domains would predictedly support membrane fusion and entry particularly of enveloped viruses.

While trapping on nonlymphoid cells can support HIV transmission into CD4+ target cells, HIV entry followed by replication into these cells was highly sensitive to compounds elevating levels of ceramides.[211,224,225] Preexposure to bacterial sphingomyelinase or long-chain ceramide (C_{16}) prevented HIV uptake into T cells, monocytes, or macrophages without affecting HIV binding, overall surface levels of CD4 and chemokine receptors, or their association with detergent-resistant membrane domains, but with lateral diffusion of CD4 toward the coreceptors.[224,226] Furthermore, membrane domains enriched in dihydroxyceramide largely abolished insertion of the fusogenic gp41, thereby preventing viral access to the cytosol and fostering endocytosis into lysosomal degradative compartments.[227] Similar to HIV, bacterial sphingomyelinase-driven interference with uptake of hepatitis C virus (HCV) occurred at the level of receptor segregation. It caused partial internalization of the major entry factor CD81 and impaired its cosegregation with the other components required for entry, scavenger receptor B1 and claudin-1, into detergent-resistant microdomains.[228]

Ceramide accumulation may, however, also support viral uptake into target cells, and this particularly applies to the uptake of viruses that involves endocytosis eventually followed by vesicular acidification. If supportive for their uptake, viruses can induce formation of ceramide-enriched platforms themselves as first revealed for major and minor subgroup picornavirus rhinovirus (RV). ASM activation after attachment of RV to epithelial cells followed by formation of large membrane platforms enriched in ceramides and GSLs was important for viral binding and uptake.[63,68] Apparently, GSLs are involved in RV trafficking because they were codetected with endocytosed virus in membrane-proximal and perinuclear vesicles. It is unknown how SLs communicate in RV internalization and if they affect recruitment or concentration of the RV receptors, ICAM-1, or low-density lipoprotein family members.

More recently, a crucial role of the endo/lysosomal cholesterol transporter Niemann–Pick C protein 1 (NPC1) in Ebola virus uptake became apparent. Access to the cytosol after viral particle endocytosis depended on NPC1 and recruitment of the homotypic fusion and vacuole protein sorting (HOPS) complex.[229,230] NPC1 binds to the proteolytically activated viral gp and thus serves as a bona fide entry receptor for Ebola virus within an intracellular compartment.[231] SM and ASM were implicated in early steps of Ebola virus infection, too. Viral attachment to the plasma membrane was SM dependent, and viral particles associated with surface displayed ASM, indicating that interaction may occur in SM-enriched domains followed by ASM activation.[70]

MV interaction activates NSM and ASM upon ligation of an unknown receptor on T cells[66] and of DC-SIGN on immature DCs.[61] In DCs, sphingomyelinase activation was required for a NEM-sensitive surface recruitment of the MV entry receptor CD150 from an intracellular compartment also containing the ASM. In ceramide-enriched platforms, CD150 was transiently codisplayed with DC-SIGN, and this explained why this molecule enhanced MV uptake. DC-SIGN binds and signals in response to a variety of pathogens, and the ability of mannan- and DC-SIGN-specific antibodies to mediate sphingomyelinase activation adds DC-SIGN into the list of surface receptors generally involved in SM turnover. If gp120, which also binds DC-SIGN, were to promote this as well, one would expect inhibition of lateral CD4 mobility and favored endocytosis, which would be in line with HIV being partially internalized into nondegradative invaginated compartments in DCs where it is stored for subsequent transmission to T cells.[232–234] DC-SIGN is a signaling molecule and can modify TLR signaling to shape adaptive immunity.[235,236] As shown for other sphingomyelinase-activating conditions (see above), activation of DC-SIGN signaling components Raf-1 and ERK relied on ASM activation, thereby linking SL turnover to DC functions and, eventually, polarization of T cell responses.[61]

7.7.1.2.3 SL-Enriched Domains in Viral Maturation and Budding

Though implicated for a number of viruses mainly based on cholesterol depletion approaches, direct evidence for the role of defined lipid domains in the production of enveloped viral particles by virion lipidomes is only available for HCV, HIV, and HCMV.[237–239] Comparative analyses with the respective host cell lipidomes showed that these are modified by viral infection and that the lipid composition of viral budding sites differs from that of the host cell membrane and varies between the viruses analyzed. Lipid composition of HIV particles varies with regard to the producer cell, and SM and dihydroSM are selectively enriched while ceramides represent a very minor virion SL component.[237,240] Budding site selection at membranes is mediated by interaction of viral envelope proteins. This has been well documented for matrix proteins of RNA viruses that interact with phospholipids at the inner leaflet of the plasma membrane beneath the outer membrane raft domain. They generally oligomerize into lattices that, per se, do have the propensity to promote outward membrane curvature as required for particle formation. This has been studied in detail for HIV Gag protein, which has been suggested to associate with raft-like domains in its multimerized form specifically linked to saturated acyl chains.[241] How the transbilayer communication induced by viruses (modulation of the outer leaflet lipid composition) is exerted, however, has not been resolved. In addition to the matrix proteins, association of viral glycoproteins with membrane microdomains is also crucial to the budding process. Not surprisingly, cosedimentation of viral glycoproteins with detergent-resistant membrane microdomains in flotation gradients was revealed in many systems. The importance of

SM-enriched domains in viral budding has, for example, been revealed upon abrogation of SM production (both pharmacologically and in cells deficient for SMS-1). This effciently impaired partitioning of influenza virus HA and NA proteins both to the cell surface and into TX-100-insoluble membrane fractions and, thereby, production of virus particles.[242]

7.8 SPHINGOMYELINASES AS MODULATORS OF PATHOGENESIS: REGULATION OF IMMUNE CELL ACTIVITY

As referred to above, genetic Asm or Nsm deficiency is associated with severe disease processes, but does not detectably affect the architecture of secondary immune tissues and the composition of the peripheral blood compartment in mice. It has, however, clearly been shown that clearance of viral and bacterial pathogens is affected in Asm-deficient animals.[71,118,243–245]

7.8.1 CERAMIDES REGULATING T CELL SIGNALING, EXPANSION, AND EFFECTOR FUNCTIONS

Microcluster organization is of central importance to TCR signaling. Once the existence of self-associating, phase-separating lipid membrane microdomains mainly consisting of cholesterol and SM was revealed, it was—and partially continues to be—an ongoing discussion about the relative contribution of the lipid or protein environment as the driving force for association of the TCR and other microclusters essential for signal propagation. With the availability of suitable reagents and high-resolution microscopy detection protocols, it became clear that even in the resting state, TCR subcomponents partitioned into l_o phases, and this was crucial for signal initiation. Indeed, preassembled TCR oligomers (owing to their limited size also referred to as nanoclusters) segregated with and appeared to be stabilized by cholesterol[246] and most likely associate with preassembled LAT and SLP-76 nanoclusters early after TCR ligation as elegantly documented by hsPALM.[247,248] Apparently, TCR nanocluster size and number in antigen-experienced T cells exceeds that in naive T cells,[249] which is consistent with their responsiveness to lower antigen doses. Again, the lipid composition of membrane microdomains is thought to be at least one of the driving forces to promote TCR oligomerization into nanoclusters.[250] Cholesterol was recently shown to bind specifically the TCRβ chain in vivo and, in conjunction with SM, TCR nanoclusters formed ligand-independently in artificial unilamellar vesicles, lending further support to the importance of l_o domains in this process.[251] It is also with regard to early relay of TCR signaling that the integrity of lipid raft domains appears to be crucial as, for instance, revealed by their requirement for Lck and PKCθ recruitment.[13,248,252]

Having established the requirement for l_o domains composed of "inactive" components such as cholesterol and SM in patterning and activity of the TCR and the membrane-proximal signalosome, SM turnover into ceramides and phosphocholine would predictably strongly affect these processes. It is as yet unknown as to whether formation of TCR nanoclusters and their condensation might be affected in membrane domains where cholesterol is excluded and SM is converted into ceramide. It may be taken as evidence that ceramide accumulation might not support IS function that SM and its ceramide metabolites are of low abundance in TCR activation domains immuno-isolated after CD3 ligation.[107]

A number of studies centered around the question which receptors might elicit SM hydrolysis on T cells and what would be their downstream effectors.

Among the most prominent T cell surface receptors, CD3,[253] CD28,[59,254,255] CD4,[256] CD40L,[257] L-selectin,[258] CD5,[60] CD95,[141] TNFR1,[140] transferrin receptor,[259] and LFA-1[260] have been shown to activate NSM or ASM upon ligation. Among those, sphingomyelinase activation through CD3 or its costimulator CD28 would be expected to primarily affect T cell activation. CD3 ligation on primary and Jurkat T cells activated NSM/Nsm, but not ASM, and this was essential for both TCR-induced apoptosis and IL-2 production.[253] Strikingly, however, ablation of NSM by antisense DNA did not affect CD3-induced tyrosine phosphorylation of Cbl, ZAP-70, and LAT, but rather abrogated MAPK activation.

Whether this is counter-regulated through CD28, which activates ASM/Asm rather than NSM, has not been directly investigated. In vitro, CD28-mediated Asm activation was required for splenic T cell proliferation and IL-2 production (which could be also induced by C_6 ceramide and bacterial sphingomyelinase)[255] and NF-κB activation.[59,254] Surprisingly, exogenous C_2 or bacterial sphingomyelinase were unable to costimulate but rather inhibited CD3 ligation-induced T cell proliferation, indicating that ceramides released in response to CD28 ligation might not be required for but rather prevent costimulation.[261] In line with this, phorbol ester-stimulated activation of PKCθ (a major effector of CD28 signaling) and NF-kB (but not NF-AT or AP-1) activation and subsequent IL-2 production were found impaired in Jurkat cells exposed to C_6 ceramide or bacterial sphingomyelinase.[200] Finally, in mouse spleen cells, Asm ablation affected release, but not CD28-dependent production of IL-2.[262] Selective secretion defects were also reported in CD8+ T cells of Asm-deficient mice, indicating that the secretory system rather than CD28 signaling per se may require ASM activity in T cells.

Several studies addressed consequences and targets of receptor-catalzyed ceramide release in affecting TCR signaling. The antitumor activity of a CD4 antibody was shown to involve ASM activation, which caused segregation of ZAP-70 (and thereby its downstream effectors Vav-1, PLC-γ, and SLP-76) from rafts, thereby destroying platforms required for signal propagation.[256] Exposure to bacterial sphingomyelinase resulted in raft exclusion of Lck and inhibition of proliferation in one[263] and in retention of Lck and LAT in rafts in another study.[264] It was also at the level of raft depletion of SM that choleratoxin B treatment acted to inhibit proliferation of human CD4+ T cells activated by PMA or CD3/CD28 ligation. Both inhibition of SM synthesis and activation of NSM (but not ASM) were reported as were ceramide release, inhibition of PKCα, and NF-κB activation.[265] CD5, which interferes with TCR signaling and regulates apoptosis, activates ASM and, classically, PKCζ and MAPK, but interestingly, not NF-κB in B and T cells. Its targets in ASM-dependent T cell suppression are as yet unknown.[60,266] Finally, ligation of TNF-R1 or CD95 abrogated CRAC channel activation in Jurkat and primary T cells after TCR triggering by ASM-catalyzed ceramide release, and this prevented store-operated calcium entry, NF-AT activation, and IL-2 synthesis.[140,141] Though the contribution of sphin-gomyelinases in this context has not been directly addressed, coligation of CD95 and CD3/CD28 in naive T cells inhibited TCR signaling at the level of ZAP-70, PLC-γ, and PKCθ redistribution as well as Ca^{2+} mobilization and nuclear translocation of NF-AT, AP-1, and NF-κB.[267]

7.8.2 PROFESSIONAL ANTIGEN-PRESENTING CELLS OR PHAGOCYTES

Mycobacterial species, for example, *Mycobacterium tuberculosis*, *Mycobacterium avium*, or *Mycobacterium smegmatis*, infect macrophages and induce the formation of epithelioid macrophages and multinucleated giant cells in granulomas in infected tissues.[268] The formation of multinucleated giant cells was shown to require Asm expression, and Asm-deficient mice failed to form giant cells upon infection with *M. avium*. Further, Asm-deficient mice are less sensitive to lethal infections with *M. avium* than wild-type mice.[74]

Ceramide among other lipids also triggers actin nucleation on phagosomes con-taining *M. avium* and *M. smegmatis*,[269] an event required for phagosomal–lysosomal fusion and thereby killing of the pathogen. Likewise, expression of Asm is prereq-uisite for macrophage-mediated killing of *Salmonella typhimurium*. Asm deficiency resulted in reduced activation of NADPH oxidase and release of reactive oxygen spe-cies and thereby in failure to kill the pathogen. This translated into a very high sus-ceptibility of Asm-deficient mice to infection with *S. typhimurium*.[270] Asm-released ceramide forms ceramide-enriched membrane domains in macrophages, which serve the clustering of subunits of NADPH oxidases, the activation of NADPH oxi-dases, and the release of reactive oxygen species.[271] The latter are a key component of the immediate innate response to pathogens and are central for killing bacteria as revealed in humans lacking a key subunit of NADPH oxidases, that is, gp91. Thus, ASM and ceramide play important roles in maturation of phagosomes and the release of reactive oxygen species, that is, central components of the innate immune system.

Though less well studied, there is also a role of sphingomyelinases in modulating the activity of DCs. As for other cell types, ASM activation can cause apoptosis in these cells, the efficiency of which can vary depending on the DC differentiation status.[272–274] When induced to differentiate, DCs respond to exposure of IL-1β or ligation of CD40 with ceramide release and, concomitantly, loss of the capacity to take up, as well as to process antigens.[275] The ability of DC-SIGN to activate sphingo-myelinases not only in the context of viral capture but also in mediating membrane-proximal Raf and ERK activation and modulation of TLR-induced NF-κB activation has been referred to already above.[61]

ACKNOWLEDGMENTS

We apologize to all colleagues whose excellent contributions to the subject could not be cited because of space constraints. We thank the Deutsche Forschungsgemeinschaft (SPP1267) for financial support of laboratory work.

REFERENCES

1. Simons, K., and M. J. Gerl. "Revitalizing Membrane Rafts: New Tools and Insights." *Nat Rev Mol Cell Biol* 11, no. 10 (2010): 688–99.
2. Mukherjee, S., and F. R. Maxfield. "Membrane Domains." *Annu Rev Cell Dev Biol* 20 (2004): 839–66.
3. Brown, D. A., and E. London. "Functions of Lipid Rafts in Biological Membranes." *Annu Rev Cell Dev Biol* 14 (1998): 111–36.
4. Harder, T., and K. Simons. "Caveolae, Digs, and the Dynamics of Sphingolipid-Cholesterol Microdomains." *Curr Opin Cell Biol* 9, no. 4 (1997): 534–42.
5. Brown, D. A., and E. London. "Structure and Origin of Ordered Lipid Domains in Biological Membranes." *J Membr Biol* 164, no. 2 (1998): 103–14.
6. Hammond, A. T., F. A. Heberle, T. Baumgart et al. "Crosslinking a Lipid Raft Component Triggers Liquid Ordered-Liquid Disordered Phase Separation in Model Plasma Membranes." *Proc Natl Acad Sci U S A* 102, no. 18 (2005): 6320–5.
7. Pabst, G., B. Boulgaropoulos, E. Gander et al. "Effect of Ceramide on Nonraft Proteins." *J Membr Biol* 231, no. 2–3 (2009): 125–32.
8. Ernst, A. M., F. X. Contreras, C. Thiele, F. Wieland, and B. Brugger. "Mutual Recognition of Sphingolipid Molecular Species in Membranes." *Biochim Biophys Acta* 1818, no. 11 (2012): 2616–22.
9. Gaus, K., E. Chklovskaia, B. Fazekas de St Groth, W. Jessup, and T. Harder. "Condensation of the Plasma Membrane at the Site of T Lymphocyte Activation." *J Cell Biol* 171, no. 1 (2005): 121–31.
10. Harder, T., C. Rentero, T. Zech, and K. Gaus. "Plasma Membrane Segregation During T Cell Activation: Probing the Order of Domains." *Curr Opin Immunol* 19, no. 4 (2007): 470–5.
11. Ludford-Menting, M. J., B. Crimeen-Irwin, J. Oliaro et al. "The Reorientation of T-Cell Polarity and Inhibition of Immunological Synapse Formation by CD46 Involves Its Recruitment to Lipid Rafts." *J Lipids* 2011 (2011): 521863.
12. Magenau, A., C. Benzing, N. Proschogo et al. "Phagocytosis of IgG-Coated Polystyrene Beads by Macrophages Induces and Requires High Membrane Order." *Traffic* 12, no. 12 (2011): 1730–43.
13. Owen, D. M., D. J. Williamson, A. Magenau, and K. Gaus. "Sub-Resolution Lipid Domains Exist in the Plasma Membrane and Regulate Protein Diffusion and Distribution." *Nat Commun* 3 (2012): 1256.
14. Bielawski, J., J. S. Pierce, J. Snider et al. "Sphingolipid Analysis by High Performance Liquid Chromatography-Tandem Mass Spectrometry (HPLC-MS/MS)." *Adv Exp Med Biol* 688 (2010): 46–59.
15. Lingwood, D., J. Ries, P. Schwille, and K. Simons. "Plasma Membranes Are Poised for Activation of Raft Phase Coalescence at Physiological Temperature." *Proc Natl Acad Sci U S A* 105, no. 29 (2008): 10005–10.
16. van Zanten, T. S., J. Gomez, C. Manzo et al. "Direct Mapping of Nanoscale Compositional Connectivity on Intact Cell Membranes." *Proc Natl Acad Sci U S A* 107, no. 35 (2010): 15437–42.
17. Pinaud, F., X. Michalet, G. Iyer et al. "Dynamic Partitioning of a Glycosyl-Phosphatidylinositol-Anchored Protein in Glycosphingolipid-Rich Microdomains Imaged by Single-Quantum Dot Tracking." *Traffic* 10, no. 6 (2009): 691–712.
18. Kaiser, R. D., and E. London. "Determination of the Depth of BODIPY Probes in Model Membranes by Parallax Analysis of Fluorescence Quenching." *Biochim Biophys Acta* 1375, no. 1–2 (1998): 13–22.
19. Kuerschner, L., C. S. Ejsing, K. Ekroos et al. "Polyene-Lipids: A New Tool to Image Lipids." *Nat Methods* 2, no. 1 (2005): 39–45.

20. Raghuraman, H., S. Shrivastava, and A. Chattopadhyay. "Monitoring the Looping up of Acyl Chain Labeled NBD Lipids in Membranes as a Function of Membrane Phase State." *Biochim Biophys Acta* 1768, no. 5 (2007): 1258–67.
21. Kusumi, A., T. K. Fujiwara, R. Chadda et al. "Dynamic Organizing Principles of the Plasma Membrane That Regulate Signal Transduction: Commemorating the Fortieth Anniversary of Singer and Nicolson's Fluid-Mosaic Model." *Annu Rev Cell Dev Biol* 28 (2012): 215–50.
22. Marks, D. L., R. Bittman, and R. E. Pagano. "Use of Bodipy-Labeled Sphingolipid and Cholesterol Analogs to Examine Membrane Microdomains in Cells." *Histochem Cell Biol* 130, no. 5 (2008): 819–32.
23. Tyteca, D., L. D'Auria, P. V. Der Smissen et al. "Three Unrelated Sphingomyelin Analogs Spontaneously Cluster into Plasma Membrane Micrometric Domains." *Biochim Biophys Acta* 1798, no. 5 (2010): 909–27.
24. Frisz, J. F., K. Lou, H. A. Klitzing et al. "Direct Chemical Evidence for Sphingolipid Domains in the Plasma Membranes of Fibroblasts." *Proc Natl Acad Sci U S A* 110, no. 8 (2013): E613–22.
25. Fujiwara, T., K. Ritchie, H. Murakoshi, K. Jacobson, and A. Kusumi. "Phospholipids Undergo Hop Diffusion in Compartmentalized Cell Membrane." *J Cell Biol* 157, no. 6 (2002): 1071–81.
26. Gowrishankar, K., S. Ghosh, S. Saha et al. "Active Remodeling of Cortical Actin Regulates Spatiotemporal Organization of Cell Surface Molecules." *Cell* 149, no. 6 (2012): 1353–67.
27. Gault, C. R., L. M. Obeid, and Y. A. Hannun. "An Overview of Sphingolipid Metabolism: From Synthesis to Breakdown." *Adv Exp Med Biol* 688 (2010): 1–23.
28. Hannun, Y. A., and L. M. Obeid. "Principles of Bioactive Lipid Signalling: Lessons from Sphingolipids." *Nat Rev Mol Cell Biol* 9, no. 2 (2008): 139–50.
29. Gault, C. R., L. M. Obeid, and Y. A. Hannun. "Many Ceramides." *J Biol Chem* 286, no. 32 (2011): 27855–62.
30. Pinto, S. N., L. C. Silva, A. H. Futerman, and M. Prieto. "Effect of Ceramide Structure on Membrane Biophysical Properties: The Role of Acyl Chain Length and Unsaturation." *Biochim Biophys Acta* 1808, no. 11 (2011): 2753–60.
31. Boudker, O., and A. H. Futerman. "Detection and Characterization of Ceramide-1-Phosphate Phosphatase Activity in Rat Liver Plasma Membrane." *J Biol Chem* 268, no. 29 (1993): 22150–5.
32. Brindley, D. N., J. Xu, R. Jasinska, and D. W. Waggoner. "Analysis of Ceramide 1-Phosphate and Sphingosine-1-Phosphate Phosphatase Activities." *Methods Enzymol* 311 (2000): 233–44.
33. Okino, N., X. He, S. Gatt et al. "The Reverse Activity of Human Acid Ceramidase." *J Biol Chem* 278, no. 32 (2003): 29948–53.
34. Ishibashi, Y., T. Nakasone, M. Kiyohara et al. "A Novel Endoglycoceramidase Hydrolyzes Oligogalactosylceramides to Produce Galactooligosaccharides and Ceramides." *J Biol Chem* 282, no. 15 (2007): 11386–96.
35. Takuwa, Y., Y. Okamoto, K. Yoshioka, and N. Takuwa. "Sphingosine-1-Phosphate Signaling in Physiology and Diseases." *Biofactors* 38, no. 5 (2012): 329–37.
36. Pyne, N. J., and S. Pyne. "Sphingosine 1-Phosphate and Cancer." *Nat Rev Cancer* 10, no. 7 (2010): 489–503.
37. Gulbins, E. and I. Petrache (Eds.). Sphingolipids in disease. In: *Handbook of Experimental Pharmacology,* vol. 216 (2013). Springer Verlag, Wien, Austria.
38. Schulze, H., and K. Sandhoff. "Lysosomal Lipid Storage Diseases." *Cold Spring Harb Perspect Biol* 3, no. 6 (2011): a004804, doi: 10.1101/cshperspect.a004804.
39. Futerman, A. H., and G. van Meer. "The Cell Biology of Lysosomal Storage Disorders." *Nat Rev Mol Cell Biol* 5, no. 7 (2004): 554–65.

40. Ginzburg, L., Y. Kacher, and A. H. Futerman. "The Pathogenesis of Glycosphingolipid Storage Disorders." *Semin Cell Dev Biol* 15, no. 4 (2004): 417–31.

41. Ryland, L. K., T. E. Fox, X. Liu, T. P. Loughran, and M. Kester. "Dysregulation of Sphingolipid Metabolism in Cancer." *Cancer Biol Ther* 11, no. 2 (2011): 138–49.

42. Jenkins, R., D. Canals, and Y. A. Hannun. "Roles and Regulation of Secretory and Lysosomal Acid Sphingomyelinase." *Cell Signal* 21, no. 6 (2009): 836–46.

43. Niemann, A. "Ein unbekanntes Krankheitsbild." *Jahrbuch für Kinderheilkunde* 97 (1914): 1–10.

44. Horinouchi, K., S. Erlich, D. P. Perl et al. "Acid Sphingomyelinase Deficient Mice: A Model of Types A and B Niemann-Pick Disease." *Nat Genet* 10, no. 3 (1995): 288–93.

45. Otterbach, B., and W. Stoffel. "Acid Sphingomyelinase-Deficient Mice Mimic the Neurovisceral Form of Human Lysosomal Storage Disease (Niemann-Pick Disease)." *Cell* 81, no. 7 (1995): 1053–61.

46. Zeidan, Y. H., B. X. Wu, R. W. Jenkins, L. M. Obeid, and Y. A. Hannun. "A Novel Role for Protein Kinase Cdelta-Mediated Phosphorylation of Acid Sphingomyelinase in UV Light-Induced Mitochondrial Injury." *FASEB J* 22, no. 1 (2008): 183–93.

47. Edelmann, B., U. Bertsch, V. Tchikov et al. "Caspase-8 and Caspase-7 Sequentially Mediate Proteolytic Activation of Acid Sphingomyelinase in TNF-R1 Receptosomes." *EMBO J* 30, no. 2 (2011): 379–94.

48. Zeidan, Y. H., R. W. Jenkins, and Y. A. Hannun. "Remodeling of Cellular Cytoskeleton by the Acid Sphingomyelinase/Ceramide Pathway." *J Cell Biol* 181, no. 2 (2008): 335–50.

49. Li, X., E. Gulbins, and Y. Zhang. "Oxidative Stress Triggers Ca-Dependent Lysosome Trafficking and Activation of Acid Sphingomyelinase." *Cell Physiol Biochem* 30, no. 4 (2012): 815–26.

50. Rotolo, J. A., J. Zhang, M. Donepudi et al. "Caspase-Dependent and -Independent Activation of Acid Sphingomyelinase Signaling." *J Biol Chem* 280, no. 28 (2005): 26425–34.

51. Charruyer, A., S. Grazide, C. Bezombes et al. "UV-C Light Induces Raft-Associated Acid Sphingomyelinase and JNK Activation and Translocation Independently on a Nuclear Signal." *J Biol Chem* 280, no. 19 (2005): 19196–204.

52. Dumitru, C. A., and E. Gulbins. "Trail Activates Acid Sphingomyelinase Via a Redox Mechanism and Releases Ceramide to Trigger Apoptosis." *Oncogene* 25, no. 41 (2006): 5612–25.

53. Bertsch, U., B. Edelmann, V. Tchikov, S. Winoto-Morbach, and S. Schutze. "Compartmentalization of TNF-Receptor 1 Signaling: TNF-R1-Associated Caspase-8 Mediates Activation of Acid Sphingomyelinase in Late Endosomes." *Adv Exp Med Biol* 691 (2011): 605–16.

54. Gulbins, E., and R. Kolesnick. "Acid Sphingomyelinase-Derived Ceramide Signaling in Apoptosis." *Subcell Biochem* 36 (2002): 229–44.

55. Kirschnek, S., F. Paris, M. Weller et al. "CD95-Mediated Apoptosis In Vivo Involves Acid Sphingomyelinase." *J Biol Chem* 275, no. 35 (2000): 27316–23.

56. Grassme, H., A. Cremesti, R. Kolesnick, and E. Gulbins. "Ceramide-Mediated Clustering Is Required for CD95-DISC Formation." *Oncogene* 22, no. 35 (2003): 5457–70.

57. Adam, D., K. Wiegmann, S. Adam-Klages, A. Ruff, and M. Kronke. "A Novel Cytoplasmic Domain of the p55 Tumor Necrosis Factor Receptor Initiates the Neutral Sphingomyelinase Pathway." *J Biol Chem* 271, no. 24 (1996): 14617–22.

58. Grassme, H., V. Jendrossek, J. Bock, A. Riehle, and E. Gulbins. "Ceramide-Rich Membrane Rafts Mediate CD40 Clustering." *J Immunol* 168, no. 1 (2002): 298–307.

59. Boucher, L. M., K. Wiegmann, A. Futerer et al. "CD28 Signals through Acidic Sphingomyelinase." *J Exp Med* 181, no. 6 (1995): 2059–68.

60. Simarro, M., J. Calvo, J. M. Vila et al. "Signaling through CD5 Involves Acidic Sphingomyelinase, Protein Kinase C-Zeta, Mitogen-Activated Protein Kinase Kinase, and C-Jun NH2-Terminal Kinase." *J Immunol* 162, no. 9 (1999): 5149–55.

61. Avota, E., E. Gulbins, and S. Schneider-Schaulies. "DC-SIGN Mediated Sphingomyelinase-Activation and Ceramide Generation Is Essential for Enhancement of Viral Uptake in DCs." *PLoS Pathog* 7, no. 2 (2011): e1001290.

62. Becker, K. A., H. Grassme, Y. Zhang, and E. Gulbins. "Ceramide in *Pseudomonas Aeruginosa* Infections and Cystic Fibrosis." *Cell Physiol Biochem* 26, no. 1 (2010): 57–66.

63. Dreschers, S., P. Franz, C. Dumitru et al. "Infections with Human Rhinovirus Induce the Formation of Distinct Functional Membrane Domains." *Cell Physiol Biochem* 20, no. 1–4 (2007): 241–54.

64. Dumitru, C. A., S. Dreschers, and E. Gulbins. "Rhinoviral Infections Activate p38MAP-Kinases Via Membrane Rafts and RhoA." *Cell Physiol Biochem* 17, no. 3–4 (2006): 159–66.

65. Esen, M., H. Grassme, J. Riethmuller et al. "Invasion of Human Epithelial Cells by *Pseudomonas Aeruginosa* Involves Src-Like Tyrosine Kinases p60src and p59fyn." *Infect Immun* 69, no. 1 (2001): 281–7.

66. Gassert, E., E. Avota, H. Harms et al. "Induction of Membrane Ceramides: A Novel Strategy to Interfere with T Lymphocyte Cytoskeletal Reorganisation in Viral Immuno-suppression." *PLoS Pathog* 5, no. 10 (2009): e1000623.

67. Grassme, H., E. Gulbins, B. Brenner et al. "Acidic Sphingomyelinase Mediates Entry of *N. Gonorrhoeae* into Nonphagocytic Cells." *Cell* 91, no. 5 (1997): 605–15.

68. Grassme, H., A. Riehle, B. Wilker, and E. Gulbins. "Rhinoviruses Infect Human Epithelial Cells Via Ceramide-Enriched Membrane Platforms." *J Biol Chem* 280, no. 28 (2005): 26256–62.

69. Hauck, C. R., H. Grassme, J. Bock et al. "Acid Sphingomyelinase Is Involved in CEACAM Receptor-Mediated Phagocytosis of *Neisseria Gonorrhoeae*." *FEBS Lett* 478, no. 3 (2000): 260–6.

70. Miller, M. E., S. Adhikary, A. A. Kolokoltsov, and R. A. Davey. "Ebola Virus Requires Acid Sphingomyelinase Activity and Plasma Membrane Sphingomyelin for Infection." *J Virol* 86, no. 14 (2012): 7473–83.

71. Herz, J., J. Pardo, H. Kashkar et al. "Acid Sphingomyelinase Is a Key Regulator of Cytotoxic Granule Secretion by Primary T Lymphocytes." *Nat Immunol* 10, no. 7 (2009): 761–8.

72. Zeidan, Y. H., and Y. A. Hannun. "Activation of Acid Sphingomyelinase by Protein Kinase Cd-Mediated Phosphorylation." *J Biol Chem* 282, no. 15 (2007): 11549–61.

73. Perrotta, C., L. Bizzozero, D. Cazzato et al. "Syntaxin 4 Is Required for Acid Sphingomyelinase Activity and Apoptotic Function." *J Biol Chem* 285, no. 51 (2010): 40240–51.

74. Utermohlen, O., J. Herz, M. Schramm, and M. Kronke. "Fusogenicity of Membranes: The Impact of Acid Sphingomyelinase on Innate Immune Responses." *Immunobiology* 213, no. 3–4 (2008): 307–14.

75. Schramm, M., J. Herz, A. Haas, M. Kronke, and O. Utermohlen. "Acid Sphingomyelinase Is Required for Efficient Phago-Lysosomal Fusion." *Cell Microbiol* 10, no. 9 (2008): 1839–53.

76. Tchikov, V., U. Bertsch, J. Fritsch, B. Edelmann, and S. Schutze. "Subcellular Compartmentalization of TNF Receptor-1 and CD95 Signaling Pathways." *Eur J Cell Biol* 90, no. 6–7 (2011): 467–75.

77. Feig, C., V. Tchikov, S. Schutze, and M. E. Peter. "Palmitoylation of CD95 Facilitates Formation of SDS-Stable Receptor Aggregates That Initiate Apoptosis Signaling." *EMBO J* 26, no. 1 (2007): 221–31.

78. Lee, K. H., C. Feig, V. Tchikov et al. "The Role of Receptor Internalization in CD95 Signaling." *EMBO J* 25, no. 5 (2006): 1009–23.

79. Akazawa, Y., J. L. Mott, S. F. Bronk et al. "Death Receptor 5 Internalization Is Required for Lysosomal Permeabilization by Trail in Malignant Liver Cell Lines." *Gastroenterology* 136, no. 7 (2009): 2365–76.

80. Qin, J., and G. Dawson. "Evidence for Coordination of Lysosomal (Asmase) and Plasma Membrane (Nsmase2) Forms of Sphingomyelinase from Mutant Mice." *FEBS Lett* 586, no. 22 (2012): 4002–9.

81. Wu, B. X., C. J. Clarke, and Y. A. Hannun. "Mammalian Neutral Sphingomyelinases: Regulation and Roles in Cell Signaling Responses." *Neuromolecular Med* 12, no. 4 (2010): 320–30.

82. Clarke, C. J., C. F. Snook, M. Tani et al. "The Extended Family of Neutral Sphingomyelinases." *Biochemistry* 45, no. 38 (2006): 11247–56.

83. Chipuk, J. E., G. P. McStay, A. Bharti et al. "Sphingolipid Metabolism Cooperates with BAK and BAX to Promote the Mitochondrial Pathway of Apoptosis." *Cell* 148, no. 5 (2012): 988–1000.

84. Tani, M., and Y. A. Hannun. "Analysis of Membrane Topology of Neutral Sphingomyelinase 2." *FEBS Lett* 581, no. 7 (2007): 1323–8.

85. Tani, M., and Y. A. Hannun. "Neutral Sphingomyelinase 2 Is Palmitoylated on Multiple Cysteine Residues. Role of Palmitoylation in Subcellular Localization." *J Biol Chem* 282, no. 13 (2007): 10047–56.

86. Corcoran, C. A., Q. He, S. Ponnusamy et al. "Neutral Sphingomyelinase-3 Is a DNA Damage and Nongenotoxic Stress-Regulated Gene That Is Deregulated in Human Malignancies." *Mol Cancer Res* 6, no. 5 (2008): 795–807.

87. Krut, O., K. Wiegmann, H. Kashkar, B. Yazdanpanah, and M. Kronke. "Novel Tumor Necrosis Factor-Responsive Mammalian Neutral Sphingomyelinase-3 Is a C-Tail-Anchored Protein." *J Biol Chem* 281, no. 19 (2006): 13784–93.

88. Trajkovic, K., C. Hsu, S. Chiantia et al. "Ceramide Triggers Budding of Exosome Vesicles into Multivesicular Endosomes." *Science* 319, no. 5867 (2008): 1244–7.

89. Filosto, S., W. Fry, A. A. Knowlton, and T. Goldkorn. "Neutral Sphingomyelinase 2 (Nsmase2) Is a Phosphoprotein Regulated by Calcineurin (PP2b)." *J Biol Chem* 285, no. 14 (2010): 10213–22.

90. Marchesini, N., C. Luberto, and Y. A. Hannun. "Biochemical Properties of Mammalian Neutral Sphingomyelinase 2 and Its Role in Sphingolipid Metabolism." *J Biol Chem* 278, no. 16 (2003): 13775–83.

91. Philipp, S., M. Puchert, S. Adam-Klages et al. "The Polycomb Group Protein EEd Couples TNF Receptor 1 to Neutral Sphingomyelinase." *Proc Natl Acad Sci U S A* 107, no. 3 (2010): 1112–7.

92. Adam-Klages, S., D. Adam, K. Wiegmann et al. "FAN, a Novel WD-Repeat Protein, Couples the p55 TNF-Receptor to Neutral Sphingomyelinase." *Cell* 86, no. 6 (1996): 937–47.

93. Boecke, A., D. Sieger, C. D. Neacsu, H. Kashkar, and M. Kronke. "Factor Associated with Neutral Sphingomyelinase Activity Mediates Navigational Capacity of Leukocytes Responding to Wounds and Infection: Live Imaging Studies in Zebrafish Larvae." *J Immunol* 189, no. 4 (2012): 1559–66.

94. Abe, M., A. Makino, F. Hullin-Matsuda et al. "A Role for Sphingomyelin-Rich Lipid Domains in the Accumulation of Phosphatidylinositol-4, 5-Bisphosphate to the Cleavage Furrow During Cytokinesis." *Mol Cell Biol* 32, no. 8 (2012): 1396–407.

95. Stoffel, W., B. Jenke, B. Block, M. Zumbansen, and J. Koebke. "Neutral Sphingomyelinase 2 (Smpd3) in the Control of Postnatal Growth and Development." *Proc Natl Acad Sci U S A* 102, no. 12 (2005): 4554–9.

96. Aubin, I., C. P. Adams, S. Opsahl et al. "A Deletion in the Gene Encoding Sphingomyelin Phosphodiesterase 3 (Smpd3) Results in Osteogenesis and Dentinogenesis Imperfecta in the Mouse." *Nat Genet* 37, no. 8 (2005): 803–5.

97. Nurminen, T. A., J. M. Holopainen, H. Zhao, and P. K. Kinnunen. "Observation of Topical Catalysis by Sphingomyelinase Coupled to Microspheres." *J Am Chem Soc* 124, no. 41 (2002): 12129–34.

98. Kolesnick, R. N., F. M. Goni, and A. Alonso. "Compartmentalization of Ceramide Signaling: Physical Foundations and Biological Effects." *J Cell Physiol* 184, no. 3 (2000): 285–300.

99. Megha, and E. London. "Ceramide Selectively Displaces Cholesterol from Ordered Lipid Domains (Rafts): Implications for Lipid Raft Structure and Function." *J Biol Chem* 279, no. 11 (2004): 9997–10004.

100. Goni, F. M., and A. Alonso. "Effects of Ceramide and Other Simple Sphingolipids on Membrane Lateral Structure." *Biochim Biophys Acta* 1788, no. 1 (2009): 169–77.

101. Grassme, H., A. Jekle, A. Riehle et al. "CD95 Signaling Via Ceramide-Rich Membrane Rafts." *J Biol Chem* 276, no. 23 (2001): 20589–96.

102. Veiga, M. P., J. L. Arrondo, F. M. Goni, and A. Alonso. "Ceramides in Phospholipid Membranes: Effects on Bilayer Stability and Transition to Nonlamellar Phases." *Biophys J* 76, no. 1 Pt 1 (1999): 342–50.

103. Zhang, Y., X. Li, K. A. Becker, and E. Gulbins. "Ceramide-Enriched Membrane Domains—Structure and Function." *Biochim Biophys Acta* 1788, no. 1 (2009): 178–83.

104. He, Q., G. Wang, S. Dasgupta et al. "Characterization of an Apical Ceramide-Enriched Compartment Regulating Ciliogenesis." *Mol Biol Cell* 23, no. 16 (2012): 3156–66.

105. Wang, G., K. Krishnamurthy, and E. Bieberich. "Regulation of Primary Cilia Formation by Ceramide." *J Lipid Res* 50, no. 10 (2009): 2103–10.

106. Owen, D. M., A. Magenau, D. Williamson, and K. Gaus. "The Lipid Raft Hypothesis Revisited—New Insights on Raft Composition and Function from Super-Resolution Fluorescence Microscopy." *Bioessays* 34, no. 9 (2012): 739–47.

107. Zech, T., C. S. Ejsing, K. Gaus et al. "Accumulation of Raft Lipids in T-Cell Plasma Membrane Domains Engaged in TCR Signalling." *EMBO J* 28, no. 5 (2009): 466–76.

108. Huang, H. W., E. M. Goldberg, and R. Zidovetzki. "Ceramide Induces Structural Defects into Phosphatidylcholine Bilayers and Activates Phospholipase A2." *Biochem Biophys Res Commun* 220, no. 3 (1996): 834–8.

109. Chiantia, S., J. Ries, N. Kahya, and P. Schwille. "Combined AFM and Two-Focus SFCS Study of Raft-Exhibiting Model Membranes." *Chemphyschem* 7, no. 11 (2006): 2409–18.

110. Holopainen, J. M., M. I. Angelova, and P. K. Kinnunen. "Vectorial Budding of Vesicles by Asymmetrical Enzymatic Formation of Ceramide in Giant Liposomes." *Biophys J* 78, no. 2 (2000): 830–8.

111. Kosaka, N., H. Iguchi, Y. Yoshioka et al. "Secretory Mechanisms and Intercellular Transfer of MicroRNAs in Living Cells." *J Biol Chem* 285, no. 23 (2010): 17442–52.

112. Kosaka, N., H. Iguchi, K. Hagiwara et al. "Neutral Sphingomyelinase 2 (Nsmase2)-Dependent Exosomal Transfer of Angiogenic Micrornas Regulate Cancer Cell Metastasis." *J Biol Chem* 288, no. 15 (2013): 10849–59.

113. Mittelbrunn, M., C. Gutierrez-Vazquez, C. Villarroya-Beltri et al. "Unidirectional Transfer of Microrna-Loaded Exosomes from T Cells to Antigen-Presenting Cells." *Nat Commun* 2 (2011): 282.

114. Dreux, M., U. Garaigorta, B. Boyd et al. "Short-Range Exosomal Transfer of Viral RNA from Infected Cells to Plasmacytoid Dendritic Cells Triggers Innate Immunity." *Cell Host Microbe* 12, no. 4 (2012): 558–70.

115. Li, J., K. Liu, Y. Liu et al. "Exosomes Mediate the Cell-to-Cell Transmission of IFN-Alpha-Induced Antiviral Activity." *Nat Immunol* 14, no. 8 (2013): 793–803.

116. Neufeld, E., A. Cooney, J. Pitha et al. "Intracellular Trafficking of Cholesterol Monitored with a Cyclodextrin." *J Biol Chem* 271, no. 35 (1996): 21604–13.

117. Bianco, F., C. Perrotta, L. Novellino et al. "Acid Sphingomyelinase Activity Triggers Microparticle Release from Glial Cells." *EMBO J* 28, no. 8 (2009): 1043–54.

118. Ng, C. G., and D. E. Griffin. "ASM Deficiency Increases Susceptibility to Fatal Alphavirus Encephalomyelitis." *J Virol* 80, no. 22 (2006): 10989–99.

119. Grassme, H., V. Jendrossek, A. Riehle et al. "Host Defense against *Pseudomonas Aeruginosa* Requires Ceramide-Rich Membrane Rafts." *Nat Med* 9, no. 3 (2003): 322–30.

120. Babiychuk, E. B., K. Monastyrskaya, S. Potez, and A. Draeger. "Intracellular Ca(2+) Operates a Switch between Repair and Lysis of Streptolysin O-Perforated Cells." *Cell Death Differ* 16, no. 8 (2009): 1126–34.

121. Babiychuk, E. B., K. Monastyrskaya, S. Potez, and A. Draeger. "Blebbing Confers Resistance against Cell Lysis." *Cell Death Differ* 18, no. 1 (2011): 80–9.

122. Tam, C., V. Idone, C. Devlin et al. "Exocytosis of Acid Sphingomyelinase by Wounded Cells Promotes Endocytosis and Plasma Membrane Repair." *J Cell Biol* 189, no. 6 (2010): 1027–38.

123. Draeger, A., K. Monastyrskaya, and E. B. Babiychuk. "Plasma Membrane Repair and Cellular Damage Control: The Annexin Survival Kit." *Biochem Pharmacol* 81, no. 6 (2011): 703–12.

124. Barrera, N. P., M. Zhou, and C. V. Robinson. "The Role of Lipids in Defining Membrane Protein Interactions: Insights from Mass Spectrometry." *Trends Cell Biol* 23, no. 1 (2013): 1–8.

125. Haberkant, P., O. Schmitt, F. X. Contreras et al. "Protein-Sphingolipid Interactions within Cellular Membranes." *J Lipid Res* 49, no. 1 (2008): 251–62.

126. Haberkant, P., R. Raijmakers, M. Wildwater et al. "In Vivo Profiling and Visualization of Cellular Protein–Lipid Interactions Using Bifunctional Fatty Acids." *Angew Chem Int Ed Engl* 52, no. 14 (2013): 4033–8.

127. Contreras, F. X., A. M. Ernst, P. Haberkant et al. "Molecular Recognition of a Single Sphingolipid Species by a Protein's Transmembrane Domain." *Nature* 481, no. 7382 (2012): 525–9.

128. Cremesti, A., F. Paris, H. Grassme et al. "Ceramide Enables Fas to Cap and Kill." *J Biol Chem* 276, no. 26 (2001): 23954–61.

129. Grassme, H., H. Schwarz, and E. Gulbins. "Molecular Mechanisms of Ceramide-Mediated CD95 Clustering." *Biochem Biophys Res Commun* 284, no. 4 (2001): 1016–30.

130. Vidalain, P. O., O. Azocar, C. Servet-Delprat et al. "CD40 Signaling in Human DCs Is Initiated within Membrane Rafts." *EMBO J* 19, no. 13 (2000): 3304–13.

131. Kaykas, A., K. Worringer, and B. Sugden. "CD40 and LMP-1 Both Signal from Lipid Rafts but LMP-1 Assembles a Distinct, More Efficient Signaling Complex." *EMBO J* 20, no. 11 (2001): 2641–54.

132. Bock, J., and E. Gulbins. "The Transmembranous Domain of CD40 Determines CD40 Partitioning into Lipid Rafts." *FEBS Lett* 534, no. 1–3 (2003): 169–74.

133. Bock, J., I. Szabo, N. Gamper, C. Adams, and E. Gulbins. "Ceramide Inhibits the Potassium Channel Kv1.3 by the Formation of Membrane Platforms." *Biochem Biophys Res Commun* 305, no. 4 (2003): 890–7.

134. Gulbins, E., I. Szabo, K. Baltzer, and F. Lang. "Ceramide-Induced Inhibition of T Lymphocyte Voltage-Gated Potassium Channel Is Mediated by Tyrosine Kinases." *Proc Natl Acad Sci U S A* 94, no. 14 (1997): 7661–6.

135. Huwiler, A., J. Brunner, R. Hummel et al. "Ceramide-Binding and Activation Defines Protein Kinase C-Raf as a Ceramide-Activated Protein Kinase." *Proc Natl Acad Sci U S A* 93, no. 14 (1996): 6959–63.

136. Bourbon, N. A., L. Sandirasegarane, and M. Kester. "Ceramide-Induced Inhibition of Akt Is Mediated through Protein Kinase Czeta: Implications for Growth Arrest." *J Biol Chem* 277, no. 5 (2002): 3286–92.

137. Ghosh, N., N. Patel, K. Jiang et al. "Ceramide-Activated Protein Phosphatase Involvement in Insulin Resistance Via Akt, Serine/Arginine-Rich Protein 40, and Ribonucleic Acid Splicing in L6 Skeletal Muscle Cells." *Endocrinology* 148, no. 3 (2007): 1359–66.

138. Canals, D., P. Roddy, and Y. A. Hannun. "Protein Phosphatase 1a Mediates Ceramide-Induced ERM Protein Dephosphorylation: A Novel Mechanism Independent of Phosphatidylinositol 4, 5-Biphosphate (PIP2) and Myosin/ERM Phosphatase." *J Biol Chem* 287, no. 13 (2012): 10145–55.
139. Gupta, N., E. Nodzenski, N. N. Khodarev et al. "Angiostatin Effects on Endothelial Cells Mediated by Ceramide and RhoA." *EMBO Rep* 2, no. 6 (2001): 536–40.
140. Church, L. D., G. Hessler, J. E. Goodall et al. "TNFR1-Induced Sphingomyelinase Activation Modulates TCR Signaling by Impairing Store-Operated Ca2+ Influx." *J Leukoc Biol* 78, no. 1 (2005): 266–78.
141. Lepple-Wienhues, A., C. Belka, T. Laun et al. "Stimulation of CD95 (Fas) Blocks T Lymphocyte Calcium Channels through Sphingomyelinase and Sphingolipids." *Proc Natl Acad Sci U S A* 96, no. 24 (1999): 13795–800.
142. Huwiler, A., B. Johansen, A. Skarstad, and J. Pfeilschifter. "Ceramide Binds to the Calb Domain of Cytosolic Phospholipase A2 and Facilitates Its Membrane Docking and Arachidonic Acid Release." *FASEB J* 15, no. 1 (2001): 7–9.
143. Yin, X., M. Zafrullah, H. Lee et al. "A Ceramide-Binding C1 Domain Mediates Kinase Suppressor of Ras Membrane Translocation." *Cell Physiol Biochem* 24, no. 3–4 (2009): 219–30.
144. Wang, G., K. Krishnamurthy, N. S. Umapathy, A. D. Verin, and E. Bieberich. "The Carboxyl-Terminal Domain of Atypical Protein Kinase Czeta Binds to Ceramide and Regulates Junction Formation in Epithelial Cells." *J Biol Chem* 284, no. 21 (2009): 14469–75.
145. Wang, G., J. Silva, K. Krishnamurthy et al. "Direct Binding to Ceramide Activates Protein Kinase Czeta before the Formation of a Pro-Apoptotic Complex with Par-4 in Differentiating Stem Cells." *J Biol Chem* 280, no. 28 (2005): 26415–24.
146. Sentelle, R. D., C. E. Senkal, W. Jiang et al. "Ceramide Targets Autophagosomes to Mitochondria and Induces Lethal Mitophagy." *Nat Chem Biol* 8, no. 10 (2012): 831–8.
147. Zafrullah, M., X. Yin, A. Haimovitz-Friedman, Z. Fuks, and R. Kolesnick. "Kinase Suppressor of Ras Transphosphorylates C-Raf-1." *Biochem Biophys Res Commun* 390, no. 3 (2009): 434–40.
148. Zhang, Y., B. Yao, S. Delikat et al. "Kinase Suppressor of Ras Is Ceramide-Activated Protein Kinase." *Cell* 89, no. 1 (1997): 63–72.
149. Zhang, H., A. Photiou, A. Grothey, J. Stebbing, and G. Giamas. "The Role of Pseudokinases in Cancer." *Cell Signal* 24, no. 6 (2012): 1173–84.
150. Hildt, E., and S. Oess. "Identification of Grb2 as a Novel Binding Partner of Tumor Necrosis Factor (TNF) Receptor I." *J Exp Med* 189, no. 11 (1999): 1707–14.
151. Bieberich, E. "Ceramide in Stem Cell Differentiation and Embryo Development: Novel Functions of a Topological Cell-Signaling Lipid and the Concept of Ceramide Compartments." *J Lipids* 2011 (2011): 610306.
152. Ganesan, V., and M. Colombini. "Regulation of Ceramide Channels by Bcl-2 Family Proteins." *FEBS Lett* 584, no. 10 (2010): 2128–34.
153. Stiban, J., L. Caputo, and M. Colombini. "Ceramide Synthesis in the Endoplasmic Reticulum Can Permeabilize Mitochondria to Proapoptotic Proteins." *J Lipid Res* 49, no. 3 (2008): 625–34.
154. Perera, M. N., V. Ganesan, L. J. Siskind et al. "Ceramide Channels: Influence of Molecular Structure on Channel Formation in Membranes." *Biochim Biophys Acta* 1818, no. 5 (2012): 1291–301.
155. Ganesan, V., M. N. Perera, D. Colombini et al. "Ceramide and Activated Bax Act Synergistically to Permeabilize the Mitochondrial Outer Membrane." *Apoptosis* 15, no. 5 (2010): 553–62.
156. Kim, H., J. Y. Mun, Y. Chun, K. Choi, and M. Kim. "Bax-Dependent Apoptosis Induced by Ceramide in HL-60 Cells." *FEBS Lett* 505, no. 2 (2001): 264–8.

157. von Haefen, C., T. Wieder, B. Gillissen et al. "Ceramide Induces Mitochondrial Activation and Apoptosis Via a Bax-Dependent Pathway in Human Carcinoma Cells." *Oncogene* 21, no. 25 (2002): 4009–19.

158. Lee, H., J. A. Rotolo, J. Mesicek et al. "Mitochondrial Ceramide-Rich Macrodomains Functionalize Bax Upon Irradiation." *PLoS One* 6, no. 6 (2011): e19783.

159. Beverly, L. J., L. A. Howell, M. Hernandez-Corbacho et al. "Bak Activation Is Necessary and Sufficient to Drive Ceramide Synthase-Dependent Ceramide Accumulation Following Inhibition of Bcl2-Like Proteins." *Biochem J* 452, no. 1 (2013): 111–9.

160. Krishnamurthy, K., G. Wang, J. Silva, B. G. Condie, and E. Bieberich. "Ceramide Regulates Atypical PKCz/l-Mediated Cell Polarity in Primitive Ectoderm Cells. A Novel Function of Sphingolipids in Morphogenesis." *J Biol Chem* 282, no. 5 (2007): 3379–90.

161. Babiychuk, E. B., K. Monastyrskaya, and A. Draeger. "Fluorescent Annexin A1 Reveals Dynamics of Ceramide Platforms in Living Cells." *Traffic* 9, no. 10 (2008): 1757–75.

162. Lasserre, R., X. J. Guo, F. Conchonaud et al. "Raft Nanodomains Contribute to Akt/PKB Plasma Membrane Recruitment and Activation." *Nat Chem Biol* 4, no. 9 (2008): 538–47.

163. Santana, P., L. A. Pena, A. Haimovitz-Friedman et al. "Acid Sphingomyelinase-Deficient Human Lymphoblasts and Mice Are Defective in Radiation-Induced Apoptosis." *Cell* 86, no. 2 (1996): 189–99.

164. Kashkar, H., K. Wiegmann, B. Yazdanpanah, D. Haubert, and M. Kronke. "Acid Sphingomyelinase Is Indispensable for UV Light-Induced Bax Conformational Change at the Mitochondrial Membrane." *J Biol Chem* 280, no. 21 (2005): 20804–13.

165. Gajate, C., E. Del Canto-Janez, A. Ulises Acuna et al. "Intracellular Triggering of Fas Aggregation and Recruitment of Apoptotic Molecules into Fas-Enriched Rafts in Selective Tumor Cell Apoptosis." *J Exp Med* 200, no. 3 (2004): 353–65.

166. Gajate, C., and F. Mollinedo. "Edelfosine and Perifosine Induce Selective Apoptosis in Multiple Myeloma by Recruitment of Death Receptors and Downstream Signaling Molecules into Lipid Rafts." *Blood* 109, no. 2 (2007): 711–9.

167. Zhu, Q. Y., Z. Wang, C. Ji et al. "C6-Ceramide Synergistically Potentiates the Anti-Tumor Effects of Histone Deacetylase Inhibitors Via Akt Dephosphorylation and a-Tubulin Hyperacetylation Both In Vitro and In Vivo." *Cell Death Dis* 2 (2011): e117.

168. Kim, S. W., H. J. Kim, Y. J. Chun, and M. Y. Kim. "Ceramide Produces Apoptosis through Induction of p27(Kip1) by Protein Phosphatase 2a-Dependent Akt Dephosphorylation in PC-3 Prostate Cancer Cells." *J Toxicol Environ Health A* 73, no. 21–2 (2010): 1465–76.

169. Fox, T. E., K. L. Houck, S. M. O'Neill et al. "Ceramide Recruits and Activates Protein Kinase C zeta (PKC zeta) within Structured Membrane Microdomains." *J Biol Chem* 282, no. 17 (2007): 12450–7.

170. Blouin, C. M., C. Prado, K. K. Takane et al. "Plasma Membrane Subdomain Compartmentalization Contributes to Distinct Mechanisms of Ceramide Action on Insulin Signaling." *Diabetes* 59, no. 3 (2010): 600–10.

171. Hajduch, E., S. Turban, X. Le Liepvre et al. "Targeting of PKCzeta and PKB to Caveolin-Enriched Microdomains Represents a Crucial Step Underpinning the Disruption in PKB-Directed Signalling by Ceramide." *Biochem J* 410, no. 2 (2008): 369–79.

172. Scarlatti, F., C. Bauvy, A. Ventruti et al. "Ceramide-Mediated Macroautophagy Involves Inhibition of Protein Kinase B and Up-Regulation of Beclin 1." *J Biol Chem* 279, no. 18 (2004): 18384–91.

173. Pattingre, S., C. Bauvy, S. Carpentier et al. "Role of JNK1-Dependent Bcl-2 Phosphorylation in Ceramide-Induced Macroautophagy." *J Biol Chem* 284, no. 5 (2009): 2719–28.

174. Canals, D., R. W. Jenkins, P. Roddy et al. "Differential Effects of Ceramide and Sphingosine 1-Phosphate on ERM Phosphorylation: Probing Sphingolipid Signaling at the Outer Plasma Membrane." *J Biol Chem* 285, no. 42 (2010): 32476–85.

175. Fehon, R. G., A. I. McClatchey, and A. Bretscher. "Organizing the Cell Cortex: The Role of ERM Proteins." *Nat Rev Mol Cell Biol* 11, no. 4 (2010): 276–87.

176. Neisch, A. L., and R. G. Fehon. "ERM: Key Regulators of Membrane-Cortex Interactions and Signaling." *Curr Opin Cell Biol* 23, no. 4 (2011): 377–82.

177. Faure, S., L. I. Salazar-Fontana, M. Semichon et al. "ERM Proteins Regulate Cytoskeleton Relaxation Promoting T Cell-APC Conjugation." *Nat Immunol* 5, no. 3 (2004): 272–9.

178. Takeuchi, K., N. Sato, H. Kasahara et al. "Perturbation of Cell Adhesion and Microvilli Formation by Antisense Oligonucleotides to ERM Family Members." *J Cell Biol* 125, no. 6 (1994): 1371–84.

179. Bonilha, V. L., S. C. Finnemann, and E. Rodriguez-Boulan. "Ezrin Promotes Morphogenesis of Apical Microvilli and Basal Infoldings in Retinal Pigment Epithelium." *J Cell Biol* 147, no. 7 (1999): 1533–48.

180. Gajate, C., and F. Mollinedo. "Cytoskeleton-Mediated Death Receptor and Ligand Concentration in Lipid Rafts Forms Apoptosis-Promoting Clusters in Cancer Chemotherapy." *J Biol Chem* 280, no. 12 (2005): 11641–7.

181. Nelson, J. B., S. P. O'Hara, A. J. Small et al. "Cryptosporidium Parvum Infects Human Cholangiocytes Via Sphingolipid-Enriched Membrane Microdomains." *Cell Microbiol* 8, no. 12 (2006): 1932–45.

182. Montfort, A., B. de Badts, V. Douin-Echinard et al. "FAN Stimulates TNF(Alpha)-Induced Gene Expression, Leukocyte Recruitment, and Humoral Response." *J Immunol* 183, no. 8 (2009): 5369–78.

183. Montfort, A., P. G. Martin, T. Levade, H. Benoist, and B. Segui. "FAN (Factor Associated with Neutral Sphingomyelinase Activation), a Moonlighting Protein in TNF-R1 Signaling." *J Leukoc Biol* 88, no. 5 (2010): 897–903.

184. Haubert, D., N. Gharib, F. Rivero et al. "Ptdins(4, 5)P-Restricted Plasma Membrane Localization of FAN Is Involved in TNF-Induced Actin Reorganization." *EMBO J* 26, no. 14 (2007): 3308–21.

185. Kim, S. S., H.-S. Chae, J.-H. Bach et al. "P53 Mediates Ceramide-Induced Apoptosis in Skn-Sh Cells." *Oncogene* 21, no. 13 (2002): 2020–8.

186. Smith, E. L., and E. H. Schuchman. "The Unexpected Role of Acid Sphingomyelinase in Cell Death and the Pathophysiology of Common Diseases." *FASEB J* 22, no. 10 (2008): 3419–31.

187. Paris, F., Z. Fuks, A. Kang et al. "Endothelial Apoptosis as the Primary Lesion Initiating Intestinal Radiation Damage in Mice." *Science (New York, N Y)* 293, no. 5528 (2001): 293–7.

188. Shirakabe, K., K. Yamaguchi, H. Shibuya et al. "Tak1 Mediates the Ceramide Signaling to Stress-Activated Protein Kinase/C-Jun N-Terminal Kinase." *J Biol Chem* 272, no. 13 (1997): 8141–4.

189. Brenner, B., U. Koppenhoefer, C. Weinstock et al. "Fas- or Ceramide-Induced Apoptosis Is Mediated by a Rac1-Regulated Activation of Jun N-Terminal Kinase/P38 Kinases and GADD153." *J Biol Chem* 272, no. 35 (1997): 22173–81.

190. Verheij, M., R. Bose, X. H. Lin et al. "Requirement for Ceramide-Initiated Sapk/Jnk Signalling in Stress-Induced Apoptosis." *Nature* 380, no. 6569 (1996): 75–9.

191. Procyk, K. J., M. R. Rippo, R. Testi et al. "Distinct Mechanisms Target Stress and Extracellular Signal-Activated Kinase 1 and Jun N-Terminal Kinase During Infection of Macrophages with Salmonella." *J Immunol* 163, no. 9 (1999): 4924–30.

192. Wang, Y. M., M. L. Seibenhener, M. L. Vandenplas, and M. W. Wooten. "Atypical PKC zeta Is Activated by Ceramide, Resulting in Coactivation of NF-kappaB/JNK Kinase and Cell Survival." *J Neurosc Res* 55, no. 3 (1999): 293–302.

193. Zumbansen, M., and W. Stoffel. "Tumor Necrosis Factor Alpha Activates NF-kappaB in Acid Sphingomyelinase-Deficient Mouse Embryonic Fibroblasts." *J Biol Chem* 272, no. 16 (1997): 10904–9.

194. Katsuyama, K., M. Shichiri, F. Marumo, and Y. Hirata. "Role of NF-kappaB Activation in Cytokine- and Sphingomyelinase-Stimulated Inducible Nitric Oxide Synthase Gene Expression in Vascular Smooth Muscle Cells." *Endocrinology* 139, no. 11 (1998): 4506–12.

195. Chen, B.-C., H.-M. Chang, M.-J. Hsu et al. "Peptidoglycan Induces Cyclooxygenase-2 Expression in Macrophages by Activating the Neutral Sphingomyelinase-Ceramide Pathway." *J Biol Chem* 284, no. 31 (2009): 20562–73.

196. Chen, C. C., Y. T. Sun, J. J. Chen, and Y. J. Chang. "Tumor Necrosis Factor-Alpha-Induced Cyclooxygenase-2 Expression Via Sequential Activation of Ceramide-Dependent Mitogen-Activated Protein Kinases, and IkappaB Kinase 1/2 in Human Alveolar Epithelial Cells." *Mol Pharmacol* 59, no. 3 (2001): 493–500.

197. Colell, A., O. Coll, M. Mari, J. C. Fernandez-Checa, and C. Garcia-Ruiz. "Divergent Role of Ceramide Generated by Exogenous Sphingomyelinases on NF-kappaB Activation and Apoptosis in Human Colon Ht-29 Cells." *FEBS Lett* 526, no. 1–3 (2002): 15–20.

198. Machleidt, T., K. Wiegmann, T. Henkel et al. "Sphingomyelinase Activates Proteolytic I Kappa B-Alpha Degradation in a Cell-Free System." *J Biol Chem* 269, no. 19 (1994): 13760–5.

199. Signorelli, P., C. Luberto, and Y. A. Hannun. "Ceramide Inhibition of NF-kappaB Activation Involves Reverse Translocation of Classical Protein Kinase C (PKC) Isoenzymes: Requirement for Kinase Activity and Carboxyl-Terminal Phosphorylation of PKC for the Ceramide Response." *FASEB J* 15, no. 13 (2001): 2401–14.

200. Abboushi, N., A. El-Hed, W. El-Assaad et al. "Ceramide Inhibits Il-2 Production by Preventing Protein Kinase C-Dependent NF-kappaB Activation: Possible Role in Protein Kinase Ctheta Regulation." *J Immunol* 173, no. 5 (2004): 3193–200.

201. Alayoubi, A. M., J. C. Wang, B. C. Au, S. Carpentier, V. Garcia, S. Dworski et al. "Systemic Ceramide Accumulation Leads to Severe and Varied Pathological Consequences." *EMBO Mol Med* 5, no. 6 (2013): 827–42.

202. Gulbins, E., M. Palmada, M. Reichel, A. Lüth, C. Böhmer, D. Amato et al. "Acid sphingomyelinase-Ceramide System Mediates Effects of Antidepressant Drugs." *Nat Med* 19, no. 7 (2013): 934–8.

203. Dhami, R., and E. H. Schuchman. "Mannose 6-Phosphate Receptor-Mediated Uptake Is Defective in Acid Sphingomyelinase-Deficient Macrophages: Implications for Niemann-Pick Disease Enzyme Replacement Therapy." *J Biol Chem* 279, no. 2 (2004): 1526–32.

204. Esen, M., B. Schreiner, V. Jendrossek et al. "Mechanisms of *S. Aureus* Induced Apoptosis of Human Endothelial Cells." *Apoptosis* 6, no. 6 (2001): 431–9.

205. Hanada, K., N. M. Palacpac, P. A. Magistrado et al. "Plasmodium Falciparum Phospholipase C Hydrolyzing Sphingomyelin and Lysocholinephospholipids Is a Possible Target for Malaria Chemotherapy." *J Exp Med* 195, no. 1 (2002): 23–34.

206. Brand, V., S. Koka, C. Lang et al. "Influence of Amitriptyline on Eryptosis, Parasitemia and Survival of Plasmodium Berghei-Infected Mice." *Cell Physiol Biochem* 22, no. 5–6 (2008): 405–12.

207. Majumder, S., R. Dey, S. Bhattacharjee et al. "Leishmania-Induced Biphasic Ceramide Generation in Macrophages Is Crucial for Uptake and Survival of the Parasite." *J Infect Dis* 205, no. 10 (2012): 1607–16.

208. Cosset, F. L., and D. Lavillette. "Cell Entry of Enveloped Viruses." *Adv Genet* 73 (2011): 121–83.

209. Hammache, D., N. Yahi, G. Pieroni et al. "Sequential Interaction of CD4 and HIV-1 gp120 with a Reconstituted Membrane Patch of Ganglioside GM3: Implications for the Role of Glycolipids as Potential HIV-1 Fusion Cofactors." *Biochem Biophys Res Commun* 246, no. 1 (1998): 117–22.

210. Lingwood, D., B. Binnington, T. Rog et al. "Cholesterol Modulates Glycolipid Conformation and Receptor Activity." *Nat Chem Biol* 7, no. 5 (2011): 260–2.

211. Puri, A., S. Rawat, H. Lin et al. "An Inhibitor of Glycosphingolipid Metabolism Blocks HIV-1 Infection of Primary T-Cells." *AIDS* 18, no. 6 (2004): 849–58.
212. Rawat, S. S., S. A. Gallo, J. Eaton et al. "Elevated Expression of GM3 in Receptor-Bearing Targets Confers Resistance to HIV-1 Fusion." *J Virol* 78, no. 14 (2004): 7360–8.
213. Mahfoud, R., A. Manis, and C. A. Lingwood. "Fatty Acid-Dependent Globotriaosyl Ceramide Receptor Function in Detergent Resistant Model Membranes." *J Lipid Res* 50, no. 9 (2009): 1744–55.
214. Lingwood, C. A., B. Binnington, A. Manis, and D. R. Branch. "Globotriaosyl Ceramide Receptor Function—Where Membrane Structure and Pathology Intersect." *FEBS Lett* 584, no. 9 (2010): 1879–86.
215. Hammache, D., G. Pieroni, N. Yahi et al. "Specific Interaction of HIV-1 and HIV-2 Surface Envelope Glycoproteins with Monolayers of Galactosylceramide and Ganglioside GM3." *J Biol Chem* 273, no. 14 (1998): 7967–71.
216. Cook, D. G., J. Fantini, S. L. Spitalnik, and F. Gonzalez-Scarano. "Binding of Human Immunodeficiency Virus Type I (HIV-1) gp120 to Galactosylceramide (GalCer): Relationship to the V3 Loop." *Virology* 201, no. 2 (1994): 206–14.
217. Lund, N., D. R. Branch, M. Mylvaganam et al. "A Novel Soluble Mimic of the Glycolipid, Globotriaosyl Ceramide Inhibits HIV Infection." *AIDS* 20, no. 3 (2006): 333–43.
218. Lund, N., D. R. Branch, D. Sakac et al. "Lack of Susceptibility of Cells from Patients with Fabry Disease to Productive Infection with R5 Human Immunodeficiency Virus." *AIDS* 19, no. 14 (2005): 1543–6.
219. Ramkumar, S., D. Sakac, B. Binnington, D. R. Branch, and C. A. Lingwood. "Induction of HIV-1 Resistance: Cell Susceptibility to Infection Is an Inverse Function of Globotriaosyl Ceramide Levels." *Glycobiology* 19, no. 1 (2009): 76–82.
220. Alfsen, A., and M. Bomsel. "HIV-1 gp41 Envelope Residues 650–685 Exposed on Native Virus Act as a Lectin to Bind Epithelial Cell Galactosyl Ceramide." *J Biol Chem* 277, no. 28 (2002): 25649–59.
221. Yu, H., A. Alfsen, D. Tudor, and M. Bomsel. "The Binding of HIV-1 gp41 Membrane Proximal Domain to Its Mucosal Receptor, Galactosyl Ceramide, Is Structure-Dependent." *Cell Calcium* 43, no. 1 (2008): 73–82.
222. Dorosko, S. M., and R. I. Connor. "Primary Human Mammary Epithelial Cells Endocytose HIV-1 and Facilitate Viral Infection of CD4+ T Lymphocytes." *J Virol* 84, no. 20 (2010): 10533–42.
223. Magerus-Chatinet, A., H. Yu, S. Garcia et al. "Galactosyl Ceramide Expressed on Dendritic Cells Can Mediate HIV-1 Transfer from Monocyte Derived Dendritic Cells to Autologous T Cells." *Virology* 362, no. 1 (2007): 67–74.
224. Finnegan, C., S. Rawat, E. Cho et al. "Sphingomyelinase Restricts the Lateral Diffusion of CD4 and Inhibits HIV Fusion." *J Virol* 81, no. 10 (2007): 5294–304.
225. Finnegan, C. M., S. S. Rawat, A. Puri et al. "Ceramide, a Target for Antiretroviral Therapy." *Proc Natl Acad Sci U S A* 101, no. 43 (2004): 15452–7.
226. Rawat, S. S., C. Zimmerman, B. T. Johnson et al. "Restricted Lateral Mobility of Plasma Membrane Cd4 Impairs HIV-1 Envelope Glycoprotein Mediated Fusion." *Mol Membr Biol* 25, no. 1 (2008): 83–94.
227. Vieira, C. R., J. M. Munoz-Olaya, J. Sot et al. "Dihydrosphingomyelin Impairs HIV-1 Infection by Rigidifying Liquid-Ordered Membrane Domains." *Chem Biol* 17, no. 7 (2010): 766–75.
228. Voisset, C., M. Lavie, F. Helle et al. "Ceramide Enrichment of the Plasma Membrane Induces CD81 Internalization and Inhibits Hepatitis C Virus Entry." *Cell Microbiol* 10, no. 3 (2008): 606–17.
229. Carette, J. E., M. Raaben, A. C. Wong et al. "Ebola Virus Entry Requires the Cholesterol Transporter Niemann-Pick C1." *Nature* 477, no. 7364 (2011): 340–3.

230. Cote, M., J. Misasi, T. Ren et al. "Small Molecule Inhibitors Reveal Niemann-Pick C1 Is Essential for Ebola Virus Infection." *Nature* 477, no. 7364 (2011): 344–8.

231. Miller, E. H., G. Obernosterer, M. Raaben et al. "Ebola Virus Entry Requires the Host-Programmed Recognition of an Intracellular Receptor." *EMBO J* 31, no. 8 (2012): 1947–60.

232. Blanchet, F., A. Moris, J. P. Mitchell, and V. Piguet. "A Look at HIV Journey: From Dendritic Cells to Infection Spread in CD4+ T Cells." *Curr Opin HIV AIDS* 6, no. 5 (2011): 391–7.

233. Izquierdo-Useros, N., M. Naranjo-Gomez, J. Archer et al. "Capture and Transfer of HIV-1 Particles by Mature Dendritic Cells Converges with the Exosome-Dissemination Pathway." *Blood* 113, no. 12 (2009): 2732–41.

234. Izquierdo-Useros, N., M. Naranjo-Gomez, I. Erkizia et al. "HIV and Mature Dendritic Cells: Trojan Exosomes Riding the Trojan Horse?" *PLoS Pathog* 6, no. 3 (2010): e1000740.

235. Geijtenbeek, T. B., and S. I. Gringhuis. "Signalling through C-Type Lectin Receptors: Shaping Immune Responses." *Nat Rev Immunol* 9, no. 7 (2009): 465–79.

236. Gringhuis, S. I., J. den Dunnen, M. Litjens, M. van der Vlist, and T. B. Geijtenbeek. "Carbohydrate-Specific Signaling through the DC-SIGN Signalosome Tailors Immunity to Mycobacterium Tuberculosis, HIV-1 and Helicobacter Pylori." *Nat Immunol* 10, no. 10 (2009): 1081–8.

237. Brugger, B., B. Glass, P. Haberkant et al. "The HIV Lipidome: A Raft with an Unusual Composition." *Proc Natl Acad Sci U S A* 103, no. 8 (2006): 2641–6.

238. Merz, A., G. Long, M. S. Hiet et al. "Biochemical and Morphological Properties of Hepatitis C Virus Particles and Determination of Their Lipidome." *J Biol Chem* 286, no. 4 (2011): 3018–32.

239. Liu, S. T., R. Sharon-Friling, P. Ivanova et al. "Synaptic Vesicle-Like Lipidome of Human Cytomegalovirus Virions Reveals a Role for SNARE Machinery in Virion Egress." *Proc Natl Acad Sci U S A* 108, no. 31 (2011): 12869–74.

240. Lorizate, M., T. Sachsenheimer, B. Glass et al. "Comparative Lipidomics Analysis of HIV-1 Particles and Their Producer Cell Membrane in Different Cell Lines." *Cell Microbiol* 15, no. 2 (2013): 292–304.

241. Sundquist, W. I., and H. G. Krausslich. "HIV-1 Assembly, Budding, and Maturation." *Cold Spring Harb Perspect Med* 2, no. 7 (2012): a006924.

242. Tafesse, F. G., S. Sanyal, J. Ashour et al. "Intact Sphingomyelin Biosynthetic Pathway Is Essential for Intracellular Transport of Influenza Virus Glycoproteins." *Proc Natl Acad Sci U S A* 110, no. 16 (2013): 6406–11.

243. Teichgraber, V., M. Ulrich, N. Endlich et al. "Ceramide Accumulation Mediates Inflammation, Cell Death and Infection Susceptibility in Cystic Fibrosis." *Nat Med* 14, no. 4 (2008): 382–91.

244. Gulbins, E., S. Dreschers, B. Wilker, and H. Grassme. "Ceramide, Membrane Rafts and Infections." *J Mol Med* 82, no. 6 (2004): 357–63.

245. Gulbins, E., and R. Kolesnick. "Raft Ceramide in Molecular Medicine." *Oncogene* 22, no. 45 (2003): 7070–7.

246. Schamel, W. W., I. Arechaga, R. M. Risueno et al. "Coexistence of Multivalent and Monovalent TCRs Explains High Sensitivity and Wide Range of Response." *J Exp Med* 202, no. 4 (2005): 493–503.

247. Sherman, E., V. Barr, S. Manley et al. "Functional Nanoscale Organization of Signaling Molecules Downstream of the T Cell Antigen Receptor." *Immunity* 35, no. 5 (2011): 705–20.

248. Williamson, D. J., D. M. Owen, J. Rossy et al. "Pre-Existing Clusters of the Adaptor LAT Do Not Participate in Early T Cell Signaling Events." *Nat Immunol* 12, no. 7 (2011): 655–62.

249. Kumar, R., M. Ferez, M. Swamy et al. "Increased Sensitivity of Antigen-Experienced T Cells through the Enrichment of Oligomeric T Cell Receptor Complexes." *Immunity* 35, no. 3 (2011): 375–87.

250. Tani-ichi, S., K. Maruyama, N. Kondo et al. "Structure and Function of Lipid Rafts in Human Activated T Cells." *Int Immunol* 17, no. 6 (2005): 749–58.

251. Molnar, E., M. Swamy, M. Holzer et al. "Cholesterol and Sphingomyelin Drive Ligand-Independent T-Cell Antigen Receptor Nanoclustering." *J Biol Chem* 287, no. 51 (2012): 42664–74.

252. Rossy, J., D. J. Williamson, C. Benzing, and K. Gaus. "The Integration of Signaling and the Spatial Organization of the T Cell Synapse." *Front Immunol* 3 (2012): 352.

253. Tonnetti, L., M. C. Veri, E. Bonvini, and L. D'Adamio. "A Role for Neutral Sphingomyelinase-Mediated Ceramide Production in T Cell Receptor-Induced Apoptosis and Mitogen-Activated Protein Kinase-Mediated Signal Transduction." *J Exp Med* 189, no. 10 (1999): 1581–9.

254. Edmead, C. E., Y. I. Patel, A. Wilson et al. "Induction of Activator Protein (Ap)-1 and NF-KappaB by CD28 Stimulation Involves Both Phosphatidylinositol 3-Kinase and Acidic Sphingomyelinase Signals." *J Immunol* 157, no. 8 (1996): 3290–7.

255. Chan, G., and A. Ochi. "Sphingomyelin-Ceramide Turnover in CD28 Costimulatory Signaling." *Eur J Immunol* 25, no. 7 (1995): 1999–2004.

256. Chentouf, M., M. Rigo, S. Ghannam et al. "The Lipid-Modulating Effects of a CD4-Specific Recombinant Antibody Correlate with Zap-70 Segregation Outside Membrane Rafts." *Immunol Lett* 133, no. 2 (2010): 62–9.

257. Koppenhoefer, U., B. Brenner, F. Lang, and E. Gulbins. "The CD40-Ligand Stimulates T-Lymphocytes Via the Neutral Sphingomyelinase: A Novel Function of the CD40-Ligand as Signalling Molecule." *FEBS Lett* 414, no. 2 (1997): 444–8.

258. Brenner, B., H. U. Grassme, C. Muller et al. "L-Selectin Stimulates the Neutral Sphingomyelinase and Induces Release of Ceramide." *Exp Cell Res* 243, no. 1 (1998): 123–8.

259. Abdel Shakor, A. B., M. M. Atia, K. Kwiatkowska, and A. Sobota. "Cell Surface Ceramide Controls Translocation of Transferrin Receptor to Clathrin-Coated Pits." *Cell Signal* 24, no. 3 (2012): 677–84.

260. Ni, H. T., M. J. Deeths, W. Li, D. L. Mueller, and M. F. Mescher. "Signaling Pathways Activated by Leukocyte Function-Associated Ag-1-Dependent Costimulation." *J Immunol* 162, no. 9 (1999): 5183–9.

261. O'Byrne, D., and D. Sansom. "Lack of Costimulation by Both Sphingomyelinase and C2 Ceramide in Resting Human T Cells." *Immunology* 100, no. 2 (2000): 225–30.

262. Stoffel, B., P. Bauer, M. Nix, K. Deres, and W. Stoffel. "Ceramide-Independent CD28 and TCR Signaling but Reduced Il-2 Secretion in T Cells of Acid Sphingomyelinase-Deficient Mice." *Eur J Immunol* 28, no. 3 (1998): 874–80.

263. Diaz, O., S. Mebarek-Azzam, A. Benzaria et al. "Disruption of Lipid Rafts Stimulates Phospholipase D Activity in Human Lymphocytes: Implication in the Regulation of Immune Function." *J Immunol* 175, no. 12 (2005): 8077–86.

264. Rouquette-Jazdanian, A. K., C. Pelassy, J. P. Breittmayer, and C. Aussel. "Full CD3/TCR Activation through Cholesterol-Depleted Lipid Rafts." *Cell Signal* 19, no. 7 (2007): 1404–18.

265. Rouquette-Jazdanian, A. K., A. Foussat, L. Lamy et al. "Cholera Toxin B-Subunit Prevents Activation and Proliferation of Human CD4+ T Cells by Activation of a Neutral Sphingomyelinase in Lipid Rafts." *J Immunol* 175, no. 9 (2005): 5637–48.

266. Howie, D., M. Simarro, J. Sayos et al. "Molecular Dissection of the Signaling and Costimulatory Functions of CD150 (SLAM): CD150/Sap Binding and CD150-Mediated Costimulation." *Blood* 99, no. 3 (2002): 957–65.

267. Strauss, G., J. A. Lindquist, N. Arhel et al. "CD95 Co-Stimulation Blocks Activation of Naive T Cells by Inhibiting TCR Signaling." *J Exp Med* 206, no. 6 (2009): 1379–93.

268. Russell, M., M. Iskandar, O. Mykytczuk et al. "A Reduced Antigen Load In Vivo, Rather Than Weak Inflammation, Causes a Substantial Delay in CD8+ T Cell Priming against *M. Bovis* (Bacillus Calmette-Guerin)." *J Immunol* 179, no. 1 (2007): 211–20.

269. Anes, E., M. P. Kuhnel, E. Bos et al. "Selected Lipids Activate Phagosome Actin Assembly and Maturation Resulting in Killing of Pathogenic Mycobacteria." *Nat Cell Biol* 5, no. 9 (2003): 793–802.

270. Utermohlen, O., U. Karow, J. Lohler, and M. Kronke. "Severe Impairment in Early Host Defense against Listeria Monocytogenes in Mice Deficient in Acid Sphingomyelinase." *J Immunol* 170, no. 5 (2003): 2621–8.

271. Zhang, A. Y., F. Yi, S. Jin et al. "Acid Sphingomyelinase and Its Redox Amplification in Formation of Lipid Raft Redox Signaling Platforms in Endothelial Cells." *Antioxid Redox Signal* 9, no. 7 (2007): 817–28.

272. Xuan, N. T., E. Shumilina, D. S. Kempe, E. Gulbins, and F. Lang. "Sphingomyelinase Dependent Apoptosis of Dendritic Cells Following Treatment with Amyloid Peptides." *J Neuroimmunol* 219, no. 1–2 (2010): 81–9.

273. Falcone, S., C. Perrotta, C. De Palma et al. "Activation of Acid Sphingomyelinase and Its Inhibition by the Nitric Oxide/Cyclic Guanosine 3',5'-Monophosphate Pathway: Key Events in Escherichia Coli-Elicited Apoptosis of Dendritic Cells." *J Immunol* 173, no. 7 (2004): 4452–63.

274. Franchi, L., F. Malisan, B. Tomassini, and R. Testi. "Ceramide Catabolism Critically Controls Survival of Human DCs." *J Leukoc Biol* 79, no. 1 (2006): 166–72.

275. Sallusto, F., C. Nicolo, R. De Maria, S. Corinti, and R. Testi. "Ceramide Inhibits Antigen Uptake and Presentation by DCs." *J Exp Med* 184, no. 6 (1996): 2411–6.

8 Domains of Phosphoinositides in the Plasma Membrane

Geert van den Bogaart and Martin ter Beest

CONTENTS

8.1 SYNOPSIS

Inositol phospholipids are a class of lipids characterized by the presence of a *myo*-inositol monosaccharide moiety in the headgroup. In addition to the phosphate group that connects this inositol ring at the 1-position to the diacylglycerol (DAG) backbone of the lipid, the inositol ring can be phosphorylated at positions 3, 4, and 5 (Figure 8.1).

This gives rise to a total of seven possible phosphoinositides that are all present in eukaryotic cells: phosphatidylinositol 3-phosphate [PI(3)P], phosphatidylinositol 4-phosphate [PI(4)P], phosphatidylinositol 5-phosphate [PI(5)P], phosphatidylinositol 3,4-bisphosphate [PI(3,4)P$_2$], phosphatidylinositol 4,5-bisphosphate [PI(4,5)P$_2$], phosphatidylinositol 3,5-bisphosphate [PI(3,5)P$_2$], and phosphatidylinositol 3,4,5-trisphosphate [PI(3,4,5)P$_3$]. Phosphoinositides are commonly believed to be only present in the cytoplasmic leaflets of organellar membranes and, although they constitute only a small fraction of the total pool of cellular lipids (see Figure 8.2 for the composition of the plasma membrane), they are involved in a plethora of cellular functions. In fact, as stated in a recent review (Balla et al. 2009): "it might be easier at this time to list the processes that are not regulated by inositides in a eukaryotic cell than those that are clearly inositide dependent." Dysregulation of cellular phosphoinositide levels has been related to a wide variety of diseases and disorders, such as cardiovascular diseases (reviewed by Ghigo et al. 2012), diabetes (reviewed by Bridges and Saltiel 2012), cancer (reviewed by Bunney and Katan 2010), and neuronal disorders and diseases (reviewed by Wen et al. 2011). It is therefore not surprising that the

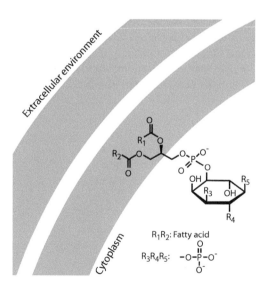

FIGURE 8.1 Structure and orientation of PI(3,4,5)P$_3$ in the plasma membrane. If all phosphate groups are completely deprotonated (as shown), the total charge of PI(3,4,5)P$_3$ would be −7. For PI(4,5)P$_2$, the PI of the hydroxyl groups of the 4′ and 5′ phosphates has been estimated at 6.7 and 7.7, respectively; see McLaughlin et al. (2002) for a discussion of the charge of phosphoinositides.

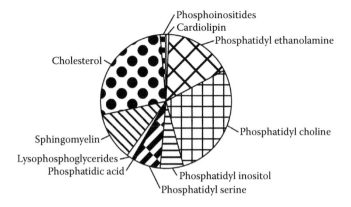

FIGURE 8.2 Lipid membrane composition of the plasma membrane of cells isolated from rat liver. (Data from Daum, G., *Biochim. Biophys. Acta.*, 822, 1–42, 1985.)

database of scientific publications *PubMed* currently lists tens of thousands of papers on the subject of phosphoinositides. In this chapter, we provide an overview of the functions of phosphoinositides in the plasma membrane and focus on their localization in membrane gradients as well as discrete membrane domains.

8.2 PHOSPHOINOSITIDES IN THE PLASMA MEMBRANE

The earliest discovered (Grado and Ballou 1960) phosphoinositides, PI(4,5)P$_2$ and PI(4)P, are generally considered the most abundant phosphoinositides in the plasma membrane. It is estimated that the plasma membrane contains approximately 1% to 1.5% of PI(4,5)P$_2$ (Ferrell and Huestis 1984; Hagelberg and Allan 1990; Mitchell et al. 1986), which would translate to approximately 5000 to 10,000 molecules/μm^2 plasma membrane (or 10,000 to 20,000 molecules/μm^2 in the inner leaflet) (Suh and Hille 2008). Phosphoinositides are often quantified by metabolic labeling of cells with radioisotopes (^{32}[P]-ATP or ^{3}[H]-inositol) followed by extraction and purification of the lipids with chromatic columns (thin layer chromatography or high-pressure liquid chromatography) and finally quantification of the radioactivity by scintillation counting (Christie and Han 2010). Table 8.1 lists estimated fractions of the various phosphoinositides in the plasma membrane that are primarily obtained with this technique. These phosphoinositide concentrations need to be interpreted with caution for the following reasons.

First, the accuracy of quantitative phosphoinositide determinations is usually limited by the low abundance and high charges of phosphoinositides that hinder a quantitative extraction from cells and the acid that is required for solubilization of phosphoinositides may lead to hydrolysis of the phosphate groups (Christie and Han 2010; Clark et al. 2011). As a consequence of these technical limitations, pools of low abundant phosphoinositides may go undetected. In order to overcome some of these problems, more sensitive approaches based on phosphate methylation coupled

TABLE 8.1

Estimated Concentrations of Phosphoinositides in the Plasma Membrane

	% of PM Lipid	Lipid per μm^{2a}	Total in PM^b
$PI(4,5)P_2$	$0.9–1.6^{c,d}$	$1.3–2.2 \times 10^4$	$0.6–1.0 \times 10^7$
$PI(4)P$	$0.6–1.2^{c,d}$	$0.8–1.7 \times 10^4$	$3.8–7.7 \times 10^6$
$PI(3)P$	$0.03^d–0.075^e$	$0.4–1.0 \times 10^3$	$1.9–4.8 \times 10^5$
$PI(5)P$	0.03^f	4.2×10^2	1.9×10^5
$PI(3,4)P_2$	0.003^d	4.2×10^1	1.9×10^4
$PI(3,4,5)P_3$	$0.001^d–0.002^g$	$1.4–2.8 \times 10^1$	$0.6–1.3 \times 10^4$
$PI(3,5)P_2$	0^h	0	0

[a] Assuming an average area per lipid of 72 Å^2 (Tristram-Nagle and Nagle 2004; see also Suh and Hille 2008).

[b] Assuming a total surface area of the plasma membrane of 460 μm^2, as determined for PC12 cells (Sieber et al. 2007).

[c] Data for erythrocytes (Ferrell and Huestis 1984; Hagelberg and Allan 1990; Mitchell et al. 1986).

[d] Data from unactivated neutrophils (Stephens et al. 1993) and converted to percentage of total phospholipids by assuming a density of the plasma membrane of 1 g ml^{-1}, an average molecular weight for a phospholipid of 750, and a phospholipid content of 50%. By following these assumptions, the values for $PI(4,5)P_2$ and $PI(4)P$ are comparable to those of erythrocytes.

[e] Assuming PI(3)P is 5% of $PI(4,5)P_2$ as shown for fibroblasts in Rameh et al. (1997).

[f] Assuming PI(5)P is 2% of $PI(4,5)P_2$ as shown for fibroblasts in Rameh et al. (1997).

[g] From Clark et al. (2011) for unactivated neutrophils.

[h] See Section 8.2.6 for details.

to high-performance liquid chromatography and mass spectrometry have recently been developed (Clark et al. 2011).

Second, quantitative data on phosphoinositides are still scarce and are only available for a small number of cell types and not all studies differentiate between cellular organelles (e.g., Pettitt et al. 2006). The concentration of phosphoinositides in the plasma membrane is best characterized for erythrocytes (e.g., Ferrell and Huestis 1984; Hagelberg and Allan 1990; Mitchell et al. 1986). Erythrocytes are a convenient system because they lack a nucleus and most organelles, which bypass the need for subsequent plasma membrane purification steps. However, because erythrocytes are terminally differentiated cells with no Golgi complex and little synthesis of new proteins, they have unusual trafficking requirements and may not be considered "typical" eukaryotic cells. Nevertheless, the scarce quantitative studies on cell types other than erythrocytes (primarily neutrophils) show a similar PI(4)P and $PI(4,5)P_2$ content in the plasma membrane compared to erythrocytes.

Third, reports of average concentrations of phosphoinositides in resting cells often do not take into account that the concentrations of particular phosphoinositides in the plasma membrane can differ by orders of magnitude during the lifetime of a cell, especially upon the triggering of cellular signaling events (see Sections 8.2.4 and 8.2.5) (Clark et al. 2011; Stephens et al. 1991).

Finally, when considering average concentrations of phosphoinositides, known clustering of phosphoinositides in membrane gradients and domains needs to be taken into account. The enrichment of phosphoinositides in membrane domains can lead to local surface concentrations that can easily reach up to three orders of magnitude higher compared to a uniform distribution of the lipids (McLaughlin et al. 2002), as further discussed in Sections 8.3 and 8.4.

8.2.1 PI(4,5)P$_2$

As already mentioned above, PI(4,5)P$_2$ is the most abundant phosphoinositide in the plasma membrane (Table 8.1). The first and best described function of plasma membrane pools of PI(4,5)P$_2$ is as a precursor to the second messengers DAG and inositol 1,4,5-triphosphate (IP$_3$) (Berridge 1983; Creba et al. 1983). Here, activation of various forms of phospholipase C by, for instance, Ca^{2+}-mobilizing hormones (e.g., vasopressin, angiotensin, adrenalin) results in cleavage of PI(4,5)P$_2$ (and possibly of PI(4)P; see Section 8.5) and the formation of DAG and IP$_3$. IP$_3$ is a soluble second messenger and (among other functions) results in release of intracellular calcium pools. DAG remains associated to the membrane and (among other functions) activates protein kinase C, which triggers a wide range of cellular events (see Vines 2012 for a recent review of phospholipase C activity). Another early discovered (Auger et al. 1989; Stephens et al. 1991) function of PI(4,5)P$_2$ is as a precursor for PI(3,4,5)P$_3$ by phosphorylation by PI 3-kinases (further discussed in Section 8.2.4). More recently, many more functions of PI(4,5)P$_2$ have been described, including (but not limited to) the regulation of membrane proteins, the actin cytoskeleton, and intracellular trafficking events.

It is now well established that PI(4,5)P$_2$ itself directly mediates activity of an astonishing number of membrane proteins, especially ion channels and transporters. Because the regulation of membrane proteins by PI(4,5)P$_2$ and other phosphoinositides has been recently reviewed in several papers (Balla et al. 2009; Gamper and Shapiro 2007; Rohacs 2009; Suh and Hille 2008), we will only summarize the basic principles of how PI(4,5)P$_2$ (and other phosphoinositides, see below) modulates protein activity. First, proteins may directly bind to one or more phosphoinositides, and this binding does not need to be stoichiometric. Second, PI(4,5)P$_2$ can both inhibit and stimulate protein activity, and this modulation can be either "permissive," where protein activity is strictly dependent on the presence or absence of PI(4,5)P$_2$, or "progressive," where a decreasing or increasing abundance of PI(4,5)P$_2$ gradually alters protein activity. A recent example of permissive modulation of protein activity was recently described for Kv7.1 ion channels, where PI(4,5)P$_2$ is essential to couple voltage sensing to channel opening (Zaydman et al. 2013). Third, the regulatory effect either can be very specific for PI(4,5)P$_2$ or can also be observed for other phosphoinositides. When, as for most membrane proteins, the effect of phosphoinositides is not very specific for PI(4,5)P$_2$, this lack of specificity is typically caused by the modulation of protein activity via nonstereospecific electrostatic interactions of the polyanionic phosphoinositides with patches of polybasic amino acids on the protein (Balla et al. 2009). When, as for some membrane proteins, the regulatory effect of PI(4,5)$_2$ is highly specific and not observed for other phosphoinositides, these proteins must contain folded domains where the interacting residues form a structured binding pocket for PI(4,5)P$_2$ (Suh and Hille 2008). Finally, PI(4,5)P$_2$ may not directly regulate membrane protein function but act via recruitment of other regulatory proteins such as calmodulin and small GTPases (reviewed by Balla et al. 2009).

PI(4,5)P$_2$ is also involved in organization of the cytoskeleton and can directly associate with the majority of adapter proteins that connect the cytoskeleton to the plasma membrane, including talin (Isenberg et al. 1996; Martel et al. 2001), vinculin, alpha-actinin (Fukami et al. 1994), profilin (Lassing and Lindberg 1985), gelsolin (Janmey et al. 1987), cofilin (Yonezawa et al. 1990), N-WASP (Miki et al. 1996), and members of the ERM (ezrin, radixin, moesin) family (Hirao et al. 1996). In general, an increase of PI(4,5)P$_2$ levels (or of other phosphoinositide species; see below) in the plasma membrane promotes actin filament formation, whereas a decrease of PI(4,5)P$_2$ results in increased actin depolymerization, and for further details, we refer to several reviews (Saarikangas et al. 2010; Takenawa and Itoh 2001; Zhang et al. 2012a). Interestingly, not only the actin cytoskeleton but also the microtubular network is affected by PI(4,5)P$_2$, which can bind to the plus-ends of microtubules via adapter proteins (IQGAP1) (Golub and Caroni 2005).

Finally, plasma membrane PI(4,5)P$_2$ (and other phosphoinositides; see below) is involved in both exo- and endocytosis. Like the other functions of PI(4,5)P$_2$ described above, the role of phosphoinositides in intracellular membrane trafficking is extensively discussed in a number of recent review papers (Czech 2003; Koch and Holt 2012; Martin 2001, 2012; Wen et al. 2011) and we will again limit ourselves to the basic principles. Regarding exocytosis, PI(4,5)P$_2$ is essential for (calcium) regulated exocytosis (Milosevic et al. 2005) and is involved in constitutive exocytosis (Wang et al. 2003). Here, PI(4,5)P$_2$ seems to be involved in vesicle tethering/docking of secretory vesicles to the plasma membrane upstream of the actual membrane fusion step. For instance, PI(4,5)P$_2$-enriched membrane domains define sites for docking of dense core granules in PC12 cells (a neuroendocrine cell line) (Aoyagi et al. 2005; James et al. 2008) and many proteins that play a role in vesicle docking bind directly to PI(4,5)P$_2$, such as CAPS (James et al. 2008) and synaptotagmin-1 (De Wit et al. 2009; Honigmann et al. 2013). PI(4,5)P$_2$ may also be involved in the final membrane fusion step, for instance, by increasing the sensitivity of the calcium sensor synaptotagmin-1 for calcium (van den Bogaart et al. 2012). In addition to exocytosis, PI(4,5)P$_2$ plays a role in endocytosis and is enriched at clathrin-assisted membrane patches (Fujita et al. 2009; Huang et al. 2004). Here, the clathrin adapter AP-2 binds directly to PI(4,5)P$_2$ (but also to other phosphoinositides such as PI(3,4,5)P$_3$; see Section 8.2.4), and this is essential for clathrin-coated pit formation (Gaidarov and Keen 1999; Höning et al. 2005; Owen et al. 2004; Rohde et al. 2002). Many other endocytotic clathrin adaptor proteins also bind to PI(4,5)P$_2$, including epsin, AP180/CALM, and arrestin (reviewed in Czech 2003; Di Paolo and De Camilli 2006; Koch and Holt 2012; Owen et al. 2004).

8.2.2   PI(4)P

Although the Golgi apparatus (which has little PI(4,5)P$_2$ compared to the plasma membrane) accounts for the largest pool of PI(4)P in the cell (Godi et al. 2004), PI(4)P is also present in the plasma membrane (Table 8.1). The classic role of PI(4)P in the plasma membrane is as a precursor for PI(4,5)P$_2$ where PI(4)P gets phosphorylated by PI 5-kinases on the Golgi apparatus or travels first to the plasma membrane and then gets phosphorylated (Balla et al. 2009; Czech 2003; Wang et al. 2003). Nevertheless, it is increasingly clear that PI(4)P does not merely act as a precursor for PI(4,5)P$_2$ but actually contributes itself to the pool of polyanionic lipids that define the plasma membrane. In fact, many of the functions traditionally associated with PI(4,5)P$_2$ (see Section 8.2.1) may in fact be (at least partly) attributed to other phosphoinositides such as PI(4)P. For instance, PI(4)P may play a role in organizing the cytoskeleton, because several adapter proteins such as gelsolin (Janmey et al. 1987) and cofilin (Yonezawa et al. 1990) bind directly not only to PI(4,5)P$_2$ but also to PI(4)P.

The most direct evidence for a distinct role of plasma membrane pools of PI(4)P comes from a recent study (Hammond et al. 2012), where it was demonstrated that most plasma membrane-localized PI(4)P was not required for the synthesis or functions of PI(4,5)P$_2$. In this study, depletion of both PI(4)P and PI(4,5)P$_2$ was required to prevent the targeting of peripheral proteins that interact with phosphoinositides (such as MARCKS [myristoylated alanine-rich C kinase substrate]; see Section 8.4.5) or to block activation of the transient receptor potential vanilloid 1 cation channel (TRPV1). Interestingly, the activity of another channel (the TRPM8 channel) was specifically dependent on PI(4,5)P$_2$ and not on PI(4)P, indicating that these two phosphoinositides may have distinct and only partially overlapping functions in the plasma membrane (Hammond et al. 2012).

8.2.3   PI(5)P

Because of its low abundance in the cell and technical difficulties in separating it from PI(4)P, the phosphoinositide PI(5)P was only recently identified in cells (Rameh et al. 1997). PI(5)P is present in various cellular membrane compartments, such as the nucleus, the endoplasmic reticulum, and the Golgi apparatus (Coronas et al. 2007; Grainger et al. 2012; Nunes and Guittard 2013; Sarkes and Rameh 2010). The plasma membrane also contains a small fraction of PI(5)P where it serves as a precursor to PI(4,5)P$_2$ by phosphorylation by PI 5-kinases (Rameh et al. 1997; Sarkes and Rameh 2010). In addition to this, PI(5)P is a signaling molecule that influences cell signaling pathways and may be involved in vesicular transport and organization of the cytoskeleton (Coronas et al. 2007; Grainger et al. 2012; Wilcox and Hinchliffe 2008). Plasma membrane pools of PI(5)P can increase upon cellular activation as, for instance, shown for T-cells where it is thought to play a role in T-cell signaling (reviewed in Nunes and Guittard 2013).

8.2.4   PI(3,4,5)P$_3$

Plasma membrane pools of PI(3,4,5)P$_3$ (Auger et al. 1989; Vadnal et al. 1989) were already identified in the 1980s (reviewed in Stephens et al. 1993). Resting cells contain only very little of PI(3,4,5)P$_3$ (Table 8.1), but, similar to PI(3,4)P$_2$ (Section 8.2.5), the concentration of PI(3,4,5)P$_3$ can rapidly increase in response to activation of almost all known cell-surface receptors (reviewed in Cantley 2002; Czech 2003;

Katso et al. 2001; Stephens et al. 1993). Here, PI 3-kinases are brought to the plasma membrane upon activation of, for example, growth factor receptors, protein tyrosine kinases, integrins, and G protein-coupled receptors and this results in synthesis of $PI(3,4,5)P_3$. For instance, activation of neutrophils by N-formyl-methionyl-leucyl-phenylalanine (a cytokine) results in an increase of the plasma membrane concentration of $PI(3,4,5)P_3$ by approximately 40- to 100-fold as determined by radioactive phosphate labeling (Stephens et al. 1991) and recently confirmed by phosphate methylation coupled to high-performance liquid chromatography and mass spectrometry (Clark et al. 2011). $PI(3,4,5)P_3$ functions as a membrane anchor, and the increase in plasma membrane pools of $PI(3,4,5)P_3$ triggers the recruitment of a large subset of signaling molecules to the membrane. This initiates complex sets of signaling cascades that control the organization of the cytoskeleton, gene transcription and translation, and cell cycle entry and ultimately mediates a variety of cellular activities such as cell proliferation, differentiation, migration, and survival (reviewed in Cantley 2002; Czech 2003; Katso et al. 2001; Stephens et al. 1993).

Similar to $PI(4,5)P_2$, $PI(3,4,5)P_3$ is also involved in constitutive exocytosis (reviewed in Czech 2003) and in Ca^{2+}-regulated exocytosis. $PI(3,4,5)P_3$ is locally enriched at the SNARE-enriched sites of dense core granule release in PC12 cells (a rat neuroendocrine cell line) and at the neuromuscular synaptic boutons of *Drosophila melanogaster* (Khuong et al. 2013). Shielding the headgroup of $PI(3,4,5)P_3$ (but not of $PI(4,5)P_2$) by overexpressing the $PI(3,4,5)P_3$-binding pleckstrin homology domain of GRP_1 resulted in a reduced release of neurotransmitter and in temperature-sensitive paralysis of *D. melanogaster*, directly demonstrating a role of $PI(3,4,5)P_3$ in Ca^{2+}-regulated neurotransmitter release. In addition to exocytosis, $PI(3,4,5)P_3$ might also play a role in endocytosis, and for instance, the clathrin adapter AP2 binds with higher affinity to $PI(3,4,5)P_3$ than to $PI(4,5)P_2$ (Gaidarov et al. 1996) (see also Czech 2003 for discussion).

8.2.5   PI(3,4)P₂

Similar to $PI(3,4,5)P_3$, $P(3,4)P_2$ is barely detectable in the plasma membrane of resting mammalian cells (Table 8.1) but is produced by PI 3-kinases in response to activation of almost all known cell-surface receptors (Czech 2003; Stephens et al. 1993). Similar to $PI(3,4,5)P_3$, $PI(3,4)P_2$ selectively recruits various proteins to the plasma membrane and thereby triggers downstream signaling cascades. These $PI(3,4)P_2$-triggered signaling pathways likely differ from that of $PI(3,4,5)P_3$ (Section 8.2.4), as indicated by the finding that some proteins specifically bind to $PI(3,4)P_2$ and not to $PI(3,4,5)P_3$ (Manna et al. 2007). Other evidence for distinct roles of $PI(3,4)P_2$ and $PI(3,4,5)P_3$ comes from the finding that activation of the thrombin receptor of blood platelets results in a biphasic response where first the concentration of $PI(3,4,5)P_3$ increases and later the concentration of $PI(3,4)P_2$ (Banfić et al. 1998). $PI(3,4)P_2$ is an intermediate in the conversion of $PI(4,5)P_2$ to $PI(3)P$ that occurs during endocytosis, and a function of $PI(3,4)P_2$ in the plasma membrane was recently demonstrated in constitutive clathrin-mediated endocytosis (Posor et al. 2013). Here, $PI(3,4)P_2$ was required for maturation of late-stage clathrin-coated pits prior to fission and for selective recruitment of the BAR domain protein SNX9 at late-stage endocytic intermediates.

8.2.6 PI(3,5)P$_2$

PI(3,5)P$_2$ is generally considered to be predominantly present in the cytoplasmic leaflets of late endosomal and lysosomal membranes (reviewed in Czech 2003) and the plasma membrane contains only very little PI(3,5)P$_2$. In fact, the plasma membrane may contain no PI(3,5)P$_2$ at all, as suggested in a recent study where they found that exogenous addition of PI(3,5)P$_2$ robustly stimulated activity of the cation channel mucolipin-1 in the plasma membrane of HEK293 cells, whereas addition of PI(4,5)P$_2$ decreased channel activity (Zhang et al. 2012b). Since mucolipin-1 is a lysosomal channel and is inactive in the plasma membrane, the antagonistic effects of PI(3,5)P$_2$ and PI(4,5)P$_2$ might ensure that this protein only functions in its correct cellular compartment (i.e., PI(3,5)P$_2$-containing lysosomes) (Zhang et al. 2012b).

8.2.7 PI(3)P

PI(3)P is predominantly present in early and recycling endosomal compartments (Czech 2003), and only a very small fraction of PI(3)P is present in the plasma membrane. In contrast to other 3-phosphorylated phosphoinositides (Sections 8.2.4 and 8.2.5), the cellular pool of PI(3)P does not change significantly upon receptor activation (Auger et al. 1989). This is probably related to the role of PI(3)P in constitutive endosomal trafficking, which requires a sustained synthesis and turnover of this phosphoinositide in the cell (Czech 2003; Katso et al. 2001).

8.3 UNIQUE PROPERTIES OF PHOSPHOINOSITIDES

As we discussed in Section 8.2, plasma membrane pools of phosphoinositides are involved in a wide range of cellular functions. This multifunctionality of phosphoinositides can be attributed to three unique properties that distinguish them from many other phospholipids: (a) the large size of their headgroups, (b) the high anionic charge of their headgroups, and (c) the partitioning in membrane gradients as well as discrete membrane domains.

8.3.1 SIZE OF THE HEADGROUP

As shown in Figure 8.1, the headgroup of phosphoinositides consists of a *myo*-inositol ring connected to one or more phosphate groups. This makes the headgroups of phosphoinositides approximately two to three times larger than that of other phospholipids such as phosphatidylcholine. Because of this large size, phosphoinositides may be able to protrude further into the aqueous phase than most other lipids (McLaughlin et al. 2002). Indeed, it was estimated that PI(4,5)P$_2$ extended approximately 5 Å further from the membrane surface compared to other phospholipids by molecular dynamics simulations (Lupyan et al. 2010).

8.3.2 CHARGE OF THE HEADGROUP

The presence of multiple phosphate groups makes phosphoinositides strongly anionic, and the charge of $PI(4,5)P_2$ has been estimated (McLaughlin et al. 2002) somewhere between −3 and −5 dependent on the precise molecular environment such as local pH and interactions with proteins and other lipids. Accordingly, mono-phosphatic $PI(3)P$, $PI(4)P$, and $PI(5)P$ might be expected to carry charges between −2 and −3 and the triphosphatic $PI(3,4,5)P_3$ could even have charges anywhere from −4 to −7 (see also Figure 8.1). Because of these high anionic charges, phosphoinositides are relatively soluble and only poorly form micelles compared to other lipids. The solubility of $PI(4,5)P_2$ in water is approximately 9 mM (Chu and Stefani 1991). Estimates of the critical micelle concentration for $PI(4,5)P_2$ range between 10 and 30 μM (see Moens and Bagatolli 2007 and references therein), which is more than three orders of magnitude higher than that of other phospholipids (for instance, 0.46 nM for C16:0 PC as determined by Avanti Polar Lipids). The large size and high charge of the headgroup make phosphoinositides ideal binding partners for many integral and peripheral membrane proteins.

8.3.3 MEMBRANE ORGANIZATION

Phosphoinositides are not randomly dispersed in the plasma membrane but are present in membrane gradients or enriched in discrete membrane domains. Such a non-homogeneous distribution in the plasma membrane has been reported for $PI(4,5)P_2$ for many different cell types, as demonstrated by microscopy where $PI(4,5)P_2$ was selectively labeled with antibodies (Aoyagi et al. 2005; Laux et al. 2000; van den Bogaart et al. 2011; Wang and Richards 2012), specific $PI(4,5)P_2$-binding domains (Garrenton et al. 2010; Huang et al. 2004; James et al. 2008; van den Bogaart et al. 2011), or fluorescently labeled $PI(4,5)P_2$ (Cho et al. 2005; Honigmann et al. 2013). A similar organization in discrete domains or gradients in the plasma membrane was shown for $PI(3,4,5)P_3$ by staining with antibodies (Wang and Richards 2012) and specific $PI(3,4,5)P_3$-binding domains (Khuong et al. 2013; Langille et al. 1999). Phosphoinositides are mobile in the plasma membrane, as suggested in a fluorescence recovery after photobleaching (FRAP) study employing $PI(4,5)P_2$ and $PI(3,4,5)P_3$ binding protein reporters (Brough et al. 2005). When phosphoinositides are sequestered in membrane domains, they can retain their mobility, as demonstrated for $PI(4,5)P_2$, which was fully mobile within the nascent cup of forming phagosomes (as determined by fluorescence correlation spectroscopy [FCS]) (Golebiewska et al. 2011). $PI(4,5)P_2$ was also mobile in membrane domains that were induced by electrostatic interactions with the SNARE protein syntaxin-1 in artificial membranes (by FRAP; see Section 8.4.5) (van den Bogaart et al. 2011).

    Although the asymmetric distribution and clustering of phosphoinositides in membrane domains may seem surprising given their high anionic charge (see Section 8.3.2), which would lead to a strong electrostatic repulsion, it offers two clear advantages for the regulation of cellular functions (see Section 8.2).

    First, the local concentration and confined orientation of phosphoinositides in membrane domains will result in a much (easily three orders of magnitude) higher effective concentration than if the phosphoinositides were randomly dispersed over the plasma membrane (see McLaughlin et al. 2002 for discussion). This effect, which is also called a "reduction of dimensionality," results in a very high local accumulation of charge in these domains (high charge density), and this could favor electrostatic interactions.

Second, the domain partitioning allows localization as well as confined regulation of the wide variety of cellular functions in which phosphoinositides are involved (see Section 8.2). The segregation of phosphoinositides in distinct and functionally different membrane domains helps explain why single molecular species of phosphoinositides (such as PI(4,5)P$_2$, discussed in Section 8.2.1) can participate in so many different cellular functions (Martin 2001; McLaughlin et al. 2002; Simonson et al. 2001). Indeed, there is now plenty of evidence for different metabolic pools of phosphoinositides. For instance, radioisotope-labeled PI(4,5)P$_2$ pools were found to be not completely identical to those that were accessible to the PI(4,5)P$_2$-binding pleckstrin homology domain of phospholipase C delta subunit in COS-7 and NIH-3T3 cells (Várnai and Balla 1998). Accordingly, two members of the PI 5-kinase family had opposite effects (stimulation and inhibition) on antigen-stimulated release of calcium from the endoplasmic reticulum in mast cells (Vasudevan et al. 2009). Targeting the catalytic domain of the PI(4,5)P$_2$ phosphatase Ins54P to the plasma membrane by two different membrane targeting domains resulted in different effects on Jurkat T-cell morphology and PI(4,5)P$_2$ content (Johnson et al. 2008), suggesting the presence of functionally distinct pools of PI(4,5)P$_2$ at the plasma membrane. Finally, in a cryo-electron microscopy study, PI(4,5)P$_2$ located in caveolae and clathrin-coated pits and free in the plasma membrane were all found to respond differently to angiotensin II treatment in cultured fibroblasts and mouse smooth muscle cells (Fujita et al. 2009).

Membrane gradients or domains enriched in phosphoinositides can be very heterogeneous in terms of size and can range from local gradients that span the entire cell to discrete submicrometer small membrane domains. Examples of large membrane gradients include the enrichment of PI(3,4,5)P$_3$ at the leading edge of migrating *Dictyostelium discoideum* during chemotaxis (Iijima et al. 2002) and the exclusive localization of PI(3,4,5)P$_3$ at the basolateral membrane in polarized epithelial cells (Gassama-Diagne et al. 2006). In epithelial cells, exogenous addition of PI(3,4,5)P$_3$ to the apical membrane led to loss of cellular polarity and recruitment of typical basolateral proteins (such as p58, sec8, and syntaxin-4) to the apical membrane, indicating that PI(3,4,5)P$_3$ is a critical determinant for the identity of the basolateral membrane (Gassama-Diagne et al. 2006). Phosphoinositides can be also partitioned to discrete membrane regions, such as to the micrometer-sized focal adhesions and membrane ruffles (Golub and Caroni 2005; Hirao et al. 1996; Honda et al. 1999; Tall et al. 2000). Here, PI(4,5)P$_2$ may induce membrane curvature and modulate the dynamics of the cortical actin cytoskeleton (see Sections 8.2.1 and 8.4.3) and the local accumulation in membrane domains might mediate the regulation of protrusive motility (Golub and Caroni 2005). PI(4,5)P$_2$ is also found in cleavage furrows of dividing fibroblasts where it mediates cell division and might rearrange the contractile fission ring (Emoto et al. 2005; Field et al. 2005). Finally, phosphoinositide-enriched membrane domains can be only a few tens of nanometers in size, as in PI(4,5)P$_2$-enriched clathrin-coated pits where PI(4,5)P$_2$ plays a role in the recruitment of the clathrin coat and in the selection of cargo molecules (see Section 8.2.1). In neuroendocrine PC12 cells, PI(4,5)P$_2$ is enriched in the plasma membrane at the sites of docked vesicles (Aoyagi et al. 2005; James et al. 2008), and these domains are only ~70 nm in diameter as shown by super-resolution microscopy (van den Bogaart et al. 2011). Interestingly, membrane domains that contain PI(4,5)P$_2$ do not overlap with domains enriched in PI(3,4,5)P$_3$ in the plasma membrane of PC12 cells (Wang and Richards 2012). Thus, phosphoinositides can partition in many different types of membrane gradients and domains with distinct sizes and compositions. This raises the question how these phosphoinositides are sequestered to such different membrane domains.

8.4 PARTITIONING MECHANISMS OF PHOSPHOINOSITIDE SEQUESTERING

Several mechanisms have been described to account for the organization of phosphoinositides in membrane domains (Figure 8.3). These include (Section 8.4.1) localized synthesis (or delivery) and degradation of phosphoinositides, (Section 8.4.2) enrichment of phosphoinositides in cholesterol-enriched raft-like domains, (Section 8.4.3) enrichment of phosphoinositides at highly curved membrane domains, (Section 8.4.4) trapping in membrane domains by molecular "fences," (Section 8.4.5) sequestration by electrostatic interactions with polycationic peptides, (Section 8.4.6) formation of hydrogen bond networks, and (Section 8.4.7) complexing of phosphoinositides with polyvalent cations.

8.4.1 LOCAL SYNTHESIS AND DEGRADATION

It is well established that the local production and degradation of phosphoinositides can result in significant gradients in the plasma membrane. Here, local synthesis and breakdown are controlled by the specific membrane recruitment of phosphatidylinositol phosphate kinases or phosphatases that generate or hydrolyze phosphoinositides, respectively. One of the best described examples is the enrichment of PI(4,5)P$_2$ at focal adhesions by local synthesis by type I phosphatidylinositol phosphate kinase isoform-g 661 (PIPKIg661) that is specifically targeted to focal adhesions via interactions with talin (Di Paolo et al. 2002; Ling et al. 2002). Membrane gradients by local phosphoinositide synthesis and degradation play a role in cell polarity, epithelial morphology, chemoreception, and cell migration and are extensively reviewed elsewhere (Doughman et al. 2003; McLaughlin et al. 2002; Sun et al. 2013; Swaney et al. 2010).

Whereas local synthesis and hydrolysis of phosphoinositides can account for membrane gradients at large spatial distances and the sequestering in larger domains, the phosphoinositides will readily diffuse away from their sites of synthesis and it alone does not suffice to explain the partitioning of phosphoinositides in small and discrete domains (see McLaughlin et al. 2002 for discussion). Thus, although phosphatidylinositol phosphate kinases are often present at discrete membrane domains that are enriched in specific phosphoinositides, such as at the cleavage furrow in

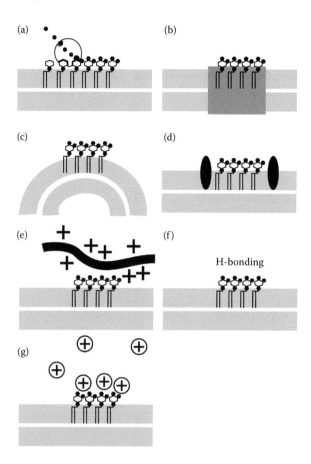

FIGURE 8.3 Mechanisms of sequestering of phosphoinositides in membrane domains. (a) Localized synthesis and hydrolysis (or alternatively localized delivery by exocytosis). (b) Partitioning to membrane lipid rafts. (c) Partitioning to curved membrane regions (either positive curvature as shown or negative curvature). (d) Trapping in domains by hindered diffusion though molecular fences. (e) Membrane sequestering by (peripheral or integral) membrane proteins with stretches of cationic residues. (f) Formation of hydrogen bond networks (H-bonding). (g) Membrane sequestering by polyvalent cations such as calcium.

dividing fibroblasts (Emoto et al. 2005), additional sequestering mechanisms need to be present in order to prevent phosphoinositides from diffusing away and explain their localization in small and discrete membrane domains (see Sections 8.4.2 through 8.4.7).

8.4.2 RAFTS

"Membrane rafts" were originally defined as membrane domains enriched in cholesterol and (sphingo)lipids with unsaturated acyl chains and certain protein species and are in the liquid ordered state instead of the (fluid) liquid crystalline state (reviewed by Lingwood and Simons 2010). Historically, the partitioning of proteins in "detergent-resistant membranes" (DRMs) that cannot be solubilized by nonionic detergents (typically Triton X-100) was considered evidence for partitioning in membrane rafts, although this is currently no longer accepted. Several studies demonstrate that (a fraction of) phosphoinositides partition in DRMs (Pike and Miller 1998; Taverna et al. 2007; Waugh et al. 1998), and this was suggested to reflect raft partitioning. More direct evidence for such a raft partitioning comes from immunofluorescence microscopy where a fraction of $PI(4,5)P_2$ was found to colocalize in membrane domains with well-known raft protein markers (Aoyagi et al. 2005; Laux et al. 2000). Accordingly, the pleckstrin homology domain of phospholipase C delta subunit (which specifically binds $PI(4,5)P_2$; Section 8.3.3) coclustered in membrane domains with heterogeneously expressed double palmitoylated RFP, further suggesting that some $PI(4,5)P_2$ located in membrane rafts (Golub and Caroni 2005).

The localization of $PI(4,5)P_2$ in membrane rafts seems surprising, given that rafts are thought to primarily contain lipids with saturated acyl chains and the major form of $PI(4,5)P_2$ contains a polyunsaturated arachidonic acid (C20:4) (Clark et al. 2011; Pettitt et al. 2006). How $PI(4,5)P_2$ would be enriched in such membrane rafts is therefore unclear, especially when considering that $PI(4,5)P_2$ clearly prefers the liquid disordered phase over the cholesterol-enriched liquid ordered phase in artificial membranes (Levental et al. 2009). One possibility is that membrane rafts are asymmetric and only present in the outer (but not inner) leaflet of $PI(4,5)P_2$-enriched domains. Such an asymmetry would be in agreement with the finding that the sphingomyelin-specific probe lysenin specifically binds to the outer leaflet of cleavage furrow during cell division that is enriched in $PI(4,5)P_2$ in the inner leaflet (Abe et al. 2012).

8.4.3 CURVATURE

The shape of the plasma membrane is very complicated and comprises a broad range of different membrane curvatures. This membrane shaping and remodeling is regulated by phosphoinositides that connect the plasma membrane to the cytoskeleton (see Section 8.2.1) and bind to proteins that shape the membrane, such as BAR-domain containing proteins (reviewed by Takenawa 2010). Because of the large size and high charges of their headgroups (Sections 8.3.1 and 8.3.2), phosphoinositides may preferentially localize to highly curved membrane regions or induce membrane curvature themselves without any interacting proteins, as shown by small-angle x-ray diffraction (Mulet et al. 2008). Indeed, phosphoinositides such as $PI(4,5)P_2$ and $PI(3,4,5)P_3$ are well known to localize to and are essential for the formation of highly curved membrane regions, such as membrane ruffles and phagocytotic cups (Czech 2003; Huang et al. 2004; Langille et al. 1999).

8.4.4 MOLECULAR FENCES

The domain partitioning of phosphoinositides has also been attributed to their trapping in membrane compartments by molecular fences. Combined with other clustering mechanisms such as local synthesis (Section 8.4.1), the spatially constrained mobility would lead to the local accumulation of the phosphoinositides. Direct evidence for such a molecular fencing comes from a recent study (Golebiewska et al. 2011) where it was demonstrated that even though PI(4,5)P$_2$ was fully mobile within the nascent cup of forming phagosomes (as demonstrated by FCS), it could not exchange with other (plasma membrane) pools of PI(4,5)P$_2$ (by FRAP). This indicates that PI(4,5)P$_2$ is trapped in the phagosomes by a molecular fence and led the authors to speculate on a role for septins in the trapping (Golebiewska et al. 2011). Septins directly interact with phosphoinositides and form filaments on artificial membranes (reviewed by Mostowy and Cossart 2012) and have also been proposed to block PI(4,5)P$_2$ diffusion in yeast (Garrenton et al. 2010).

Alternatively or complementary to septins, phosphoinositide diffusion may be blocked by the cortical actin network as suggested in a FRAP study where the confined motion of fluorescently labeled PI(4,5)P$_2$ analogs in mouse atrial myocytes was dependent on filamentous actin (Cho et al. 2005). Indeed, the cortical actin skeleton is well known to act as a semipermeable barrier, hindering the diffusion of membrane components (reviewed by Kusumi et al. 2012), and the majority of adapter proteins that connect the cytoskeleton to the plasma membrane bind to phosphoinositides such as PI(4,5)P$_2$ (see Section 8.2.1).

8.4.5 PROTEIN SEQUESTERING

Because of its high negative charge (Section 8.3.2), phosphoinositides interact with positively charged residues on proteins. In the plasma membrane, polybasic protein motifs that contain a high density of cationic residues can bind to multiple phosphoinositides to form an electrostatically neutral complex. As elaborately reviewed (McLaughlin et al. 2002), many proteins contain such clusters of basic residues that are located near the membrane interface and thereby could be involved in sequestering polyanionic phosphoinositides laterally. This is best described for the protein MARCKS, which is proposed to regulate the amount of free PI(4,5)P$_2$ in the plasma membrane (reviewed by McLaughlin et al. 2002; Suh and Hille 2008). MARCKS is a 331-residue peripheral membrane protein that contains an effector region of 25 residues with 13 clustered basic charges. This effector region is unstructured and can sequester several PI(4,5)P$_2$ molecules in the membrane (McLaughlin et al. 2002). Phosphorylation of the polybasic effector region by protein kinase C or engagement by calmodulin may result in the release of PI(4,5)P$_2$ molecules from MARCKS; hence, they can interact with other proteins.

Integral membrane proteins can also sequester phosphoinositides, as is best shown for the SNARE protein syntaxin-1 that interacts with PI(4,5)P$_2$ via five conserved positive charges located at its juxtamembrane interface (Murray and Tamm 2009). Indeed, syntaxin-1 can form clusters with PI(4,5)P$_2$ and PI(3,4,5)P$_3$ in artificial membranes, and these phosphoinositides are important for clustering of syntaxin-1 in the plasma membrane (Khuong et al. 2013; van den Bogaart et al. 2011). Here, the polyanionic phosphoinositides act as "charge bridges" and cluster the polybasic proteins together. Polybasic patches on structured (folded) protein domains can also sequester phosphoinositides, as suggested by recent molecular dynamics simulations where the C2 domain of auxilin-1 (which contains a structured PI(4,5)P$_2$-binding pocket) was found to sequester multiple PI(4,5)P$_2$ molecules (Kalli et al. 2013).

Binding to polybasic effector is often not specific for a specific species of phosphoinositides. Such a lack of specificity is also indicated by the finding that depletion of only $PI(4,5)P_2$ is not sufficient to abolish recruitment of positively targeted proteins to the plasma membrane, and other phosphoinositides are also involved in this process (Hammond et al. 2012; Heo et al. 2006). The binding of polybasic effector protein motifs to phosphoinositides is a purely electrostatic interaction, and the strength of this interaction is determined by the charge density (McLaughlin et al. 2002). Because $PI(3,4,5)P_3$ has a higher charge density than $PI(4,5)P_2$, polybasic effector motifs can be expected to bind stronger to $PI(3,4,5)P_3$ than to $PI(4,5)P_2$, as shown for syntaxin-1 by Förster resonance energy transfer (Khuong et al. 2013). Finally, the headgroups of phosphoinositides that are engaged with polybasic effector motifs may still be accessible to other (stereospecific) binding partners, as shown for pleckstrin homology domains that can still bind to $PI(4,5)P_2$ when engaged with MARCKS (McLaughlin et al. 2002) and to $PI(4,5)P_2$ and $PI(3,4,5)P_3$ engaged with syntaxin-1 (Khuong et al. 2013; van den Bogaart et al. 2011).

8.4.6 SEQUESTRATION BY HYDROGEN BONDING

Phosphoinositides are capable of hydrogen bond formation. By a variety of optical spectroscopy techniques and area-pressure measurements, phosphoinositides were shown to form hydrogen bond networks in artificial membranes through their polar lipid headgroups, leading to clustering in microdomains (Levental et al. 2008; Redfern and Gericke 2004, 2005). Clustering by hydrogen bonding was observed for all tested phosphoinositides (PI(3)P, PI(4)P, PI(5)P, $PI(3,5)P_2$, $PI(4,5)P_2$, and $PI(3,4)P_2$), although the extent of clustering was dependent on the precise molecular species of phosphoinositide. Whereas hydrogen bond networks of phosphoinositides can be readily observed in artificial membranes, it still remains to be elucidated if and to what extent such hydrogen bonding contributes to clustering of phosphoinositides in the plasma membrane of cells.

8.4.7 SEQUESTRATION BY POLYVALENT CATIONS

Physiological concentrations of Ca^{2+} (in the micromolar range) can lead to clustering of $PI(4,5)P_2$ and other phosphoinositides in artificial membranes as demonstrated by a wide variety of techniques: area-pressure measurements, fluorescence, atomic force microscopy, and electron microscopy (Carvalho et al. 2008; Levental et al. 2009; Wang et al. 2012). Here, and similar to clustering by polycationic peptides (Section 8.4.5), polyvalent cations form charge bridges that connect multiple phosphoinositides in microdomains. Clustering of $PI(4,5)P_2$ is selective for Ca^{2+}, and much higher concentrations of other polyvalent cations such as Mg^{2+} are required to induce $PI(4,5)P_2$ clustering compared to Ca^{2+}. Despite this preference for Ca^{2+} over Mg^{2+}, the clustering of $PI(4,5)P_2$ (and other phosphoinositides) by Mg^{2+} may be physiologically relevant given that intracellular Mg^{2+} concentrations in resting cells are two to three orders of magnitude higher (millimolar) than Ca^{2+} concentrations (micromolar). Such a role of Mg^{2+} in the clustering of phosphoinositides is also indicated by the finding that phosphoinositides display a specificity for certain cations:

$PI(4,5)P_2$ and $PI(3,4)P_2$ bind with a higher affinity to Ca^{2+} compared to Mg^{2+}, whereas $PI(3,5)P_2$ has a preference for Mg^{2+} over Ca^{2+} (Wang et al. 2012). It has been suggested that this opposite preference for Ca^{2+} or Mg^{2+} between $PI(3,4)P_2/PI(4,5)P_2$ and $PI(3,5)P_2$ may relate to their different physiological functions (see Section 8.2) and might help explain how different phosphoinositides can segregate into distinct membrane domains (Wang et al. 2012). Nevertheless, the clustering of phosphoinositides by polyvalent cations has hitherto only been observed in artificial membranes, and it still remains unknown if and to what extent phosphoinositides cluster by interactions with polyvalent cations in the plasma membrane of cells.

8.5 CONCLUSIONS AND OUTLOOK

We started this chapter by providing an overview of the functions of phosphoinositides in the plasma membranes (Section 8.2). Six out of seven phosphoinositides are present at the plasma membrane. Only $PI(3,5)P_2$ seems not present at the plasma membrane but might be exclusively present at intracellular membranes. $PI(4)P$ and $PI(4,5)P_2$ are constitutively present in comparatively high concentrations (~1%; see Table 8.1) and $PI(5)P$ and $PI(3)P$ are present at much lower concentrations (<0.1%) in the plasma membrane. $PI(3,4)P_2$ and $PI(3,4,5)P_3$ are also present at low concentrations in the plasma membrane of a resting cell but can dramatically increase upon cellular stimulation. Whereas all these plasma membrane phosphoinositides have some unique cellular functions, in many cases, their functions overlap and specific functions cannot be assigned to a single molecular species of phosphoinositide. For instance, $PI(4,5)P_2$, $PI(3,4,5)P_3$, $PI(4)P$, and $PI(5)P$ all affect the cytoskeleton (Sections 8.2.1 through 8.2.4) and both $PI(4,5)P_2$ and $PI(3,4,5)P_3$ seem to regulate endocytosis as well as exocytosis (Sections 8.2.1 and 8.2.4). Thus, many of the cellular functions of the phosphoinositides in the plasma membrane seem to at least partially overlap.

The overlap of many of the cellular functions of phosphoinositides can be attributed to the promiscuity of many effector proteins that can bind to multiple species of phosphoinositides. As explained in Sections 8.2.1 and 8.4.5, many proteins interact with the highly charged headgroups of phosphoinositides via polybasic effector domains, and these interactions are typically purely electrostatic and not stereoselective. Also in the case of many phosphoinositide-binding proteins that do contain folded binding pockets, their interactions are often not very specific, such as for pleckstrin homology domains that are often able to bind to multiple species of phosphoinositide (Lemmon and Ferguson 2000; Yu et al. 2004). Interestingly, phospholipase C that cleaves $PI(4,5)P_2$ into DAG and inositol 1,4,5-trisphosphate (IP_3) (Section 8.2.1) is also not specific for $PI(4,5)P_2$ but binds to and hydrolyzes other phosphoinositides as well such as $PI(4)P$ (Balla et al. 2009). In fact, several of the original studies on phospholipase C activity demonstrate not only a decrease of $PI(4,5)P_2$ and an increase of IP_3 but also a decrease of $IP(4)P$ and an increase of inositol 1,4-bisphosphate (for instance, Berridge 1983 and Creba et al. 1983). Just as it is increasingly clear that many of the functions that were originally assigned to $PI(4,5)P_2$ can also be attributed to other phosphoinositides in the plasma membrane (see Section 8.2), it might be that other inositol phosphates (such as inositol 1,4-bisphosphate) have functions comparable to IP_3.

As we described in Sections 8.3 and 8.4, phosphoinositides are not uniformly distributed over the plasma membrane but are organized in membrane domains and gradients that show a surprising diversity not only in the phosphoinositides they contain but also in their sizes, lifetimes, and molecular compositions. These phosphoinositide-enriched membrane domains constitute functional platforms for a wide range of cellular functions, for instance, clathrin-coated pits, sites of exocytosis, the cleavage furrow during cell division, and focal adhesions. Phosphoinositide clustering in membrane domains and gradients is explained by the combination of several (probably seven) different clustering effects that cooperate in a synergistic manner: localized synthesis (or delivery) and degradation of phosphoinositides, enrichment of phosphoinositides in cholesterol-enriched raft-like domains, enrichment of phosphoinositides at highly curved membrane domains, trapping in membrane domains by molecular "fences," sequestration by electrostatic interactions with polycationic peptides, formation of hydrogen bond networks, and complexing of phosphoinositides with polyvalent cations (Figure 8.3). Considering the large variety in size, lifetime, and composition among phosphoinositide-enriched membrane domains, the precise contribution of each of these clustering mechanisms likely differs for different membrane domains.

Since (i) the same molecular species of phosphoinositide is involved in a wide range of different cellular functions and (ii) the functions of phosphoinositides often overlap and do not seem specific for a particular molecular species of phosphoinositide, the function of a phosphoinositide-enriched membrane domain seems not (or at least not solely) determined by the species of phosphoinositide but rather by other effector molecules present in these domains. Indeed, phosphoinositide-enriched membrane domains often contain effector proteins required for their functions, such as kinases, phosphatases, trafficking proteins, receptors, integrins, and proteins that connect the plasma membrane to the cortical cytoskeleton. Given the multifunctionality of phosphoinositides and the promiscuity of their binding proteins, this coenrichment of specific effector molecules in phosphoinositide-enriched membrane domains must explain how these domains can specifically act in particular cellular functions.

Thus, we reach the final conclusion that the functionality of phosphoinositides in the plasma membrane cannot (or not only) be attributed to their precise molecular configuration but is primarily governed by the effector molecules they copartition with in membrane domains. Thereby, the capacity of phosphoinositides to localize in diverse plasma membrane domains and gradients that contain specific sets of effector molecules explains the multifunctionality of phosphoinositides. Understanding the mechanisms that drive the clustering and segregation of phosphoinositides in such structurally and functionally diverse membrane domains is therefore critical for understanding the cellular functions of phosphoinositides.

ACKNOWLEDGMENTS

We thank Mirjam M.P. Zegers and Annemiek B. van Spriel (Radboud University Medical Centre, the Netherlands) for comments. Geert van den Bogaart is a recipient of a Starting Grant from the European Research Council.

REFERENCES

Abe, M., Makino, A., Hullin-Matsuda, F., Kamijo, K., Ohno-Iwashita, Y., Hanada, K. et al. "A role for sphingomyelin-rich lipid domains in the accumulation of phosphatidylinositol-4,5-bisphosphate to the cleavage furrow during cytokinesis." *Mol. Cell. Biol.* 23 (2012): 1396–1407.

Aoyagi, K., Sugaya, T., Umeda, M., Yamamoto, S., Terakawa, S., and Takahashi, M. "The activation of exocytotic sites by the formation of phosphatidylinositol 4,5-bisphosphate microdomains at syntaxin clusters." *J. Biol. Chem.* 280 (2005): 17346–17352.

Auger, K.R., Serunian, L.A., Soltoff, S.P., Libby, P., and Cantley, L.C. "PDGF-dependent tyrosine phosphorylation stimulates production of novel polyphosphoinositides in intact cells." *Cell.* 57 (1989): 167–175.

Balla, T., Szentpetery, Z., and Kim, Y.J. "Phosphoinositide signaling: New tools and insights." *Physiology (Bethesda).* 24 (2009): 231–244.

Banfić, H., Downes, C.P., and Rittenhouse, S.E. "Biphasic activation of PKBalpha/Akt in platelets. Evidence for stimulation both by phosphatidylinositol 3,4-bisphosphate, produced via a novel pathway, and by phosphatidylinositol 3,4,5-trisphosphate." *J. Biol. Chem.* 273 (1998): 11630–11637.

Berridge, M.J. "Rapid accumulation of inositol trisphosphate reveals that agonists hydrolyse polyphosphoinositides instead of phosphatidylinositol." *Biochem. J.* 212 (1983): 849–858.

Bridges, D., and Saltiel, A.R. "Phosphoinositides in insulin action and diabetes." *Curr. Top. Microbiol. Immunol.* 362 (2012): 61–85.

Brough, D., Bhatti, F., and Irvine, R.F. "Mobility of proteins associated with the plasma membrane by interaction with inositol lipids." *J. Cell Sci.* 118 (2005): 3019–3025.

Bunney, T.D., and Katan, M. "Phosphoinositide signalling in cancer: Beyond PI3K and PTEN." *Nat. Rev. Cancer.* 10 (2010): 342–352.

Cantley, L.C. "The phosphoinositide 3-kinase pathway." *Science.* 296 (2002): 1655–1657.

Carvalho, K., Ramos, L., Roy, C., and Picart, C. "Giant unilamellar vesicles containing phosphatidylinositol(4,5)bisphosphate: Characterization and functionality." *Biophys. J.* 95 (2008): 4348–4360.

Cho, H., Kim, Y.A., Yoon, J-Y., Lee, D., Kim, J.H., Lee, S.H., and Ho, W-K. "Low mobility of phosphatidylinositol 4,5-bisphosphate underlies receptor specificity of Gq-mediated ion channel regulation in atrial myocytes." *Proc. Natl. Acad. Sci. USA.* 102 (2005): 15241–15246.

Christie, W.W., and Han, X. Lipid Analysis. *Isolation, Separation, Identification, and Lipidomic Analysis.* Bridgwater UK: The Oily Press Lipid Library, 2010.

Chu, A., and Stefani, E. "Phosphatidylinositol 4,5-bisphosphate-induced Ca^{2+} release from skeletal muscle sarcoplasmic reticulum terminal cisternal membranes. Ca^{2+} flux and single channel studies." *J. Biol. Chem.* 266 (1991): 7699–7705.

Clark, J., Anderson, K.E., Juvin, V., Smith, T.S., Karpe, F., Wakelam, M.J. et al. "Quantification of PtdInsP3 molecular species in cells and tissues by mass spectrometry." *Nat. Methods.* 8 (2011): 267–272.

Coronas, S., Ramel, D., Pendaries, C., Gaits-Iacovoni, F., Tronchere, H., and Payrastre, B. "PtdIns5P: A little phosphoinositide with big functions?" *Biochem. Soc. Symp.* 74 (2007): 117–128.

Creba, J.A., Downes, C.P., Hawkins, P.T., Brewster, G., Michell, R.H., and Kirk, C.J. "Rapid breakdown of phosphatidylinositol 4-phosphate and phosphatidylinositol 4,5-bisphosphate in rat hepatocytes stimulated by vasopressin and other Ca^{2+}-mobilizing hormones." *Biochem. J.* 212 (1983): 733–747.

Czech, M.P. "Dynamics of phosphoinositides in membrane retrieval and docking." *Annu. Rev. Physiol.* 65 (2003): 791–815.

Daum, G. "Lipids of mitochondria." *Biochim. Biophys. Acta.* 822 (1985): 1–42.

De Wit, H., Walter, A.M., Milosevic, I., Gulyás-Kovács, A., Riedel, D., Sørensen, J.B., and Verhage, M. "Synaptotagmin-1 docks secretory vesicles to syntaxin-1/SNAP-25 acceptor complexes." *Cell.* 138 (2009): 935–946.

Di Paolo, G., Pellegrini, L., Letinic, K., Cestra, G., Zoncu, R., Voronov, S. et al. "Recruitment and regulation of phosphatidylinositol phosphate kinase type 1 gamma by the FERM domain of talin." *Nature.* 420 (2002): 85–89.

Di Paolo, G., and De Camilli, P. "Phosphoinositides in cell regulation and membrane dynamics." *Nature.* 443 (2006): 651–657.

Doughman, R.L., Firestone, A.J., and Anderson, R.A. "Phosphatidylinositol phosphate kinases put PI4,5P(2) in its place." *J. Membr. Biol.* 194 (2003): 77–89.

Emoto, K., Inadome, H., Kanaho, Y., Narumiya, S., and Umeda, M. "Local change in phospholipid composition at the cleavage furrow is essential for completion of cytokinesis." *J Biol Chem.* 280 (2005): 37901–37907.

Ferrell, J.E. Jr., and Huestis, W.H. "Phosphoinositide metabolism and the morphology of human erythrocytes." *J. Cell Biol.* 98 (1984): 1992–1998.

Field, S.J., Madson, N., Kerr, M.L., Galbraith, K.A., Kennedy, C.E., Tahiliani, M. et al. "PtdIns(4,5)P$_2$ functions at the cleavage furrow during cytokinesis." *Curr. Biol.* 15 (2005): 1407–1412.

Fujita, A., Cheng, J., Tauchi-Sato, K., Takenawa, T., and Fujimoto, T. "A distinct pool of phosphatidylinositol 4,5-bisphosphate in caveolae revealed by a nanoscale labeling technique." *Proc. Natl. Acad. Sci. USA.* 106 (2009): 9256–9261.

Fukami, K., Endo, T., Imamura, M., and Takenawa, T. "Alpha-actinin and vinculin are PIP2-binding proteins involved in signaling by tyrosine kinase." *J. Biol. Chem.* 269 (1994): 1518–1522.

Gaidarov, I., Chen, Q., Falck, J.R., Reddy, K.K., and Keen, J.H. "A functional phosphatidylinositol 3,4,5-trisphosphate/phosphoinositide binding domain in the clathrin adaptor AP-2 alpha subunit. Implications for the endocytic pathway." *J. Biol. Chem.* 271 (1996): 20922–20929.

Gaidarov, I., and Keen, J.H. "Phosphoinositide-AP-2 interactions required for targeting to plasma membrane clathrin-coated pits." *J. Cell Biol.* 146 (1999): 755–764.

Gamper, N., and Shapiro, M.S. "Regulation of ion transport proteins by membrane phosphoinositides." *Nat. Rev. Neurosci.* 8 (2007): 921–934.

Garrenton, L.S., Stefan, C.J., McMurray, M.A., Emr, S.D., and Thorner, J. "Pheromone-induced anisotropy in yeast plasma membrane phosphatidylinositol-4,5-bisphosphate distribution is required for MAPK signaling." *Proc. Natl. Acad. Sci. USA.* 107 (2010): 11805–11810.

Gassama-Diagne, A., Yu, W., ter Beest, M., Martin-Belmonte, F., Kierbel, A., Engel, J., and Mostov, K. "Phosphatidylinositol-3,4,5-trisphosphate regulates the formation of the basolateral plasma membrane in epithelial cells." *Nat. Cell. Biol.* 8 (2006): 963–970.

Ghigo, A., Perino, A., and Hirsch, E. "Phosphoinositides and cardiovascular diseases." *Curr. Top. Microbiol. Immunol.* 362 (2012): 43–60.

Godi, A., Di Campli, A., Konstantakopoulos, A., Di Tullio, G., Alessi, D.R., Kular, G.S. et al. "FAPPs control Golgi-to-cell-surface membrane traffic by binding to ARF and PtdIns(4)P." *Nat. Cell Biol.* 6 (2004): 393–404.

Golebiewska, U., Kay, J.G., Masters, T., Grinstein, S., Im, W., Pastor, R.W. et al. "Evidence for a fence that impedes the diffusion of phosphatidylinositol 4,5-bisphosphate out of the forming phagosomes of macrophages." *Mol. Biol. Cell.* 22 (2011): 3498–3507.

Golub, T., and Caroni, P. "PI(4,5)P$_2$-dependent microdomain assemblies capture microtubules to promote and control leading edge motility." *J. Cell Biol.* 169 (2005): 151–165.

Grado, C., and Ballou, C.E. "Myo-inositol phosphates from beef brain phosphoinositide." *J. Biol. Chem.* 235 (1960): PC23–24.

Grainger, D.L., Tavelis, C., Ryan, A.J., and Hinchliffe, K.A. "The emerging role of PtdIns5P: Another signaling phosphoinositide takes its place." *Biochem. Soc. Trans.* 40 (2012): 257–261.

Hagelberg, C., and Allan, D. "Restricted diffusion of integral membrane proteins and polyphosphoinositides leads to their depletion in microvesicles released from human erythrocytes." *Biochem. J.* 271 (1990): 831–834.

Hammond, G.R., Fischer, M.J., Anderson, K.E., Holdich, J., Koteci, A., Balla, T., and Irvine, R.F. "PI4P and PI(4,5)P$_2$ are essential but independent lipid determinants of membrane identity." *Science.* 337 (2012): 727–730.

Heo, W.D., Inoue, T., Park, W.S., Kim, M.L., Park, B.O., Wandless, T.J., and Meyer, T. "PI(3,4,5)P$_3$ and PI(4,5)P$_2$ lipids target proteins with polybasic clusters to the plasma membrane." *Science.* 314 (2006): 1458–1461.

Hirao, M., Sato, N., Kondo, T., Yonemura, S., Monden, M., Sasaki, T. et al. "Regulation mechanism of ERM (ezrin/radixin/moesin) protein/plasma membrane association: Possible involvement of phosphatidylinositol turnover and Rho-dependent signaling pathway." *J. Cell Biol.* 135 (1996): 37–51.

Honda, A., Nogami, M., Yokozeki, T., Yamazaki, M., Nakamura, H., Watanabe, H. et al. "Phosphatidylinositol 4-phosphate 5-kinase alpha is a downstream effector of the small G protein ARF6 in membrane ruffle formation." *Cell.* 99 (1999): 521–532.

Honigmann, A., van den Bogaart, G., Iraheta, E., Risselada, H.J., Milovanovic, D., Mueller, V. et al. "Phosphatidylinositol 4,5-bisphosphate clusters act as molecular beacons for vesicle recruitment." *Nat. Struct. Mol. Biol.* 20 (2013): 679–686.

Höning, S., Ricotta, D., Krauss, M., Späte, K., Spolaore, B., Motley, A. et al. "Phosphatidylinositol-(4,5)-bisphosphate regulates sorting signal recognition by the clathrin-associated adaptor complex AP2." *Mol. Cell.* 18 (2005): 519–531.

Huang, S., Lifshitz, L., Patki-Kamath, V., Tuft, R., Fogarty, K., and Czech, M.P. "Phosphatidylinositol-4,5-bisphosphate-rich plasma membrane patches organize active zones of endocytosis and ruffling in cultured adipocytes." *Mol. Cell Biol.* 24 (2004): 9102–9123.

Iijima, M., Huang, Y.E., and Devreotes, P. "Temporal and spatial regulation of chemotaxis." *Dev. Cell.* 3 (2002): 469–478.

Isenberg, G., Niggli, V., Pieper, U., Kaufmann, S., and Goldmann, W.H. "Probing phosphatidylinositolphosphates and adenosinenucleotides on talin nucleated actin polymerization." *FEBS Lett.* 397 (1996): 316–320.

James, D.J., Khodthong, C., Kowalchyk, J.A., and Martin, T.F. "Phosphatidylinositol 4,5-bisphosphate regulates SNARE-dependent membrane fusion." *J. Cell Biol.* 182 (2008): 355–366.

Janmey, P.A., Iida, K., Yin, H.L., and Stossel, T.P. "Polyphosphoinositide micelles and polyphosphoinositide-containing vesicles dissociate endogenous gelsolin-actin complexes and promote actin assembly from the fast-growing end of actin filaments blocked by gelsolin." *J. Biol. Chem.* 262 (1987): 12228–12236.

Johnson, C.M., Chichili, G.R., and Rodgers, W. "Compartmentalization of phosphatidylinositol 4,5-bisphosphate signaling evidenced using targeted phosphatases." *J. Biol. Chem.* 283 (2008): 29920–29928.

Kalli, A.C., Morgan, G., and Sansom M.S. "Interactions of the auxilin-1 PTEN-like domain with model membranes result in nanoclustering of phosphatidyl inositol phosphates." *Biophys. J.* 105 (2013): 137–145.

Katso, R., Okkenhaug, K., Ahmadi, K., White, S., Timms, J., and Waterfield, M.D. "Cellular function of phosphoinositide 3-kinases: Implications for development, homeostasis, and cancer." *Annu. Rev. Cell Dev. Biol.* 17 (2001): 615–675.

Khuong, T.M., Habets, R.L., Kuenen, S., Witkowska, A., Kasprowicz, J., Swerts, J. et al. "Synaptic PI(3,4,5)P$_3$ is required for syntaxin1A clustering and neurotransmitter release." *Neuron.* 77 (2013): 1097–1108.

Koch, M., and Holt, M. "Coupling exo- and endocytosis: An essential role for PIP$_2$ at the synapse." *Biochim. Biophys. Acta.* 1821 (2012): 1114–1132.

Kusumi, A., Fujiwara, T.K., Morone, N., Yoshida, K.J., Chadda, R., Xie, M. et al. "Membrane mechanisms for signal transduction: The coupling of the meso-scale raft domains to membrane-skeleton-induced compartments and dynamic protein complexes." *Semin. Cell. Dev. Biol.* 23 (2012): 126–144.

Langille, S.E., Patki, V., Klarlund, J.K., Buxton, J.M., Holik, J.J., Chawla, A. et al. "ADP ribosylation factor 6 as a target of guanine nucleotide exchange factor GRP1." *J. Biol. Chem.* 274 (1999): 27099–27104.

Lassing, I., and Lindberg, U. "Specific interaction between phosphatidylinositol 4,5-bisphosphate and profilactin." *Nature.* 314 (1985): 472–474.

Laux, T., Fukami, K., Thelen, M., Golub, T., Frey, D., and Caroni, P. "GAP43, MARCKS, and CAP23 modulate PI(4,5)P2 at plasmalemmal rafts, and regulate cell cortex actin dynamics through a common mechanism." *J. Cell Biol.* 149 (2000): 1455–1472.

Lemmon, M.A., and Ferguson, K.M. "Signal-dependent membrane targeting by pleckstrin homology (PH) domains." *Biochem. J.* 350 (2000): 1–18.

Leventhal, I., Cebers, A., and Janmey, P.A. "Combined electrostatics and hydrogen bonding determine intermolecular interactions between polyphosphoinositides." *J. Am. Chem. Soc.* 130 (2008): 9025–9030.

Leventhal, I., Christian, D.A., Wang, Y.H., Madara, J.J., Discher, D.E., and Janmey, P.A. "Calcium-dependent lateral organization in phosphatidylinositol 4,5-bisphosphate (PIP2)- and cholesterol-containing monolayers." *Biochemistry.* 48 (2009): 8241–8248.

Ling, K., Doughman, R.L., Firestone, A.J., Bunce, M.W., and Anderson, R.A. "Type I g phosphatidylinositol phosphate kinase targets and regulates focal adhesions." *Nature* 420 (2002): 89–93.

Lingwood, D., and Simons, K. "Lipid rafts as a membrane-organizing principle." *Science.* 327 (2010): 46–50.

Lupyan, D., Mezei, M., Logothetis, D.E., and Osman, R. "A molecular dynamics investigation of lipid bilayer perturbation by PIP2." *Biophys. J.* 98 (2010): 240–247.

Manna, D., Albanese, A., Park, W.S., and Cho, W. "Mechanistic basis of differential cellular responses of phosphatidylinositol 3,4-bisphosphate- and phosphatidylinositol 3,4,5-trisphosphate-binding pleckstrin homology domains." *J. Biol. Chem.* 282 (2007): 32093–32105.

Martel, V., Racaud-Sultan, C., Dupe, S., Marie, C., Paulhe, F., Galmichei, A. et al. "Conformation, localization, and integrin binding of Talin depend on its interaction with phosphoinositides." *J. Biol. Chem.* 276 (2001): 21217–21227.

Martin, T.F. "PI(4,5)P$_2$ regulation of surface membrane traffic." *Curr. Opin. Cell Biol.* 13 (2001): 493–499.

Martin, T.F. "Role of PI(4,5)P(2) in vesicle exocytosis and membrane fusion." *Subcell. Biochem.* 59 (2012): 111–130.

McLaughlin, S., Wang, J., Gambhir, A., and Murray, D. "PIP(2) and proteins: Interactions, organization, and information flow." *Annu. Rev. Biophys. Biomol. Struct.* 31 (2002): 151–175.

Miki, H., Miura, K., and Takenawa, T. "NWASP, a novel actin-depolymerizing protein, regulates the cortical cytoskeletal rearrangement in a PIP2-dependent manner downstream of tyrosine kinases." *EMBO J.* 15 (1996): 5326–5335.

Milosevic, I., Sørensen, J.B., Lang, T., Krauss, M., Nagy, G., Haucke, V. et al. "Plasmalemmal phosphatidylinositol-4,5-bisphosphate level regulates the releasable vesicle pool size in chromaffin cells." *J. Neurosci.* 25 (2005): 2557–2565.

Mitchell, K.T., Ferrell, J.E. Jr., and Huestis, W.H. "Separation of phosphoinositides and other phospholipids by two-dimensional thin-layer chromatography." *Anal. Biochem.* 158 (1986): 447–453.

Moens, P.D., and Bagatolli, L.A. "Profilin binding to sub-micellar concentrations of phosphatidylinositol (4,5) bisphosphate and phosphatidylinositol (3,4,5) trisphosphate." *Biochim. Biophys. Acta.* 1768 (2007): 439–449.

Mostowy, S., and Cossart, P. "Septins: The fourth component of the cytoskeleton." *Nat. Rev. Mol. Cell Biol.* 13 (2012): 183–194.

Mulet, X., Templer, R.H., Woscholski, R., and Ces, O. "Evidence that phosphatidylinositol promotes curved membrane interfaces." *Langmuir.* 24 (2008): 8443–8447.

Murray, D.H., and Tamm, L.K. "Clustering of syntaxin-1A in model membranes is modulated by phosphatidylinositol 4,5-bisphosphate and cholesterol." *Biochemistry.* 48 (2009): 4617–4625.

Nunes, J.A., and Guittard, G. "An emerging role for PI5P in T cell biology." *Front. Immunol.* 4 (2013): 80.

Owen, D.J., Collins, B.M., and Evans, P.R. "Adaptors for clathrin coats: Structure and function." *Annu. Rev. Cell Dev. Biol.* 20 (2004): 153–191.

Pettitt, T.R., Dove, S.K., Lubben, A., Calaminus, S.D., and Wakelam, M.J. "Analysis of intact phosphoinositides in biological samples." *J. Lipid Res.* 47 (2006): 1588–1596.

Pike, L.J., and Miller, J.M. "Cholesterol depletion delocalizes phosphatidylinositol bisphosphate and inhibits hormone-stimulated phosphatidylinositol turnover." *J. Biol. Chem.* 273 (1998): 22298–22304.

Posor, Y., Eichhorn-Gruenig, M., Puchkov, D., Schöneberg, J., Ullrich, A., Lampe, A. et al. "Spatiotemporal control of endocytosis by phosphatidylinositol-3,4-bisphosphate." *Nature.* 499 (2013): 233–237.

Rameh, L.E., Tolias, K.F., Duckworth, B.C., and Cantley, L.C. "A new pathway for synthesis of phosphatidylinositol-4,5-bisphosphate." *Nature.* 390 (1997): 192–196.

Redfern, D.A., and Gericke, A. "Domain formation in phosphatidylinositol monophosphate/phosphatidylcholine mixed vesicles." *Biophys. J.* 86 (2004): 2980–2992.

Redfern, D.A., and Gericke, A. "pH-dependent domain formation in phosphatidylinositol polyphosphate/phosphatidylcholine mixed vesicles." *J. Lipid Res.* 46 (2005): 504–515.

Rohacs, T. "Phosphoinositide regulation of non-canonical transient receptor potential channels." *Cell Calcium.* 45 (2009): 554–565.

Rohde, G., Wenzel, D., and Haucke, V. "A phosphatidylinositol (4,5)-bisphosphate binding site within mu2-adaptin regulates clathrin-mediated endocytosis." *J. Cell Biol.* 158 (2002): 209–214.

Saarikangas, J., Zhao, H., and Lappalainen, P. "Regulation of the actin cytoskeleton-plasma membrane interplay by phosphoinositides." *Physiol. Rev.* 90 (2010): 259–289.

Sarkes, D., and Rameh, L.E. "A novel HPLC-based approach makes possible the spatial characterization of cellular PtdIns5P and other phosphoinositides." *Biochem. J.* 428 (2010): 375–384.

Sieber, J.J., Willig, K.I., Kutzner, C., Gerding-Reimers, C., Harke, B., Donnert, G. et al. "Dynamics of a supramolecular membrane protein cluster." *Science.* 317 (2007): 1072–1076.

Simonson, A., Wurmser, A.E., Emr, S.D., and Stenmark, H. "The role of phosphoinositides in membrane transport." *Curr. Opin. Cell Biol.* 13 (2001): 485–492.

Stephens, L.R., Hughes, K.T., and Irvine, R.F. "Pathway of phosphatidylinositol(3,4,5)-trisphosphate synthesis in activated neutrophils." *Nature.* 351 (1991): 33–39.

Stephens, L.R., Jackson, T.R., and Hawkins, P.T. "Agonist-stimulated synthesis of phosphatidylinositol(3,4,5)-trisphosphate: A new intracellular signalling system?" *Biochim. Biophys. Acta.* 1179 (1993): 27–75.

Suh, B., and Hille, B. "PIP2 is a necessary cofactor for ion channel function: How and why?" *Annu. Rev. Biophys.* 37 (2008): 175–195.

Sun, Y., Thapa, N., Hedman, A.C., and Anderson, R.A. "Phosphatidylinositol 4,5-bisphosphate: Targeted production and signaling." *Bioessays.* 35 (2013): 513–522.

Swaney, K.F., Huang, C.H., and Devreotes, P.N. "Eukaryotic chemotaxis: A network of signaling pathways controls motility, directional sensing, and polarity." *Annu. Rev. Biophys.* 39 (2010): 265–289.

Takenawa, T. "Phosphoinositide-binding interface proteins involved in shaping cell membranes." *Proc. Jpn. Acad. Ser. B Phys. Biol. Sci.* 86 (2010): 509–523.

Takenawa, T., and Itoh, T. "Phosphoinositides, key molecules for regulation of actin cytoskeletal organization and membrane traffic from the plasma membrane." *Biochim. Biophys. Acta.* 1533 (2001): 190–206.

Tall, E., Spector, I., Pentyala, S.N., Bitter, I., and Rebecchi, M.J. "Dynamics of phosphatidylinositol 4,5-bisphosphate in actin-supported structures." *Curr. Biol.* 10 (2000): 743–746.

Taverna, E., Saba, E., Linetti, A., Longhi, R., Jeromin, A., Righi, M., Clementi, F., and Rosa, P. "Localization of synaptic proteins involved in neurosecretion in different membrane microdomains." *J. Neurochem.* 100 (2007): 664–677.

Tristram-Nagle, S., and Nagle, J.F. "Lipid bilayers: Thermodynamics, structure, fluctuations, and interactions." *Chem. Phys. Lipids.* 127 (2004): 3–14.

Vadnal, R.E., and Parthasarathy, R. "The identification of a novel inositol lipid, phosphatidylinositol trisphosphate (PIP3), in rat cerebrum using in vivo techniques." *Biochem. Biophys. Res. Commun.* 163 (1989): 995–1001.

van den Bogaart, G., Meyenberg, K., Risselada, H.J., Amin, H., Willig, K.I., Hubrich, B.E. et al. "Membrane protein sequestering by ionic protein-lipid interactions." *Nature.* 479 (2011): 552–555.

van den Bogaart, G., Meyenberg, K., Diederichsen, U., and Jahn, R. "Phosphatidylinositol 4,5-bisphosphate increases the Ca^{2+} affinity of synaptotagmin-1 40-fold." *J. Biol. Chem.* 287 (2012): 16447–16453.

Várnai, P., and Balla, T. "Visualization of phosphoinositides that bind pleckstrin homology domains: Calcium- and agonist-induced dynamic changes and relationship to myo-[^{3}H] inositol-labeled phosphoinositide pools." *J. Cell Biol.* 143 (1998): 501–510.

Vasudevan, L. "The β- and γ-isoforms of type I PIP5K regulate distinct stages of Ca^{2+} signaling in mast cells." *J. Cell. Sci.* 122 (2009): 2567–2574.

Vines, C.M. "Phospholipase C." *Adv. Exp. Med. Biol.* 740 (2012): 235–254.

Wang, J., and Richards, D.A. "Segregation of PIP2 and PIP3 into distinct nanoscale regions within the plasma membrane." *Biol. Open.* 1 (2012): 857–862.

Wang, Y.H., Collins, A., Guo, L., Smith-Dupont, K.B., Gai, F., Svitkina, T., and Janmey, P.A. "Divalent cation-induced cluster formation by polyphosphoinositides in model membranes." *J. Am. Chem. Soc.* 134 (2012): 3387–3395.

Wang, Y.J., Wang, J., Sun, H.Q., Martinez, M., Sun, Y.X., Macia, E. et al. "Phosphatidylinositol 4 phosphate regulates targeting of clathrin adaptor AP-1 complexes to the Golgi." *Cell.* 114 (2003): 299–310.

Waugh, M.G., Lawson, D., Tan, S.K., and Hsuan, J.J. "Phosphatidylinositol 4-phosphate synthesis in immunoisolated caveolae like vesicles and low buoyant density non-caveolar membranes." *J. Biol. Chem.* 273 (1998): 17115–17121.

Wen, P.J., Osborne, S.L., and Meunier, F.A. "Dynamic control of neuroexocytosis by phosphoinositides in health and disease." *Prog. Lipid Res.* 50 (2011): 52–61.

Wilcox, A., and Hinchliffe, K.A. "Regulation of extranuclear PtdIns5P production by phosphatidylinositol phosphate 4-kinase 2α." *FEBS Lett.* 582 (2008): 1391–1394.

Yonezawa, N., Nishida, E., Iida, K., Yahara, I., and Sakai, H. "Inhibition of the interactions of cofilin, destrin, and deoxyribonuclease I with actin by phosphoinositides." *J. Biol. Chem.* 265 (1990): 8382–8386.

Yu, J.W., Mendrola, J.M., Audhya, A., Singh, S., Keleti, D., DeWald, D.B. et al. "Genome-wide analysis of membrane targeting by *S. cerevisiae* pleckstrin homology domains." *Mol. Cell.* 13 (2004): 677–688.

Zaydman, M.A., Silva, J.R., Delaloye, K., Li, Y., Liang, H., Larsson, H.P. et al. "Kv7.1 ion channels require a lipid to couple voltage sensing to pore opening." *Proc. Natl. Acad. Sci. USA.* 110 (2013): 13180–13185.

Zhang, L., Mao, Y.S., Janmey, P.A., and Yin, H.L. "Phosphatidylinositol 4,5 bisphosphate and the actin cytoskeleton." *Subcell. Biochem.* 59 (2012a): 177–215.

Zhang, X., Li, X., and Xu, H. "Phosphoinositide isoforms determine compartment-specific ion channel activity." *Proc. Natl. Acad. Sci. USA.* 109 (2012b): 11384–11389.

9 Signaling Phagocytosis
Role of Specialized Lipid Domains

Sharon Eisenberg and Sergio Grinstein

CONTENTS

The plasma membrane bilayer plays a central role in cellular signaling: it not only establishes the spatial segregation between the extracellular and cytosolic compartments but also harbors transmembrane receptors, adaptors, and effectors, and serves to anchor membrane-associated scaffolds that are involved in many signal transduction pathways.[1–4] It is now clear that, far from being disordered, the plasma membrane is a complex, highly organized yet dynamic structure, whose components are continuously reorganized. Proteins and lipids are spatially segregated in defined micrometer- and nanometer-scale regions of the cell membrane.[5,6]

Data collected during the past years suggest that, in all likelihood, not only the plasmalemma but also endomembranes are segregated into dynamic nanodomains. Notably, previous studies have shown that endosomes act as intracellular signal transduction hubs with distinct subdomains.[7,8] In addition, proteins that leave the endoplasmic reticulum emerge as export complexes at specialized exit sites, where they accumulate in transport carriers. These structures then transit from the reticulum intermediate compartment to the Golgi apparatus, where they fuse with the *cis* cisternae.[9] While such endomembrane nanodomains are increasingly appreciated, the plasmalemmal nanodomains are by far the best studied, in part because they are more readily accessible. The lateral segregation within the plasma membrane is caused by a variety of lipid–lipid, lipid–protein, and protein–protein associations, as well as by interactions of membrane components with the cytoskeleton.[2] The net result of these interactions is the nonrandom distribution of lipids and proteins across different types of nanodomains. One important function ascribed to these structures is the concentration of proteins or lipids to generate transport stations or signaling complexes (signalosomes). Examples of such nanodomains are the lateral assemblies of cholesterol and sphingolipids, which are termed *lipid rafts*,[1,10,11] as well as caveolae and clathrin-coated pits.[12]

The stability of the nanodomains varies: some are relatively permanent or at least long lived, while others are metastable. In the plasma membrane, the reported lifetimes of nanodomains can vary greatly: from tens of seconds—as in the case of clathrin clusters[13]—down to milliseconds in the case of small rafts.[14,15] The transient small rafts can be stabilized when assembled into larger structures by clustering their constituent proteins.[16–18] However, in most of these studies, clustering was achieved by cross-linking raft components with antibodies and the physiological significance of these observations is questionable. Yet, recent studies have shown that cross-linking of GM1 gangliosides with natural ligands such as cholera toxin resulted in the formation of comparable raft aggregates.[19,20]

In addition to the nanodomains present in the steady state, unique novel complexes can be generated transiently during signaling. One such instance was described by Tian et al.,[21] who reported that small and dynamic K-Ras nanoclusters are formed in response to stimulation, acting like "nano-switches" that function as high-gain signal amplifiers of the Raf kinase pathway.

A particularly interesting and extensively studied membrane subdomain is the nascent phagosome, which forms de novo in the plasma membrane during the process of particle engulfment by professional phagocytes such as macrophages or neutrophils. This receptor-mediated internalization process provides unique opportunities for the study of signaling by optical methods. The key events occur in comparably large structures, well above the diffraction limit of the optical microscope. Importantly, the size of the active zone where signals are generated and conveyed, termed the *phagocytic cup*, can be manipulated experimentally by supplying cells with phagocytic targets of the desired diameter. In addition, phagocytosis develops relatively slowly and persists for many seconds to minutes. Together, these convenient features enable the application of three-dimensional confocal imaging and other advanced biophysical techniques to the study of an important biological process.

9.1 PHAGOCYTOSIS: A PRIMER

Phagocytosis is defined as the ingestion by cells of large (≥ 0.5 μm in diameter) particles. It is a critical event in the elimination of invading microorganisms and other foreign particles and in the subsequent presentation of antigens for development of acquired immunity. Moreover, the phagocytosis of effete (apoptotic or necrotic) cells, termed *efferocytosis*, is key to tissue homeostasis and remodeling. Phagocytosis can be conceptually divided into two sequential steps: phagosome formation and maturation. The former refers to the engulfment process, whereby the target particles are initially recognized by surface receptors and subsequently internalized by the phagocytic cell, becoming enclosed within a membrane-bound vacuole, the nascent phagosome. Maturation refers to the progressive conversion of the nascent phagosome from an inert vacuole into an effective microbicidal and degradative organelle, the phagolysosome. Over the course of an hour, the phagosome transforms thoroughly, ultimately resembling a lysosome; its lumen becomes markedly acidic and rich in hydrolases and in a variety of bacteriostatic and microbicidal agents.

Phagocytosis contributes to the first line of defense against infection. Foreign bodies such as bacteria or fungi can be eliminated at infection sites by professional phagocytes such as neutrophils, macrophages, and dendritic cells. By generating antigens from such microorganisms and presenting them to lymphoid cells, phagocytosis also plays a key role in the initiation of the adaptive immune response. Interestingly, phagocytes attract lymphoid cells by releasing proinflammatory cytokines, which are released upon engagement of phagocytic targets.[22,23] Notably, whereas professional phagocytes unleash an inflammatory reaction when engulfing foreign bodies, they respond differently when confronted with apoptotic bodies. In this instance, phagocytosis is accompanied by the release of anti-inflammatory mediators, which prevent tissue damage and contribute to healing.

Owing to the number of different phagocytic cell types and receptors, the variety of their targets, and the complexity of their interactions, the engulfment processes are not always identical. Indeed, phagocytosis is an umbrella term that encompasses a diversity of related, yet distinct phenomena that likely differ considerably at the molecular level. Both phagosome formation and maturation are complex and sophisticated processes that involve signaling, cytoskeleton remodeling, and membrane traffic and restructuring.

Phagocytosis can be triggered by a wide variety of receptors that, judging from the limited evidence available to date, differ in their mode of signaling and in the eventual outcome. The most studied are the Fcγ receptors, which recognize the Fc region of antibodies. Internalization of IgG-coated particles by Fcγ receptors is by far the best understood model of phagocytosis. The majority of the results discussed below were obtained by triggering phagocytosis via these receptors. Though highly informative, data obtained from Fcγ receptor-mediated engulfment may not be applicable to other forms of phagocytosis. Moreover, most of the experiments described in this chapter were performed using macrophages—the phagocytic cell par excellence—as a model system and may not apply to neutrophils, dendritic cells, or nonprofessional phagocytes. In fact, much of the information was derived from studies of the murine macrophage line RAW264.7. These cells have an insatiable appetite and are moderately transfectable, making them an attractive experimental model. However, it is clear that RAW264.7 cells are an imperfect mimic of the primary macrophage; generalization of the concepts derived from their use will require future validation using bona fide primary phagocytes.

Fc receptors in general, and Fcγ receptors in particular, are activated by multivalent ligands that induce receptor clustering, forcing the de novo formation of signaling nanodomains.[24,25] The lateral aggregation of the Fc receptors by extracellular ligands forces the local accumulation of their cytosolic domains, which possess a unique region known as the immunoreceptor tyrosine-based activation motif (ITAM). This activation motif is characterized by tandem YxxI/L sequences that can be phosphorylated by tyrosine kinases such as Hck, Lyn,[26,27] Fgr,[28] and probably other kinases of the Src family,[29] and also by Syk. Depending on the type of Fcγ receptor, the ITAM can be part of the same polypeptidic chain that engages the ligand, as in the case of Fcγ receptor IIA and Fcγ receptor IIC, or of a separate γ subunit that associates noncovalently with the ligand-binding subunit of the receptor, as in the case of Fcγ receptor I and Fcγ receptor IIIA. Importantly, phosphorylation of both tyrosines of the ITAM is required for optimal signaling and phagocytosis.[30,31]

Despite extensive study, the precise mechanism whereby receptor clustering leads to the ITAM tyrosine phosphorylation remains unclear. One model suggests that clustering stabilizes the association between the receptors and cholesterol-enriched nanodomains, where Src-family kinases are concentrated, thereby generating a signaling-platform nanodomain. Accordingly, a number of studies have shown that Fcγ receptor II becomes associated with detergent-resistant membranes upon cross-linking.[32,33] This association was shown to depend, in the case of Fcγ IIA, on receptor palmitoylation;[34] introduction of a palmitate moiety is known to promote association of membrane proteins with lipid rafts. In addition, it has been reported that cholesterol depletion with methyl-β-cyclodextrin inhibits Fcγ receptor IIA phosphorylation in response to clustering,[32] but this is not a universal observation and may reflect nonselective membrane alterations. Despite this suggestive evidence, several caveats must be considered: (a) among the Fcγ receptors, Fcγ IIA is the only isoform that undergoes palmitoylation. Therefore, other Fcγ receptors may not associate with lipid rafts or would do so by a different mechanism; (b) it is not clear whether the detergent-resistant membranes indeed reflect the segregation of lipids in biological membranes, or are artificially induced by the nonionic detergents used in their isolation; (c) since methyl-β-cyclodextrin is suspected to have additional effects on membrane organization unrelated to cholesterol removal,[35] conclusions based on this treatment are increasingly being questioned. Taken together, the lipid raft model of Fc receptor activation must be considered with caution.

Once the Fcγ receptor ITAM is doubly phosphorylated (primarily via Src kinases), a different tyrosine kinase, Syk, can bind firmly via its two Src-homology 2 (SH2) domains.[36] This cytosolic kinase is expressed mostly in hematopoietic cells and becomes activated by phosphorylation upon Fcγ receptor clustering.[36,37] Studies in macrophages from $syk^{-/-}$ mice demonstrated that Syk is absolutely required for Fcγ receptor-mediated phagocytosis.[38,39] Remarkably, however, the actin polymerization that normally accompanies phagocytosis is not totally eliminated, and the cells form incipient phagocytic cups that become arrested at an early stage.[38] This observation suggests that, whereas Syk is essential for completion of phagocytosis, some early signaling can be triggered independently of this kinase. Interestingly, phosphorylation of the Fcγ receptor γ chain is greatly reduced in $syk^{-/-}$ macrophages, and Syk can phosphorylate the receptor ITAM in vitro.[39] Thus, it is possible that once some ITAM tyrosines are phosphorylated by Src-family kinases, Syk is recruited and can phosphorylate additional tyrosine residues within the same or in neighboring ITAMs, thereby amplifying the signaling cascade.

Syk phosphorylation leads to additional recruitment or phosphorylation of adaptor or signaling proteins to the activated Fcγ receptor complex, including growth factor receptor-bound protein 2 (Grb2), the linker of activated T cells (LAT), class I phosphatidylinositol-3-phosphate kinase (PI3K), phospholipase Cγ (PLCγ), and Vav isoforms.[40,41] This signaling cascade induces a biphasic actin remodeling response. Like construction scaffolding, actin filaments at the phagosomal cup are initially assembled and then disassembled as the pseudopod progresses around the target particle. The spike in actin polymerization is tied to the recruitment of multiple guanine nucleotide-exchange factors such as Vav and DOCK180, which recruit the actin nucleator Arp2/3 via one or more Rho-family small GTPases. Rac and Cdc42 are activated by Fc receptors and in turn activate the Wiskott–Aldrich syndrome family proteins WAVE and WASP[42] that finally recruit Arp2/3. Inhibition of actin polymerization causes an inability of the membrane to protrude, envelop, and ultimately engulf the particle.[43] Importantly, after the particle is surrounded by the phagocytic pseudopods, the opposite reaction is needed: in order to allow the nascent phagosome to enter the cell, the actin filaments that normally line the plasma membrane must disassemble. In contrast to the intensive analysis of the mechanism of actin polymerization, the molecular basis of the subsequent depolymerization has not been studied directly. Likely candidates involved in this process include actin-severing proteins and Rho family GTPase-activating proteins. Clearly, the actin polarization/depolarization cycle must be timed accurately to ensure optimal engulfment. Yet, the coordination of these events is poorly understood. How phagosomes undergo scission from the plasma membrane is also unclear.

9.2   LIPID REMODELING AND PHAGOCYTOSIS

Despite these gaping holes in our knowledge, it is becoming apparent that phospholipids play a critical role in orchestrating the signaling events that trigger phagosome formation, scission, and maturation. During the early stages of the process, the plasma membrane undergoes extensive remodeling by lipid alteration and formation of specialized domains.[44] For a long time, studies of lipid dynamics were hampered by the poor sensitivity and very limited spatial and temporal resolution of the methods available. Lipids and lipid-derived second messengers are often scarce, short lived, and chemically unstable, hence difficult to detect. They are susceptible to hydrolysis, oxidation, or other irreversible alterations in the course of cell lysis and fractionation, complicating precise quantification by conventional biochemical methods. Analysis by immunological methods is sometimes available but poses another set of unique challenges. Suitable, specific antibodies to defined lipids are rare. In addition, the methods commonly used for immunodetection of intracellular proteins, which utilize fixation followed by permeabilization with detergents or solvents, are not directly applicable to lipids. Unlike proteins, lipids are not readily fixable and often undergo extensive removal or massive distortion of their architecture when cells are permeabilized.

These considerations brought to the fore the urgent need for new techniques to assess lipid distribution and dynamics in intact cells. The field was pioneered by the laboratories of Tamas Balla and Tobias Meyer,[45–48] who introduced a series of genetically encoded lipid-specific probes. The fundamental concept underlying the design of practically all such probes is similar: the sequence of a fluorescent protein, such as GFP or RFP, is fused to the sequence encoding a domain derived from a cellular protein previously established to interact selectively with the head-group of a defined lipid, in the context of its physiological function. Thus, PH (pleckstrin homology), FYVE (named after Fab 1, YOTB, Vac 1, and EEA1), and PX (*phox* or phagocyte oxidase) domains, which had been appreciated to bind to specific phosphoinositides, have been exploited to monitor the distribution and metabolism of their cognate lipids. In addition, C1 domains are now extensively used to monitor diacylglycerol (DAG), and discoidin C2 domains recognize phosphatidylserine (PS) and are now used for its detection in live cells. The ever-increasing availability of fluorescent proteins with varying spectral properties[49] enables researchers to monitor two, and potentially more, different probes simultaneously.

One such biosensor containing the PH domain of PLCδ binds selectively to phosphatidylinositol 4,5-bisphosphate [PI(4,5)P$_2$].[50] This phosphoinositide is of particular interest in the context of phagocytosis, because of its well-known role in actin remodeling. PI(4,5)P$_2$ binds to a range of actin-capping, severing, and monomer-binding proteins and can thereby influence actin filament formation, extension, and fragmentation.[51] Using the fluorescent PH-PLCδ probe, it was shown that, as in other cells, the plasma membrane of resting macrophages is rich in PI(4,5)P$_2$.[52] In response to Fcγ receptor clustering by IgG-coated particles, Botelho et al.[52] reported a modest, transient enrichment of PI(4,5)P$_2$ at the early stages of phagocytosis, followed by a marked reduction in the PI(4,5)P$_2$ levels at the base of the phagosomal cup. This phenomenon is even more pronounced in the case of *Candida*, which forms long hyphae that are engulfed slowly and often incompletely (Figure 9.1). PI(4,5)P$_2$ becomes undetectable when the nascent phagosome undergoes scission from the plasma membrane. As illustrated in Figure 9.1a, the elimination of PI(4,5)P$_2$ begins even before phagosome closure is completed, first around the base of the phagocytic cup and then extending along the pseudopods. Remarkably, the loss of PI(4,5)P$_2$

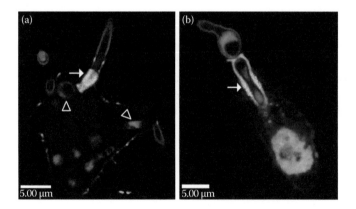

FIGURE 9.1 Distribution of PI(4,5)P$_2$ and PI(3,4,5)P$_3$ during phagocytosis. RAW264.7 macrophages were transfected with a chimeric construct consisting of the pleckstrin homology domain of PLCδ (a) or Akt (b) fused to GFP. These constructs are biosensor for PI(4,5)P$_2$ or PI(3,4,5)P$_3$, respectively. The cells were then exposed to hyphae of *Candida* that expressed blue fluorescent protein. After 60 min, extracellular *Candida* or portions thereof were identified by addition of rhodamine-labeled concanavalin A. Finally, F-actin was stained using labeled phalloidin (shown white in the figure). The solid arrow indicates actin structure at the neck of the unsealed phagosome formed around an incompletely internalized hypha. (a) Open arrowheads point to internalized portions of *Candida* that reside within PI(4,5)P$_2$-depleted vacuoles. (b) Note the accumulation of PI(3,4,5)P$_3$ in the phagocytic cup to concentrations greater than those detectable in the adjacent plasma membrane. (Images acquired and kindly provided by Drs. Xenia Naj and Michelle Maxson.)

does not extend to the bulk membrane abutting the forming phagosome. More recent FCS (fluorescence correlation spectroscopy) and FRAP (fluorescence recovery after photobleaching) studies support the hypothesis that there is a barrier or fence around the forming phagosome that impedes the diffusion of $PI(4,5)P_2$ into and out of the phagosomal cup. This putative fence allows the surface concentration of $PI(4,5)P_2$ in the cup to first increase and then decrease locally during phagocytosis.[53] The site of actin accumulation at the neck of *Candida* coincides with the diffusional divide. We speculate that a specialized actin structure underpins the formation of a stable diffusional barrier composed of a dense cluster of transmembrane proteins anchored to the cortical cytoskeleton.

The mechanism accounting for the initial transient elevation of $PI(4,5)P_2$ is not well understood. It most likely involves the local stimulation of phosphatidylinositol 4-phosphate 5 kinases (PIP5K),[54] but this remains to be verified experimentally. By contrast, much more is known about the processes that mediate the disappearance of $PI(4,5)P_2$ from the membrane of the forming phagosome. Elimination of $PI(4,5)P_2$ appears to involve a combination of several concomitant events: conversion to phosphatidylinositol 3,4,5-trisphosphate [$PI(3,4,5)P_3$] by activation of PI3K (Figure 9.1b), hydrolysis to DAG and inositol 3,4,5-trisphosphate by PLCγ, recruitment of the 5-phosphatases OCRL and Inpp5b that convert $PI(4,5)P_2$ back to $PI(4)P$, and a net reduction in $PI(4,5)P_2$ synthesis caused by dissociation of the kinases from the membrane.[52,54,55]

These early changes in lipid metabolism are required for the progression of phagocytosis. Inhibition of $PI(4,5)P_2$ phosphorylation by PI3K (e.g., using wortmannin or PI-103) or of its hydrolysis (e.g., using the PLC inhibitor U73122) arrests phagocytosis. A similar result is obtained when PIP5K is overexpressed or when its retention at the phagosomal cup is enforced by changing its targeting determinants.[54] It is generally believed that $PI(3,4,5)P_3$ and possibly also DAG provide essential signals to promote phagocytosis. In addition, $PI(4,5)P_2$ disappearance itself is likely required for cytoskeletal remodeling, presumably favoring actin dissociation from the base of the cup.[56]

DAG can directly activate protein kinase C (PKC) or other proteins with C1 domains. However, it may also serve as the substrate for the formation of phosphatidic acid (PA), through the action of DAG kinase.[57] Indeed, PA accumulates at the phagocytic cup and on nascent phagosomes in response to Fcγ receptor clustering. It is not clear, however, whether this PA is generated primarily by DAG-kinases or through hydrolysis of phosphatidylcholine by phospholipase D (PLD).[58,59] In macrophages, the PLD1 isoform is localized in the late endosomal and lysosomal compartments, while PLD2 is found on the plasma membrane, including the phagocytic cup and the extending pseudopods.[59] It is noteworthy that both isoforms of PLD require $PI(4,5)P_2$ for optimal activity, but they differ in their requirement for other cofactors: PLD1 is markedly stimulated by GTPases like Rho, Ral, and Arf, or by PKC.[59,60] PA can also be formed de novo through the acylation of glycerol-3-phosphate, by acylation of lysophosphatidic acid (LPA) by LPA acyltransferase, or, as stated above, by phosphorylation of DAG by DAG kinases.[61–63]

Because the cross-sectional area of its negatively charged head-group is very small compared with that of its acyl chains, which are often unsaturated, PA is a cone-shaped (type II) lipid. As such, it can confer negative (concave) curvature on membranes.[64] Because of this bilayer-curving property, PA has been suggested to promote membrane fission and may be required for scission of nascent phagosomes from the surface membrane. Moreover, PA may contribute to phagocytosis also through its ability to stimulate PIP5K. These speculative notions merit experimental testing.

PI(3,4,5,)P$_3$ and DAG remain at the phagosomal membrane for approximately 1 to 2 min after sealing of the nascent vacuole is completed and rapidly disappear afterward.[52,65] Two distinct phosphatases have been proposed to account for the hydrolysis of PI(3,4,5,)P$_3$: the SH2 domain-containing inositol phosphatase (SHIP) and phosphatase and tensin homolog (PTEN). SHIP has been documented to accumulate at sites of phagocytosis, attracted at least in part by the immunoreceptor tyrosine–based inhibitory motif of inhibitory Fc receptors. Recruitment or activation of PTEN during phagocytosis, to our knowledge, has not been reported. The basal activity of this largely soluble phosphatase could contribute to the disappearance of PI(3,4,5,)P$_3$, but this remains to be ascertained experimentally. DAG may conceivably be removed from sealed phagosomes by lipases or by continued conversion to PA by kinases.

Remodeling of lipids appears to be critical in timing protein recruitment and activation during phagocytosis. PI(3,4,5,)P$_3$ and DAG act as second messengers capable of recruiting and activating a variety of downstream effectors. DAG has the ability to bind proteins with C1 domains, including DAG kinases and many PKC isoforms.[66] By binding anionic phospholipids—mostly phosphoinositides and PS—the C2 domain of PKC also contributes to association of the kinase with the membrane,[67] usually in a calcium-dependent manner. A variety of other proteins attach to the membrane via PH, ENTH (epsin NH-terminal homology), FERM (band 4.1/ezrin/radixin/moesin), and other similar domains that recognize the head-group of PI(4,5)P$_2$ stereospecifically.[68,69] Some of these proteins influence cytoskeletal structure by capping or severing actin filaments,[70] while others, like PLD, can generate second messengers or modulate the activity of GTPases.[71] PI(3,4,5)P$_3$ can also be recognized selectively by proteins with PH or PX domain,[72] such as PLCγ, Akt, Vav, and PKD isoforms that are attracted to the membrane, where they contribute to phagocytosis and its associated responses.

In addition to the stereospecific recognition events described in the preceding paragraph, the anionic phospholipids of the membrane contribute to protein recruitment and activation by electrostatic means. Because of their anionic character, PS and the phosphoinositides—mostly PI(4,5)P$_2$—confer a net negative charge to the inner leaflet of the plasma membrane.[73] This charge attracts and retains cationic proteins and other cationic species at or near the membrane. Importantly, the local alterations in lipid composition that take place during phagocytosis are, by necessity, associated with changes in the surface charge and hence the electrostatic potential of the membrane. As such, the remodeling of lipids can, in principle, cause redistribution of proteins that associate with the membrane (at least in part) by means of cationic domains. Using fluorescent probes of surface charge—coincidence detectors consisting of a polycationic sequence and a hydrophobic determinant—Yeung et al.[74] found that the disappearance of PI(4,5)P$_2$ from the phagosomal membrane is associated with, and likely causes, a marked reduction in the surface charge of the membrane of the nascent vacuole.

PS is the most abundant anionic phospholipid in the plasma membrane.[75] Because it is asymmetrically distributed, virtually confined to the inner leaflet, PS is thought to be a major contributor to the negative charge of the surface of the membrane facing the cytosol.[76] Despite its abundance and importance, no probes were available until recently to detect PS inside live cells. Annexin V, widely used as a probe for exofacial PS, is ineffective inside cells, because it requires high (supraphysiological) concentrations of calcium. To overcome this deficiency, Yeung et al.[77] developed a fluorescent biosensor that binds PS selectively, based on the use of discoidin-type C2 domains. These β-barreled structures have exquisite selectivity for the phosphoserine head-group of PS. Applying these novel probes to live macrophages engulfing particles revealed that PS persists on the phagosomal membrane throughout the phagosome formation and maturation stages.

By retaining PS, the nascent phagosome membrane maintains a degree of residual negativity, despite the depletion of $PI(4,5)P_2$ and $PI(3,4,5)P_3$.[74] The reduced, yet nevertheless significant negative charge of sealed phagosomes promotes the recruitment of signaling molecules with moderately cationic charge. One such protein, c-Src, is relevant to phagocytosis and phagolysosome fusion;[78,79] its association with the phagosomal membrane shows strong correlation with the presence of PS.[74] The distribution of small GTPases of the Rab and Rho superfamilies, which have been shown to be guided electrostatically to cellular membranes,[80] is also affected by the changes associated with lipid remodeling. As discussed above and elsewhere, these GTPases play crucial roles in phagosome formation and maturation. Importantly, PIP5K, the kinase responsible for generation of $PI(4,5)P_2$ at the membrane, also associates electrostatically with the resting plasmalemma and dissociates from the phagosome as the surface charge drops.[54] This in turn terminates the biosynthesis of $PI(4,5)P_2$ after scission of the phagosome from the surface membrane.

To date, the studies of lipid dynamics and surface charge during the course of phagocytosis have all been limited to the microscale, as opposed to the nanoscale. Clearly, there is an urgent need for the application of super-resolution imaging tools capable of defining and tracking nanodomains and even single molecules. The coming years will surely see the application of modern imaging approaches to break the diffraction barrier. Basic observations of cells performing phagocytosis have been made by electron microscopy, but these have been largely descriptive and are, by necessity, stationary. We anticipate dedicated use of atomic force microscopy, near-field scanning optical microscopy, stimulated emission depletion (STED) microscopy, FCS, and nanoclustering-based Forster resonance energy transfer (FRET) (detailed in Refs. 81–84) to the analysis of phagosome formation and maturation. Even electron microscopy should be revisited with the aim of analyzing the heterogeneity of lipids in the membrane during the course of phagocytosis. This approach was recently used to provide quantitative information on the subcellular distribution of PS in cells at rest.[85] Lipid nanodomains have also been studied by STED microscopy, which showed that $PI(4,5)P_2$ can accumulate in neuronal membranes in nanodomains of ~73 nm in size. These nanodomains, which are distinct from rafts, are generated electrostatically as a result of clustering of syntaxin.[86]

In summary, phagocytosis offers an ideal paradigm to study receptor-initiated changes in membrane domain structure. The ability to dictate the time and site of stimulation, together with the comparatively slow development of the responses, makes it possible to direct analytical tools to regions of the membrane where marked, progressive changes take place. While conventional optical methods have been used for the most part to date, single-particle tracking and other super-resolution approaches are beginning to be applied to this fascinating phenomenon and will surely yield many invaluable insights.

REFERENCES

1. Edidin, M. "The State of Lipid Rafts: From Model Membranes to Cells." *Annu Rev Biophys Biomol Struct* 32 (2003): 257–83.
2. Hancock, J. F. "Lipid Rafts: Contentious Only from Simplistic Standpoints." *Nat Rev Mol Cell Biol* 7, no. 6 (2006): 456–62.
3. Kusumi, A., H. Ike, C. Nakada, K. Murase, and T. Fujiwara. "Single-Molecule Tracking of Membrane Molecules: Plasma Membrane Compartmentalization and Dynamic Assembly of Raft-Philic Signaling Molecules." *Semin Immunol* 17, no. 1 (2005): 3–21.
4. Munro, S. "Lipid Rafts: Elusive or Illusive?" *Cell* 115, no. 4 (2003): 377–88.
5. Jacobson, K., E. D. Sheets, and R. Simson. "Revisiting the Fluid Mosaic Model of Membranes." *Science* 268, no. 5216 (1995): 1441–2.
6. Maxfield, F. R. "Plasma Membrane Microdomains." *Curr Opin Cell Biol* 14, no. 4 (2002): 483–7.
7. Fehrenbacher, N., D. Bar-Sagi, and M. Philips. "Ras/MAPK Signaling from Endo-membranes." *Mol Oncol* 3, no. 4 (2009): 297–307.
8. Schenck, A., L. Goto-Silva, C. Collinet et al. "The Endosomal Protein Appl1 Mediates Akt Substrate Specificity and Cell Survival in Vertebrate Development." *Cell* 133, no. 3 (2008): 486–97.
9. Murshid, A., and J. F. Presley. "ER-to-Golgi Transport and Cytoskeletal Interactions in Animal Cells." *Cell Mol Life Sci* 61, no. 2 (2004): 133–45.
10. Simons, K., and E. Ikonen. "Functional Rafts in Cell Membranes." *Nature* 387, no. 6633 (1997): 569–72.
11. Simons, K., and W. L. Vaz. "Model Systems, Lipid Rafts, and Cell Membranes." *Annu Rev Biophys Biomol Struct* 33 (2004): 269–95.
12. Kirchhausen, T., W. Boll, A. van Oijen, and M. Ehrlich. "Single-Molecule Live-Cell Imaging of Clathrin-Based Endocytosis." *Biochem Soc Symp*, 72 (2005): 71–6.
13. Ehrlich, M., W. Boll, A. Van Oijen et al. "Endocytosis by Random Initiation and Stabilization of Clathrin-Coated Pits." *Cell* 118, no. 5 (2004): 591–605.
14. Kenworthy, A. K., N. Petranova, and M. Edidin. "High-Resolution FRET Microscopy of Cholera Toxin B-Subunit and GPI-Anchored Proteins in Cell Plasma Membranes." *Mol Biol Cell* 11, no. 5 (2000): 1645–55.
15. Kawasaki, K., J. J. Yin, W. K. Subczynski, J. S. Hyde, and A. Kusumi. "Pulse EPR Detection of Lipid Exchange between Protein-Rich Raft and Bulk Domains in the Membrane: Methodology Development and Its Application to Studies of Influenza Viral Membrane." *Biophys J* 80, no. 2 (2001): 738–48.
16. Suzuki, K. G., T. K. Fujiwara, M. Edidin, and A. Kusumi. "Dynamic Recruitment of Phospholipase C gamma at Transiently Immobilized GPI-Anchored Receptor Clusters Induces IP3-Ca^{2+} Signaling: Single-Molecule Tracking Study 2." *J Cell Biol* 177, no. 4 (2007): 731–42.
17. Suzuki, K. G., T. K. Fujiwara, F. Sanematsu et al. "GPI-Anchored Receptor Clusters Transiently Recruit Lyn and G alpha for Temporary Cluster Immobilization and Lyn Activation: Single-Molecule Tracking Study 1." *J Cell Biol* 177, no. 4 (2007): 717–30.

18. Kusumi, A., I. Koyama-Honda, and K. Suzuki. "Molecular Dynamics and Interactions for Creation of Stimulation-Induced Stabilized Rafts from Small Unstable Steady-State Rafts." *Traffic* 5, no. 4 (2004): 213–30.

19. van Zanten, T. S., J. Gomez, C. Manzo et al. "Direct Mapping of Nanoscale Compositional Connectivity on Intact Cell Membranes." *Proc Natl Acad Sci U S A* 107, no. 35 (2010): 15437–42.

20. Stefl, M., R. Sachl, J. Humpolickova et al. "Dynamics and Size of Cross-Linking-Induced Lipid Nanodomains in Model Membranes." *Biophys J* 102, no. 9 (2012): 2104–13.

21. Tian, T., A. Harding, K. Inder et al. "Plasma Membrane Nanoswitches Generate High-Fidelity Ras Signal Transduction." *Nat Cell Biol* 9, no. 8 (2007): 905–14.

22. Yeung, T., B. Ozdamar, P. Paroutis, and S. Grinstein. "Lipid Metabolism and Dynamics During Phagocytosis." *Curr Opin Cell Biol* 18, no. 4 (2006): 429–37.

23. Vieira, O. V., R. J. Botelho, and S. Grinstein. "Phagosome Maturation: Aging Gracefully." *Biochem J* 366, no. Pt 3 (2002): 689–704.

24. Odin, J. A., J. C. Edberg, C. J. Painter, R. P. Kimberly, and J. C. Unkeless. "Regulation of Phagocytosis and [Ca2+]i Flux by Distinct Regions of an Fc Receptor." *Science* 254, no. 5039 (1991): 1785–8.

25. Holowka, D., D. Sil, C. Torigoe, and B. Baird. "Insights into Immunoglobulin E Receptor Signaling from Structurally Defined Ligands." *Immunol Rev* 217 (2007): 269–79.

26. Ghazizadeh, S., J. B. Bolen, and H. B. Fleit. "Physical and Functional Association of Src-Related Protein Tyrosine Kinases with Fc Gamma RII in Monocytic THP-1 Cells." *J Biol Chem* 269, no. 12 (1994): 8878–84.

27. Wang, A. V., P. R. Scholl, and R. S. Geha. "Physical and Functional Association of the High Affinity Immunoglobulin G Receptor (Fc Gamma RI) with the Kinases Hck and Lyn." *J Exp Med* 180, no. 3 (1994): 1165–70.

28. Hamada, F., M. Aoki, T. Akiyama, and K. Toyoshima. "Association of Immunoglobulin G Fc Receptor II with Src-Like Protein-Tyrosine Kinase Fgr in Neutrophils." *Proc Natl Acad Sci U S A* 90, no. 13 (1993): 6305–9.

29. Fitzer-Attas, C. J., M. Lowry, M. T. Crowley et al. "Fcgamma Receptor-Mediated Phagocytosis in Macrophages Lacking the Src Family Tyrosine Kinases Hck, Fgr, and Lyn." *J Exp Med* 191, no. 4 (2000): 669–82.

30. Mitchell, M. A., M. M. Huang, P. Chien et al. "Substitutions and Deletions in the Cytoplasmic Domain of the Phagocytic Receptor Fc Gamma RIIA: Effect on Receptor Tyrosine Phosphorylation and Phagocytosis." *Blood* 84, no. 6 (1994): 1753–9.

31. Ibarrola, I., P. J. Vossebeld, C. H. Homburg et al. "Influence of Tyrosine Phosphorylation on Protein Interaction with FcgammaRIIa." *Biochim Biophys Acta* 1357, no. 3 (1997): 348–58.

32. Kwiatkowska, K., and A. Sobota. "The Clustered Fcgamma Receptor II Is Recruited to Lyn-Containing Membrane Domains and Undergoes Phosphorylation in a Cholesterol-Dependent Manner." *Eur J Immunol* 31, no. 4 (2001): 989–98.

33. Rollet-Labelle, E., S. Marois, K. Barbeau, S. E. Malawista, and P. H. Naccache. "Recruitment of the Cross-Linked Opsonic Receptor CD32a (FcgammaRIIa) to High-Density Detergent-Resistant Membrane Domains in Human Neutrophils." *Biochem J* 381, no. Pt 3 (2004): 919–28.

34. Garcia-Garcia, E., E. J. Brown, and C. Rosales. "Transmembrane Mutations to FcgammaRIIa Alter Its Association with Lipid Rafts: Implications for Receptor Signaling." *J Immunol* 178, no. 5 (2007): 3048–58.

35. Shvartsman, D. E., O. Gutman, A. Tietz, and Y. I. Henis. "Cyclodextrins but Not Compactin Inhibit the Lateral Diffusion of Membrane Proteins Independent of Cholesterol." *Traffic* 7 (2006): 917–26.

36. Johnson, S. A., C. M. Pleiman, L. Pao et al. "Phosphorylated Immunoreceptor Signaling Motifs (ITAMs) Exhibit Unique Abilities to Bind and Activate Lyn and Syk Tyrosine Kinases." *J Immunol* 155, no. 10 (1995): 4596–603.

37. Ghazizadeh, S., J. B. Bolen, and H. B. Fleit. "Tyrosine Phosphorylation and Association of Syk with Fc Gamma RII in Monocytic THP-1 Cells." *Biochem J* 305 (Pt 2) (1995): 669–74.

38. Crowley, M. T., P. S. Costello, C. J. Fitzer-Attas et al. "A Critical Role for Syk in Signal Transduction and Phagocytosis Mediated by Fcgamma Receptors on Macrophages." *J Exp Med* 186, no. 7 (1997): 1027–39.

39. Kiefer, F., J. Brumell, N. Al-Alawi et al. "The Syk Protein Tyrosine Kinase Is Essential for Fcgamma Receptor Signaling in Macrophages and Neutrophils." *Mol Cell Biol* 18, no. 7 (1998): 4209–20.

40. Tridandapani, S., T. W. Lyden, J. L. Smith et al. "The Adapter Protein LAT Enhances Fcgamma Receptor-Mediated Signal Transduction in Myeloid Cells." *J Biol Chem* 275, no. 27 (2000): 20480–7.

41. Yu, M., C. A. Lowell, B. G. Neel, and H. Gu. "Scaffolding Adapter Grb2-Associated Binder 2 Requires Syk to Transmit Signals from FcepsilonRI." *J Immunol* 176, no. 4 (2006): 2421–9.

42. May, R. C., E. Caron, A. Hall, and L. M. Machesky. "Involvement of the Arp2/3 Complex in Phagocytosis Mediated by FcgammaR or CR3." *Nat Cell Biol* 2, no. 4 (2000): 246–8.

43. Araki, N., M. T. Johnson, and J. A. Swanson. "A Role for Phosphoinositide 3-Kinase in the Completion of Macropinocytosis and Phagocytosis by Macrophages." *J Cell Biol* 135, no. 5 (1996): 1249–60.

44. Botelho, R. J., C. C. Scott, and S. Grinstein. "Phosphoinositide Involvement in Phagocytosis and Phagosome Maturation." *Curr Top Microbiol Immunol* 282 (2004): 1–30.

45. Oancea, E., M. N. Teruel, A. F. Quest, and T. Meyer. "Green Fluorescent Protein (GFP)-Tagged Cysteine-Rich Domains from Protein Kinase C as Fluorescent Indicators for Diacylglycerol Signaling in Living Cells." *J Cell Biol* 140, no. 3 (1998): 485–98.

46. Stauffer, T. P., S. Ahn, and T. Meyer. "Receptor-Induced Transient Reduction in Plasma Membrane PtdIns(4, 5)P2 Concentration Monitored in Living Cells." *Curr Biol* 8, no. 6 (1998): 343–6.

47. Varnai, P., K. I. Rother, and T. Balla. "Phosphatidylinositol 3-Kinase-Dependent Membrane Association of the Bruton's Tyrosine Kinase Pleckstrin Homology Domain Visualized in Single Living Cells." *J Biol Chem* 274, no. 16 (1999): 10983–9.

48. Varnai, P., and T. Balla. "Visualization of Phosphoinositides That Bind Pleckstrin Homology Domains: Calcium- and Agonist-Induced Dynamic Changes and Relationship to Myo-[3H]Inositol-Labeled Phosphoinositide Pools." *J Cell Biol* 143, no. 2 (1998): 501–10.

49. Giepmans, B. N., S. R. Adams, M. H. Ellisman, and R. Y. Tsien. "The Fluorescent Toolbox for Assessing Protein Location and Function." *Science* 312, no. 5771 (2006): 217–24.

50. Raucher, D., T. Stauffer, W. Chen et al. "Phosphatidylinositol 4,5-Bisphosphate Functions as a Second Messenger That Regulates Cytoskeleton-Plasma Membrane Adhesion." *Cell* 100, no. 2 (2000): 221–8.

51. Takenawa, T., and T. Itoh. "Phosphoinositides, Key Molecules for Regulation of Actin Cytoskeletal Organization and Membrane Traffic from the Plasma Membrane." *Biochim Biophys Acta* 1533, no. 3 (2001): 190–206.

52. Botelho, R. J., M. Teruel, R. Dierckman et al. "Localized Biphasic Changes in Phosphatidylinositol-4,5-Bisphosphate at Sites of Phagocytosis." *J Cell Biol* 151, no. 7 (2000): 1353–68.

53. Golebiewska, U., J. G. Kay, T. Masters et al. "Evidence for a Fence That Impedes the Diffusion of Phosphatidylinositol 4,5-Bisphosphate out of the Forming Phagosomes of Macrophages." *Mol Biol Cell* 22, no. 18 (2011): 3498–507.

54. Fairn, G. D., K. Ogata, R. J. Botelho et al. "An Electrostatic Switch Displaces Phosphatidylinositol Phosphate Kinases from the Membrane During Phagocytosis." *J Cell Biol* 187, no. 5 (2009): 701–14.

55. Marshall, J. G., J. W. Booth, V. Stambolic et al. "Restricted Accumulation of Phosphatidylinositol 3-Kinase Products in a Plasmalemmal Subdomain During Fc Gamma Receptor-Mediated Phagocytosis." *J Cell Biol* 153, no. 7 (2001): 1369–80.

56. Scott, C. C., W. Dobson, R. J. Botelho et al. "Phosphatidylinositol-4,5-Bisphosphate Hydrolysis Directs Actin Remodeling During Phagocytosis." *J Cell Biol* 169, no. 1 (2005): 139–49.

57. Kent, C. "Eukaryotic Phospholipid Biosynthesis." *Annu Rev Biochem* 64 (1995): 315–43.

58. Kusner, D. J., C. F. Hall, and S. Jackson. "Fc Gamma Receptor-Mediated Activation of Phospholipase D Regulates Macrophage Phagocytosis of IgG-Opsonized Particles." *J Immunol* 162, no. 4 (1999): 2266–74.

59. Corrotte, M., S. Chasserot-Golaz, P. Huang et al. "Dynamics and Function of Phospholipase D and Phosphatidic Acid During Phagocytosis." *Traffic* 7, no. 3 (2006): 365–77.

60. Ktistakis, N. T., C. Delon, M. Manifava et al. "Phospholipase D1 and Potential Targets of Its Hydrolysis Product, Phosphatidic Acid." *Biochem Soc Trans* 31, no. Pt 1 (2003): 94–7.

61. Moolenaar, W. H., L. A. van Meeteren, and B. N. Giepmans. "The Ins and Outs of Lysophosphatidic Acid Signaling." *Bioessays* 26, no. 8 (2004): 870–81.

62. Kooijman, E. E., K. M. Carter, E. G. van Laar et al. "What Makes the Bioactive Lipids Phosphatidic Acid and Lysophosphatidic Acid So Special?" *Biochemistry* 44, no. 51 (2005): 17007–15.

63. Kooijman, E. E., V. Chupin, N. L. Fuller et al. "Spontaneous Curvature of Phosphatidic Acid and Lysophosphatidic Acid." *Biochemistry* 44, no. 6 (2005): 2097–102.

64. Kooijman, E. E., V. Chupin, B. de Kruijff, and K. N. Burger. "Modulation of Membrane Curvature by Phosphatidic Acid and Lysophosphatidic Acid." *Traffic* 4, no. 3 (2003): 162–74.

65. Vieira, O. V., R. J. Botelho, L. Rameh et al. "Distinct Roles of Class I and Class III Phosphatidylinositol 3-Kinases in Phagosome Formation and Maturation." *J Cell Biol* 155, no. 1 (2001): 19–25.

66. Larsen, E. C., T. Ueyama, P. M. Brannock et al. "A Role for PKC-Epsilon in Fc GammaR-Mediated Phagocytosis by Raw 264.7 Cells." *J Cell Biol* 159, no. 6 (2002): 939–44.

67. Igarashi, K., M. Kaneda, A. Yamaji et al. "A Novel Phosphatidylserine-Binding Peptide Motif Defined by an Anti-Idiotypic Monoclonal Antibody. Localization of Phosphatidylserine-Specific Binding Sites on Protein Kinase C and Phosphatidylserine Decarboxylase." *J Biol Chem* 270, no. 49 (1995): 29075–8.

68. Hao, J. J., Y. Liu, M. Kruhlak et al. "Phospholipase C-Mediated Hydrolysis of PIP2 Releases ERM Proteins from Lymphocyte Membrane." *J Cell Biol* 184, no. 3 (2009): 451–62.

69. Lemmon, M. A. "Membrane Recognition by Phospholipid-Binding Domains." *Nat Rev Mol Cell Biol* 9, no. 2 (2008): 99–111.

70. Saarikangas, J., H. Zhao, and P. Lappalainen. "Regulation of the Actin Cytoskeleton-Plasma Membrane Interplay by Phosphoinositides." *Physiol Rev* 90, no. 1 (2010): 259–89.

71. Oude Weernink, P. A., M. Lopez de Jesus, and M. Schmidt. "Phospholipase D Signaling: Orchestration by PIP2 and Small GTPases." *Naunyn Schmiedebergs Arch Pharmacol* 374, no. 5–6 (2007): 399–411.

72. Flannagan, R. S., G. Cosio, and S. Grinstein. "Antimicrobial Mechanisms of Phagocytes and Bacterial Evasion Strategies." *Nat Rev Microbiol* 7, no. 5 (2009): 355–66.

73. Yeung, T., M. Terebiznik, L. Yu et al. "Receptor Activation Alters Inner Surface Potential During Phagocytosis." *Science* 313, no. 5785 (2006): 347–51.

74. Yeung, T., B. Heit, J. F. Dubuisson et al. "Contribution of Phosphatidylserine to Membrane Surface Charge and Protein Targeting During Phagosome Maturation." *J Cell Biol* 185, no. 5 (2009): 917–28.

75. Vance, J. E., and R. Steenbergen. "Metabolism and Functions of Phosphatidylserine." *Prog Lipid Res* 44, no. 4 (2005): 207–34.

76. Leventis, R., and J. R. Silvius. "Lipid-Binding Characteristics of the Polybasic Carboxy-Terminal Sequence of K-Ras4B." *Biochemistry* 37, no. 20 (1998): 7640–8.

77. Yeung, T., G. E. Gilbert, J. Shi et al. "Membrane Phosphatidylserine Regulates Surface Charge and Protein Localization." *Science* 319, no. 5860 (2008): 210–3.

78. Majeed, M., E. Caveggion, C. A. Lowell, and G. Berton. "Role of Src Kinases and Syk in Fcgamma Receptor-Mediated Phagocytosis and Phagosome-Lysosome Fusion." *J Leukoc Biol* 70, no. 5 (2001): 801–11.

79. Peyron, P., I. Maridonneau-Parini, and T. Stegmann. "Fusion of Human Neutrophil Phagosomes with Lysosomes In Vitro: Involvement of Tyrosine Kinases of the Src Family and Inhibition by Mycobacteria." *J Biol Chem* 276, no. 38 (2001): 35512–7.

80. Heo, W. D., T. Inoue, W. S. Park et al. "Pi(3, 4, 5)P$_3$ and Pi(4, 5)P$_2$ Lipids Target Proteins with Polybasic Clusters to the Plasma Membrane." *Science* 314, no. 5804 (2006): 1458–61.

81. Hinterdorfer, P., M. F. Garcia-Parajo, and Y. F. Dufrene. "Single-Molecule Imaging of Cell Surfaces Using Near-Field Nanoscopy." *Acc Chem Res* 45, no. 3 (2012): 327–36.

82. Muller, T., C. Schumann, and A. Kraegeloh. "STED Microscopy and Its Applications: New Insights into Cellular Processes on the Nanoscale." *Chemphyschem* 13, no. 8 (2012): 1986–2000.

83. Kohnke, M., S. Schmitt, N. Ariotti et al. "Design and Application of In Vivo FRET Biosensors to Identify Protein Prenylation and Nanoclustering Inhibitors." *Chem Biol* 19, no. 7 (2012): 866–74.

84. He, H. T., and D. Marguet. "Detecting Nanodomains in Living Cell Membrane by Fluorescence Correlation Spectroscopy." *Annu Rev Phys Chem* 62 (2011): 417–36.

85. Fairn, G. D., N. L. Schieber, N. Ariotti et al. "High-Resolution Mapping Reveals Topologically Distinct Cellular Pools of Phosphatidylserine." *J Cell Biol* 194, no. 2 (2011): 257–75.

86. van den Bogaart, G., K. Meyenberg, H. J. Risselada et al. "Membrane Protein Sequestering by Ionic Protein-Lipid Interactions." *Nature* 479, no. 7374 (2011): 552–5.

Section II

Advanced Ensemble Imaging Techniques

10 Fluctuation Spectroscopy Methods for the Analysis of Membrane Processes

Michelle A. Digman

CONTENTS

10.1 INTRODUCTION

In the field of membrane lipid and protein dynamics, fluorescence recovery after photobleaching (FRAP) and single-particle tracking methods have provided ample evidence that lipids and proteins could have their motion restricted by interaction with other lipids and with the cell cytoskeleton.[1–8] Fluorescence correlation spectroscopy (FCS) is a relatively new method in this field that has received particular attention recently because of the possible combination with super-resolution microscopy methods.[9–14] In this context, the use of very small volumes of excitation or variable volumes of excitation[15] was considered necessary to unravel to transport of molecules at the nanoscale. However, most of the FCS studies done so far are based on the original idea of measuring temporal correlation at a single point in the membrane. Measuring a single location in the membrane is restrictive since the temporal fluctuations at one point cannot reveal local microstructures or the anisotropic molecular transport in membranes. In this contribution, we discuss fluctuation methods based on spatial correlation that reveal the dynamics of membrane lipids and proteins at the nanoscale.[16–27] We show here that spatial correlations intrinsically contain more information than the classical temporal correlation first introduced with the single-point FCS. Spatiotemporal correlation approaches have the potential to shift the paradigm in the use and kind of information that can be derived from fluctuation methods for membrane studies. Also, spatiotemporal correlation can complement single-particle tracking experiments with much higher sensitivity and faster time scale.

One way to introduce the basic concepts in FCS is to emphasize the spatial distribution that arises owing to the diffusion of molecules. For example, if a molecule is at a given location at time $\tau = 0$, as the time evolves, the probability of finding the same molecule at a given distance from the original point can be described by a three-dimensional (3D) Gaussian function in which the variance σ^2 of the Gaussian increases with time according to the following expression:

$$\sigma^2 = 4D\tau, \tag{10.1}$$

where D is the diffusion coefficient and τ is the time. Figure 10.1 schematically illustrates this idea.

We use the concept depicted in Figure 10.1 to illustrate in Figure 10.2 some of the methods used to measure the diffusion of particles in 3D and also in the cell membrane.

As shown in Figure 10.2 at time $\tau = 0$, the particle is at the origin. The variance of the Gaussian describing the spatial distribution is zero at this time. Then, at a later time, the particle can be found at different locations as shown in Figure 10.2 for panels a through c. As illustrated in Figure 10.2a, the probability to find the particle at the location indicated by the dark gray circle, or observation volume, decreases with time. The reason to use a circle in this schematic representation of the process in Figure 10.2 is to account for the way the fluctuations are measured, generally by focusing a laser beam to a diffraction-limited spot. At very long time, the probability for the same particle to be within the circle in Figure 10.2a becomes very small. If we multiply the probability to find the particle in the circle at time $t = 0$ multiplied by the probability at a later time t, this product will start high and then will become small at long times. This schematic representation of the spatial and temporal evolution of the probability density of finding

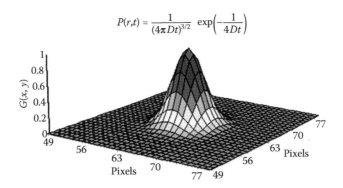

$$P(r,t) = \frac{1}{(4\pi Dt)^{3/2}} \exp\left(-\frac{1}{4Dt}\right)$$

FIGURE 10.1   Fick's law for diffusion describes the evolution of the probability to find a particle at a location r at time t if the particle was at the origin at $t = 0$. This figure emphasizes the concept that the spatial distribution of this probability is Gaussian in a uniform medium. The width of the Gaussian increases linearly with time while the amplitude of the Gaussian decreases with time.

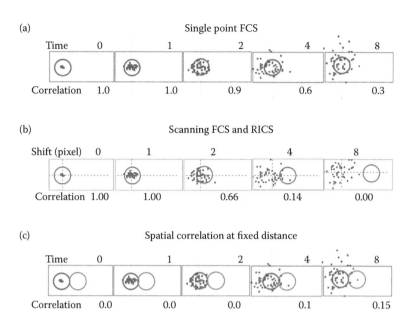

FIGURE 10.2 Schematic representation of different FCS techniques. In all cases, a particle is at the origin at time = 0 and then the particle diffuses so that the probability of finding a particle at a larger distance increases with time. The small dots graphically indicate this probability. The positions of the dots are identical in the three parts of the figure to emphasize that the physical process is the same but what is different is the way we observe the diffusion. (a) In the single-point FCS, we observe the system always at the same point and we measure the decay of the probability of finding the particle within the volume of observation indicated by the circle at the origin. (b) In the scanning FCS and RICS technique, we gradually move the volume of observation. If the movement is fast, we rapidly decrease the probability to observe the same particle. (c) In the spatial cross-correlation technique, we simultaneously observe different volumes and then we calculate the probability that a particle that was in the circle at the origin at $t = 0$ will appear in the shifted circle at a later time. This probability is initially zero, increases with time, and then finally decays to zero.

a particle at a given location gives us the opportunity to put the different techniques under a common scenario used for fluctuation spectroscopy and to introduce the concept of spatially correlated fluctuations. The simplest implementation of the correlation methods is when the intensity fluctuations are measured at the same point. This method is commonly known as single-point FCS (Figure 10.2a). Another variant is when the point of observation is moved systematically as in line (or circular) scan FCS or in a raster scan motion as in the raster image correlation spectroscopy (RICS) method (Figure 10.2b). Finally, other methods measure the intensity fluctuation at two or more points simultaneously such as the method called pCF (pair correlation function). Alternatively, measuring fluctuations of many points simultaneously can be done with the image mean square displacement (iMSD) method (Figure 10.2c). There are other variants of the FCS technique that are included in Table 10.1 with a short description.

All the techniques mentioned in Table 10.1 can have additional prefixes such as "cc" for cross-correlation.

TABLE 10.1

Technique Comments

spFCS	Single-point FCS, the original method
lsFCS	Line scanning FCS, used to analyze many points along a line
ICS	Image correlation spectroscopy, used to measure protein aggregation
tICS	Time ICS, calculates the time ACF at each point in an image
RICS	Raster scan ICS, temporally correlates adjacent points in an image
STICS	Spatiotemporal ICS, correlates points in subsequent frames
kICS	K-space ICS, computes correlations in the k-transformed space
PICS	Particle ICS, fits particle positions and correlates in subsequent frames
iMSD	Image mean square displacement, uses STICS correlations for spatial probabilities
pCF	Pair correlation function, calculates cross-correlation between points at a given distance p
pCH	Photon counting histogram, analyzes brightness of particles at a single point
N&B	Number and brightness analysis, calculates number and brightness from first and second moments of intensity fluctuations

10.2 THE AUTOCORRELATION FUNCTION

The spectrum of the fluctuations at a given location is generally represented by the autocorrelation function (ACF). Starting from an expression of the fluorescence intensity as indicated in Figure 10.3, we define the ACF as shown in the logical scheme of Figure 10.3.

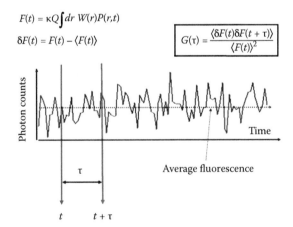

$$F(t) = \kappa Q \int dr\, W(r)P(r,t)$$

$$\delta F(t) = F(t) - \langle F(t)\rangle$$

$$G(\tau) = \frac{\langle \delta F(t)\delta F(t+\tau)\rangle}{\langle F(t)\rangle^2}$$

FIGURE 10.3 The fluorescence intensity $F(t)$ is proportional to instrument factors indicated by κ, the molecule quantum yield Q, and the convolution of the probability $P(r,t)$ that a molecule is in the profile of illumination $W(r)$ where t is the time and r is the spatial coordinate. The fluorescence fluctuation $\delta F(t)$ is defined as the fluorescence at times t subtracted by the average fluorescence $\langle F(t)\rangle$. The brackets $\langle\rangle$ indicate temporal average. The normalized correlation function $G(\tau)$ is defined in the figure that also shows schematically the intensity fluctuations, the average intensity, and the delay τ between points at which the correlation function is computed.

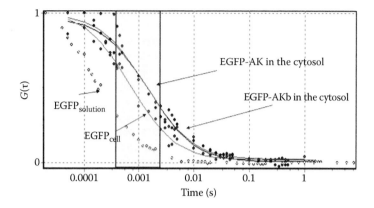

FIGURE 10.4   Typical ACF curves for proteins in solution and in cells as indicated in the figure. All correlation functions are normalized to 1 at very short correlation times. The gray area indicates the region where the major changes in the ACF occur for proteins in cells.

If the profile of illumination is Gaussian in all dimensions and if the changes in concentration follow Fick's law described in Figure 10.1, then the correlation function can be calculated by simple integration of the definition given in Figure 10.3.

$$G(\tau) = \frac{\gamma}{N}\left(1 + \frac{4D\tau}{w_{3DG}^2}\right)^{-1}\left(1 + \frac{4D\tau}{z_{3DG}^2}\right)^{-1/2} \tag{10.2}$$

This is the common form of the ACF for temporal fluctuations owing to diffusion in 3D. Some typical measurements of the ACF are shown in Figure 10.4 for proteins in solutions and in cells.

The fluorescence fluctuations measurement at a single point or more points also contains information about the amplitude of the fluctuation. Several approaches were proposed to statistically analyze the amplitude of the fluctuations. In the single-point approach, the method is called PCH, which stands for photon count histogram,[28–30] and in the contest of image analysis, it is known as N&B, which stands for number and brightness analysis.[19,31,32]

In this chapter, we will discuss the application of the fluctuation methods that are more relevant for the studies of membrane systems, which have particular requirements.

10.3   THE PRINCIPLE OF SCANNING FCS

Scanning FCS can be performed with a commercial confocal microscope with analog detectors or a homebuilt two-photon laser scanning system with photon counting detectors. If we can move the point at which we acquire FCS data fast enough to other points and then *return* to the original point "before" the particle had left the volume of excitation, then we can "multiplex the time" and collect FCS data at several points simultaneously as schematically shown in Figure 10.5a.[33]

(a)   (b)

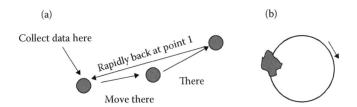

FIGURE 10.5 (a) Schematic representation of the scanning FCS principle. The method measures the intensity at several points in very rapid sequence and returns to the first point before the fluctuation has decayed. (b) The fastest time to return to the original position using the galvo scanner, which is common in commercial laser scanning microscopes, is achieved by performing an orbital trajectory.

The fastest way to scan several points in a confocal microscope and then return to the original point is to perform a circular orbit using the scanner galvos (Figure 10.5b). For this motion to occur, two galvos for the x and y axis, respectively, are driven by two sine waves shifted by 90°, thereby obtaining a projected circular orbit on the sample. Using current conventional technology, one orbit could be performed in times of less than 1 to 0.5 ms, or in 0.15 to 0.1 ms using acousto-optic deflectors. What is the minimum time required for an orbit so that we will not miss the "fastest" diffusion process in a cell? As shown in Figure 10.4, enhanced green fluorescent protein diffuses in the cytoplasm with an apparent diffusion coefficient of approximately 20 μm^2/s. The transit across the laser beam (assuming a w_0 of 0.35 mm) is approximately 1.5 ms (formula used: time = $w_0^2/4D$). Therefore, if we could perform a full orbit in approximately 0.5 to 1 ms, we should be able to return to the same position before a molecule of green fluorescent protein (GFP) should have moved away from the original volume of excitation. Instead, for the same protein in solution, the motion is too fast and diffusing molecules will be partially missed. This scenario is shown in Figure 10.4 where the gray band indicates the region of change of the amplitude of the fluctuation. For all cases of proteins in cells, a characteristics sampling time of approximately 1 ms is sufficient to see the same protein within the same volume of illumination (PSF, point spread function). The separation between sampled points along the orbit depends on the orbit radius and the sampling time. For an orbit radius of 5 μm, the length of the orbit is approximately 32 μm. Light is collected along the orbit, generally in the range 64 to 256 points. At 64 points per orbit, the average distance is approximately 0.5 μm or 0.125 μm for 256 points. If the orbit period is 1 ms, the dwell time at each point along the orbit is approximately 16 μs (64 points) or 4 μs (256 points), respectively.

Why is the distance between points important? As illustrated in Figure 10.6, if the orbit radius is larger than 5 μm, the points are separated by more than the width of the PSF (assuming 64 points per orbit: $2\pi R/64$ ~500 nm). Setting the conditions of the instrument for no overlap has the result of making the measurements at the different points partially independent, but it limits the capability of obtaining spatial correlations along the orbit.

Once the data along the orbits have been measured for approximately 1000 to 10,000 orbits (1 to 10 s), the data stream is presented as a "carpet" in which the

(a) (b)

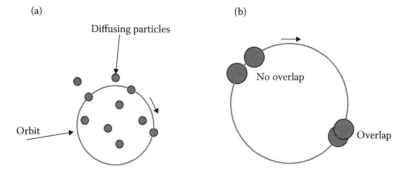

FIGURE 10.6 (a) Particles can be detected at different points along the orbit. (b) If the observation of the fluctuations is done at well-separated points, we can calculate the ACF at each point independently. If the points are overlapping, we can obtain additional information regarding the motions of molecules from one point to adjacent points.

horizontal coordinate represents data along the orbit and the vertical coordinate represents data at successive orbits (kymographs) (Figure 10.7).

There are different approaches that we can use to extract the diffusion of particles, the number of particles, and their brightness at each point along the orbit. If we consider the intensity at each point of the orbit and in the carpet representation we select a column of the carpet, we obtain a time sequence at a specific point of the orbit. Using this time sequence, we calculate the ACF as shown in Figure 10.8. The sampling time in this time sequence is equal to the orbit time; the ACF can then be used to extract the local (to the

(a) (b)

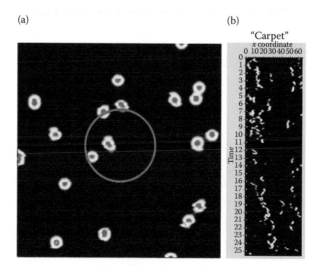

FIGURE 10.7 (a) Simulation of particles diffusing on a membrane superimposed with the orbit along which the measurements are taken. (b) In the carpet representation, we plot the intensity along each orbit (x coordinate) as a function of the orbit number or time (y coordinate). A vertical line in the carpet represents measurements done at the same position of the image.

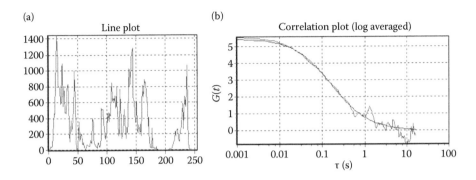

FIGURE 10.8 (a) For the carpet in Figure 10.7b, one line is extracted. Only a portion of the line is shown. (b) The ACF is calculated for the time sequence in (a). The continuous line corresponds to the best fit that recovers the value of 10 $\mu m^2/s$ used for the simulations.

orbit location) diffusion coefficient. The simulation shown in Figure 10.8 corresponds to particles diffusing randomly with a diffusion coefficient of 10 $\mu m^2/s$.

For a homogeneous sample, every column should be equivalent, so that we can calculate the ACF for every column and then fit all the columns either globally or individually as shown in Figure 10.9.

In this example, the $G(0)$ changes from line to line, because the statistics is poor (Figure 10.9b, dark gray line), but the diffusion coefficient (Figure 10.9b, light gray line) is pretty constant at the expected value of $D = 0.1$ $\mu m^2/s$. Using the scanning principle and the carpet ACF, it seems that we are unable to analyze cases where the fluctuations are fast since we cannot come back at the same location before the fluctuation dissipates. However, if the molecule that has caused the fluctuation moves to adjacent pixels, we could capture the fluctuation by correlating the fluctuation at adjacent pixels. Using spatial correlations, we gain in the detection of fast dynamics at the expense of spatial resolution.

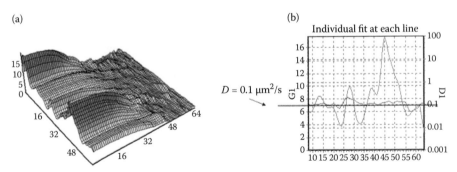

FIGURE 10.9 (a) Carpet surface obtained by extracting each column of Figure 10.7b and calculating the ACF. (b) Carpet fit of each of the ACF functions in (a) to extract the amplitude $G(0)$ and the diffusion constant from the fit (continuous smooth line). The expected value of the diffusion constant for this simulation is recovered at each line, while the amplitude (which is inversely proportional to the number of particles) has much more noise owing to the small number of particles used in this simulation.

10.4 THE RICS PRINCIPLE

The RICS method explicitly takes into account the spatial correlation among adjacent points (Figure 10.10).[17,24] Since adjacent points are needed to extract dynamics, we can have a combination of very high time resolution with sufficient spatial resolution. A major benefit of RICS is that it can be done using the raster scan pattern (rather than the circular pattern) that is usually available in commercial laser scanning microscopes. Another significant advantage is that it can be done with analog detection, as well as with photon counting systems, although the characteristic of the detector must be carefully characterized owing to possible time correlations at very short times attributed to the analog filter found in some microscope electronics. More importantly, RICS provides an intrinsic method to separate the immobile fraction and can reveal the different spatial distribution that arises from processes such as weak binding form true diffusion.

The principle of RICS is schematically depicted in Figure 10.10. Briefly, in a raster scan image, points are measured at different positions and at different times simultaneously. If we consider the time sequence, it is not continuous in time; instead, if we consider the pixel sequence, it is contiguous in space. In the RICS approach, we calculate the two-dimensional (2D) spatial correlation function (similarly to the ICS method of Petersen and Wiseman[34,35]):

$$G_{RICS}(\xi, \psi) = \frac{\langle I(x,y)I(x+\xi, y+\psi)\rangle}{\langle I(x,y)\rangle^2} - 1. \tag{10.3}$$

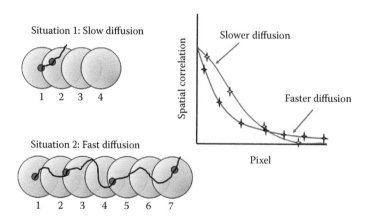

FIGURE 10.10 In situation 1, we schematically show the laser beam moving along a line in the raster scan pattern. If a particle indicated by the dot moves slowly, as the laser is moved, the particle can only be found in the very adjacent pixels. In these pixels, the spatial correlation of the fluctuations is high as shown by the line in the graph. In situation 2, the particle is diffusing fast. The probability of finding the particle in the very adjacent pixels decreases, but it increases at distant pixels. The spatial correlation decreases at the closest pixels, but it increases at distant pixels (line in the graph).

In Equation 10.3, the variables ξ and ψ represent spatial increments in the x and y directions, respectively. 2D spatial correlation can be computed very efficiently using fast Fourier transform methods.

To introduce the "RICS concept," we must account for the relationship between time and position of the laser beam so that x and y are explored in a specific time sequence according to the raster scan pattern. The RICS correlation function is generally written as the product of two or more terms. One term accounts for the temporal fluctuations caused by the diffusion and the other term account for the spatial distribution owing to Fick's law:

$$G_{RICS}(\xi, \psi) = S(\xi, \psi) \times G(\xi, \psi) \tag{10.4}$$

For any diffusion value, the amplitude decreases as a function of time and the width of the Gaussian increases as a function of time according to the following relationship also illustrated in Figure 10.11.

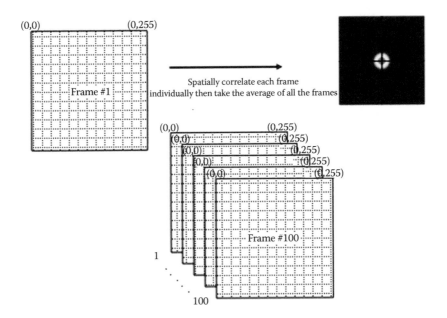

FIGURE 10.11 Schematic illustration of the spatial correlation operation. Each pixel in frame #1 is multiplied by itself and all the products are added. The result of this addition (normalized to the total number of points) is plotted at the (0,0) location in the spatial correlation function. Then, the pixels of frame #1 are shifted by 1 in the x direction, and the product of those pixels with the unshifted frame are added, normalized, and plotted in position (1,0) of the spatial correlation function. This process is repeated for each pixel shifted in the x and y direction, giving the correlation function schematically shown in the right part of the image. Many frames can be collected, and the spatial correlation function for each frame is calculated. All the correlation functions obtained can be averaged to increase the S/N.

The temporal correlation of fluctuations caused by diffusion has the same overall expression as in Equation 10.1 with the notable difference that the time of pixel sampling depends on the raster scan pattern.

$$G(\xi,\psi) = \frac{\gamma}{N}\left(1 + \frac{4D(\tau_p\xi + \tau_l\psi)}{w_0^2}\right)^{-1}\left(1 + \frac{4D(\tau_p\xi + \tau_l\psi)}{w_z^2}\right)^{-1/2} \quad (10.5)$$

τ_p and τ_l indicate the pixel time and the line time. The correlation owing to the spatial term in the diffusion is given by Equation 10.6:

$$S(\xi,\psi) = \exp\left(-\frac{\left[\left(\frac{2\xi\delta r}{w_0}\right)^2 + \left(\frac{2\psi\delta r}{w_0}\right)^2\right]}{\left(1 + \frac{4D(\tau_p\xi + \tau_l\psi)}{w_0^2}\right)}\right), \quad (10.6)$$

where δr is the pixel size. For $D = 0$, the spatial correlation gives the autocorrelation of the PSF, with an amplitude equal to γ/N. As D increases, the correlation (G term) becomes narrower and the width of the S term increases. Figure 10.12 and the caption describe how an experiment is performed using simulated data.

Until now, we have only discussed the principle of the spatial correlation method. When we apply the RICS approach to cells, we must account for the immobile fraction, since the spatial correlation of the image contains all the spatial features of the cell rather than just the fluctuations attributed to motion of the molecules. We need to separate this immobile fraction from the mobile part before calculating the spatial correlation function. This is achieved by subtracting the average image pixel by pixel. Furthermore, we need to disregard the correlation at time zero and at shift (0,0); the correlation at this point contains the noise of the detector. The detector noise does not propagate to adjacent pixel; it neither has a time memory. If we subtract the average intensity and disregard the zero time–space point, the immobile bright region totally disappears from the correlation function.

Figure 10.13 shows schematically the procedure to subtract the immobile part before calculating the RICS correlation function.

As a take-home message for this first part of our contribution, the RICS approach either along a line or in entire images can be used to measure dynamic rates from the microsecond-to-millisecond time scale. Anyone with a commercially available instrument can use it. Immobile structures can be filtered out and fast fluctuations can be detected. The range of processes that can be measured include the diffusion of small molecules in solutions and cytosolic diffusion of proteins and can be used to discriminate other types of processes and interactions such as weak binding, blinking, and conformational transitions.

Although RICS is a quite powerful technique, in the context of membrane biophysics, there are other fundamental processes that are difficult if not impossible.

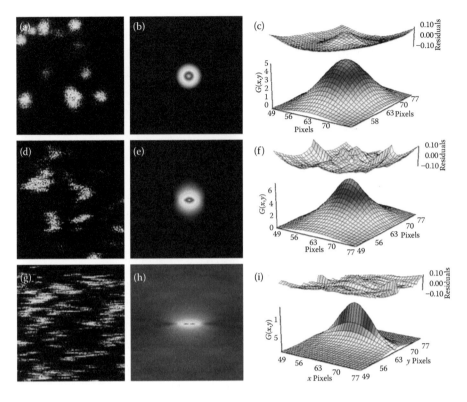

FIGURE 10.12 All frames are acquired at the same raster scan speed. (a) Particles diffusing at $D = 0.1$ μm²/s appear relatively round at the scanning speed used. (b) The resulting spatial correlation function mostly reflects the roundness of the particle in the image. (c) The lower surface is the fit of the spatial correlation function corresponding to $D = 0.1$ μm²/s. The upper surface is the plot of the residues of the fit. (d) Raster scan image of particles diffusing at $D = 5.0$ μm²/s. The particles appear defocused because they move while they are being measured. (e) The resulting spatial correlation function mostly reflects the partially elongated shape of each particle in the image. (f) The lower surface is the fit of the spatial correlation function corresponding to $D = 5.0$ μm²/s. (g) Raster scan image of particles diffusing at $D = 90$ μm²/s. The particles appear very elongated because they move away before the next line is scanned. (h) The resulting spatial correlation function shows a very elongated pattern. (i) The lower surface is the fit of the spatial correlation function corresponding to $D = 90$ μm²/s.

RICS is based on correlating fluctuation among adjacent pixels, but the RICS correlation function does not calculate correlations among fluctuations occurring at longer times corresponding to different frames in a time stack acquisition. Using this more general approach, we could address questions related to the diffusion as well as the confinement of the diffusing molecules and measurement of active transport, which are commonly studied using single-particle tracking.

Spatial correlation

Spatial correlation
before subtracting
background

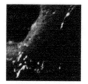

Subtract the average

Spatial correlation
of entire image after
subtracting image

FIGURE 10.13 Logical representation of the algorithm to subtract the immobile structures in order to obtain the correlation function of only the moving particles. A stack of images is acquired in rapid succession (approximately 50 to 100 frames). If we calculate the spatial correlation of the image, we will see a characteristic pattern that reflects the spatial structures of the images rather than the intensity fluctuations. We then calculate the average of all frames in the stack and subtract this average from each of the frames. Finally, we calculated the spatial correlation function of the images after subtraction of the average, immobile fraction.

10.5 THE iMSD CONCEPT AND THE GENERALIZATION OF FLUCTUATION CORRELATION EXPERIMENTS

Molecules on biological membranes move according to an underlying spatial structure that has been shown by single-particle tracking.[1,36] However, single-particle tracking requires labeling molecules with large probes and a concentration in which each particle is separated from the other. Particle tracking experiments were quite important because they have given us information about the structure and dynamics of membranes at the 100–200 nm scale that are not amenable to other structural methods (x-rays, etc.). The algorithms for determining the trajectory of particles require the motion to be essentially in 2D and that the particles should not disappear/reappear during tracking. The advantage of single-particle tracking is the detailed information that can be obtained through the analysis of the mean square displacement (MSD). The MSD provides information about directed motion, flows, and directionality. However, this is obtained one particle at a time at a long time range (several seconds per particle) (Table 10.2).

The method that we discuss here (iMSD) provides the value of the MSD similarly to single-particle tracking but using single-particle fluctuations in an ensemble analysis approach based on correlation functions.[37] This method can be applied to entire images or parts of images and it is done using fast cameras (in the TIRF configuration for membrane studies) at a relatively high concentration of fluorescent particles. To calculate the spatiotemporal correlation function, we acquire a stack of images, generally approximately 1000. The STICS correlation function is given by the following expression[38]:

$$G_{STICS}(\xi, \psi, \tau) = \frac{\langle I(x, y, t)I(x+\xi, y+\psi, t+\tau)\rangle}{\langle I(x, y, t)\rangle^2} - 1. \tag{10.7}$$

TABLE 10.2

Advantages and Limitations of Common Dynamic Techniques Employed to Measure Molecular Diffusion and Aggregation in Cells

Technique	Advantages	Limitations
FRAP, iFRAP, FLIP	Well established, high signal-to-noise ratio	Only measures populations, limited spatial and temporal resolution, difficult to do in multicolor mode
Single-point FCS/PCH/ ccFCS/ccPCH	Well established, measures single molecular fluctuations	Difficult to obtain diffusion and interaction in every position in the cell, difficult to obtain molecular interaction and stoichiometry of aggregates
RICS/ccRICS/N&B/ccN&B	Provides a map of molecular diffusion and aggregates in the entire cell, provides stoichiometry information	Works better with fast diffusion and fast binding (on and off rates)
Single-particle tracking	Provides detailed information about directional motion, diffusion in restricted space	One particle at a time, the particles must be bright and isolated from each other

The correlation function can be calculated using the principles already outlined in Figure 10.2, based on the excitation profile and a model for the diffusion, in our case, Fick's law:

$$G(\xi, \psi, \tau) = g_0 p(\xi, \psi, \tau) \times W(\xi, \psi) \tag{10.8}$$

The general expression for the correlation function takes the following form:

$$G(\xi, \psi, \tau) = g(\tau) \times \exp\left(-\frac{\xi^2 + \psi^2}{\sigma_r^2(\tau)}\right) + g_\infty(\tau). \tag{10.9}$$

The term $g(\tau)$ corresponds to a decay function that is indicative of the lack of correlation at a long time. Figure 10.14 shows the general concepts behind the iMSD approach.

The variance of the Gaussian term can be modeled according to (i) free diffusion, (ii) confined diffusion, and (iii) transient confinement, with a probability to escape from confinement.

$$\sigma_r^2(\tau) = 4D\tau + \sigma_0^2 \tag{10.10}$$

$$\sigma_r^2(\tau) \cong \frac{L^2}{3}\left(1 - \exp\left(-\frac{\tau}{\tau_c}\right)\right) + \sigma_0^2 \tag{10.11}$$

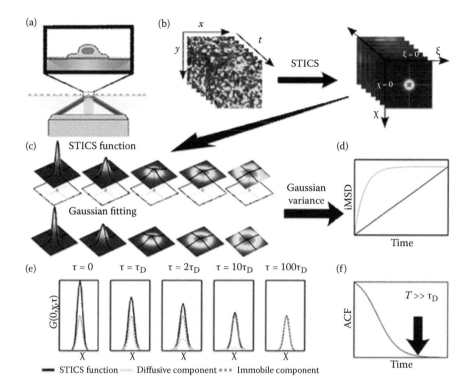

FIGURE 10.14 (a) Starting from a TIRF (total internal reflection) microscope, a time stack of images (b) is collected at relatively high speed, generally in the order of 100 frames/s. (c) The STICS correlation function (Equation 10.7) is applied to the stack. Either a fit of the correlation function or an estimation of the variance of the distribution is used to construct the iMSD plot. (e) The function will tend to the immobile part, which is generally subtracted in this analysis so that only the diffuse component is analyzed (line in e). Under this condition, the ACF will go to zero at long correlation times as shown in (f). (Image reproduced from Di Rienzo, C. et al., *Proc Natl Acad Sci*, 110, 12307–12, 2013.)

$$\sigma_r^2(\tau) \cong \frac{L^2}{3}\left(1 - \exp\left(-\frac{\tau}{\tau_c}\right)\right) + 4D_{\text{macro}}\tau + \sigma_0^2 \qquad (10.12)$$

The three situations are illustrated in Figure 10.15.

One crucial characteristic of the iMSD approach is that the iMSD at time $t = 0$ converges to σ_0^2. This is the size of the PSF. If we determine the size of the PSF with great precision and we subtract it from the iMSD, then the limiting value should tend to the size of the particle. Since in our measurements we use molecules that are of negligible size compared to the PSF, any excess value of iMSD above zero must be due to a fast motion within the exposure time of the camera (Figure 10.16).

A distinct advantage of the iMSD technique is that we can measure the iMSD using a line scan. The iMSD is based on correlation rather than tracking, so we do

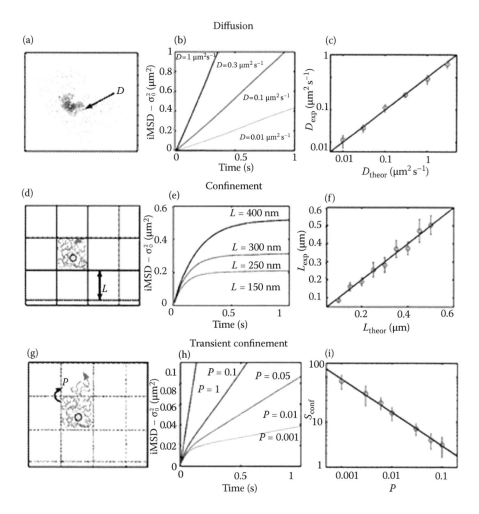

FIGURE 10.15 Simulations of different diffusion behaviors typically found in biological membranes. (a) Free diffusion. (b) For free diffusion, the iMSD increases linearly with the correlation time. (c) From the slope of the iMSD, we can recover the value used for the simulation over a broad range. (d) Simulation of confined motion in a confinement zone of size $L \times L$. (e) The iMSD saturates as the correlation time increases. (f) From the saturation value, we can directly extract the value of L used for the simulations. (g) Simulation of transient confinement shows that the iMSD has a mixed behavior as shown in (h). (i) Fit of the iMSD curve provides both the value of the local diffusion and the confinement strength parameter. (Image reproduced from Di Rienzo, C. et al., *Proc Natl Acad Sci*, 110, 12307–12, 2013.)

not need to exactly follow the particle for many frames. If the particle disappears and then reappears like in a line scan, the correlation function will "fill the dots" and the iMSD could be measured at very high speed in the microsecond range, which is not attainable yet using cameras. This point will be further discussed in connection with experimental results.

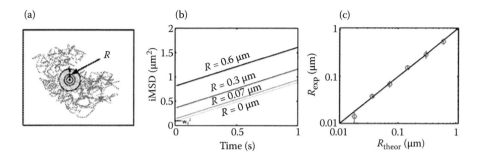

FIGURE 10.16 Simulations of diffusion of particles of different size. (a) The size of the particles was varied from zero to 600 nm. (b) In all cases, the intercepts of the iMSD at $t = 0$ gives the radius of the particle. (c) The recovery of the simulated value always corresponds to the value used for the simulation. (Image reproduced from Di Rienzo, C. et al., *Proc Natl Acad Sci*, 110, 12307–12, 2013.)

10.6 EXAMPLE OF STUDIES OF MEMBRANE LATERAL DIFFUSION THAT EMPHASIZE THE SPATIAL CORRELATION METHOD

In this example, we show an application of the iMSD spatial correlation method to determine transient confinement in cell membranes. The original work by Kusumi's laboratory[36] using single-particle tracking demonstrated that the transferrin receptor (TfR) is transiently confined and that the confinement is due to interactions of the receptor with the underlying cytoskeleton as schematically shown in Figure 10.17a. Images of cells transfected with TfR-GFP are shown in Figure 10.17b. In the TIRF microscope, images were acquired at 100 frames/s and the iMSD correlation function was calculated and shown at different delays τ (Figure 10.17c). The correlation decays as a function of time and the amplitude of the correlation function is shown in Figure 10.17d. The iMSD is calculated as described in Figure 10.14 and plotted in Figure 10.17e (light gray curve). In accordance with the work of Kusumi et al.,[36] we can clearly see the transient confinement of the TfR. We then treated the cells with latrunculin, which is known to disorganize the actin cytoskeleton (Figure 10.17f). After treatment, the receptor moves almost unobstructed as shown in Figure 10.17e (dark gray curve). We note that this experiment was done with a relatively small added part to the TfR receptor (the GFP), which better reproduces the biological situation than the gold particles or antibodies used by Kusumi. Furthermore, in our experiment, we have a relatively large density of receptors; still, the iMSD can be obtained with great accuracy.

To further investigate if the barrier that causes the confinement is due to a simple mechanical obstruction, we performed experiments as a function of temperature in a relatively narrow temperature range not to affect the cell membrane. We found that an increase in temperature causes an increase in the rate of hopping over the barrier. An Arrhenius analysis allowed us to determine the barrier height at the origin of the confinement. Figure 10.18a shows the iMSD as two temperatures and Figure 10.18b shows the iMSD at very short time delays. In Figure 10.18c, we show that

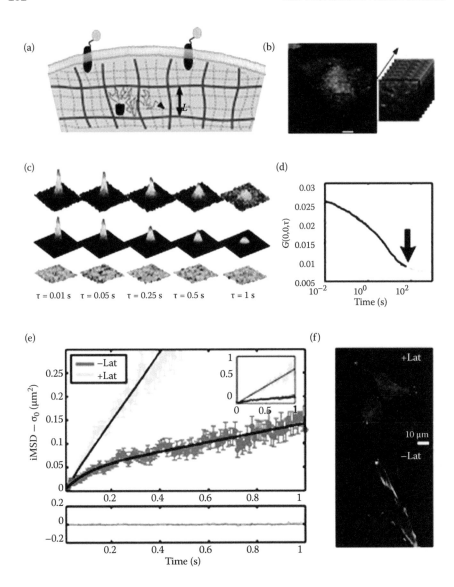

FIGURE 10.17 Motion of the TfR in cell membranes. (a) Schematic representation of the membrane and underlying actin network. (b) CHO-K1 cells transfected with TfR-GFP. (c) The stack of images collected in the TIRF microscope is used to compute the STICS correlation function. (d) The amplitude of the correlation decreases as a function of the delay time. (e) The iMSD for the TfR is affected by the treatment with latrunculin. (f) Cells treated with latrunculin lose their shape after 30 min. (Image reproduced from Di Rienzo, C. et al., *Proc Natl Acad Sci*, 110, 12307–12, 2013.)

Transient confinement if TfR is due to an Arrhenius barrier

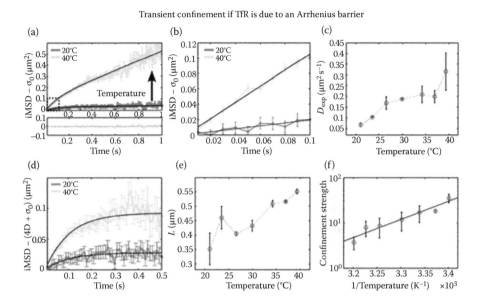

FIGURE 10.18 Temperature effect on the motion of the TfR in cell membranes. (a) As the temperature increases, the iMSD plot shows a marked increase in the mobility of the receptor. (b) Detail of the behavior at short times. (c) Calculation of the apparent diffusion coefficient as a function of temperature. (d) Subtracting the PSF value clearly shows the confinement. (e) Determination of the confinement parameter L as a function of temperature. (f) Arrhenius analysis to determine the barrier height (1.4 ± 0.5 eV). (Image reproduced from Di Rienzo, C. et al., *Proc Natl Acad Sci*, 110, 12307–12, 2013.)

the apparent diffusion increases with temperature. We paid particular attention to the behavior of the iMSD at very short times, and after subtracting the value of the PSF, we realized that the iMSD shows a confinement effect from which we determined the confinement parameter L (Figure 10.18e). In Figure 10.18f, we show the Arrhenius analysis that shows a single slope. We also observed that the iMSD was not going to zero, as predicted by the theory.

We hypothesized that the minimum frame time of 0.01 s allowed by our camera is still too long and that during that time, the protein could diffuse in within the confinement zone, producing a spot of a given size that is due to motion rather than to the real size of the molecule (Figure 10.19a).

We then exploited the property of the iMSD that allows us to use a very fast line scan to explore the very beginning of the iMSD curve (Figure 10.19b). The iMSD analysis of line scan shows that at very short times, the iMSD goes to zero, as predicted by the theory. We then determine directly the transition point and we were able to find independently the size of the confinement zone. This latter result is quite intriguing because it suggests that only at very fast times can we observe the "true" behavior of the TfR and that at very short times, the protein diffuses relatively fast.

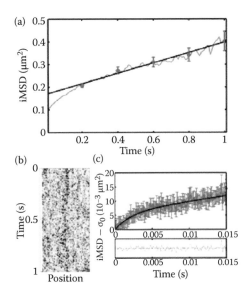

FIGURE 10.19 iMSD behavior at very short correlation times. (a) The values of the iMSD determined with the camera do not extrapolate to zero. (b) Line scan analysis is used to determine the behavior at very short times. (c) Line iMSD shows that the iMSD goes to zero at very short times as predicted by the theory. (Image reproduced from Di Rienzo, C. et al., *Proc Natl Acad Sci*, 110, 12307–12, 2013.)

10.7 CONCLUSIONS

The development of the concept of spatial correlation in the FCS approach is particularly important for membrane studies. The concept shifts the focus from the measurements of intensity fluctuations caused by the passage of the molecule in the volume of illumination to the spatial path taken by the molecule. Given the intrinsic structural and dynamical nano- and macrostructure of biological membranes, this shift of paradigm could be very significant. The development of the spatial correlation of the fluctuations requires a more complex mathematical approach but produces simple and intuitive results that can be inferred directly from the shape and behavior of the spatial correlation function. The concept of the iMSD method was key for the discovery of membrane domains and confinement and, in general macrostructures, comes naturally from mathematical derivation. More importantly, measurements of fluctuations are done using relatively small fluorescence tags and on single molecules. There are no large particles attached to lipids or proteins. The measurement of the spatial correlation can be done either using confocal techniques or using fast, commercially available cameras. Camera measurements can be supplemented with fast line scans to interrogate a time range that is still not reachable with current camera technologies. Data analysis is very simple and fast as opposed to single-particle tracking that requires sophisticated algorithms for determining the regions of confinement.

A topic not discussed in this contribution is that the iMSD approach can be done using multiple detection channels similarly to the cross-correlation fluctuation techniques. This still unexploited capability could reveal the formation of molecular complexes and their transport in the membrane. Another subject that is not discussed here is the measurement of molecular flows, as proposed originally by the Wiseman laboratory upon the introduction of the STICS technique. The current RICS or iMSD analysis allows dividing the image in small subimages so that the behavior of a large portion of the plasma membrane of cells could be studied and compared. Another interesting topic that is enabled by the RICS technique is the quantification of aggregation and binding. The N&B methods are currently used to analyze the distribution of the amplitude of the fluctuations, to determine membrane receptor aggregations and other biologically significant processes.

The fluctuation correlation approach is a powerful method used to determine several membrane properties such as local structure, molecular interactions, and protein and lipid transport. Although the principles of the method have been known for some time, only recently has the fluctuation approach been applied to the study of membrane systems in great detail. As originally conceived, the FCS method provides information about the rate of fluorescence intensity fluctuations at a single point. During the last few years, the fluctuation analysis has been enhanced to account for spatially correlated fluctuations. In the context of membrane studies, this evolution of the fluctuation correlation method has opened new possibilities that have brought notable insight about the dynamic structures of membranes, both in model systems and in the membranes of living cells. Since spatial correlation methods are relatively new, here we review the conceptual framework that has allowed us to develop and apply the notion of spatial correlation to cellular systems. First, we describe the spatial correlation approach using schematic graphical representations and then we show a recent application of image correlation analysis to membrane systems in live cells.

ACKNOWLEDGMENTS

This work is supported in part by NIH-P41 GM103540 and NIH-P50 GM076516.

REFERENCES

1. Kusumi, A., and K. Suzuki. "Toward Understanding the Dynamics of Membrane-Raft-Based Molecular Interactions." *Biochim Biophys Acta* 1746, no. 3 (2005): 234–51.
2. Jacobson, K., O. G. Mouritsen, and R. G. Anderson. "Lipid Rafts: At a Crossroad between Cell Biology and Physics." *Nat Cell Biol* 9, no. 1 (2007): 7–14.
3. Dietrich, C., L. A. Bagatolli, Z. N. Volovyk et al. "Lipid Rafts Reconstituted in Model Membranes." *Biophys J* 80, no. 3 (2001): 1417–28.
4. Dietrich, C., B. Yang, T. Fujiwara, A. Kusumi, and K. Jacobson. "Relationship of Lipid Rafts to Transient Confinement Zones Detected by Single Particle Tracking." *Biophys J* 82, no. 1 Pt 1 (2002): 274–84.
5. Bagatolli, L. A. "To See or Not to See: Lateral Organization of Biological Membranes and Fluorescence Microscopy." *Biochim Biophys Acta* 1758, no. 10 (2006): 1541–56.
6. Kapustina, M., E. Vitriol, T. C. Elston, L. M. Loew, and K. Jacobson. "Modeling Capping Protein Frap and Cali Experiments Reveals In Vivo Regulation of Actin Dynamics." *Cytoskeleton (Hoboken)* 67, no. 8 (2010): 519–34.
7. Magnusson, K. E., J. Wojcieszyn, C. Dahlgren et al. "Lateral Diffusion of Wheat Germ Agglutinin-Labeled Glycoconjugates in the Membrane of Differentiating HL-60 and

U-937 Cells Assessed with Fluorescence Recovery after Photobleaching (FRAP)." *Cell Biophys* 5, no. 2 (1983): 119–28.

8. Axelrod, D., P. Ravdin, D. E. Koppel et al. "Lateral Motion of Fluorescently Labeled Acetylcholine Receptors in Membranes of Developing Muscle Fibers." *Proc Natl Acad Sci U S A* 73, no. 12 (1976): 4594–8.

9. Ries, J., and P. Schwille. "Studying Slow Membrane Dynamics with Continuous Wave Scanning Fluorescence Correlation Spectroscopy." *Biophys J* 91, no. 5 (2006): 1915–24.

10. Schwille, P., J. Korlach, and W. W. Webb. "Fluorescence Correlation Spectroscopy with Single-Molecule Sensitivity on Cell and Model Membranes." *Cytometry* 36, no. 3 (1999): 176–82.

11. Honigmann, A., V. Mueller, S. W. Hell, and C. Eggeling. "STED Microscopy Detects and Quantifies Liquid Phase Separation in Lipid Membranes Using a New Far-Red Emitting Fluorescent Phosphoglycerolipid Analogue." *Faraday Discuss* 161 (2013): 77–89; discussion 113–50.

12. Leutenegger, M., C. Ringemann, T. Lasser, S. W. Hell, and C. Eggeling. "Fluorescence Correlation Spectroscopy with a Total Internal Reflection Fluorescence STED Microscope (Tirf-Sted-Fcs)." *Opt Express* 20, no. 5 (2012): 5243–63.

13. Mueller, V., A. Honigmann, C. Ringemann et al. "FCS in STED Microscopy: Studying the Nanoscale of Lipid Membrane Dynamics." *Methods Enzymol* 519 (2013): 1–38.

14. Sezgin, E., I. Levental, M. Grzybek et al. "Partitioning, Diffusion, and Ligand Binding of Raft Lipid Analogs in Model and Cellular Plasma Membranes." *Biochim Biophys Acta* 1818, no. 7 (2012): 1777–84.

15. Wawrezinieck, L., H. Rigneault, D. Marguet, and P. F. Lenne. "Fluorescence Correlation Spectroscopy Diffusion Laws to Probe the Submicron Cell Membrane Organization." *Biophys J* 89, no. 6 (2005): 4029–42.

16. Brown, C. M., R. B. Dalal, B. Hebert et al. "Raster Image Correlation Spectroscopy (RICS) for Measuring Fast Protein Dynamics and Concentrations with a Commercial Laser Scanning Confocal Microscope." *J Microsc* 229, no. Pt 1 (2008): 78–91.

17. Digman, M. A., C. M. Brown, P. Sengupta et al. "Measuring Fast Dynamics in Solutions and Cells with a Laser Scanning Microscope." *Biophys J* 89, no. 2 (2005): 1317–27.

18. Digman, M. A., and E. Gratton. "Analysis of Diffusion and Binding in Cells Using the Rics Approach." *Microsc Res Tech* 72, no. 4 (2009): 323–32.

19. Digman, M. A., M. Stakic, and E. Gratton. "Raster Image Correlation Spectroscopy and Number and Brightness Analysis." *Methods Enzymol* 518 (2013): 121–44.

20. Gielen, E., N. Smisdom, M. vandeVen et al. "Measuring Diffusion of Lipid-Like Probes in Artificial and Natural Membranes by Raster Image Correlation Spectroscopy (RICS): Use of a Commercial Laser-Scanning Microscope with Analog Detection." *Langmuir* 25, no. 9 (2009): 5209–18.

21. Rossow, M. J., J. M. Sasaki, M. A. Digman, and E. Gratton. "Raster Image Correlation Spectroscopy in Live Cells." *Nat Protoc* 5, no. 11 (2010): 1761–74.

22. Bachir, A. I., D. L. Kolin, K. G. Heinze, B. Hebert, and P. W. Wiseman. "A Guide to Accurate Measurement of Diffusion Using Fluorescence Correlation Techniques with Blinking Quantum Dot Nanoparticle Labels." *J Chem Phys* 128, no. 22 (2008): 225105.

23. Brandao, H. B., H. Sangji, E. Pandzic et al. "Measuring Ligand-Receptor Binding Kinetics and Dynamics Using K-Space Image Correlation Spectroscopy." *Methods* 66, no. 2 (2014): 273–82.

24. Digman, M. A., P. Sengupta, P. W. Wiseman et al. "Fluctuation Correlation Spectroscopy with a Laser-Scanning Microscope: Exploiting the Hidden Time Structure." *Biophys J* 88, no. 5 (2005): L33–6.

25. Digman, M. A., P. W. Wiseman, A. R. Horwitz, and E. Gratton. "Detecting Protein Complexes in Living Cells from Laser Scanning Confocal Image Sequences by the Cross Correlation Raster Image Spectroscopy Method." *Biophys J* 96, no. 2 (2009): 707–16.

26. Kolin, D. L., and P. W. Wiseman. "Advances in Image Correlation Spectroscopy: Measuring Number Densities, Aggregation States, and Dynamics of Fluorescently Labeled Macromolecules in Cells." *Cell Biochem Biophys* 49, no. 3 (2007): 141–64.

27. Sergeev, M., A. G. Godin, L. Kao et al. "Determination of Membrane Protein Transporter Oligomerization in Native Tissue Using Spatial Fluorescence Intensity Fluctuation Analysis." *PLoS One* 7, no. 4 (2012): e36215.

28. Chen, Y., J. D. Muller, Q. Ruan, and E. Gratton. "Molecular Brightness Characterization of EGFP In Vivo by Fluorescence Fluctuation Spectroscopy." *Biophys J* 82, no. 1 Pt 1 (2002): 133–44.

29. Muller, J. D., Y. Chen, and E. Gratton. "Resolving Heterogeneity on the Single Molecular Level with the Photon-Counting Histogram." *Biophys J* 78, no. 1 (2000): 474–86.

30. Muller, J. D., Y. Chen, and E. Gratton. "Fluorescence Correlation Spectroscopy." *Methods Enzymol* 361 (2003): 69–92.

31. Digman, M. A., P. W. Wiseman, C. Choi, A. R. Horwitz, and E. Gratton. "Stoichiometry of Molecular Complexes at Adhesions in Living Cells." *Proc Natl Acad Sci U S A* 106, no. 7 (2009): 2170–5.

32. Ossato, G., M. A. Digman, C. Aiken et al. "A Two-Step Path to Inclusion Formation of Huntingtin Peptides Revealed by Number and Brightness Analysis." *Biophys J* 98, no. 12 (2010): 3078–85.

33. Berland, K. M., P. T. So, Y. Chen, W. W. Mantulin, and E. Gratton. "Scanning Two-Photon Fluctuation Correlation Spectroscopy: Particle Counting Measurements for Detection of Molecular Aggregation." *Biophys J* 71, no. 1 (1996): 410–20.

34. Petersen, N. O., C. Brown, A. Kaminski et al. "Analysis of Membrane Protein Cluster Densities and Sizes In Situ by Image Correlation Spectroscopy." *Faraday Discuss*, 111 (1998): 289–305; discussion 31–43.

35. Petersen, N. O., P. L. Hoddelius, P. W. Wiseman, O. Seger, and K. E. Magnusson. "Quantitation of Membrane Receptor Distributions by Image Correlation Spectroscopy: Concept and Application." *Biophys J* 65, no. 3 (1993): 1135–46.

36. Kusumi, A., C. Nakada, K. Ritchie et al. "Paradigm Shift of the Plasma Membrane Concept from the Two-Dimensional Continuum Fluid to the Partitioned Fluid: High-Speed Single-Molecule Tracking of Membrane Molecules." *Annu Rev Biophys Biomol Struct* 34 (2005): 351–78.

37. Di Rienzo, C., E. Gratton, F. Beltram, and F. Cardarelli. "Fast Spatiotemporal Correlation Spectroscopy to Determine Protein Lateral Diffusion Laws in Live Cell Membranes." *Proc Natl Acad Sci U S A* 110, no. 30 (2013): 12307–12.

38. Hebert, B., S. Costantino, and P. W. Wiseman. "Spatiotemporal Image Correlation Spectroscopy (STICS) Theory, Verification, and Application to Protein Velocity Mapping in Living CHO Cells." *Biophys J* 88, no. 5 (2005): 3601–14.

11 Spatial Intensity Distribution Analysis (SpIDA)

A Method to Probe Membrane Receptor Organization in Intact Cells

Antoine G. Godin, Benjamin Rappaz,
Laurent Potvin-Trottier, Yves De Koninck,
and Paul W. Wiseman

CONTENTS

11.1 INTRODUCTION

A quantitative description of protein interactions and organization is key to understanding the initial steps in cell signaling mechanisms, but measuring interactions directly in intact cellular environments has remained a daunting challenge owing to the molecular scale of these events and the resolution limit of conventional optical microscopy imposed by the diffraction of light. Changes in the oligomerization state of many classes of receptors are linked to function[1–8] and activation in cellular signaling; hence, the ability to follow such changes is a prerequisite for building accurate models that reflect the molecular mechanisms that regulate these processes. Furthermore, receptor protein distribution and clustering state vary spatially throughout the cell during intracellular shuttling, membrane residency, and finally internalization (turnover) from the plasma membrane; thus, it is important to be able to measure the processes in different regions of the cell.

Recent years have witnessed many advances in fluorescence microscopy, the introduction of new biophysical tools to study cells along with developments of new fluorescent probes that allow specific labeling of receptors in living cells. Indeed, for the last two decades, the impact of the green fluorescent protein (GFP) and its derivatives (e.g., CFP, YFP, and mCherry)[9,10] on progress in cell biology has been tremendous. The sequencing of GFP[11] created the opportunity to create fusion constructs with many proteins, thereby making fluorescent proteins (FPs) the tool of choice to study receptor organization in single cells. Fusion protein expression systems provide highly flexible environments where different pharmacological paradigms could be tested using fluorescence microscopy. Genetic modifications were systematically studied to provide brighter GFP variants in addition to monomeric constructs (monomeric GFP [mGFP])[12] along with mutants yielding a palette of FPs emitting in most parts of the visible spectrum.[10] Concurrently, fluorescence microscopy was developed and refined to the point where confocal laser scanning microscopy (CLSM)[13,14] is now a universal tool accessible to most biology laboratories.

Many quantitative fluorescence methods have also been developed to study receptor trafficking, mobility, and interactions. Fluorescence correlation spectroscopy (FCS)[15,16] measures temporal fluorescence intensity fluctuations arising from time-dependent changes in the number of fluorescent molecules within the fixed focus of a laser beam within a sample. Autocorrelation analysis of the intensity fluctuation record in time is used in FCS to measure the concentration and diffusion coefficient of the fluorescent molecules. FCS has been used to successfully discriminate fluorescent species in mixtures by measuring their diffusion coefficients.[17]

The photon counting histogram (PCH)[18] technique is complementary to FCS as it relies on the same temporal fluctuations in fluorescence, but the difference is that it can discriminate oligomerization states (e.g., monomers and dimers) in a mixture of two fluorescent species with different molecular brightness values. In the limit of small oligomer size and in the absence of quenching, most fluorescence measurement approaches are linear; hence, the detected oligomerization state of the labeled protein assemblies is proportional to the total collected signal counts per independent complex (e.g., a dimer appears twice as bright as a monomer). The quantal brightness is defined as the average photon count collected per unit time from the effective laser beam focal volume per fluorescent entity present. However, PCH cannot distinguish whether the labeled proteins are part of a larger complex containing nonfluorescent molecules (e.g., hetero-oligomerization). In PCH, time-binned histograms of photon counts collected from a single fixed laser beam focus within the sample are iteratively fit for different distributions of molecules in focus, converging to obtain concentrations and mean quantal brightness of diffusing fluorescent molecules. Applications of these approaches have provided important information about molecular oligomerization for rapidly diffusing species in the nucleus and the cytoplasm. Number and brightness (N&B)[19] was also developed to obtain density and oligomerization averages from calculation of the mean and variance of temporal fluctuations from single-pixel stacks from image time series. High-order correlation analysis[20,21] was also developed to obtain information on the number of membrane receptors and their aggregation states and has proven to be especially useful for studying large clusters (>10 molecules).

Image correlation spectroscopy (ICS),[22–25] the imaging analog of FCS, measures membrane receptor densities from single images by exploiting fluorescence intensity fluctuations sampled in space rather than in time. Several ICS family derivatives were developed, including image cross-correlation spectroscopy,[26] temporal ICS,[22] spatial temporal ICS,[27,28] raster-scanned ICS,[29] k-space ICS,[30,31] and nu-space ICS,[32] which differ in the precise details of correlation function analysis of the fluorescence fluctuations for different types of protein dynamics and imaging conditions. Each of these approaches has its advantages and taps different molecular properties; however, none of these techniques can accurately discriminate different oligomeric species in a mixture from single images.

Spatial intensity distribution analysis (SpIDA)[33–36] was developed to address the need to measure mixtures of oligomers from single images, that is, with spatial fluorescence fluctuations only. With a single image as an input, SpIDA is able to reliably detect and measure mixtures of fluorescently labeled receptor oligomer distributions by fitting fluorescence intensity histograms. The technique was first validated by measuring the dimerization of the epidermal growth factor receptor (EGFR) after activation by its ligand, the epidermal growth factor.[33–35] We also monitored signaling transactivation of EGFRs by measuring its dimerization in response to activation of a series of G-protein-coupled receptors with their cognate ligands.[34,35] SpIDA was then applied to different types of cell systems and using many types of fluorescent probes.[20,33,34,37,38] SpIDA has been applied to quantify the oligomerization states of receptors fused to fluorescent proteins in expression systems,[33,34,38] to study the organization of endogenous receptors in primary culture neurons,[37,34] and directly in intact tissue samples[20,33] using fluorescently tagged antibodies. In these applications, SpIDA was restricted to the study of single species of receptors in order to measure their distribution as monomers and dimers.

In this chapter, we present the theoretical background of SpIDA and show how we can extend it to analyze high-order oligomers from images collected using fluorescence microscopy. We will also define its limitations. An important technical challenge faced by all fluorescence microscopy based oligomerization measurement techniques is the fidelity of labeling of the receptors, where the ideal case would involve every subunit being labeled with a single emitting and detectable fluorophore. In practice, imperfect labeling or stochastic probe emission introduces systematic errors that widen the distribution of oligomeric states measured from the actual oligomeric system. For example, in a cellular system with uniform expression of tetramers, fractional labeling of the receptor subunits will entail the presence of fluorescent monomers, dimers, trimers (respectively clustered with three, two, or one nonlabeled subunit), and fully labeled tetramers that will be detected with different probabilities. This labeling artifact will generate a discrepancy between the true biological and the observed fluorescent oligomeric distributions. Using fluorescently tagged antibodies, the proportion of labeled antigen varies with the concentration of antibodies used and their affinity toward the antigen. But even in the saturation regime, nothing ensures that all targeted proteins are revealed and some sites might not be accessible owing to different protein conformations, phosphorylation, association, fixation, or permeabilization effects. This artifact not only is present with immunocytochemistry labeling but also can be observed when using genetically encoded FPs to reveal receptors. Even if by construction all receptors are fused with the genetically encoded FP, it has been reported that at least 20% of them are misfolded and, consequently, cannot emit fluorescence.[39,40]

We will present an algorithm that can correct for the stochastic mislabeling artifact and that allows the measurement of the oligomerization state of some receptors that are organized in higher oligomeric states.

11.2   SPATIAL INTENSITY DISTRIBUTION ANALYSIS

In this section, an overview of SpIDA is presented while the theory and derivation of SpIDA will be explained in full detail in the Appendix. The first step in SpIDA is the calculation of an intensity histogram from pixels in a region of interest (ROI) from a single fluorescence microscopy image of a cell.[33,34] The intensity histogram of an image ROI is calculated by counting the number of pixels for each intensity value or intensity bin within the selected ROI. The intensity of each pixel in a CLSM image is the integrated fluorescence intensity collected from fluorescence originating within the region of the sample excited by the laser beam focal volume. The pixel intensity histograms for different ROIs are fit with super-Poissonian distributions.

A super-Poissonian distribution is defined as the intensity distribution of randomly (Poisson) distributed particles in space convolved with the optical point spread function (PSF) of the microscope. SpIDA outputs information on the densities of the underlying fluorescent molecules and their quantal brightness values, which are fitting parameters in the analysis. In SpIDA, the quantal brightness is defined as the average intensity unit (iu) (which is not a photon count) collected over the whole effective volume of the PSF for a distinct fluorescent entity (monomer or oligomer). SpIDA was inspired by the temporal PCH method,[18] but the key difference being that it is applied in the spatial domain, enabling measurements on subregions within single images collected on conventional fluorescence microscopes equipped with analog photomultiplier tube (PMT) detectors. Examples of intensity histogram generation and SpIDA analyses are presented in Figure 11.1. The fluorescence signal of mGFP-f expressed on the cell membrane can be observed (Figure 11.1a) with the intensity histograms of two selected regions with their corresponding SpIDA fit values in Figure 11.1b and c.

In the theoretical discussion in the Appendix, various SpIDA models for different distribution scenarios are described in detail. The first is a model for one-population SpIDA for imaged regions that contain particles with the same (i.e., uniform) oligomeric state (Equation 11.4). The histogram fitting functions of SpIDA are numerically calculated in an iterative manner. The first step is to calculate the intensity (k) distribution probability when exactly one single emitter of quantal brightness ε is randomly positioned in the PSF-defined focal volume [$\rho^1(\varepsilon;k) = \int \delta(\varepsilon \cdot I(\mathbf{r}) - k)\,d\mathbf{r}$; Equation 11.1 and Figure 11.2].

Then iteratively, the intensity distribution probability, $\rho^n(\varepsilon;k)$, when exactly n emitters, each of brightness ϵ, are randomly positioned in the PSF focus, which is

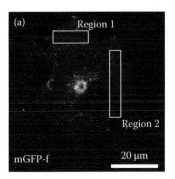

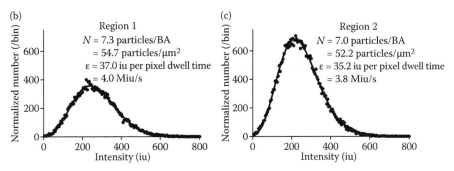

FIGURE 11.1 Example of histogram generation and SpIDA analysis. (a) Sample CLSM image of mGFP expressed at the membrane of cos7 cells. Image of size 1024 × 1024 pixels with a pixel size of 0.058 μm and a pixel dwell time of 9.2 μs. Two selected rectangular ROIs with their histograms and recovered fit from SpIDA are shown in parts (b) and (c). The fit values obtained for regions 1 and 2 are, respectively, 54.7 particles/μm² with a quantal brightness of 4.0 Miu/s and 52.2 particles/μm² with a quantal brightness of 3.8 Miu/s.

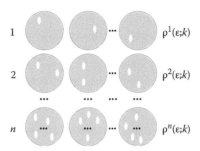

FIGURE 11.2 Schematic overview of the iterative histogram generation. Schematic overview of the iterative histogram generation for 1, 2,..., n fluorescent particles (oval "receptors") in the PSF illumination profile (circular regions). Each configuration contributes a certain number of photons that are measured as an intensity brightness k, and the histogram $\rho^n(\varepsilon;k)$ is, then, generated for all configurations containing n particles.

determined recursively from $\rho^1(\varepsilon;k)$ [$\rho^2(\varepsilon;k) = \rho^1(\varepsilon;k) \otimes \rho^1(\varepsilon;k)$ and $\rho^n(\varepsilon;k) = \rho^1(\varepsilon;k) \otimes \rho^{n-1}(\varepsilon;k)$; Equations 11.2 and 11.3 and Figure 11.2]. In summary, the fluorescence intensity distribution of all possible configurations of n particles of quantal brightness ε in the beam focal volume is calculated from $\rho^1(\varepsilon;k)$.

Then, the intensity distribution for a single population in an ROI, with an average of N particles per focal volume and quantal brightness ϵ, can be calculated by adding all the n-particle distributions, $\rho^n(\varepsilon;k)$, weighted by their respective probabilities, assuming a Poisson distribution of particles in space with mean N, of having n particles in the focus [$H(\varepsilon,N;k) = \sum_n \rho^n(\varepsilon;k) \cdot poi(n,N)$ with $\rho^0(\varepsilon;k) = \delta_{k,0}$, Equation 11.4].

Using this model, an intensity histogram of a single population in an ROI can be used to recover its density and quantal brightness, which is proportional to the number of photons emitted by each of the distinct moieties in the population. In order to model the reality of labeling and emission artifacts, we have previously shown the impact of having nonperfect emission from probes (e.g., a distribution of the quantal brightness) on the accuracy of SpIDA measurements.[33]

Iteratively, we derived the expression for the two-population [$H(\varepsilon_1, N_1, \varepsilon_2, N_2, A;k) = A \cdot H(\varepsilon_1, N_1;k) \otimes H(\varepsilon_2, N_2;k)$; Equation 11.5] and the three-population [$H(\varepsilon_1, N_1, \varepsilon_2, N_2, \varepsilon_3 N_3 A;k) = A \cdot H(\varepsilon_1, N_1;k) \otimes H(\varepsilon_2, N_2;k) \otimes H(\varepsilon_3 N_3;k)$; Equation 11.7] cases. In short, if a mixture of populations of different oligomerization states is spatially present and randomized in space, the intensity distribution can be calculated by convolving the distributions for the independent one-population distributions (Equations 11.5 and 11.7).

As the number of distinct oligomer populations increases, the number of fitting variables necessarily increases and the fit model will not converge to unique solutions. For this reason, reducing the number of variables in a fit is essential for the accuracy of the analysis. For example, if only a fraction of the subunits forming tetramers are labeled, then fluorescent monomers, dimers, trimers, and tetramers will contribute to the resulting intensity histogram with different probability weights. Fitting for the densities of the monomers, dimers, trimers, and tetramers independently will not yield accurate results (five variables: four densities and one quantal brightness). However, by employing a simpler model that fits for only the number of tetramers and the probability that a single subunit will be fluorescent (three variables: one density, one quantal brightness, and a subunit emission probability) can provide more accurate fitting convergence. Therefore, we can also reduce the number of fitting variables owing to the presence of mislabeling for all of the SpIDA fitting cases introduced (Equations 11.4, 11.5, and 11.7).

11.3 RESULTS AND DISCUSSION

11.3.1 Limits of SpIDA for a Single Population and for Mixtures of Monomers and Dimers

The accuracy and precision of SpIDA for a single population and for a two-population mixture of monomers and dimers have been reported previously[33] so we will focus this chapter on mixtures containing multiple populations. Figure 11.3 presents three examples of computer-simulated images containing monomer–dimer mixtures of different ratios (Figure 11.3a through c) with the corresponding intensity histogram and fit (Figure 11.3d). Details on how the simulation images were generated are given in the Materials and methods section of the Appendix. The results show that, with appropriate sampling, SpIDA can accurately discriminate between images containing a single population of either monomers or dimers from another image containing a mixture of monomers and dimers (Figure 11.3e, which illustrates different ratios of monomers/dimers set in the simulations and measured by SpIDA).

In summary, assuming reasonable signal-to-noise ratio (~3:1) for a single oligomer population and a mixture of monomers and dimers, if the image ROI is large enough to provide sufficient sampling of fluorescence fluctuations (~50 beam focus areas [BAs] or ~6 μm^2 for our confocal microscope), SpIDA can give accurate results (<20% error on all fit parameters).

11.3.2 Measuring Three Populations of Oligomers in Single Images

To test whether SpIDA can be applied to resolve three-population mixtures of oligomers, we generated large simulated images containing different numbers of dimers and tetramers and we varied the number of monomers. To generate Figure 11.4, we assumed that the oligomeric states of the populations present are known a priori (e.g., only monomers, dimers, and tetramers can be present); thus, only the population densities are fit in this case. We considered the assembly hierarchy scheme where monomers form dimers and then dimers group together to form tetramers since it is common in cell biology (e.g., glutamate receptors[41,42] and GABAB[3]).

Figure 11.4a through c shows that when we apply a three-population fitting model (Equation 11.7) for cases where only two populations were actually present, SpIDA still converges to give reliable results, demonstrating that the analysis indicates if an overcomplete model is used (e.g., three-population model when only two populations are present). However, as shown in Figure 11.4c and d, the results are not accurate for the monomeric population, because the monomers in this case correspond to a small proportion of the total intensity. The same explanation holds for the fit of the monomeric population in Figure 11.4d where the numbers of dimers and tetramers are

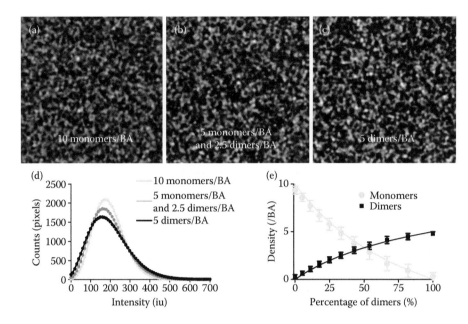

FIGURE 11.3 Precision of SpIDA applied to a monomer–dimer mixture. Computer-simulated images of different mixtures of monomers and dimers. (a through c) The monomers and dimers have densities N1 and N2 per beam area (BA), respectively, in the images while the percentage of dimers in this figure is defined as N2/(N1 + N2). (a) Monomers only; a mixture of (b) 5 monomers/BA and 2.5 dimers/BA, and (c) 5 dimers/BA. The intensity histograms presented in part (d) were measured from the three simulated images showed in parts (a) through (c). The two-population SpIDA best fits (solid lines) are also presented in part (d). For part (a), the results were 9.8 monomers/BA and 0.07 dimers/BA; for part (b), 4.8 monomers/BA and 2.5 dimers/BA; and, finally, for part (c), 0.1 monomers/BA and 4.9 dimers/BA. Part (e) illustrates the accuracy of the technique and shows how SpIDA could discriminate mixtures of monomers and dimers. The monomeric quantal brightness was set to 20 iu, the e^{-2} convolution radius was set to 3 pixels, and the image size was 200×200 pixels. Each point in the graph corresponds to 100 simulations and the error bars correspond to standard deviations (SDs).

higher than the monomers. For this reason, for each fitted distribution, it is important to consider the density-weighted contribution of each of the oligomer populations to the total intensity.

A single-population SpIDA fit model used on images in which both monomer and dimer are present will either fit a quantal brightness that is in between monomers and dimers or inaccurately fit if the quantal brightness is fixed to either the monomer or dimer quantal brightness. However, applying the two-population SpIDA fit model with fixed quantal brightness (monomers and dimers) on images containing a single population of either monomers or dimers will produce an analysis that is still accurate and reveal the presence of just a single population. These three-population simulation results also demonstrate that SpIDA can still provide accurate results when mixtures of three oligomer populations are present in single images when the signal-to-noise ratio is sufficiently high (~3:1[33]) and there is sufficient spatial

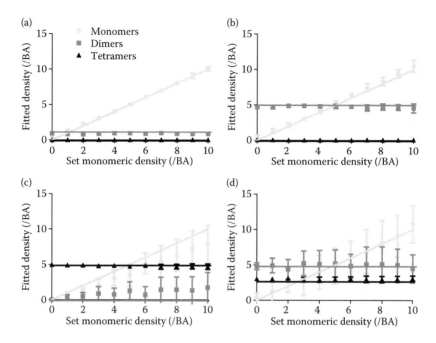

FIGURE 11.4 Three-population SpIDA analysis. SpIDA analysis was applied to simulated images containing three distinct populations (monomers, dimers, and tetramers). Here, the results are for cases where we set the density of dimers (N2) and tetramers (N4) and varied the density of monomers in the image from 0 to 10 per BA. (a) N2 = 1 dimer/BA, N4 = 0 tetramer/BA; (b) N2 = 5 dimers/BA, N4 = 0 tetramer/BA; (c) N2 = 0 dimer/BA, N4 = 5 tetramers/BA; and (d) N2 = 3 dimers/BA, N4 = 1 tetramer/BA. All the values in the graphs correspond to an average of 20 images. The lines correspond to the set values and the data points correspond to the experimentally measured values. The monomeric quantal brightness was set to 20 iu, the e^{-2} convolution radius was set to 3 pixels, and the image size was 500 × 500 pixels. The error bars correspond to SDs.

sampling in the ROI. Therefore, this more general model could be applied to all the two-population cases, while only increasing computing time requirements.

11.3.3 Effect of Mislabeling on the SpIDA-Measured Oligomerization States of Oligomers

An underlying assumption of SpIDA is that the oligomerization state is assumed to be proportional to the integrated fluorescence intensity per oligomer. In other words, if quenching between fluorophores on adjacent subunits is negligible and the detectors are in the linear regime, a dimer will be twice as bright as a monomer and, iteratively, an oligomer, made of n subunits (an n_{mer}), will be n-fold more intense than a monomer.

Mislabeling of receptors will always introduce a systematic perturbation since the integrated intensity will not represent the underlying subunit composition. This effect was previously demonstrated in studies of the oligomerization of ion channels using single molecule step photobleaching experiments.[39,40]

Incomplete labeling can influence the SpIDA measurement of oligomerization states in a variety of ways. For example, for a single population of pure monomers, only the fit density will be affected, as the monomers that are not labeled will not contribute to the fluorescence distribution. In contrast, for a single population of dimers, some fluorescent monomers will be detected (Figure 11.5a through c) since some of the dimers have nonemitting subunits. Figure 11.5c shows the binomial distribution prediction for measuring monomers and dimers for the simulated image presented in Figure 11.5b. A binomial distribution is expected if the probability of any subunit being labeled is the same (p). We assume this to be the case in the rest of the chapter.

If N2 dimers are present in an image ROI (Figure 11.5a), the number of observed dimers will be equal to p^2*N2 and the number of observed monomers, $2*(1 - p)*p*N2$ (Figure 11.5b and c). This means that if the ROI contains a mixture of N1 monomers and N2 dimers, the number of observed monomers will be equal to $p*N1 + 2*(1 - p)*p*N2$, while the number of observed dimers will still be a factor (p^2) times the real number of dimers present. This shows that relative comparison of the number of observed dimers in two different ROIs will indeed provide a valid proportionality ratio even without correcting for mislabeling (i.e., the number of dimers measured is proportional to the real number of dimers). Similarly, if only tetramers are present in

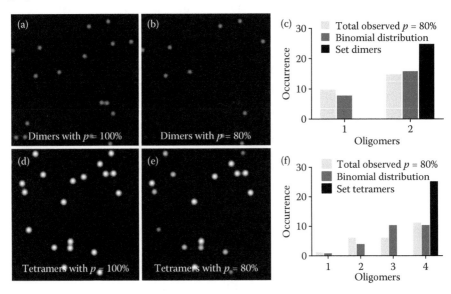

FIGURE 11.5 Effect of subunit mislabeling on the measured oligomeric distribution. Computer-simulated images showing the impact of mislabeling on sparse oligomers. Twenty-five dimers were randomly distributed in the image. Two cases are presented: (a) 100% particle labeling percentage, (b) 80% particle labeling percentage. The set oligomer distribution (a) and observed distribution when mislabeling occurs (b) are presented in part (c). Computer-simulated images in which 25 tetramers are randomly distributed in the image are presented for 100% labeling (d) and 80% labeling (e). The set oligomer distribution (d) and observed distribution when mislabeling occurs (e) are presented in part (f). The monomeric quantal brightness was set to 20 iu, the e^{-2} convolution radius was set to 50 pixels, and the image size was 1500 × 1500 pixels.

an image ROI but with some fractional mislabeling (Figure 11.5d), then a distribution of trimers, dimers, and monomers will also be observed (Figure 11.5e and f).

The phenomenon of subunit mislabeling will always introduce a systematic error when measuring densities and oligomerization states by SpIDA if not properly accounted for and corrected. Assuming an incorrect mislabeling probability will introduce a systematic error on the measured density of each population that is, to first order, proportional to the error on the assumed probability (not shown).

The recovered monomer and dimer distributions for a system with only dimers present are presented in Figure 11.6a as a function of the subunit labeling probability p. Similarly, if higher-order oligomers are mislabeled, the one-population

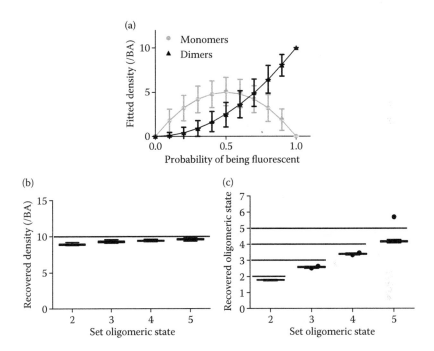

FIGURE 11.6 Effect of subunit mislabeling on SpIDA measurement of a uniform oligomeric state. (a) SpIDA results for images containing only dimers as a function of labeling probability. Ten dimers were labeled with a subunit labeling probability p, and the distribution of observed fluorescent monomers and dimers was measured via SpIDA. This step was repeated 1000 times and the distribution of monomers and dimers as a function of the labeling probability is shown. The error bars correspond to SDs. The effect on the density (b) and quantal brightness (c) fits recovered with one-population SpIDA (Equation 11.4) when only $p = 80\%$ of the oligomers are fluorescently labeled for different types of oligomers ($n_{mer} = 2$ to 5). Here, we deliberately applied the wrong one-population SpIDA model without accounting for mislabeling (i.e., $p = 100\%$ is forced in the fit). The images generated for those simulations were 250×250 pixels, e^{-2} convolution radius was set to 3 pixels, the oligomer density was set to 10 oligomers/BA, the quantal brightness was set to 20 iu, and $p = 80\%$. The box and whiskers correspond to the Tukey method. The top and bottom of the box correspond to the 25th and 75th percentiles, respectively, and the whiskers correspond to the 75th percentile plus 1.5-fold the interquartile distance.

SpIDA analysis (Equation 11.4) will not provide the exact densities (Figure 11.6b) or oligomeric states (Figure 11.6c) and the recovered values will be systematically underestimated.

11.3.4 MEASURING THE LABELING PROBABILITY USING SPIDA

In Section 11.3.3, we showed the effect of mislabeling on the accuracy of SpIDA. Here, we wish to determine if we can recover the density and the labeling probability from single images containing labeled species of known oligomeric state (e.g., tetramers). To examine this, we generated computer-simulated images with 10 tetramers/BA with subunits randomly labeled with $p = 80\%$. It can be seen in Figure 11.7 that by using one-population SpIDA taking into account mislabeling (Equation 11.5) on simulated images with varying size, it is possible to recover the set densities (Figure 11.5a) and the set labeling probability (Figure 11.7b), even if detector noise is present (see the Materials and methods section of the Appendix). A precision of 20% can be obtained when analyzing images that have more than 100 BAs (~12 μm²). Example images in which all subunits are labeled (Figure 11.7c) and with mislabeling (Figure 11.7d) are shown, along with their intensity histograms (Figure 11.7e).

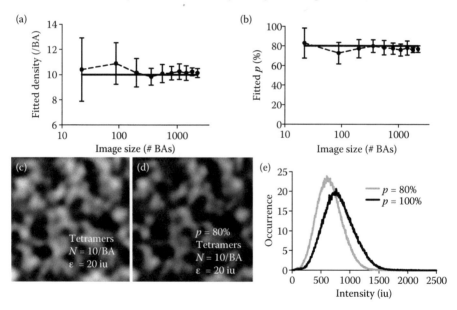

FIGURE 11.7 Measuring densities and mislabeling probability by applying SpIDA to a single oligomer population. Twenty-five simulated images containing 10 tetramers/BA were generated with varying size to measure the accuracy of one-population SpIDA in the presence of mislabeling (Equation 11.8). The set density (solid line) and SpIDA recovered densities (a) and set labeling percentage $p = 80\%$ and measured p value (b) are presented as a function of the size of the image. The error bars correspond to SDs. Example images where all subunits are labeled (c) and with mislabeling (d) with the corresponding intensity histograms (e) are shown. The monomeric quantal brightness was set to 20 iu, the e^{-2} convolution radius was set to 3 pixels, and the image size was 300 × 300 pixels.

Our results suggest that if one can prepare a sample with known fixed oligomeric states with tagged GFP (or other FPs), then the labeling constant p can be experimentally measured.

11.3.5 MEASURING THREE OLIGOMER POPULATIONS IN SINGLE IMAGES INCLUDING MISLABELING

To verify that three-population SpIDA could accurately resolve a complex distribution of monomers, dimers, and tetramers in the presence of mislabeling, we simulated images of varying size containing 10 monomers/BA, 3 dimers/BA, and 1 tetramer/BA (Figure 11.8a through c). The effect of the mislabeling can be seen in Figure 11.8a and b. These simulations show that three-population SpIDA accurately converges in the presence of mislabeling and that the precision improves as the spatial sampling of the image ROI increases (Figure 11.8c).

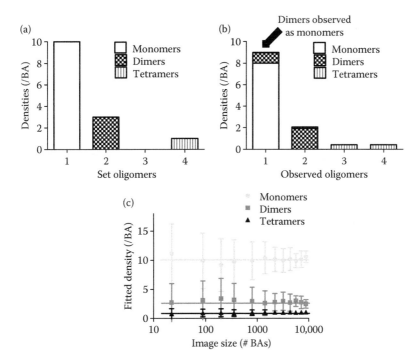

FIGURE 11.8 Effect of spatial sampling on measuring densities in images containing three population mixtures. Simulated images containing 10 monomers/BA, 3 dimers/BA, and 1 tetramer/BA were generated. The size of the images was varied to study the impact of spatial sampling on the recovered densities. The oligomer distributions when all (a) and when only $p = 80\%$ (b) of the subunits are labeled are shown. The recovered fit values for three-population SpIDA in the presence of mislabeling are presented in part (c) as a function of the image size. In the fit function, the oligomer distribution (monomers, dimers, and tetramers) and the labeling percentage was set ($p = 80\%$). The monomeric quantal brightness was set to 20 iu and the e^{-2} convolution radius was set to 3 pixels. The error bars correspond to SDs.

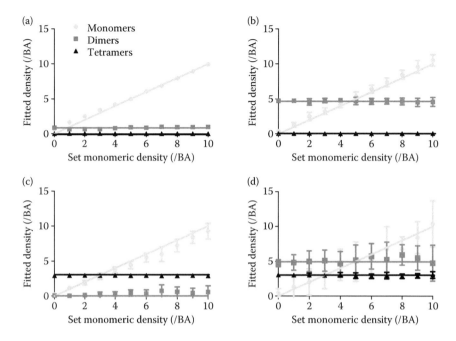

FIGURE 11.9 Three-population SpIDA analysis with subunit mislabeling ($p = 80\%$). SpIDA analysis was applied to simulated images containing three distinct populations (monomers, dimers, and tetramers) with 80% labeling of subunits. Here, the SpIDA results for many different cases where we set the density of dimers (N2) and tetramers (N4) and varied the number of monomers in the image from 0 to 10 per BA are shown. (a) N2 = 1 dimer/BA, N4 = 0 tetramer/BA; (b) N2 = 5 dimers/BA, N4 = 0 tetramer/BA; (c) N2 = 0 dimer/BA, N4 = 3 tetramers/BA; and (d) N2 = 3 dimers/BA, N4 = 1 tetramer/BA. All the data points in the graphs correspond to averages of results from 20 images. The monomeric quantal brightness was set to 20 iu, the e^{-2} convolution radius was set to 3 pixels, and the image size was 500×500 pixels. The error bars correspond to SDs.

Different densities of dimers and tetramers were generated to test the accuracy of three-population SpIDA in the presence of mislabeling (Figure 11.9a through d). The analysis was done for a range of monomer densities. Again, if only two populations are present, the three-population SpIDA model can still recover the set densities of the two populations present and reveal the absence of the third one (Figure 11.9a and b).

This demonstrates that SpIDA can resolve the densities of mixtures of three oligomer populations in the presence of mislabeling (Figure 11.9d) and that the fit parameter precision decreases for a population as a function of its decreasing density contribution.

11.4 CONCLUSION

Accurate measurement of the oligomerization states of receptors in different compartments in single cells is important to fully understand their role and molecular mechanisms in normal cellular function and disease dysfunction. To date, such measurements in intact cells have remained a challenge. SpIDA is a technique that quantitatively measures densities and oligomerization states of fluorescently tagged molecules within specific regions of cells using single images. Previous applications of SpIDA were restricted to monomer/dimer distributions, and measurements of higher oligomers were not attempted. In this chapter, we showed how mislabeling of receptor subunits will bias the results of any quantitative fluorescence approach since only emitting subunits are observed and measured. It is even more important to consider this effect when higher oligomers are present in the images. For this reason, we derived the theoretical basis for the application of three-population SpIDA in the presence of subunit mislabeling and we show how this new algorithm could be applied to both antibody-labeled protein and GFP-fusion constructs to study higher oligomerization even in the presence of mislabeling and to measure, in principle, the labeling probability if a sample of known uniform oligomerization state is measured.

ACKNOWLEDGMENTS

A.G.G. was supported by the Canadian Institutes of Health Research (CIHR) Neurophysics Training Program. A.G.G. and L.P.-T. acknowledge fellowship support from Fonds québécois de la recherche sur la nature et les technologies. L.P.-T. also acknowledges fellowship support from Natural Sciences and Engineering Research Council of Canada (NSERC). B.R. was supported by a Swiss National Science Foundation fellowship (PA00P3_131496). Y.D.K. is a Fonds de la recherche en santé du Québec Chercheur National. P.W.W. acknowledges funding support from the NSERC and the CIHR. The authors would like to also thank Prof. Paul De Koninck for the generous gift of the membrane mGFP (mGFP-f).

APPENDIX A: THEORETICAL BASIS OF SpIDA

Let $I(\mathbf{r})$ be the optical PSF (e.g., the excitation laser intensity spatial profile at focus) and ε the quantal brightness of a single fluorescent particle. The probability of observing an intensity of fluorescence k (assumed proportional to the number of photons emitted) by one particle of brightness ϵ in the focal volume is given by

$$\rho^1(\varepsilon;k) = \int \delta(\varepsilon \cdot I(\mathbf{r}) - k)\,d\mathbf{r} \qquad (11A.1)$$

δ is the Dirac delta function ($\delta(0) = 1$, and 0 otherwise). For two identical particles in the beam focus, $\rho^2(\varepsilon;k)$, which is the probability of observing an intensity of fluorescence k when exactly two particles are present in the focal volume, is the convolution of the average configuration for one particle with itself,

$$\rho^2(\varepsilon;k) = \rho^1(\varepsilon;k) \otimes \rho^1(\varepsilon;k) \qquad (11A.2)$$

and recursively for n particles in the focal volume:

$$\rho^n(\varepsilon;k) = \rho^1(\varepsilon;k) \otimes \rho^{n-1}(\varepsilon;k) \qquad (11A.3)$$

The final histogram for a single oligomeric state population of identical particles can be calculated by weighting each density configuration with its proper probability assuming a Poisson distribution of the particles in space. The fitting function becomes:

$$H(\varepsilon, N; k) = \sum_n \rho^n(\varepsilon; k) \cdot poi(n, N) \text{ with } \rho^0(\varepsilon; k) = \delta_{k,0} \qquad (11A.4)$$

The histogram H is then normalized over all the intensity values so the integral over k is unity. With the normalized functions, the two fitting parameters in Equation 11A.4 are the fluorescent particle density (N particles per PSF defined focal volume) and the particle quantal brightness (ε iu per unit of pixel integration time).

On standard CLSMs, the fluorescence intensity is measured using analog PMTs and the number of collected photoelectrons is a function of the polarization voltage. However, analog PMTs contribute additional noise to the distribution that broadens the signal variance, but this broadening can be measured and corrected for in the analysis performed on a given CLSM as shown below.

Given an input CLSM image time series, SpIDA can determine the aggregation state of the fluorescent particles in time and space. The first step is to determine the monomeric quantal brightness, ε_0, of the fluorescent label using a control experiment. We refer to a particle population with $\varepsilon = 2*\varepsilon_0$ as the dimer population (assuming no quenching). A population of true dimers can be differentiated from a population of single monomers of twice the density owing to differences in the intensity fluctuations as a function of space. Even if the mean image intensities for those two cases are equal, the histograms will differ and SpIDA will differentiate between them.

TWO-OLIGOMER-POPULATION MIXTURE

When two different particle oligomer populations are mixed within the same region in space, the total histogram simply becomes the convolution of the two individual distributions:

$$H(\varepsilon_1, N_1, \varepsilon_2, N_2, A; k) = A \cdot H(\varepsilon_1, N_1; k) \otimes H(\varepsilon_2, N_2; k) \qquad (11A.5)$$

Once the quantal brightness has been defined, Equation 11A.5, which assumes a mixture of two oligomerization states, is used to analyze the samples. If only one oligomerization state is present, the fitting routine simply yields a negligible density value for the other oligomerization state. A simplification of this model can be used if the oligomerization states present in the sample are known a priori. For example, if a sample is composed uniquely of monomers and dimers, then Equation 11A.5 can be simplified by assuming that $\varepsilon_2 = 2*\varepsilon_1$, which yields Equation 11A.6.

$$H(\varepsilon_1, N_1, N_2, N_2, A; k) = A \cdot H(\varepsilon_1, N_1; k) \otimes H(2\varepsilon_1, N_2; k) \qquad (11A.6)$$

Similarly, this model can further be simplified by using a known control sample to measure the monomeric quantal brightness.[33–35,37] In this case, Equation 11A.6 only contains two contributing density variables (N_1 and N_2).

THREE-OLIGOMER-POPULATION MIXTURE

Similar to the two-population case, if three oligomer populations are present in an image, the final histogram will be the convolution of the three individual population distributions:

$$H(\varepsilon_1, N_1, \varepsilon_2, N_2, \varepsilon_3, N_3, A;k) = A \cdot H(\varepsilon_1, N_1;k) \otimes H(\varepsilon_2, N_2;k) \otimes H(\varepsilon_3, N_3;k) \quad (11A.7)$$

In practice, Equation 11A.7, with its seven variables, does not converge readily. But here again, if the oligomeric states of the populations composing the mixture in the biological sample are known, then the model can be simplified and accurate densities can be recovered for the three populations.

MISLABELING OF SUBUNITS IN HIGHER-ORDER OLIGOMERS

When studying high-order oligomers with any biophysical fluorescence-based approach, mislabeling (i.e., when a targeted protein is not revealed by a fluorescent probe, it does not contribute emission to the total fluorescence signal) introduces a systematic error because what you observe is the fluorescent species and the true complete distribution of subunits is not represented in the integrated signal. Suppose a sample consisting of a population of oligomers, n_{mer}, and that each of the subunits in an oligomer has a probability p of being fluorescently labeled (and hence emitting). Then, the intensity distribution of a population of such an oligomer in the sample will simply be the convolution of oligomer contributions for integer increments of emitting (labeled) subunits:

$$H(n_{mer} \cdot \varepsilon_0, N, p, A; k)$$
$$= A \cdot H(\varepsilon_1^{n_{mer}}, N_1^{n_{mer}};k) \otimes \ldots \otimes H(\varepsilon_{n_{mer}-1}^{n_{mer}}, N_{n_{mer}-1}^{n_{mer}};k) \otimes H(\varepsilon_{n_{mer}}^{n_{mer}}, N_{n_{mer}}^{n_{mer}};k) \quad (11A.8)$$

where $\varepsilon_l^{n_{mer}} = l \cdot \varepsilon_0$ and $N_l^{n_{mer}} = \dfrac{n_{mer}!}{l! \cdot (n_{mer} - l)!} \cdot p^l \cdot (1-p)^{n_{mer}-l} N$.

The theoretical distribution for two- or three-oligomer-population mixtures can be obtained by convolution as for Equations 11A.5 and 11A.7, but with replacement of the one-population distribution (Equation 11A.4) by the one-population histogram with mislabeling (Equation 11A.8).

ANALOG DETECTOR CALIBRATION

As described earlier, SpIDA measures the fluorescence intensity fluctuations of the signal in the image to return information on the number of particles and their quantal brightness values. For this reason, it is important to consider only the fluctuations that originate from true signal variations of the fluorescently labeled proteins in the sample and not to include fluctuations inherent to the detector noise response. To calibrate an analog PMT detector, it is essential to empirically determine the inherent detector noise over the entire linear output range of the PMT for the microscope. To do this, one can measure the back reflection of the laser from a mirror placed at focus or by using a sample with a solution containing an extremely high concentration of fluorophores and collect the intensity from a point-scan measurement as a function of time. Using either approach, a graph of the variance of the signal versus the mean intensity is plotted. The slope of the curve of the signal versus the mean intensity can depend on many parameters (dwell time, PMT voltage, scan speed, temperature, etc.), and for each set of collection parameters, a separate calibration should be made. When performing measurements on different samples, it is, therefore, essential to maintain identical collection conditions for all samples.

Using this, the SpIDA histograms should incorporate this measured detector noise for any of the SpIDA functions (Equations 11A.4 through 11A.7). A similar calibration can be performed for a CCD camera detector by generating image time series of constant stable light source and generating a graph of the variance of each pixel as a function of the mean intensity. If the CLSM has photon counting detectors, then this calibration is not necessary.

Full details on the calibration procedures can be found in earlier publications.[20,33,35,38]

MATERIALS AND METHODS

Simulations

All of the simulated images were generated and analyzed by means of custom-written MATLAB® routines (The MathWorks Inc., Natick, MA), running on a PC, using two toolboxes (Image Processing Toolbox and Optimization Toolbox).

For single-population simulations, N particles were randomly distributed across a two-dimensional (2D) matrix. More than one particle can occupy the same matrix element and each particle contributes a value of one. Since the quantal brightness is defined as the mean number of intensity counts detected from a particle within a focal volume, each value in this integer matrix was multiplied by the product of the particle brightness, ε, and the area of a disk of radius ω_0, where ω_0 is the e^{-2} radius of the Gaussian convolution function used in the simulations. The final image matrix was obtained by convolution with a Gaussian function of user set e^{-2} radius that simulated integration with a TEM_{00} laser beam of radius ω_0 (i.e., a Gaussian intensity profile PSF in 2D).

For simulations of many mixed populations, single-population images of the same dimensions were independently generated with their corresponding densities and quantal brightness values, and then all images were convolved with the same Gaussian function. The image matrices were then summed to generate a single image matrix containing the mixed populations. To model real systems, detector shot noise was simulated by adding white noise to all simulation images presented in the manuscript; a slope for the noise of 10 iu[20,33,35,38] was arbitrarily chosen as it reflects the value we measured using our experimental setup.

Confocal Imaging

All images were obtained with an Olympus FV300-IX71 (Olympus America Inc., Melville, NY) confocal laser scanning microscope (CLSM) with a 60× plan-apochromatic Apo oil immersion objective (NA 1.4), using laser excitation with the 488 nm line of an argon ion laser and dichroic filter FV-FCBGR 488/543/633 and a BA510IF long-pass emission filter (Chroma, Rockingham, VT). For each experiment, an optimal setting of the laser power and PMT voltage was chosen to minimize pixel saturation and photobleaching. The CLSM settings were kept constant for all samples and controls (laser power, filters, dichroic mirrors, polarization voltage, scan speed) so that valid comparisons could be made between SpIDA measurements from different images taken over the course of a given experiment. Acquisition parameters were always set within the linear range of the detector, which was determined by calibration.[33,35]

Image Analysis

The ROI sizes for SpIDA analysis were carefully set by establishing an optimal trade-off between sampling different cell morphological features in the real samples (smaller ROI) and increasing the fluctuation sampling statistics (larger ROI) needed to obtain reliable results. The fitting procedure times varied from less than 1 s to 10 s depending on the model used and the bin size.

Cell Culture

COS-7 cells were maintained on untreated tissue-culture dishes (Falcon) in Dulbecco's modified Eagle's medium (DMEM) and 10% fetal bovine serum. Cells were grown at 37°C in a 5% CO_2 atmosphere, and medium was changed every third day. For passaging cells, confluent plates were washed once with phosphate-buffered saline, followed by a short trypsination with 0.05% trypsin–ethylenediaminetetraacetic acid (EDTA) (Sigma).

REFERENCES

1. Sieghart, W., K. Fuchs, V. Tretter et al. "Structure and Subunit Composition of GABA(A). Receptors." *Neurochem Int* 34, no. 5 (1999): 379–85.
2. Szidonya, L., M. Cserzo, and L. Hunyady. "Dimerization and Oligomerization of G-Protein-Coupled Receptors: Debated Structures with Established and Emerging Functions." *J Endocrinol* 196, no. 3 (2008): 435–53.
3. Comps-Agrar, L., J. Kniazeff, L. Norskov-Lauritsen et al. "The Oligomeric State Sets GABA(B) Receptor Signalling Efficacy." *EMBO J* 30, no. 12 (2011): 2336–49.
4. Galmes, R., J. L. Delaunay, M. Maurice, and T. Ait-Slimane. "Oligomerization Is Required for Normal Endocytosis/Transcytosis of a GPI-Anchored Protein in Polarized Hepatic Cells." *J Cell Sci* 126, no. Pt 15 (2013): 3409–16.
5. Conn, P. M. "Methods in Enzymology. G Protein Coupled Receptors Trafficking and Oligomerization. Preface." *Methods Enzymol* 521 (2013): xix.
6. Fatmi, M. Q., and C. E. Chang. "The Role of Oligomerization and Cooperative Regulation in Protein Function: The Case of Tryptophan Synthase." *PLoS Comput Biol* 6, no. 11 (2010): e1000994.

7. Ali, M. H., and B. Imperiali. "Protein Oligomerization: How and Why." *Bioorg Med Chem* 13, no. 17 (2005): 5013–20.

8. Bouvier, M. "Oligomerization of G-Protein-Coupled Transmitter Receptors." *Nat Rev Neurosci* 2, no. 4 (2001): 274–86.

9. Brejc, K., T. K. Sixma, P. A. Kitts et al. "Structural Basis for Dual Excitation and Photoisomerization of the Aequorea Victoria Green Fluorescent Protein." *Proc Natl Acad Sci U S A* 94, no. 6 (1997): 2306–11.

10. Day, R. N., and M. W. Davidson. "The Fluorescent Protein Palette: Tools for Cellular Imaging." *Chem Soc Rev* 38, no. 10 (2009): 2887–921.

11. Ormo, M., A. B. Cubitt, K. Kallio et al. "Crystal Structure of the Aequorea Victoria Green Fluorescent Protein." *Science* 273, no. 5280 (1996): 1392–5.

12. Zacharias, D. A., J. D. Violin, A. C. Newton, and R. Y. Tsien. "Partitioning of Lipid-Modified Monomeric GFPs into Membrane Microdomains of Live Cells." *Science* 296, no. 5569 (2002): 913–6.

13. Stephens, D. J., and V. J. Allan. "Light Microscopy Techniques for Live Cell Imaging." *Science* 300, no. 5616 (2003): 82–6.

14. Paddock, S. "Over the Rainbow: 25 Years of Confocal Imaging." *Biotechniques* 44, no. 5 (2008): 643–4, 646, 648.

15. Kim, S. A., K. G. Heinze, and P. Schwille. "Fluorescence Correlation Spectroscopy in Living Cells." *Nat Methods* 4, no. 11 (2007): 963–73.

16. Hess, S. T., S. Huang, A. A. Heikal, and W. W. Webb. "Biological and Chemical Applications of Fluorescence Correlation Spectroscopy: A Review." *Biochemistry* 41, no. 3 (2002): 697–705.

17. Lamb, D. C., A. Schenk, C. Rocker, C. Scalfi-Happ, and G. U. Nienhaus. "Sensitivity Enhancement in Fluorescence Correlation Spectroscopy of Multiple Species Using Time-Gated Detection." *Biophys J* 79, no. 2 (2000): 1129–38.

18. Chen, Y., J. D. Muller, P. T. So, and E. Gratton. "The Photon Counting Histogram in Fluorescence Fluctuation Spectroscopy." *Biophys J* 77, no. 1 (1999): 553–67.

19. Digman, M. A., P. W. Wiseman, C. Choi, A. R. Horwitz, and E. Gratton. "Stoichiometry of Molecular Complexes at Adhesions in Living Cells." *Proc Natl Acad Sci U S A* 106, no. 7 (2009): 2170–5.

20. Sergeev, M., A. G. Godin, L. Kao et al. "Determination of Membrane Protein Transporter Oligomerization in Native Tissue Using Spatial Fluorescence Intensity Fluctuation Analysis." *PLoS One* 7, no. 4 (2012): e36215.

21. Sergeev, M., S. Costantino, and P. W. Wiseman. "Measurement of Monomer-Oligomer Distributions Via Fluorescence Moment Image Analysis." *Biophys J* 91, no. 10 (2006): 3884–96.

22. Kolin, D. L., and P. W. Wiseman. "Advances in Image Correlation Spectroscopy: Measuring Number Densities, Aggregation States, and Dynamics of Fluorescently Labeled Macromolecules in Cells." *Cell Biochem Biophys* 49, no. 3 (2007): 141–64.

23. Rappaz, B., and P. W. Wiseman. "Image Correlation Spectroscopy for Measurements of Particle Densities and Colocalization." *Curr Protoc Cell Biol* Chapter 4 (2013): Unit 4.27.1–15.

24. Wiseman, P. W. "Image Correlation Spectroscopy: Mapping Correlations in Space, Time, and Reciprocal Space." *Methods Enzymol* 518 (2013): 245–67.

25. Wiseman, P. W. "Fluctuation Imaging Spiced up with a Piece of Pie." *Biophys J* 105, no. 4 (2013): 831.

26. Comeau, J. W., D. L. Kolin, and P. W. Wiseman. "Accurate Measurements of Protein Interactions in Cells Via Improved Spatial Image Cross-Correlation Spectroscopy." *Mol Biosyst* 4, no. 6 (2008): 672–85.

27. Hebert, B., S. Costantino, and P. W. Wiseman. "Spatiotemporal Image Correlation Spectroscopy (STICS) Theory, Verification, and Application to Protein Velocity Mapping in Living CHO Cells." *Biophys J* 88, no. 5 (2005): 3601–14.

28. Toplak, T., E. Pandzic, L. Chen et al. "STICCS Reveals Matrix-Dependent Adhesion Slipping and Gripping in Migrating Cells." *Biophys J* 103, no. 8 (2012): 1672–82.

29. Digman, M. A., P. W. Wiseman, A. R. Horwitz, and E. Gratton. "Detecting Protein Complexes in Living Cells from Laser Scanning Confocal Image Sequences by the Cross Correlation Raster Image Spectroscopy Method." *Biophys J* 96, no. 2 (2009): 707–16.

30. Kolin, D. L., D. Ronis, and P. W. Wiseman. "K-Space Image Correlation Spectroscopy: A Method for Accurate Transport Measurements Independent of Fluorophore Photophysics." *Biophys J* 91, no. 8 (2006): 3061–75.

31. Brandao, H. B., H. Sangji, E. Pandzic et al. "Measuring Ligand-Receptor Binding Kinetics and Dynamics Using K-Space Image Correlation Spectroscopy." *Methods* (2013).

32. Potvin-Trottier, L., L. Chen, A. R. Horwitz, and P. W. Wiseman. "A Nu-Space for Image Correlation Spectroscopy: Characterization and Application to Measure Protein Transport in Live Cells." *New J Phys* 15, no. 8 (2013): 085006.

33. Godin, A. G., S. Costantino, L. E. Lorenzo et al. "Revealing Protein Oligomerization and Densities In Situ Using Spatial Intensity Distribution Analysis." *Proc Natl Acad Sci U S A* 108, no. 17 (2011): 7010–5.

34. Swift, J. L., A. G. Godin, K. Dore et al. "Quantification of Receptor Tyrosine Kinase Transactivation through Direct Dimerization and Surface Density Measurements in Single Cells." *Proc Natl Acad Sci U S A* 108, no. 17 (2011): 7016–21.

35. Barbeau, A., A. G. Godin, J. L. Swift et al. "Quantification of Receptor Tyrosine Kinase Activation and Transactivation by G-Protein-Coupled Receptors Using Spatial Intensity Distribution Analysis (SpIDA)." *Methods Enzymol* 522 (2013): 109–31.

36. Barbeau, A., J. L. Swift, A. G. Godin et al. "Spatial Intensity Distribution Analysis (SpIDA): A New Tool for Receptor Tyrosine Kinase Activation and Transactivation Quantification." *Methods Cell Biol* 117 (2013): 1–19.

37. Doyon, N., S. A. Prescott, A. Castonguay et al. "Efficacy of Synaptic Inhibition Depends on Multiple, Dynamically Interacting Mechanisms Implicated in Chloride Homeostasis." *PLoS Comput Biol* 7, no. 9 (2011): e1002149.

38. Sergeev, M., J. L. Swift, A. G. Godin, and P. W. Wiseman. "Ligand-Induced Clustering of EGF Receptors: A Quantitative Study by Fluorescence Image Moment Analysis." *Biophys Chem* 161 (2012): 50–3.

39. Ulbrich, M. H., and E. Y. Isacoff. "Subunit Counting in Membrane-Bound Proteins." *Nat Methods* 4, no. 4 (2007): 319–21.

40. Durisic, N., A. G. Godin, C. M. Wever et al. "Stoichiometry of the Human Glycine Receptor Revealed by Direct Subunit Counting." *J Neurosci* 32, no. 37 (2012): 12915–20.

41. Rosenmund, C., Y. Stern-Bach, and C. F. Stevens. "The Tetrameric Structure of a Glutamate Receptor Channel." *Science* 280, no. 5369 (1998): 1596–9.

42. Tichelaar, W., M. Safferling, K. Keinanen, H. Stark, and D. R. Madden. "The Three-Dimensional Structure of an Ionotropic Glutamate Receptor Reveals a Dimer-of-Dimers Assembly." *J Mol Biol* 344, no. 2 (2004): 435–42.

12 Live-Cell TIRF Imaging of Molecular Assembly and Plasma Membrane Topography

Adam D. Hoppe and Shalini T. Low-Nam

CONTENTS

12.1 INTRODUCTION

Signaling by transmembrane receptors involves the coordinated assembly of macromolecular complexes under constraints imposed by the organization of the plasma membrane (PM). Signaling by receptor tyrosine kinases (RTKs) such as the epidermal growth factor receptor (EGFR or erbB1) or macrophage colony-stimulating factor receptor (MCSFR) requires rearrangements on the PM including receptor dimerization, phosphorylation, signaling complex assembly, and endocytosis (Figure 12.1).[1,2] While the protein–protein interactions of RTK signal transduction have been extensively studied, the contributions of the PM in controlling the diffusion and local concentrations of signaling components and therefore the dynamics of assembly and signal amplitudes remain poorly defined. Specifically, how do the chemical potentials that modulate the lateral diffusion in the PM influence receptor assembly?

261

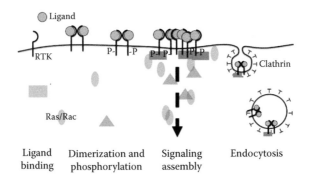

| Ligand binding | Dimerization and phosphorylation | Signaling assembly | Endocytosis |

FIGURE 12.1 Molecular rearrangements of RTK signaling at the PM. From left to right: monomeric receptors on the cell surface bind cognate ligands leading to the formation of dimers or oligomeric clusters. In these complexes, receptors undergo phosphorylation, providing docking sites that are recognized by specific domains (i.e., SH3 domains) within adaptor proteins leading to the formation of signaling complexes. Receptors and some associated signaling molecules are removed from the cell surface by endocytosis to attenuate signaling.

How do topographical features such as endocytic pits and membrane ruffles accelerate or slow these reactions? Addressing these questions requires methods capable of measuring the interplay between the formation of signaling assemblies and the dynamic organization of the PM.

Here, we describe the combination of minimally invasive, high-speed spectroscopic methods with total internal reflection fluorescence (TIRF) imaging, that can access these dynamics. Specifically, we describe how fluorescence resonance energy transfer (FRET) can be extended to image multiple fluorophores in TIRF–FRET mode and thereby capture the dynamics of molecular assembly on the surfaces of cells. Furthermore, we discuss advances in polarized TIRF (pol-TIRF) that enable imaging of the subresolution membrane topography associated with endocytic and exocytic sites on the PMs of living cells. Specific examples include imaging the activation of the cell shape-regulating proteins Rac1 and Cdc42 at the PM and the topographical changes of the PM relative to the recruitment of clathrin during endocytosis. These examples set the stage for imaging nanodomains on the PM that govern cellular signaling.

Diffusion within the PM determines the speed of the imaging approaches required to capture signaling dynamics. For most transmembrane proteins and lipids, the diffusion coefficient in the PM is ~0.1–1 $\mu m^2/s$, which is approximately two to three orders of magnitude slower than protein diffusion in the cytosol.[3-6] Thus, lateral diffusion over the expected 10–1000 nm length scale limits the rate of signaling complex assembly to the millisecond-to-second timescale. Furthermore, the recruitment of proteins from the cytosol to the PM requires a similar amount of time since the large volume of the cytosol offsets the larger cytosolic diffusion rates.[4] In the case of the MCSFR, the steps illustrated in Figure 12.1 occur over approximately 3 min. Therefore, subsecond temporal resolution for durations of 5–10 min are required to capture receptor exploration of the PM and the evolution of interactions with binding partners after ligation.

Domains that organize the PM influence the lateral distributions and diffusional transport of lipids and proteins over length scales ranging from tens to hundreds of nanometers.[7] Three well-established domain types include cytoskeletal corrals, lipid rafts, and clusters of transmembrane proteins (Figure 12.2a). While these domains have been observed by a variety of methods, much of what we know about their sizes comes from optical imaging methods on intact cells. In particular, cytoskeletal corrals are frequently observed by single-particle tracking (SPT) as the confinement of molecules within actin-dependent domains that are 100–300 nm across.[5,8–10] Lipid rafts have been defined by biochemical methods as a strong copartitioning of sphingolipids and cholesterol. Their direct observation by live-cell microscopy remains controversial.[11,12] Estimates for their size range from 50 to 200 nm[13] with nanoscopy methods suggesting that they are as small as 5–10 nm and lasting only for ~10 ms.[14] Clustering of transmembrane proteins by direct binding interactions is commonly observed by biochemical methods; however, the size and lifetimes of these assemblies range widely (10–2000 nm, milliseconds to hours). Examples of these domains include the T-cell receptors at the immune synapses that can span micrometers and last for hours and RTKs that assemble quickly into small patches (in nanometers, milliseconds).[9,15–17] It is likely that all three of these domains contribute to organization of the PM and may exert concerted effects on receptor signaling. Given their sizes, observation of these nanoscale domains and their impact on signaling by optical microscopy requires new approaches capable of accessing information below the diffraction limit.

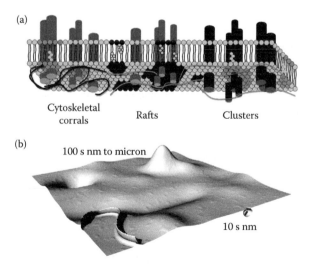

FIGURE 12.2 The lateral and topographical domains of the PM. (a) Three models for lateral membrane organization. Cytoskeletal corrals are defined by actin cytoskeletal fibers proximate to the inner leaflet that create barriers to diffusion. Lipid rafts are distinguished as cholesterol-rich, detergent-resistant membranes. Clustering of transmembrane proteins can create nanodomains. Defining features of each domain are dark gray. (b) The PM has extensive topographic features, including small regions of curvature on the scale of tens of nanometers (the example of an endocytic pit shown) to larger features up to microns in diameter (such as a cellular ruffle).

Rather than a planar sea of lipids, the cell surface is composed of dynamic peaks, pits, and valleys ranging in size from 10 to 1000 nm (Figure 12.2b). These structures may modulate receptor signaling by the recruitment of proteins that recognize membrane curvature, sorting of lipids and proteins on curved membranes, and altering the exchange of molecules between the cytoplasm and the PM.[18,19] A prominent example of a topographical nanodomain is the clathrin-coated pit and the formation of vesicles by clathrin-mediated endocytosis (CME; Figures 12.1 and 12.2b). Here, the topography of the pit itself may recruit proteins such as BAR (Bin–Amphiphysin–Rvs) domain-containing proteins and the GTPase dynamin.[20,21] Similar mechanisms of curvature recognition may influence RTK signaling.

Topographical features of the PM create diffusion barriers that may suppress or amplify signaling reactions. For example, micrometer-sized circular ruffles, which are precursors of macropinosomes, can create a diffusional barrier that confines proteins within the forming macropinocytic cup, thereby promoting interactions that amplify signaling biochemistries.[22] Such large-scale topographic features of the PM are largely driven by the dynamics in the underlying actin cytoskeleton. Thus actin-rich protrusions may concentrate membrane-associated molecules relative to the cytoplasm and thereby create a local environment for the amplification of membrane-proximal signaling.[19] Furthermore, actin-driven topographical dynamics can modulate the binding of Fcγ-receptor interactions with antibody-coated particles,[23,24] providing another mechanism by which the PM topography modulates receptor function during phagocytosis.

Fluorescence imaging provides a powerful tool for accessing the dynamic organization of the PM and biochemical signaling at the surfaces of living cells. While super-resolution approaches such as photoactivated localization microscopy (PALM) and stochastic optical reconstruction microscopy (STORM) have the ability to see at this length scale,[25,26] they lack the temporal resolution and multispectral capabilities to capture the live-cell dynamics of lipids and proteins in the PM. Here, we focus our discussion to spectroscopic imaging approaches in combination with TIRF illumination to enable multiprobe, high-speed selective imaging of the PM. Specifically, we discuss how the exponentially decaying TIRF excitation field can be combined with FRET (TIRF–FRET) to detect protein–protein interactions and clustering as well as pol-TIRF imaging of a PM-associated carbocyanine dye molecule, DiI, to image the dynamics of membrane topography. Unlike some of the super-resolution approaches, these techniques permit high-speed (tens of milliseconds) imaging over long durations (minutes) and low phototoxicity.

12.2 SELECTIVE IMAGING OF THE PM OF LIVING CELLS BY TIRF MICROSCOPY

Over the last two decades, TIRF microscopy has emerged as a preferred illumination strategy for selectively imaging fluorescent molecules on the surfaces of living cells. TIRF has seen application in a wide range of cell biology studies including single molecule movement on the surfaces of cells,[8,27] molecular reorganization at simulated cell–cell contacts,[28,29] fusion and fission of exocytic and endocytic vesicles,[30–34] signal transduction, and viral assembly.[35] The growth in popularity of TIRF is the result of numerous technical advances[36–38] including through-the-objective lens TIRF (TTO-TIRF), made possible by lenses with numerical apertures (NAs) greater than 1.45 and multilaser illumination strategies. Devising new strategies for implementing spectroscopic methods such as FRET and pol-TIRF will enable visualization of PM nanodomain dynamics and, ultimately, novel mechanistic insights into membrane organization during signal transduction.

TIRF microscopy allows for selective and minimally invasive live-cell imaging by creating a shallow illumination field at the interface between a high-refractive index glass coverslip and the lower refractive index of the cytoplasm and surrounding media (Figure 12.3a). At the point of reflection, an evanescent wave is created that propagates with an exponentially decaying intensity into the low-refractive index media,

$$I(z) = e^{-z/d}, \tag{12.1}$$

where z is the distance above the coverslip and d is the incidence angle-dependent characteristic penetration depth of the evanescent wave and can be calculated as

$$d = \frac{\lambda}{4\pi} \sqrt{\eta_g^2 \sin^2 \theta - \eta_c^2} \tag{12.2}$$

given the refractive index of the glass (η_g) and cell (η_c), the wavelength of light λ, and the angle between the incident light and the surface normal of the interface (θ). For total internal reflection to occur, θ must be greater than the critical angle (θ_C or the angle at which refraction stops and reflection begins),

$$\theta_C = \sin^{-1} \frac{\eta_1}{\eta_2}. \tag{12.3}$$

In a typical TIRF microscope, the critical angle for cells sitting on a glass coverslip, $\theta_C \sim 68°$, and the penetration depth for a 500 nm laser and incident angle of 75° produce a TIRF field with $d \sim 176$ nm.[39] The lateral resolution will be diffraction-limited corresponding to roughly 1/2 the wavelength or ~250 nm. Thus, TIRF affords approximately fivefold improvement in the z-axis resolution over confocal microscopy and orders of magnitude improvement in z-axis selectivity over wide-field microscopy.[40]

While multiple configurations for TIRF are possible, TTO-TIRF provides a convenient approach for live-cell analysis.[41] TTO-TIRF illumination works by focusing a laser onto the objective's back focal plane (BFP) to create a collimated light beam. Focusing a laser onto the outer edge of the BFP of a high NA (>1.45) will produce a collimated beam that contacts the coverglass–cell interface at an angle greater than the critical angle, thereby producing a TIRF illumination field (Figure 12.3a, 1-point TIRF). These lenses are often designed with correction collars that allow for compensation in changes of index of refraction of the immersion oil when imaging live cells at physiological temperatures. While TTO-TIRF greatly simplifies

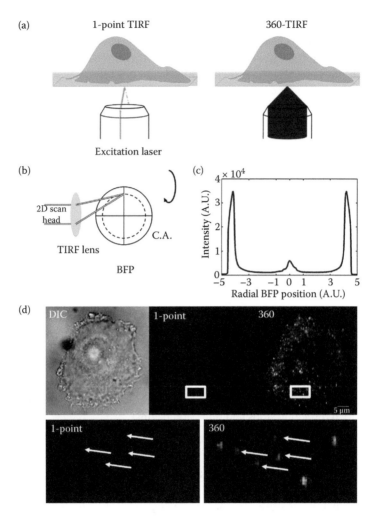

FIGURE 12.3 360-TIRF illumination improves detection of localized protein recruitment. (a) Schematic representation of illumination strategies for TIRF. In 1-point TIRF, laser excitation is introduced at a single position in the BFP of a high-NA lens. In contrast, in 360-TIRF, laser light is rotated around the BFP, creating a cone of illumination. (b) Schematic of the light path for 360-TIRF. A 2D scan head directs laser light through a motorized TIRF lens for focusing onto positions in the BFP with millisecond movement times. (c) Centering the excitation light is accomplished by measuring the intensity of light reflected at the coverglass–cell interface onto a quadrant diode. Intensity (in artificial units, A.U.) is plotted as a function of the radial position in the BFP (measured in units of the galvanometric mirror positions). We define center as the point when intensities at full-width half-maximum are matched at the positive and negative radial positions. (d) A cell expressing dynamin-GFP visualized using DIC, 1-point TIRF, and 360-TIRF. The 360-TIRF images show improved detail of protein clustering; full-field and zoomed-in regions with arrows indicating individual protein clusters (bottom row).

live-cell TIRF imaging, it also carries the disadvantage of creating a laterally non-uniform illumination field owing to imperfections in the microscope optics, such as the flatness of the dichroic reflector. The resulting coherence fringing is variable across samples and dependent on both the illumination wavelength and the angle of incidence (Figure 12.4b and c). Coherence fringing degrades the fidelity of the

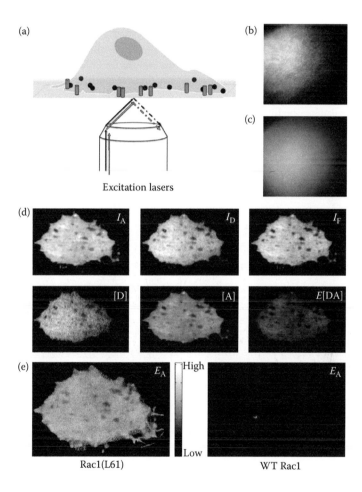

FIGURE 12.4 TIRF–FRET imaging of Rac1 activity at the PM. (a) Schematic of TIRF–FRET experiment. Two excitation lasers are used to excite the donor and acceptor FP fusions (where CFP-PBD is shown as black circles and YFP-Rac1 is shown as gray cylinders). Note that excitation is diagrammed here using 1-point TIRF for simplicity. Interference fringes are suppressed using the 360-TIRF illumination strategy. Images of a coverslip uniformly coated with YFP illustrate the strong coherence fringing observed with 1-point TIRF (b) and its suppression by 360-TIRF (c) illumination. (d) Cells expressing GTP-bound YFP-Rac1(L61) and CFP-PBD were imaged by TIRF–FRET, and the raw data (I_A, I_D, I_F) were unmixed to give the total donor and acceptor images ([D] and [A]) as well as the apparent FRET interaction (E[DA]). (e) Apparent FRET efficiency images (E_A) showed strong and uniform FRET for Rac1(L61) but not for wild-type Rac1.

TIRF image and precludes spectroscopic methods, such as FRET, that require a linear correspondence between different illumination wavelengths or polarization.[39] Coherence fringing can be overcome by rotating the illumination beam about the objective's optical axis.[42–44]

We have shown recently that a two-dimensional (2D) scan head can both reduce coherence fringing (Figure 12.4b and c) and allow combined TIRF–FRET microscopy with TTO illumination.[39] The galvanometric mirrors of the scan head focus excitation light through the TIRF lens to distinct positions in the BFP of the objective lens (Figure 12.3b). Rapid steering of the illumination beam around the BFP (within milliseconds) creates a cone of incident illumination (360-TIRF) that averages out heterogeneities introduced at discrete BFP positions (Figures 12.3a and b and 12.4b and c). For this strategy to be fully realized, the beam must be centered on the optical axis. By measuring the light reflected at the glass–cell interface on a separate detector (quadrant diode, explained in Ref. 39), a centering plot is used to calibrate the positions of the galvos in order to ensure symmetry in sampling the BFP (Figure 12.3c). When applied to cells expressing a fluorescent protein (FP)-tagged biomolecule, 360-TIRF enhances detection of protein clusters and produces images with signal-to-noise ratios several times higher than seen using 1-point illumination (Figure 12.3d). This increased sensitivity is essential for imaging the remodeling of signaling complexes.

12.3   TIRF–FRET IMAGING OF MOLECULAR INTERACTIONS

FRET microscopy is a powerful tool capable of imaging molecular interactions via a spectroscopic signature. Specifically, this signature can be observed as a decrease in the fluorescence from a higher-energy (bluer, shorter-wavelength) donor fluorophore and a corresponding increase in fluorescence from a lower-energy (redder, longer-wavelength) acceptor fluorophore. Given that FRET is mediated by a dipole–dipole coupling, the FRET efficiency scales as $1/r^6$ with a distance of 50% energy transfer corresponding to the Förster distance of approximately 5 nm (reviewed in Ref. 45). These stringent distance requirements make FRET sensitive to the appropriate length scale for measurement of molecular binding and clustering events. By appropriately calibrating the microscope, FRET can be used to measure the fractions of interacting molecules,[46,47] thereby providing a quantitative map of molecular interactions and conformations.[48–50]

FPs are potent tools for FRET analysis of protein–protein binding events. The genes encoding FPs can be fused with genes of interest and expressed as chimeric proteins. This approach affords exquisite specificity in molecular tagging and is the most efficient approach to date for labeling molecules inside living cells. FRET can be used to image the dynamics of molecular interactions when both molecules are tagged with appropriate donor–acceptor FP pairs. A useful demonstration is monitoring the activation of small GTPases such as Rac1 via FRET between YFP-Rac1 (acceptor) and its activation-dependent binding to donor-tagged effector domain (Figure 12.5a).[50,51] Likewise, FRET of FP-tagged molecules has enabled analysis of EGFR clustering and recruitment of downstream signaling molecules such as Grb2 and Cbl after addition of EGF.[52,53] These and numerous other examples in the literature indicate the tremendous potential of FP-based FRET for revealing the dynamics of molecular assembly inside living cells.

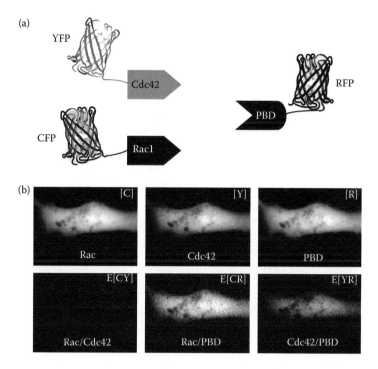

FIGURE 12.5 Simultaneous quantification of Rac and Cdc42 activation by N-Way FRET. (a) Schematic representation of FP-tagged GTPases and binding domain (PBD). GTP-bound YFP-Cdc42(V12) and CFP-Rac1(V12) can interact with RFP-PBD with comparable affinity. (b) N-Way FRET results showing the distributions of total fluorophores ([C], [Y], [R] and their apparent FRET interactions (E[CY], E[CR], E[YR]) indicate where Cdc42 and Rac1 are in complex with PBD, but not with one another.

Despite these successes, FRET microscopy has yet to see wide application in protein interactions. We can identify four main challenges that must be overcome for FRET to reach its full potential in analyzing the nanoscale organization of the PM: (1) simultaneous quantification of multiple protein interactions within the same sample, (2) detection of FRET between large full-length proteins, (3) selective imaging of the PM, and (4) imaging molecules at their native concentrations and under endogenous regulation. We describe strategies for overcoming these limitations below.

12.3.1 N-Way FRET of Multiple Interacting Proteins

Most FRET approaches can only image one pair of interacting molecules, thereby limiting their application to heterogeneous, multimeric assemblies within domains of the PM. Recently, we and others developed FRET methods for the analysis of multifluorophore data capable of measuring multiple molecular interactions.[54-56] Building on the work of Neher and colleagues,[57] we developed an improved mathematical description for correcting spectral overlap of donors and acceptors while correctly modeling the spectral signature of FRET. This led to a definition for the excitation–emission (e.g., FRET and non-FRET) couplings between any numbers of fluorophores in the system. The resulting N-Way FRET analysis[56] can be summarized as the linear mixing problem in which

$$d = Bc, \tag{12.4}$$

where d is a vector containing the data (e.g., FRET images), B is a matrix with columns containing intrafluorophore and interfluorophore excitation–emission couplings, and c is a vector that contains the relative concentrations of fluorophores and complexes scaled by their FRET efficiencies (E) (e.g., [FP1], [FP2]... $E_{1\to2}$[FP1–FP2]). Calibration of a microscope for N-Way FRET requires free FPs and FP–FP constructs that have known FRET efficiencies.[56] Once B has been defined for a set of possible interacting fluorophores, cellular images can be analyzed by computing the inverse of B to yield fluorophore concentrations and apparent FRET complexes as

$$c = B^{-1}d \tag{12.5}$$

Furthermore, the error in the measurement of c can be estimated from the uncertainty in the data (d) and expressed as a matrix Σ^d,

$$\Sigma^c = B\Sigma^d B'. \tag{12.6}$$

A simple form for the uncertainty Σ^d can be obtained by estimating the shot noise associated with detecting a limited number of photons in d.[56] Taken together, N-Way FRET provides a rigorous approach for accounting for FRET between multiple fluorophores and analysis of their error.

With N-Way FRET, it should be possible to view molecular assemblies involving multiple molecules such as the proof-of-concept experiment in which N-Way FRET was able to measure the assembly HIV viral-like particles as the association of blue, yellow, and red FP-GAG on the PMs of living cells.[56] Additionally N-Way FRET can simultaneously monitor Cdc42 and Rac1 activity in a single living cell (Figure 12.5). In this example, FRET is observed between a single effector domain, p21-binding-domain of PAK1 (PBD) and GTP-bound Cdc42 and Rac1 with similar affinity (Figure 12.5). Extension of these methods to other small GTPases that share effector domains, or by 4-Way FRET should enable simultaneous imaging of the multiple small GTPases such as Ras and Rac activation downstream of growth factor receptors in a living cell.

12.3.2 Detection of FRET between Large Full-Length Proteins

While FRET has seen much success with small proteins such as the Ras-related GTPases, it has seen limited application for lager proteins. Extension of N-Way FRET to larger proteins will require new strategies such as the hi-FRET approach that uses weak interaction domains and long tethers to bring donor and acceptor fluorophores together despite large separations in their attachment points to larger proteins.[58] Hi-FRET greatly improved the FRET signal between full-length Raf and Ras, whereas previous approaches were limited to detection of FRET between Ras and a small portion of Raf that contains the Ras binding domain.[58] Approaches such as hi-FRET should make FRET analysis of large proteins more feasible. Caution will be needed for the analysis of membrane-bound proteins, as small affinities can have significant impact on interactions at the PM.[59]

12.3.3   TIRF–FRET MICROSCOPY OF THE PM

While FRET is sensitive to nanoscale molecular rearrangements, its imaging resolution is defined by the diffraction limit. This means that FRET signals will be averaged over the volume of the microscope's point spread function (PSF). Given the large extent of widefield and confocal PSFs along the z-axis, extensive averaging with light from adjacent molecules also degrades the FRET signal.[60] This spatial averaging limits both the sensitivity and local accuracy of FRET microscopy. While spatial averaging can be significantly reversed by deconvolution or use of confocal microscopes,[60] optimal FRET imaging of PM nanodomains requires that we reduce the detection volumes and minimize spatial averaging with signals emanating from the cytoplasm. Recently, we have demonstrated that quantitative FRET imaging can be achieved during TIRF illumination.[39] This TIRF–FRET method requires reproducible and linear calibration of both the donor and acceptor excitation. Unlike widefield illumination, where this criterion is easily met with illumination corrections,[61] the coherence fringing encountered in TIRF creates heterogeneities across the excitation field that are difficult (or impossible) to reproduce and is dependent upon the wavelength of excitation (Ref. 39 and Figure 12.4b and c). Furthermore, the penetration depth also depends on the wavelength (Equation 12.2), indicating that both lateral homogeneity and matching penetration depths for multiple excitation wavelengths are needed for TIRF–FRET imaging to be realized.[62] These criteria could both be met by implementing 360-TIRF illumination to overcome coherence fringing (Figures 12.3a and 12.4c) and allow adjustment of the penetration depth by changing the incidence angle between donor and acceptor illuminations. The resulting method allows diffraction-limited TIRF–FRET imaging at frame rates of 10 Hz or faster.[39] An example of TIRF–FRET applied to imaging activated Rac1 at the PM via the interaction of YFP-PBD and CFP-Rac1(V12) is shown (Figure 12.4). The activated Rac1(V12), as expected, shows a highly uniform distribution on the PM and uniform FRET, consistent with its deregulated activity across the cell surface.[63]

Although it remains to be realized, N-Way FRET and TIRF–FRET can be combined to enable highly selective imaging of multifluorophore assemblies on the PMs of living cells. This combination should provide a potent tool for capturing assembly of proteins on the surface of living cells through the use of FP and lipid fluorophore tags.

12.3.4   GENOME EDITING FOR FRET ANALYSIS OF
ENDOGENOUSLY EXPRESSED FPS

A critical effort in the application of TIRF–FRET to analyzing dynamic molecular interactions at the PM is the careful treatment of the reduction in dimensionality effect. In other words, as molecules assemble on the PM, their effective concentration increases, which may allow for weak affinity interactions that would not be observed for molecules that are diluted within the three-dimensional volume of the cytosol. Examples of this effect in action include "FRET by crowding," in which overexpressed donor- and acceptor-tagged pleckstrin homology domains are recruited to the PM via binding to phosphorylated phospholipids and are brought close enough together to give FRET.[64–66] While these data indicate that FRET by crowding can measure the increase in concentration owing to localization at the PM, they also highlight the need to carefully control the expression levels of molecules used in the analysis of PM-associated proteins.

Recent advances in genome editing strategies such as CRISPR, TALEN, and Zinc Finger Nuclease (ZFN) systems represent an attractive possibility for regulated expression of FP fusions.[67–69] These approaches allow insertion of FP coding regions into the chromosomal locus for the protein of interest and thereby maintain native regulation of expression. Indeed, recent work using ZFNs to label the endogenous clathrin and dynamin proteins illustrates the importance of regulated expression of the FP fusions for proper function of the CME machinery.[34] Of these, the CRISPR system provides the most cost-effective and simple approach for inserting FPs and should facilitate FP-imaging studies. Specifically, CRISPR uses single-stranded RNA to guide the Cas9 DNA nuclease to a targeted site to mediate double-stranded breaks and homologous recombination with exogenous DNA constructs (such as an FP gene).[70,71] Regardless of approach, the editing of multiple genes with FP fusions has been achieved,[34] indicating that FRET analysis of endogenously tagged proteins is imminent.

12.4   pol-TIRF IMAGING OF MEMBRANE CURVATURE LEADING TO NANODOMAIN ORGANIZATION

Advances in pol-TIRF imaging have set the stage for analyzing the interplay of signaling and PM topography in living cells. Membrane topographies such as ruffles, filopodia, and sites of endocytosis and exocytosis are key topographical features that modulate receptor signaling at the PM.[19,72] The work of Axelrod, Holz, and Anantharam has shown that the dynamic changes in membrane topography associated with actin remodeling and exocytosis can be imaged by pol-TIRF using the carbocyanine dye, C-18 DiI. Specifically, the acyl chains of DiI insert into the bilayer such that its bridging double bonds and dipole moment lie parallel to the PM (Figure 12.6a).[73,74] The orientation of DiI follows the contours of the PM. DiI is preferentially excited by light with polarization matching the orientation of DiI's dipole. Thus, membrane curvature is visualized by pol-TIRF fields that are perpendicular (p-pol) or parallel (s-pol) to the PM[33] (Figure 12.6b). We have taken advantage of our scan head illumination system to create p-pol and s-pol TIRF fields by focusing laser excitation at orthogonal positions in the objective's BFP (Figure 12.6a). This strategy enables millisecond resolution of PM curvature and reduced coherence fringing by averaging across the two possible excitation directions for p-pol and s-pol. Physical theory and experiments demonstrate that membrane topography is described by the ratio of the p-pol image over the s-pol image (Figure 12.6c).[33,73]

Pol-TIRF has been used to image dynamic changes in membrane topography associated with exocytosis of secretory granules in chromaffin cells.[33,75–77] This

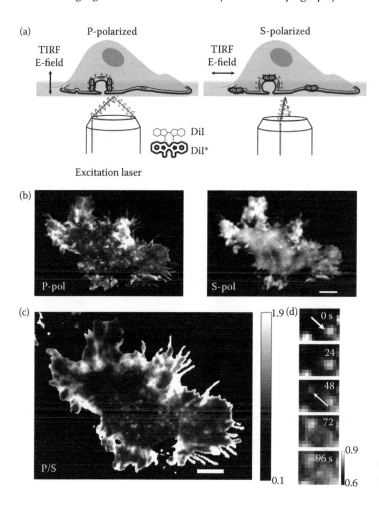

FIGURE 12.6 Pol-TIRF imaging of membrane curvature dynamics. (a) Schematics of TIRF illumination using p-polarized (p-pol) and s-polarized (s-pol) laser excitation, respectively. Lipophilic DiI molecules orient within the membrane, allowing the vertical and horizontal membrane (denoted by DiI*) to be discriminated using p-pol and s-pol excitation, respectively. (b) Individual frames of a single DiI-labeled cell visualized using p-pol and s-pol excitation, respectively. (c) The ratio of p-pol to s-pol images (P/S) indicates regions of high curvature (edge of the cell, small punctate structures). (d) Dynamics within a small region of the membrane visualized over time. Notice the disappearance of a curved feature (thick white arrow) and appearance of another curved feature (thin white arrow). Greyscale bars indicate the P/S range; the scale bar represents 5 μm.

work addressed models for vesicle fusion with the PM including full collapse, partial flattening, or recycling through endocytosis.[33] Their results demonstrated that rapid endocytosis of fusing membrane was a minor component and led to the surprising discovery that the GTPase dynamin and its GTPase activity were required for opening of the fusion pore.[77] This work demonstrated the tremendous potential of

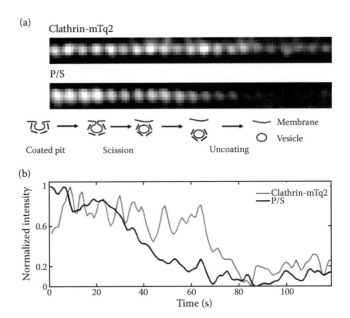

FIGURE 12.7 Combined pol-TIRF and 360-TIRF imaging of membrane curvature at sites of CME. (a) 360-TIRF (Clathrin-Tq2) and pol-TIRF (P/S) images of the curvature and clathrin uncoating of an endocytic vesicle in 293-T cells expressing CLTA-mTq2 and labeled with DiI. Below the data acquired over 120 s is a cartoon interpretation of the stages of CME captured in these data. (b) The normalized intensities of the CLTA-mTq2 and DiI signatures from the event in part (a).

pol-TIRF for discerning the mechanisms of exocytosis and provided a new avenue for analyzing receptor signaling and PM topography.

Recently, we have combined pol-TIRF and 360-TIRF for improved imaging of subresolution membrane topography and molecular recruitment. An example of this approach is imaging the final stages of CME where changes in membrane topography were imaged by pol-TIRF and clathrin uncoating by 360-TIRF (Figure 12.7a). This illustrates the ability of pol-TIRF to capture membrane curvature associated with CME vesicles (diameter, ~100 nm) that are much smaller than the previously measured exocytic granules (diameter, ~300 nm). SPT of these subresolution structures combined with nanometer accuracy image registration should allow precise characterization of multiple subresolution events.[9,78] This example demonstrates how pol-TIRF can be used to correlate membrane topography and CME machinery within PM nanodomains (Figure 12.7b) previously only accessible by electron microscopy.

12.5   OUTLOOK FOR IMAGING THE ROLE OF PM NANODOMAINS IN CONTROLLING SIGNALING

The integration of live-cell TIRF microscopy with spectroscopic imaging of protein interactions and membrane curvature opens new avenues for understanding how PM nanodomains shape receptor signaling. TIRF–FRET and pol-TIRF provide dynamic views of molecular assembly and membrane topography that together should be capable of capturing the dynamics and spatial organization of single signaling complexes relative to the PM structure. Furthermore, by expanding the number of interactions probed, N-Way TIRF–FRET should enable measurement of the order of assembly of receptor signaling complexes. While the combination of these approaches has yet to be realized, it holds the potential to capture receptor interactions, docking of signaling proteins, and membrane topography simultaneously.

A major challenge that remains for determining how receptor signaling is influenced by PM domains is connecting signaling biochemistry with membrane architecture. Meeting this challenge will require multiplexing of imaging modalities with appropriate resolution and specificity. Table 12.1 provides principal characteristics of imaging modalities commonly applied to mechanisms of protein–membrane interplay. While most techniques are amenable to live-cell imaging, the achievable resolutions and accessible cellular features vary widely. The combination of

---

TABLE 12.1

Imaging-Based Approaches to Quantifying Features of Protein–Membrane Interactions and Cell Signaling

Technique	Live Cell	Spatial Resolution	Temporal Resolution	Features Accessible
FRAP	✓	~500 nm	Milliseconds	Cytoplasmic or membrane diffusion
N-Way FRET	✓	~1 nm (molecular) ~250 nm (cellular)	Milliseconds	Protein–protein interactions Aggregation state
SPT	✓	~10–100 nm	Milliseconds	Diffusion rates; modes of motion Trajectories of movements
FCS	✓	~250 nm	Milliseconds	Diffusion rates Concentration of proteins
Localization super-resolution	✓	~10–70 nm	Milliseconds	Diffusion rates Aggregation states and protein distributions
360-TIRF	✓	~250 nm (x-y) ~50–100 nm (z)	Milliseconds	Protein clustering Distributions within the illumination volume
pTIRF	✓	~250 nm (x-y) ~50–100 nm (z)	Milliseconds	Membrane topography
EM	✓	~0.5 nm	Minutes	Ultrastructure Distributions of molecules in fixed, embedded samples
AFM	✓	~0.3–1 nm	Minutes	Membrane topography Protein aggregation
NSOM	✓	10–100 nm	Milliseconds	Membrane topography Protein aggregation

TIRF–FRET and pol-TIRF may provide details of assembly mechanisms governing signaling complexes within curved regions of the membrane while distinguishing nanodomains from endocytic invaginations. Super-resolution approaches such as PALM and STORM are easily adaptable to TIRF imaging and may enhance imaging of cellular biochemistry in fixed cells. Techniques such as SPT and AFM may also provide optimal resolution of diffusional constraints and cellular topography but will be challenging or impossible to combine with TIRF. Nonetheless, optimization of these approaches and implementation alongside TIRF illumination will continue to refine our understanding of PM nanodomains and their role in regulating signaling. This work, in turn, should lead to new mechanistic understanding of receptor signaling at the PM.

ACKNOWLEDGMENTS

We thank Brandon Scott for helping with the FRET figures and discussion and Jason Kerkvliet, M.S., for preparation of 293-T cells. Geoffrey Graff, NCAARB, LEED AP, prepared the membrane model in Figure 12.2b. We appreciate the contributions of all members of the Hoppe laboratory for suggestions to improve the text. This material is based on work supported by the National Science Foundation under Grant No. 0953561, the South Dakota Governor's 2010 Center for the Biological Control and Analysis by Applied Photonics (BCAAP) and South Dakota State University Chemistry and Biochemistry startup funds to ADH, and the National Institutes of Health Ruth L. Kirschstein National Research Service Award (1F32GM105277) to SL-N.

REFERENCES

1. Pixley, F. J., and E. R. Stanley. "CSF-1 Regulation of the Wandering Macrophage: Complexity in Action." *Trends Cell Biol* 14, no. 11 (2004): 628–38.
2. Schlessinger, J. "Ligand-Induced, Receptor-Mediated Dimerization and Activation of EGF Receptor." *Cell* 110, no. 6 (2002): 669–72.
3. Cherry, R. J. "Rotational and Lateral Diffusion of Membrane Proteins." *Biochim Biophys Acta* 559, no. 4 (1979): 289–327.
4. Kholodenko, B. N., J. B. Hoek, and H. V. Westerhoff. "Why Cytoplasmic Signalling Proteins Should Be Recruited to Cell Membranes." *Trends Cell Biol* 10, no. 5 (2000): 173–8.
5. Kusumi, A., Y. Sako, and M. Yamamoto. "Confined Lateral Diffusion of Membrane Receptors as Studied by Single Particle Tracking (Nanovid Microscopy). Effects of Calcium-Induced Differentiation in Cultured Epithelial Cells." *Biophysical Journal* 65 (1993): 2021–40.
6. Groves, J. T., and J. Kuriyan. "Molecular Mechanisms in Signal Transduction at the Membrane." *Nat Struct Mol Biol* 17, no. 6 (2010): 659–65.
7. Kusumi, A., T. K. Fujiwara, R. Chadda et al. "Dynamic Organizing Principles of the Plasma Membrane That Regulate Signal Transduction: Commemorating the Fortieth Anniversary of Singer and Nicolson's Fluid-Mosaic Model." *Annu Rev Cell Dev Biol* 28 (2012): 215–50.
8. Andrews, N. L., K. A. Lidke, J. R. Pfeiffer et al. "Actin Restricts Fcepsilonri Diffusion and Facilitates Antigen-Induced Receptor Immobilization." *Nat Cell Biol* 10, no. 8 (2008): 955–63.

9. Low-Nam, S. T., K. A. Lidke, P. J. Cutler et al. "ErbB1 Dimerization Is Promoted by Domain Co-Confinement and Stabilized by Ligand Binding." *Nat Struct Mol Biol* 18, no. 11 (2011): 1244–9.

10. Jaqaman, K., H. Kuwata, N. Touret et al. "Cytoskeletal Control of CD36 Diffusion Promotes Its Receptor and Signaling Function." *Cell* 146, no. 4 (2011): 593–606.

11. Lingwood, D., and K. Simons. "Lipid Rafts as a Membrane-Organizing Principle." *Science* 327, no. 5961 (2010): 46–50.

12. Simons, K., and J. L. Sampaio. "Membrane Organization and Lipid Rafts." *Cold Spring Harb Perspect Biol* 3, no. 10 (2011): a004697.

13. Jacobson, K., O. G. Mouritsen, and R. G. Anderson. "Lipid Rafts: At a Crossroad between Cell Biology and Physics." *Nat Cell Biol* 9, no. 1 (2007): 7–14.

14. Vicidomini, G., G. Moneron, K. Y. Han et al. "Sharper Low-Power STED Nanoscopy by Time Gating." *Nat Methods* 8, no. 7 (2011): 571–3.

15. Klammt, C., and B. F. Lillemeier. "How Membrane Structures Control T Cell Signaling." *Front Immunol* 3 (2012): 291.

16. Owen, D. M., S. Oddos, S. Kumar et al. "High Plasma Membrane Lipid Order Imaged at the Immunological Synapse Periphery in Live T Cells." *Mol Membr Biol* 27, no. 4–6 (2010): 178–89.

17. Cambi, A., and D. S. Lidke. "Nanoscale Membrane Organization: Where Biochemistry Meets Advanced Microscopy." *ACS Chem Biol* 7, no. 1 (2012): 139–49.

18. Kirchhausen, T. "Bending Membranes." *Nat Cell Biol* 14, no. 9 (2012): 906–8.

19. Rangamani, P., A. Lipshtat, E. U. Azeloglu et al. "Decoding Information in Cell Shape." *Cell* 154, no. 6 (2013): 1356–69.

20. Qualmann, B., D. Koch, and M. M. Kessels. "Let's Go Bananas: Revisiting the Endocytic Bar Code." *EMBO J* 30, no. 17 (2011): 3501–15.

21. Schmid, S. L., and V. A. Frolov. "Dynamin: Functional Design of a Membrane Fission Catalyst." *Annu Rev Cell Dev Biol* 27 (2011): 79–105.

22. Welliver, T. P., S. L. Chang, J. J. Linderman, and J. A. Swanson. "Ruffles Limit Diffusion in the Plasma Membrane During Macropinosome Formation." *J Cell Sci* 124, Pt 23 (2011): 4106–14.

23. Dale, B. M., D. Traum, H. Erdjument-Bromage, P. Tempst, and S. Greenberg. "Phagocytosis in Macrophages Lacking Cbl Reveals an Unsuspected Role for Fc Gamma Receptor Signaling and Actin Assembly in Target Binding." *J Immunol* 182, no. 9 (2009): 5654–62.

24. Flannagan, R. S., R. E. Harrison, C. M. Yip, K. Jaqaman, and S. Grinstein. "Dynamic Macrophage 'Probing' Is Required for the Efficient Capture of Phagocytic Targets." *J Cell Biol* 191, no. 6 (2010): 1205–18.

25. Janoos, F., K. Mosaliganti, X. Xu et al. "Robust 3D Reconstruction and Identification of Dendritic Spines from Optical Microscopy Imaging." *Med Image Anal* 13, no. 1 (2009): 167–79.

26. Huang, B. "Super-Resolution Optical Microscopy: Multiple Choices." *Curr Opin Chem Biol* 14, no. 1 (2010): 10–4.

27. Kasai, R. S., K. G. Suzuki, E. R. Prossnitz et al. "Full Characterization of GPCR Monomer-Dimer Dynamic Equilibrium by Single Molecule Imaging." *J Cell Biol* 192, no. 3 (2011): 463–80.

28. Dustin, M. L. "Insights into Function of the Immunological Synapse from Studies with Supported Planar Bilayers." *Curr Top Microbiol Immunol* 340 (2010): 1–24.

29. Dustin, M. L., and D. Depoil. "New Insights into the T Cell Synapse from Single Molecule Techniques." *Nat Rev Immunol* 11, no. 10 (2011): 672–84.

30. Kirchhausen, T. "Imaging Endocytic Clathrin Structures in Living Cells." *Trends Cell Biol* 19, no. 11 (2009): 596–605.

31. Rappoport, J. Z., S. M. Simon, and A. Benmerah. "Understanding Living Clathrin-Coated Pits." *Traffic* 5, no. 5 (2004): 327–37.

32. Weinberg, J., and D. G. Drubin. "Clathrin-Mediated Endocytosis in Budding Yeast." *Trends Cell Biol* 22, no. 1 (2012): 1–13.
33. Anantharam, A., B. Onoa, R. H. Edwards, R. W. Holz, and D. Axelrod. "Localized Topological Changes of the Plasma Membrane Upon Exocytosis Visualized by Polarized TIRFM." *J Cell Biol* 188, no. 3 (2010): 415–28.
34. Doyon, J. B., B. Zeitler, J. Cheng et al. "Rapid and Efficient Clathrin-Mediated Endocytosis Revealed in Genome-Edited Mammalian Cells." *Nat Cell Biol* 13, no. 3 (2011): 331–7.
35. Jouvenet, N., S. M. Simon, and P. D. Bieniasz. "Visualizing HIV-1 Assembly." *J Mol Biol* 410, no. 4 (2011): 501–11.
36. Axelrod, D., N. L. Thompson, and T. P. Burghardt. "Total Internal Inflection Fluorescent Microscopy." *J Microsc* 129, Pt 1 (1983): 19–28.
37. Martin-Fernandez, M. L., C. J. Tynan, and S. E. Webb. "A 'Pocket Guide' to Total Internal Reflection Fluorescence." *J Microsc* 252, no. 1 (2013): 16–22.
38. Axelrod, D. "Evanescent Excitation and Emission in Fluorescence Microscopy." *Biophys J* 104, no. 7 (2013): 1401–9.
39. Lin, J., and A. D. Hoppe. "Uniform Total Internal Reflection Fluorescence Illumination Enables Live Cell Fluorescence Resonance Energy Transfer Microscopy." *Microsc Microanal* 19, no. 2 (2013): 350–9.
40. Hoppe, A. D., S. Seveau, and J. A. Swanson. "Live Cell Fluorescence Microscopy to Study Microbial Pathogenesis." *Cell Microbiol* 11, no. 4 (2009): 540–50.
41. Mattheyses, A. L., S. M. Simon, and J. Z. Rappoport. "Imaging with Total Internal Reflection Fluorescence Microscopy for the Cell Biologist." *J Cell Sci* 123, Pt 21 (2010): 3621–8.
42. Mattheyses, A. L., K. Shaw, and D. Axelrod. "Effective Elimination of Laser Interference Fringing in Fluorescence Microscopy by Spinning Azimuthal Incidence Angle." *Microsc Res Tech* 69, no. 8 (2006): 642–7.
43. Fiolka, R., Y. Belyaev, H. Ewers, and A. Stemmer. "Even Illumination in Total Internal Reflection Fluorescence Microscopy Using Laser Light." *Microsc Res Tech* 71, no. 1 (2008): 45–50.
44. van 't Hoff, M., V. de Sars, and M. Oheim. "A Programmable Light Engine for Quantitative Single Molecule TIRF and HILO Imaging." *Opt Express* 16, no. 22 (2008): 18495–504.
45. Clegg, R. M. "Fluoresence Resonance Energy Transfer." In *Fluorescence Imaging Spectroscopy and Microscopy*, edited by Wang, X. F. and Herman, B., 179–252. New York: John Wiley & Sons, 1996.
46. Mattheyses, A. L., A. D. Hoppe, and D. Axelrod. "Polarized Fluorescence Resonance Energy Transfer Microscopy." *Biophys J* 87, no. 4 (2004): 2787–97.
47. Hoppe, A., K. Christensen, and J. A. Swanson. "Fluorescence Resonance Energy Transfer-Based Stoichiometry in Living Cells." *Biophys J* 83, no. 6 (2002): 3652–64.
48. Cai, D., A. D. Hoppe, J. A. Swanson, and K. J. Verhey. "Kinesin-1 Structural Organization and Conformational Changes Revealed by FRET Stoichiometry in Live Cells." *J Cell Biol* 176, no. 1 (2007): 51–63.
49. Beemiller, P., A. D. Hoppe, and J. A. Swanson. "A Phosphatidylinositol-3-Kinase-Dependent Signal Transition Regulates ARF1 and ARF6 During Fcgamma Receptor-Mediated Phagocytosis." *PLoS Biol* 4, no. 6 (2006): e162.
50. Swanson, J. A., and A. D. Hoppe. "The Coordination of Signaling During Fc Receptor-Mediated Phagocytosis." *J Leukoc Biol* 76, no. 6 (2004): 1093–103.
51. Hoppe, A. D. "FRET-Based Imaging of Rac and Cdc42 Activation During Fc-Receptor-Mediated Phagocytosis in Macrophages." *Methods Mol Biol* 827 (2012): 235–51.
52. Jiang, X., and A. Sorkin. "Coordinated Traffic of Grb2 and Ras During Epidermal Growth Factor Receptor Endocytosis Visualized in Living Cells." *Mol Biol Cell* 13, no. 5 (2002): 1522–35.

53. Sorkin, A., M. McClure, F. Huang, and R. Carter. "Interaction of EGF Receptor and Grb2 in Living Cells Visualized by Fluorescence Resonance Energy Transfer (FRET) Microscopy." *Curr Biol* 10, no. 21 (2000): 1395–8.

54. Sun, Y., H. Wallrabe, C. F. Booker, R. N. Day, and A. Periasamy. "Three-Color Spectral FRET Microscopy Localizes Three Interacting Proteins in Living Cells." *Biophys J* 99, no. 4 (2010): 1274–83.

55. Woehler, A. "Simultaneous Quantitative Live Cell Imaging of Multiple FRET-Based Biosensors." *PLoS One* 8, no. 4 (2013): e61096.

56. Hoppe, A. D., B. L. Scott, T. P. Welliver, S. W. Straight, and J. A. Swanson. "N-Way FRET Microscopy of Multiple Protein-Protein Interactions in Live Cells." *PLoS One* 8, no. 6 (2013): e64760.

57. Neher, R. A., and E. Neher. "Applying Spectral Fingerprinting to the Analysis of FRET Images." *Microsc Res Tech* 64, no. 2 (2004): 185–95.

58. Grunberg, R., J. V. Burnier, T. Ferrar et al. "Engineering of Weak Helper Interactions for High-Efficiency FRET Probes." *Nat Methods* 10, no. 10 (2013): 1021–7.

59. Axelrod, D., and M. D. Wang. "Reduction-of-Dimensionality Kinetics at Reaction-Limited Cell Surface Receptors." *Biophys J* 66, no. 3 Pt 1 (1994): 588–600.

60. Hoppe, A. D., S. L. Shorte, J. A. Swanson, and R. Heintzmann. "Three-Dimensional FRET Reconstruction Microscopy for Analysis of Dynamic Molecular Interactions in Live Cells." *Biophys J* 95, no. 1 (2008): 400–18.

61. Hoppe, A. D. "Quantitative FRET Microscopy of Live Cells." In *Imaging Cellular and Molecular Biological Functions*, edited by Shorte S. L. and Frischknecht, F., 157–80. New York: Springer, 2007.

62. Lam, A. D., S. Ismail, R. Wu et al. "Mapping Dynamic Protein Interactions to Insulin Secretory Granule Behavior with TIRF-FRET." *Biophys J* 99, no. 4 (2010): 1311–20.

63. Hoppe, A. D., and J. A. Swanson. "Cdc42, Rac1, and Rac2 Display Distinct Patterns of Activation During Phagocytosis." *Mol Biol Cell* 15, no. 8 (2004): 3509–19.

64. Varnai, P., K. I. Rother, and T. Balla. "Phosphatidylinositol 3-Kinase-Dependent Membrane Association of the Bruton's Tyrosine Kinase Pleckstrin Homology Domain Visualized in Single Living Cells." *J Biol Chem* 274, no. 16 (1999): 10983–9.

65. van der Wal, J., R. Habets, P. Varnai, T. Balla, and K. Jalink. "Monitoring Agonist-Induced Phospholipase C Activation in Live Cells by Fluorescence Resonance Energy Transfer." *J Biol Chem* 276, no. 18 (2001): 15337–44.

66. Seveau, S., T. N. Tham, B. Payrastre et al. "A FRET Analysis to Unravel the Role of Cholesterol in Rac1 and PI 3-Kinase Activation in the InlB/Met Signalling Pathway." *Cell Microbiol* 9, no. 3 (2007): 790–803.

67. Wang, H., H. Yang, C. S. Shivalila et al. "One-Step Generation of Mice Carrying Mutations in Multiple Genes by CRISPR/Cas-Mediated Genome Engineering." *Cell* 153, no. 4 (2013): 910–8.

68. Bikard, D., W. Jiang, P. Samai et al. "Programmable Repression and Activation of Bacterial Gene Expression Using an Engineered CRISPR-Cas System." *Nucleic Acids Res* 41, no. 15 (2013): 7429–37.

69. Cho, S. W., S. Kim, J. M. Kim, and J. S. Kim. "Targeted Genome Engineering in Human Cells with the Cas9 RNA-Guided Endonuclease." *Nat Biotechnol* 31, no. 3 (2013): 230–2.

70. Cong, L., F. A. Ran, D. Cox et al. "Multiplex Genome Engineering Using CRISPR/Cas Systems." *Science* 339, no. 6121 (2013): 819–23.

71. Mali, P., L. Yang, K. M. Esvelt et al. "RNA-Guided Human Genome Engineering Via Cas9." *Science* 339, no. 6121 (2013): 823–6.

72. Sorkin, A., and M. Von Zastrow. "Signal Transduction and Endocytosis: Close Encounters of Many Kinds." *Nat Rev Mol Cell Biol* 3, no. 8 (2002): 600–14.

73. Sund, S. E., J. A. Swanson, and D. Axelrod. "Cell Membrane Orientation Visualized by Polarized Total Internal Reflection Fluorescence." *Biophys J* 77, no. 4 (1999): 2266–83.

74. Axelrod, D. "Carbocyanine Dye Orientation in Red Cell Membrane Studied by Microscopic Fluorescence Polarization." *Biophys J* 26, no. 3 (1979): 557–73.

75. Anantharam, A., D. Axelrod, and R. W. Holz. "Polarized TIRFM Reveals Changes in Plasma Membrane Topology before and during Granule Fusion." *Cell Mol Neurobiol* 30, no. 8 (2010): 1343–9.

76. Anatharam, A., D. Axelrod, and R. W. Holz. "Real-Time Imaging of Plasma Membrane Deformations Reveals Pre-Fusion Membrane Curvature Changes and a Role for Dynamin in the Regulation of Fusion Pore Expansion." *J Neurochem* 122, no. 4 (2012): 661–71.

77. Anantharam, A., M. A. Bittner, R. L. Aikman et al. "A New Role for the Dynamin GTPase in the Regulation of Fusion Pore Expansion." *Mol Biol Cell* 22, no. 11 (2011): 1907–18.

78. Lidke, D. S., S. T. Low-Nam, P. J. Cutler, and K. A. Lidke. "Determining FcεR Diffusional Dynamics Via Single Quantum Dot Tracking." *Methods Mol Biol* 748 (2011): 121–32.

Section III

Expanding the Fluorescence Toolbox

13 Laurdan Identifies Different Lipid Membranes in Eukaryotic Cells

Enrico Gratton and Michelle A. Digman

CONTENTS

13.1 INTRODUCTION

13.1.1 SPECTROSCOPIC PROPERTIES OF LAURDAN

There are several commonly used approaches for the study of membrane properties of live cells based on fluorescence probes. In one approach, lipids with specific fluorescent markers are incorporated in the cell membranes. The advantage of this approach is that it is possible to study the membrane distribution of specific lipids. However, when the aim of the study is to detect membrane microdomains independently of their lipid composition, it is more useful to use a single probe that can report on the specific properties of the membrane microdomains, independently of the probe segregation in one specific domain and location in the cell. One fluorescent probe that has been successfully used for this purpose is the lipophilic probe Laurdan (2-dimethylamino-6-lauroylnaphthalene), originally synthesized by Weber and Farris.[1] Different membrane environments produce marked changes both in the spectrum and in the fluorescence lifetime of Laurdan. The sensitivity of the emission spectrum of Laurdan to the environment originates from the specific molecular structure of Laurdan in which the excited-state dipole is substantially different from the ground-state dipole (Figure 13.1).

During the absorption of the excitation photon, which lasts approximately 10^{-15} s, there is no time for reorientation of the surrounding solvent molecules, generally water in biological samples (Figure 13.2).

Depending on the nature of the environment, the reorientation of solvent molecules around the excited-state dipole of Laurdan can occur in the nanosecond time range. This time is comparable to the total duration of the excited state and, as a consequence of the solvent reorientation, the spectrum of Laurdan changes with time after excitation in a continuous way (Figure 13.3).

This property of Laurdan, which results in an "undefined" emission spectrum, since the spectrum depends on the time after excitation, must be considered with extreme care when we want to identify the emission with a particular "phase" of structural organization of the membrane. Originally, our laboratory proposed using a specific scale, the Generalized Polarization (GP) scale to quantify the degree of dipolar relaxation.[2–4] This scale is experimentally defined using the emission spectral bandwidths and measuring the normalized emission in the two bandwidths. Specifically, the two bandwidths were chosen at 440/20 nm and 490/20 nm and the GP value is calculated according to the following expression:

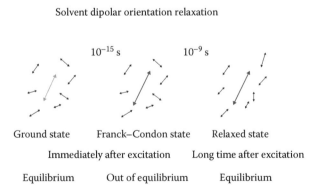

FIGURE 13.1   In the ground state, solvent molecules are partially organized around the Laurdan molecule. Upon excitation, which occurs in 10^{-15} s, the Laurdan dipole substantially increases. At this point in time, the solvent molecules start to rotate to minimize the energy with respect to the excited-state dipole until equilibrium is reached.

As the relaxation proceeds, the energy of the excited state decreases
and the emission moves toward the dotted vertical transition

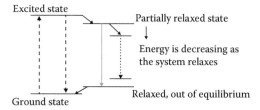

FIGURE 13.2 Jablonski diagram indicating the relative position of the excited state at the time of excitation and the shift of the level of the excited state as the energy is minimized as a result of the orientation of the solvent molecules. The colors of the different down arrows schematically show that the energy of the emitted photon decreases as a function of time after excitation.

The emission spectrum moves toward the dotted vertical transition with time

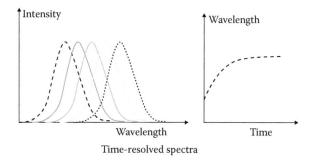

Time-resolved spectra

FIGURE 13.3 Schematic representation of the continuous shift of the wavelength of emission of the fluorescence. The first molecules to decay emit in the dashed line and the last ones emit in the dotted line. The apparent lifetime of the excited state changes with time. If one is to measure using a bandpass in the dotted part of the spectrum, initially there is no emission in this bandpass since the spectrum has not shifted yet. In the dotted part of the spectrum, the intensity starts to increase after some time and then eventually decays to zero. This delay of the emission gives rise to a very peculiar behavior of the apparent lifetime in the dotted part of the spectrum.

$$GP = \frac{(I_{440} - gI_{490})}{(I_{440} + gI_{490})}. \tag{13.1}$$

Note that the intensity in the two filters must be calibrated for each instrument and for a specific set of filters since the sensitivity of the instrument could be different from one laboratory to another. This is done by determining the value of the constant g in Equation 13.1 using as compound of known GP, generally Laurdan in dimethyl sulfoxide (DMSO). Note also that given the definition, the GP value is constrained to be between +1 and −1. While the GP is rigorously defined, the meaning of the GP must be carefully discussed. There is a general trend of the values of the GP that is very useful for the evaluation of the membrane overall properties. For example, when the dipolar relaxations are slow compared to the excited-state lifetime, most of the emission occurs in the 440 nm filter (blue filter) and the GP is positive and typically in the range 0.6 to 0.7. When the dipolar relaxations are fast (compared to the excited-state lifetime), most of the emission is in the 490 nm filter (green filter) and the GP is negative in the −0.3 range.

What is important for the discussion here is that, in principle, there are no definite values for the GP in different membrane phases since the rate of dipolar relaxation is strongly influenced by the lipid composition, membrane curvature, presence of defects, and other parameters than can affect the rate of dipolar relaxation as well as the duration of the excited-state lifetime. For example, if the excited-state lifetime is shortened because of quenching effects, the GP will increase without a change of the dipolar relaxation rate. Specifically, depending on the polarity of the solvent, the excited-state lifetime can change. In apolar solvents, the fluorescence lifetime of Laurdan can be in the range 7–8 ns, while in more polar solvents, the lifetime can be in the range 3–4 ns. Hence, by a mere change of the polarity of the membrane, the GP value can change by a relatively large factor without a corresponding change in the rate of dipolar relaxation. One notable example is the presence of cholesterol in the membrane, which increases the lifetime of Laurdan, allowing for more time for the dipolar relaxation to occur. From this discussion, it is clear that the measurement of Laurdan lifetime provides complementary information needed to properly interpret the spectral changes. Also, it is clear that the assumption that there are only two values for the Laurdan GP (or lifetime) must be carefully discussed and probed. Mainly for this reason, the GP function was initially proposed as an index that correlates with the water content of the membrane to be used to detect changes in membrane packing that influence the amount of water in the membrane.

As laser scanning fluorescence microscopy was developed in the 1990s and with the advent of femtosecond lasers that allowed two-photon excitation of Laurdan, we were able to obtain images of GP that clearly show that the GP function is different in different cells and in different membranes or part of the same membrane of the cell.[5] Then, an important issue arose about the meaning of the absolute value of the GP and whether this value could provide information about membrane composition and membrane packing. Although we could measure the entire emission spectrum and the lifetime in each emission bandwidth in a bulk experiment, this is more complicated in the microscope setup. Most of the earlier studies were done using two emission bandpasses (generally referred to as the blue and green filters) and the GP function was calculated at each pixel of the image.[2] The GP scale was used to interpret the GP "image" as regions in the cell in which the membrane was more or less permeable to water. This approach provided interesting results, and it was used mainly for producing contrast in images on the basis of the GP value.[6] The question that will be discussed next is if we could assign values of the GP to specific membrane phases such as highly packed liquid ordered phase and less packed liquid disordered phase. Since we want to fabricate a scale to determine the correlation between the Laurdan emission spectrum and the phase of the membrane, we should look at the entire emission spectrum and possibly perform lifetime measurements at selected bandpasses in the microscope setup. We also need to find a way to visualize all this information (spectrum and lifetime) in such a way that we could correlate the pixel histogram of the GP values with a specific structure in the image. Note that this procedure is different from using a fluorescent label that partitions in a specific lipid structure or cell organelle.

13.2 THE PHASOR APPROACH TO SPECTRAL AND LIFETIME ANALYSIS

For this discussion, we have developed an approach that is based on the measurement of the spectrum of Laurdan obtained in a microscope setup where a single giant unilamellar vesicle (GUV) or cell can be visualized and analyzed. As we discussed, the spectrum changes continuously in time as the excited state returns to the ground state. We are using an analysis based on the "phasor approach" in which the spectrum is characterized by a few parameters. The advantage of the phasor approach is that we can represent some spectral characteristics in a global view in the phasor plot. Another advantage is that if there are only two (or a few) discrete spectra that are typical of a type of membrane domain, then it will be possible to distinguish the combination of domains containing regions with characteristic spectra because the phasor components add linearly for two (or more) species.[7–9] Given a spectrum measured at each pixel indicated by $I(\lambda)$, according to Fereidouni et al.,[10] we define the following two quantities that we interpret as two coordinates in a Cartesian plot. The symbol n indicate the "harmonic order" and we use generally either a value of 1 (first harmonic) or 2 (for the second harmonic) for n.

$$g = \frac{\sum_{\lambda} I(\lambda)\cos(2\pi_n \lambda/L)}{\sum_{\lambda} I(\lambda)} \qquad s = \frac{\sum_{\lambda} I(\lambda)\sin(2\pi_n \lambda/L)}{\sum_{\lambda} I(\lambda)} \qquad (13.2)$$

A typical spectrum for Laurdan in the laser scanning microscope Zeiss 710NLO is shown in Figure 13.4, using two-photon excitation at 790 nm.

Unfortunately, given the limited range of the spectral detectors for commercial microscopes, we are generally limited to collect only a portion of the emission spectrum. Clearly, in the spectrum of Figure 13.4, we are cutting all the emissions below 416 nm. This is not a limitation since the g and s functions are defined only in the region of the measurement (Equation 13.2). A fundamental property of the coordinates g and s is that they behave as components of a vector. That means that if the measured spectrum is the sum of two spectra, the measured g and s are the sum of individual coordinates for each of the spectra measured independently. This is illustrated in Figure 13.5 where the phasor positions for two spectra are schematically shown with the black and gray dot. Figure 13.5 shows that the position of a phasor is determined by the phase angle and the modulus, that is, the radial position of the phasor. In Figure 13.5, the angular position in the phasor plot (counterclockwise) corresponds to the average wavelength of emission where bluer emissions have smaller phases. The radial distance from the center depends on the spectrum width with narrower spectra having larger radii. The harmonic number $n = 2$ multiplies the phases

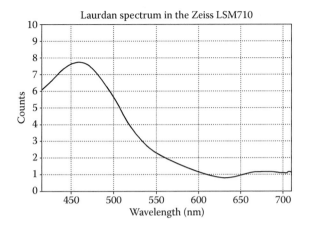

FIGURE 13.4 Typical spectrum of Laurdan in cells measured using the spectral detector of the Zeiss LSM710 laser scanning microscope. The spectrum is obtained using two-photon excitation at 790 nm. The spectral detector has 32 independent detectors equally spaced in wavelength in the region 416 to 727 nm. In this figure, the intensity of the detectors is interpolated and the spectrum is smoothed.

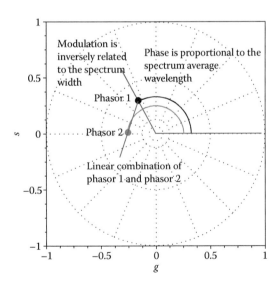

FIGURE 13.5 Spectral phasor plot indicating the position of the phasor corresponding to two different spectra. The angular position of a spectrum in the phasor plot is proportional to the average emission wavelength while the radial potion is inversely related to the spectral width. If in a pixel we have the combination of the two spectra, the phasor position must fall in the line joining the phasor of the two spectra as indicated in the figure.

approximately by a factor of 2, and it is much less sensitive to the lack of cutoff of the spectrum owing to the limited wavelength range of the microscope and more sensitive to spectral changes. In this chapter, we use $n = 2$ for all spectral analysis.

For example, if a spectrum has a shape indicated by the dot 1 and another spectrum has the shape indicated by 2, their linear combination must follow the line joining the phasor plot of the phasors of the two spectra. The assessment whether or not a spectrum is the linear combination of 2 "unknown" spectra can be made without any knowledge of the spectra.

In principle, the spectral phasor analysis is equivalent to spectral demixing. However, in spectral demixing, we need to know the basis spectra used in the demixing algorithm, which are unknown for Laurdan. More importantly, the spectra change continuously because of solvent dipolar relaxations so that any method that assumes that there are only few spectral components is inadequate.

For the lifetime analysis, the phasor approach works in the same way as that for spectral analysis with some interesting additions as explained in Section 13.3.

13.3 THE LIFETIME PHASOR TRANSFORMATION AND ITS INTERPRETATION

In a fluorescence lifetime imaging microscopy (FLIM) measurement, the fluorescence decay is obtained at each pixel generally using a photon counting system that measures the histograms of time delays between the excitation of the molecule caused by the laser pulse excitation and the emission of a photon from the excited state of the molecule. In each pixel, an average of approximately 100 to 500 photons is collected. Analysis of the decay using exponential models cannot be done accurately using such a low number of photons in the histogram, and specifically for Laurdan, as discussed in Section 13.1, an exponential decay is inadequate to describe the decay since Laurdan decay is affected by solvent relaxations. In the phasor approach, only a few moments of the delay histogram are used to determine some proprieties of the decay. The phasor approach applies a transformation (the phasor transformation) to the measured decay histogram as shown in Equations 13.3 and 13.4, where $I_{i,j}(t)$ is the histogram of photon delays measured at pixel (i,j).[7] At each pixel, the phasor transformation provides two coordinates g and s, which are plotted in a polar plot called the phasor plot.

$$g_{i,j}(\omega) = \frac{\int_0^T I_{i,j}(t)\cos(\omega t)dt}{\int_0^T I_{i,j}(t)dt} \tag{13.3}$$

$$s_{i,j}(\omega) = \frac{\int_0^T I_{i,j}(t)\sin(\omega t)dt}{\int_0^T I_{i,j}(t)dt} \tag{13.4}$$

There is a relationship between the exponential decay and points in the phasor plot (Figure 13.6). If the fluorescence decay is single exponential, the phasor transformation gives points that lay on a semicircle called the universal circle.

As we indicated earlier, the phasor transformation has the property that the coordinates g and s behave like coordinates of a vector. The consequence of this mathematical property is that if in a pixel we have molecules that decay with two different exponential constants, the phasor of each of the molecules will lay on different points on the universal circle, but their linear combination (which depends on their fractional intensity contribution to the decay in that pixel) must be on the line joining the two points on the universal circle, as shown in Figure 13.7a. This linear combination property holds even if the phasors of the two species are not on the universal circle (Figure 13.7b). Since the decay of Laurdan is nonexponential, if in one pixel we have coexistence of regions of different decay properties, the measured phasor must be on the line corresponding to these different decay properties. For example, if in one pixel we have coexistence of regions (microdomains below the pixel resolution) of

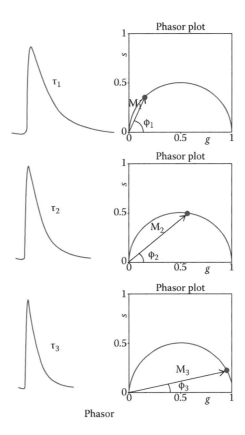

FIGURE 13.6 Schematic of the phasor transformation. Decay curves with different single-exponential lifetimes map in different position in the phasor plot with points on the universal circle. The faster is the exponential decay, the more the point is to the right.

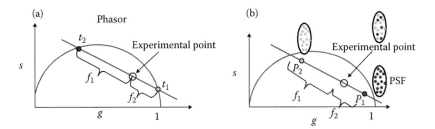

FIGURE 13.7 Linear combination property of phasors. (a) The combination in one pixel of two single exponentials gives a phasor value on the line joining the phasors corresponding to the two exponentials. (b) If in one pixel (the size of the PSF, approximately 300 nm) there are Laurdan molecules with different environments, although each environment is decaying as a complex exponential, they will combine linearly to give experimental points in the line joining the phasors of the two different environments.

liquid order and liquid disorder, then the phasor position must be along the line joining the phasor of the liquid ordered and liquid disordered membrane phases.

13.4 RESULTS OF THE ANALYSIS OF THE EMISSION OF LAURDAN USING SPECTRAL AND LIFETIME PHASORS IN GUVs MODEL SYSTEMS

We will first discuss the values of the spectral and lifetime phasors measured in GUVs composed of one lipid species (DPPC, DMPC, and DLPC).

Notably, the phasor values of the different composition and temperature GUVs follow a straight line. The colors of the circles in the phasor plot correspond to the colors in the images. As expected, Laurdan in DPPC at 20°C (T_m approximately at 41°C) is emitting in the blue (smaller phase), while Laurdan in DLPC at 20°C (T_m approximately at 8°C) has a spectrum that is in the green region (larger phase). The phasor positions of the samples at equal temperature (DPPC, DMPC, and DLPC) span a relatively large range in the phasor plot (red circle = 454 nm, green circle = 458 nm, cyan circle = 468 nm, blue circle = 480 nm). Surprisingly, the distance of the various phasor clusters from the origin varies. This distance is inversely related to the width of the spectrum, which is evidently different in the different samples. According to the linear combination rule for phasors, the samples that are in the linear segment in Figure 13.8 (not at the extreme of the segment) should contain a linear combination of the spectral properties corresponding to the extremes of the segment. For example, the cluster of phasors indicated with the color green or cyan should correspond to the linear combination of the two spectra corresponding to the red and blue clusters. However, in this particular experiment, each of the samples is composed of only one phospholipid and the samples should be homogeneous, except for the samples at temperature corresponding to the phase transition temperature for a specific phospholipid. The fact that the clusters align as shown in Figure 13.8 could imply that there are "only two" environments for the Laurdan molecule; in this case, it will be the gel and the liquid crystal. However, DMPC should be in a homogeneous

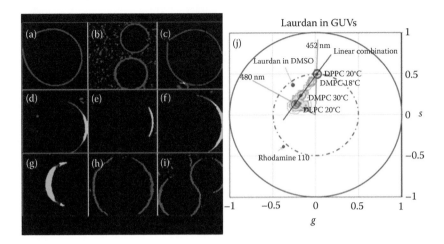

FIGURE 13.8 Spectral phasor analysis of Laurdan in GUVs made of a single phospholipid and at different temperatures. (a) DLPC at 20°C. (b and c) POPC at 20°C. (d) DMPC at 30°C. (e) DMPC at 28°C. (f) DMPC at 25°C. (g) DMPC at 21°C. (h) DMPC at 18°C. (i) DPPC at 20°C. (j) Spectral phasor plot of the GUVs samples. The underlining contour plot shows the position of the phasor for the different samples. Also, the position of the spectral phasors for Laurdan in DMSO and Rhodamine 110 in water is shown. The phasor of the GUVs apparently fall on a single line, which could be identified as the linear combination of two extreme values, for the liquid disordered phase of DLPC and DOPC at 20°C and the gel phase of DPPC at 20°C. The colors of the circles in (j) are used to paint the image with the pixels that have the phasor inside the corresponding circle in the phasor plot.

phase at least at temperatures far from the phase transition (30°C and 18°C), rather than a mixture of gel and liquid crystalline phase at all temperatures. The simplistic interpretation of the linear combination property in terms of coexistence of different phases does not hold in this case. Another possibility is that there are mainly two "environments" for the Laurdan probe, one with fast relaxation and the other with very slow relaxation, since Laurdan spectral position depends on the solvent relaxation rate. If this is the case, then the position at an intermediate value along the line between the gel and the liquid crystalline phase could just be attributed to the fraction of Laurdan molecules in the two environments. We can further elaborate on this idea and propose that the "two" environments can be identified, one with local membrane cavities with one or more molecules of water and the other with Laurdan in a tighter structure without water in the proximity. This suggestion was previously made on the basis of the observation of Laurdan spectra in a variety of conditions.[11,12]

13.5   THE LIFETIME PHASOR FOR LAURDAN IN GUVs

In regard to the lifetime, it is interesting that, in general, the lifetime of Laurdan cannot be described by only two components, but rather by a distribution of components. Depending on the emission bandwidth, the lifetime of Laurdan in the blue part of the emission spectrum is relatively long (7–8 ns) and relatively single exponential. As the lipid composition changes, the lifetime in the blue filter aligns along the universal circle while the lifetime in the green filter could be outside of the universal circle because of the dipolar relaxation effect as the relaxation time becomes comparable in time to the overall decay time (see Figure 13.9 for an explanation why the phasor in the green filter can be outside of the universal circle).

In relation to Figure 13.9, if we measure the decay in the blue emission filter, the lifetime phasor position for Laurdan in the absence of surrounding water is shown in blue (low polarity, depending on the lipid environment). As the polarity of the medium increases, the lifetime shortens and the lifetime phasor moves along the universal circle to lower lifetime values (more polar position). The line between less polar and more polar corresponds to the linear combination of the Laurdan in the two environments, that is, to the fraction of molecules in polar versus nonpolar environments. If we measure the decay in the green emission bandpass, the unrelaxed or relaxed positions in Figure 13.9 correspond to the Laurdan molecules sensing

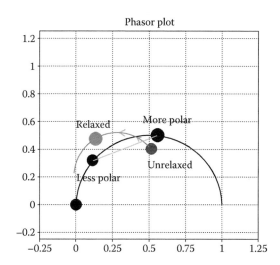

FIGURE 13.9 Schematic representation of the lifetime phasor position expected for Laurdan at two emission bandpass (gray 440/20 nm and light gray 540/40 nm, shown in black color in the figure). In the gray filter, the phasor position is on the universal circle, which indicates that Laurdan decays as a single exponential in the gray filter. The lifetime is quenched because of the polarity of the surrounding solvent. This effect should not be confused with solvent dipolar relaxation. The phasor position moves along the universal circle depending on the amount of quenching. If in one pixel there is a mixture of environments with different polarity, in this pixel, the phasor must fall in the gray line joining the two extreme values. In the light gray filter, the position of the phasor is determined by the solvent relaxation. In the absence of relaxation or if the relaxation is very fast, the position of the phasor is generally inside the universal circle owing to the heterogeneity of the decay. As the rate of dipolar relaxation increases, the phasor position moves toward the outside of the universal circle because the intensity increases with a delay with respect to the excitation. The maximum displacement toward the outside of the universal circle occurs when the rate of dipolar relaxation matches the decay rate.

different degrees of solvent dipolar relaxation. As the relaxation time increases, the phasor position in the green filter moves toward the position indicated with the dark gray toward the relaxed position (Figure 13.9). The maximum displacement along the dark gray curve is obtained when the relaxation time matches the decay time.

In Figure 13.10, we show the phasor lifetime analysis of GUVs made of a single phospholipid (DOPC and DPPC) at the same temperature (20°C) in the blue and green filters, respectively.

Figure 13.10 and the explanations given in its caption are used to construct an empirical lifetime phasor scale for the membrane fluidity. Note that the scale is very different at different wavelengths (blue vs. green) and that this scale is influenced by

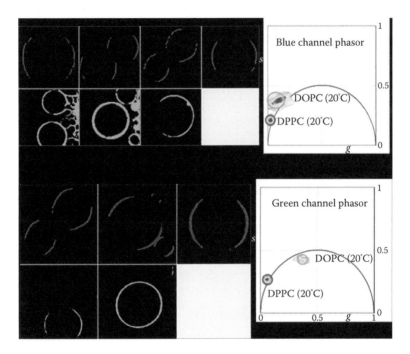

FIGURE 13.10 Empirical sensitivity scale for Laurdan lifetime phasor in two extreme phases, gel and liquid crystalline, and at two emission bandpasses (blue channel = 440/20 nm and green channel = 540/40 nm). The red cursor marks the position of the gel phase as found in the DPPC GUVs at room temperature, and the green cursor corresponds to the phasor position of DOPC at room temperature, which is in the liquid disordered phase. Excitation was obtained using a Ti:sapphire laser at 790 nm with a repetition frequency of 80 MHz. In DPPC, there are no measurable dipolar relaxations. The lifetime phasor position is largely independent of the emission wavelength. The fluorescence lifetime in this phase is approximately 8.0 ns. For DOPC, the relaxations are relatively fast and the emission in the blue channel senses the relaxations. The phasor distribution is elongated and outside the universal circle, indicating that there is lifetime heterogeneity and that the long lifetime components are sensitive to the dipolar relaxations. In the green channel, DOPC lifetime is quite short and faster than the dipolar relaxations, so that the phasor position returns inside the universal circle, according to the explanations given in Figure 13.9.

factors that change the polarity and the solvent relaxation rates. Also note that only in the green channel is the span of the fluidity scale relatively large (approximately a quarter of the phasor plot). In comparison with the spectral phasor scale in Figure 13.8, the span of the lifetime scale is reduced.

The effect of cholesterol on the spectral position and the spectral lifetime is quite interesting, and it can be understood on the basis of the spectroscopic principles outlined in the first part of this section.[13] In general, as the cholesterol concentration increases, not only does the spectrum move toward the blue, but the lifetime also becomes longer, allowing for observation of slower dipolar relaxation even in the green part of the emission spectrum. The combinations of these two effects, blue shifting but lengthening of the lifetime in the green filter, provides a characteristic signature of the presence of cholesterol. This idea has been recently presented,[13] and it is a direct consequence of the scheme shown in Figure 13.9.

As a take-home message regarding the characteristic spectroscopic properties of Laurdan, the apparent alignment of the phasors along a straight line cannot be taken as evidence that we are observing the contribution of two (or more) phases in the region of observation (pixel), but two different environments for the Laurdan molecules. Since these two (or more) environments can also be observed in phases of a single phospholipid far from the phase transition temperature, we believe that the two environments are attributed to situations in which the Laurdan molecules have no water around at the time of excitation and the other situation to Laurdan molecules with some water around. Membrane packing alone could be responsible for this effect. The same conclusion, that is, that the apparent alignment of the phasor clusters in the phasor plot does not imply that there are only two phases in the region of observation, applies to the lifetime phasor, which has a more complex behavior because the apparent lifetime is a function of the emission wavelength.

We propose, using the position along the linear combination line as a measure of water penetration, to provide an empirical scale of membrane "fluidity." To establish this empirical scale of fluidity, we measured the phasor positions of Laurdan in an artificial system composed of different lipids that at the same temperature form two different phases, liquid and gel. Of course, we do not expect these two phases to exist in biological systems, but we are using this scale as an indication of the maximum range of changes expected in lipid bilayer systems.

13.6   LIVE CELL MEMBRANE FLUIDITY

13.6.1   Spectral Phasors

A highly debated issue about biological membranes relates to the formation of membrane microdomains with specific characteristics distinct from the rest of the membranes. Since the spectrum of Laurdan reflects the water content of the membrane and, indirectly, membrane fluidity, the question arises whether it is possible, using the Laurdan probe, to distinguish different microdomains in biological membranes and characterize their size and location.

Figure 13.11 shows the phasor spectral analysis of the cancer cell line 3T3. The series of images are obtained at different z-sections spaced by 0.6 μm. The phasor distribution

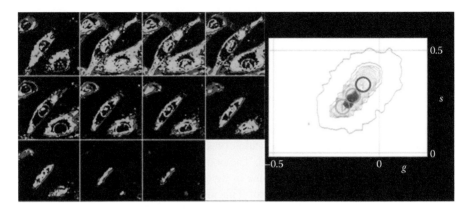

FIGURE 13.11 Z section images of 3T3 cells taken each 0.6 μm. The fluorescence was excited at 790 nm and the emission was collected using the spectral detector of the Zeiss 710LSM. In the right part of the figure, the spectral phasor plot is shown. The contour lines indicate the density of pixels with a given value of the phasor. The image on the left is colored according to the phasor position indicated with the colored circles in the phasor plot. Clearly, the phasor distribution is elongated and we can distinguish at least three different regions in the phasor plot that correspond to the plasma membrane and two regions corresponding to internal structures in the cells. The average line in this plot has a different slope from the line in Figure 13.8, indicating that the environment of the cell membrane is different from the single phospholipid environ of the GUVs used to produce Figure 13.8.

is broad and it distributes along a line, which is different from the line obtained using GUVs of different compositions. In relation to the spectra in single lipid GUVs and using the proposed empirical fluidity scale, the cell membranes corresponding to internal membranes (mitochondria, Golgi, and endoplasmic reticulum) are less packed than the plasma membrane. This observation corresponds to the common knowledge that the plasma membrane is the most rigid of the cell membranes. Instead, the spectral phasor of the plasma membrane is broader (smaller radius in Figure 13.11) than the spectrum of the gel-phase GUV. In cell membranes, the prevalent phase should be the Ld phase for the plasma membrane. Measurements of the spectral phasor of GUV composed of lipid mixture in the Lo phase (data not shown) show that the location of plasma membrane phasor is closer to the location of the Lo phase. Figure 13.12 shows higher-resolution data for the spectral phasor from a different 3T3 cell and the corresponding spectral phasor plot.

We can clearly see that the plasma membrane is relatively homogeneous and with low water content. Our measurements show that the phasor of the various membranes in a cell aligns along a common straight line, which reflects the different local environment of Laurdan in the various membranes. We could carefully examine different parts of the plasma membrane (Figure 13.12) and notice that different sections of the plasma membrane have definitely different spectra (indicated by the arrows in Figure 13.12). However, at the level of resolution of the images in these figures, it is not possible to distinguish if these regions correspond to regions where the internal membranes get closer to the plasma membrane or there are microdomains in the plasma membrane of different spectral properties.

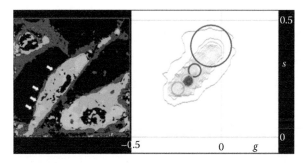

FIGURE 13.12   Single section of a 3T3 cell. The fluorescence was excited at 790 nm and the emission was collected using the spectral detector of the Zeiss 710LSM. In the right part of the figure, the spectral phasor plot is shown. The contour lines indicate the density of pixels with a given value of the phasor. The image on the left is colored according to the phasor position indicated with the colored circles in the phasor plot. As shown in Figure 13.11, the phasor distribution is elongated, and at this resolution, we can distinguish at least four different regions in the phasor plot. The violet-colored region corresponds to points with low intensity mainly at the border of the cell. The position and color coding of the other regions are the same as in Figure 13.11. Following the cell contour, we observe regions of the cell membrane indicated by white arrows with different spectra as selected by the different regions in the spectral phasor plot. This large spectral heterogeneity could indicate either that the pixels along the cell contour are contaminated by the contribution of both external and internal membranes or that the plasma membrane is made of macroscopic domains of different Laurdan spectral characteristics.

13.6.2   Lifetime Phasors in Live 3T3 Cells

The lifetime phasor analysis of 3T3 cells shows a similar behavior of the spectral phasor where the plasma membrane corresponds to higher values in our fluidity scale and the internal membranes are more fluid. Also, in this type of cells, the plasma membrane displays alternating regions of different values in the empirical fluidity scale. Figure 13.13 shows the lifetime phasor analysis in the blue and green channels. Compared to the GUVs in Figure 13.10, the location of the phasors in the blue channel is completely outside the universal circle, indicating that dipolar solvent relaxation is responsible for this effect. This observation implies that all membranes, including the plasma membrane and the internal membrane, are strongly affected by the dipolar relaxation effect. This is also shown in the green channel. As we know, dipolar relaxation is enhanced by cholesterol, which has the effect of lengthening the average lifetime and therefore better matching the decay rate with the solvent relaxation rate.

One feature of the images colored according to the phasor location is the spotted appearance of the plasma membrane. To further investigate if this spotted appearance is simply caused by noise or there is a continuation of the spots if we perform a series of three-dimensional (3D) sections, we obtained the spectral information at each section and we performed the phasor analysis at each section maintaining the selection of phasors at each section. In this way, we can obtain a 3D mask of a given color that corresponds to the empirical fluidity scale that we constructed using the data in Figures 13.11 and 13.12. The results are displayed in Figure 13.14. Figure 13.14a is the intensity

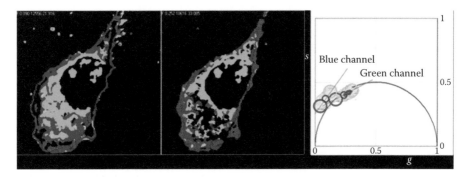

FIGURE 13.13 Lifetime phasor plot of a 3T3 cell. Excitation was at 790 nm using a Ti:sapphire laser and emission was measured at two bandpasses (440/20 nm and 540/40 nm). Images are colored according to the selection of the phasor clusters in the phasor plot. Colors are matched for the selections and the colors in the figure. The image size is 43 × 43 μm. According to the empirical fluidity scale, the plasma membrane has less fluid than the internal membrane and the contour of the cell is spotted.

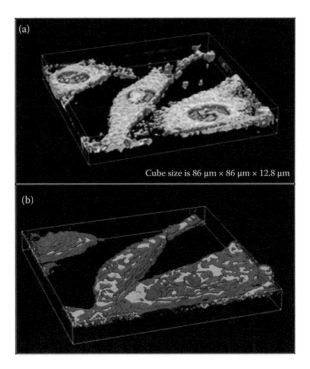

FIGURE 13.14 3D reconstruction of intensity and spectral phasor masks of a 3T3 cell. The masks were obtained using the spectral phasor positions of Figures 13.11 and 13.12. The color code is also the same used in these figures. The 3D reconstruction shows that the appearance of spots in the contours of single sections is attributed to the large domain spectral heterogeneity of the cell membrane.

image colored according to the z-section. Figure 13.14b is the same image but colored according to the phasor mask used in Figures 13.11 and 13.12. Clearly, the entire plasma membrane appears less fluid in this 3D reconstruction and the spots observed in the single images are actually sections of much larger regions of different fluidity.

13.7 CONCLUSIONS AND FURTHER CONSIDERATIONS

In conclusion, the location of a specific phasor cluster in the line of linear combination between the Lo and Ld phases cannot be interpreted as evidence of the coexistence of microdomains in these regions but only reports the fraction of very local environments of the Laurdan molecules. These local environments correspond in our opinion to membrane defects where one or more molecules of water can reside and can produce the solvent relaxation effect, which is the signature of the shifts of the emission spectrum of Laurdan and of the apparent changes of lifetime. Unless other information about the clustering of these cavities is obtained, for example, independent measurement of the size, we cannot conclude that an intermediate position of the spectrum or lifetime between two extremes is evidence of membrane microdomains, although membrane microdomains will produce this behavior. However, an analysis of the spectral and lifetime behavior of Laurdan shows a very rich scenario where relatively large domains resolved at the diffraction-limited resolution of the experiments reported in this contribution that extend in 3D. In addition, Laurdan is clearly sensitive to the relative differences in fluidity between different internal cell membranes.

From a biological point of view, membrane fluidity changes are implicated in a range of biological processes including signaling, membrane fusion, endocytosis, and many others. For example, the role of membrane fluidity during development has been discussed,[14–23] but we are still lacking a systematic study of changes in membrane fluidity during embryo development. In general, lipids and lipid domains independent of their size play a fundamental role in the structural organization of the cytoplasmic membrane of eukaryotic cells. The results described in this chapter show that Laurdan can detect the difference between the plasma membrane and the membranes of internal organelles, which are of fundamental importance for the compartmentalization of cell functions. The complexity of the membrane lipid composition has suggested the coexistence of domains characterized by different dynamic properties in the membrane plane as sites for preferential partitioning of proteins and solutes, for modulating membrane activity, and for diffusion along the plane and through the bilayer.[24–33]

Several invasive methods that use membrane isolation can be used to establish the exact lipid composition of membranes. However, when these methods are used to study membrane domains, they can be subject to localization error because lipids can migrate between different cellular compartments during the membrane isolation. Instead, fluorescence spectroscopy can be used directly in live cells and in tissues while the cells are being excited and are functioning in their natural biological environments. Using fluorescence, the information on membrane packing and dynamics is obtained from the spectroscopic properties of fluorescent probes residing in the membrane at very low concentrations, generally less than 1:100 probe-to-lipid molar ratio.

Among several fluorescent probes, the sensitivity of Laurdan to the polarity of the membrane environment presents several advantages for membrane studies. This sensitivity arises from the greater than 50 nm red shift of the emission maximum in polar versus nonpolar environments, so that simple fluorescence intensity measurements at two properly selected wavelengths provide information on the membrane polarity. Several studies have shown that Laurdan spectroscopic properties reflect local water content in the membrane and, indirectly, membrane fluidity. Laurdan is a molecule whose spectroscopic properties are influenced by both the composition and dynamics of its local surroundings.[2–4,11,13,34–45] In other words, Laurdan's fluorescence properties are dependent on two major factors: the polarity of the environment (ground state of the fluorophore) and the rate of dipolar relaxation of molecules or molecular residues that can reorient around Laurdan's fluorescent moiety during its excited-state lifetime.

In this chapter, we show that spectral and lifetime information can be analyzed in a common framework on the basis of the phasor transformation. This is important in the evaluation of the sensitivity of the two spectroscopic approaches. We show here that while spectral analysis has a larger range, lifetime analysis offers a possibility to distinguish unambiguously between changes in polarity and changes in the solvent dipolar relaxation rate.

In this chapter, we compare the use of Laurdan emission spectra and Laurdan fluorescence lifetime as a means to determine differences between membranes in eukaryotic cells, with particular emphasis on the membranes of cancer cell lines. We discuss the different information that can be extracted using spectral and lifetime measurements of Laurdan in live cells when these techniques are applied to confocal images. Using the spectral and the FLIM approach, we build a fluidity scale based on calibration with model systems of different lipid composition. Using FLIM, we show that it is possible to quantify and separate the changes in membrane water content that affect the spectral relaxation process of Laurdan from changes that are caused by polarity of the Laurdan environment, which mainly affect the emission spectrum. Both for the analysis of FLIM data and spectral data, we use a common approach based on the use of phasors. The phasor approach is a fit-less way to visually display where in the cells Laurdan has different spectroscopic properties. The relevance of the phasor approach is that it allows a simple graphical way to separate regions of the cells where we have coexistence of different environments from other regions where there are unique but different environments. The measurement of the phasor locations in GUVs made of single lipids of different transition temperatures allows us to construct a sensitivity scale that we can use to compare the spectral and the FLIM approach. An analysis of different membranes of the same cell shows marked differences in spectroscopic properties as well as in lifetime. These differences allow the use of a single probe to label different membranes. Since Laurdan easily diffuses in cell cultures and tissues and is not fluorescent in the aqueous environment, its use is particularly simple in biological samples.

13.8 METHODS

13.8.1 Preparation of the GUVs

Phospholipids (from Avanti Polar, Alabama) were diluted with chloroform to a final concentration of 0.2 mg/ml. Two platinum wires attached to a Teflon chamber were coated with 2 μl of the lipid mixture and dried under N_2 (g). The water-jacketed chamber was sealed with a No. 1.5 coverslip and was attached to a circulating water bath according to the procedure from Ruan et al.[46] Phospholipids were rehydrated with 1 mM Tris, pH 7.4. The platinum wires were attached to a frequency generator with alternating current set to 10 Hz and 2 V. A thermocouple was used to monitor the temperature of the chamber.

13.8.2 NIH3T3 CELL CULTURES

NIH/3T3 (mouse fibroblast) cell line was purchased from Sigma-Aldrich. The cells were cultured in Dulbecco's Modified Eagle's Medium, supplemented with 1.5 g/L sodium bicarbonate, 10 mM HEPES, pH 7.4, 100 U/mL penicillin G, 100 L/g/mL streptomycin, and 10% fetal calf serum at 37°C in a humidified atmosphere consisting of 95% air and 5% CO_2. Cells were passaged by removing 90% of the supernatant and replacing it with fresh medium approximately twice a week and detachment using a 0.25% trypsin–EDTA solution. For FLIM experiments, the cells were scraped and plated on glass bottom dishes (MatTek, AshLand, USA) coated with 10 µg/ml poly-D-lysine (MP Biomedicals, California, USA) and 20 µg/ml laminin (Sigma-Aldrich), 1 day before the analysis.

13.8.3 FLIM ANALYSIS

FLIM data were acquired with a Zeiss LSM710 META laser scanning microscope, coupled to a 2-Photon Ti:sapphire laser (Spectra-Physics Mai Tai, Newport Beach, CA) producing 80 fs pulses at a repetition of 80 MHz and an ISS A320 FastFLIMBox (ISS Inc., Champaign, IL) for the lifetime data. A 40× water immersion objective 1.2 N.A. (Zeiss, Oberkochen, Germany) was used for all experiments. The excitation wavelength was set at 780 nm. An SP 760 nm dichroic filter was used to separate the fluorescence signal from the laser light. For FLIM data, the fluorescence signal was directed through a 495 LP filter and the signal was split between two photo-multiplier detectors (H7422P-40, Hamamatsu, Japan), with the following bandwidth filters in front of each: blue channel 460/40 and green 540/25, respectively. For image acquisition, the pixel frame size was set to 256 × 256 and the pixel dwell time was 25.61 µs/pixel. The average laser power at the sample was maintained at the milliwatt level.

13.8.4 SPECTRAL ANALYSIS

All images were taken using a Zeiss LSM710 spectral emission microscope equipped with a two-photon laser. Laurdan was excited at 780 nm and the spectral emission was collected at 9.4 nm bands centered between 421 and 723 nm. Each data set was collected at 256 × 256 pixels at 177 µs/pixel. For cell work, 3D z-stacks were taken at 1 µm or 0.6 µm z-section steps (range, between 20 and 40 slices).

ACKNOWLEDGMENT

Funding was provided by National Institutes of Health P50 GM076516, 27-8 P41 GM103540-27.

REFERENCES

1. Weber, G., and F. J. Farris. "Synthesis and Spectral Properties of a Hydrophobic Fluorescent Probe: 6-Propionyl-2-(Dimethylamino)Naphthalene." *Biochemistry* 18, no. 14 (1979): 3075–8.

2. Parasassi, T., G. De Stasio, A. d'Ubaldo, and E. Gratton. "Phase Fluctuation in Phospholipid Membranes Revealed by Laurdan Fluorescence." *Biophys J* 57, no. 6 (1990): 1179–86.

3. Parasassi, T., G. De Stasio, G. Ravagnan, R. M. Rusch, and E. Gratton. "Quantitation of Lipid Phases in Phospholipid Vesicles by the Generalized Polarization of Laurdan Fluorescence." *Biophys J* 60, no. 1 (1991): 179–89.

4. Parasassi, T., E. Gratton, W. M. Yu, P. Wilson, and M. Levi. "Two-Photon Fluorescence Microscopy of Laurdan Generalized Polarization Domains in Model and Natural Membranes." *Biophys J* 72, no. 6 (1997): 2413–29.

5. Bagatolli, L. A., and E. Gratton. "Two Photon Fluorescence Microscopy of Coexisting Lipid Domains in Giant Unilamellar Vesicles of Binary Phospholipid Mixtures." *Biophys J* 78, no. 1 (2000): 290–305.

6. Bagatolli, L. A. "Direct Observation of Lipid Domains in Free Standing Bilayers: From Simple to Complex Lipid Mixtures." *Chem Phys Lipids* 122, no. 1–2 (2003): 137–45.

7. Digman, M. A., V. R. Caiolfa, M. Zamai, and E. Gratton. "The Phasor Approach to Fluorescence Lifetime Imaging Analysis." *Biophys J* 94, no. 2 (2008): L14–6.

8. James, N. G., J. A. Ross, M. Stefl, and D. M. Jameson. "Applications of Phasor Plots to In Vitro Protein Studies." *Anal Biochem* 410, no. 1 (2011): 70–6.

9. Jameson, D. M., E. Gratton, and R. Hall. "The Measurement and Analysis of Heterogeneous Emissions by Multifrequency Phase and Modulation Fluorometry." *Appl Spectrosc Rev* 20, no. 1 (1984): 55–106.

10. Fereidouni, F., A. N. Bader, and H. C. Gerritsen. "Spectral Phasor Analysis Allows Rapid and Reliable Unmixing of Fluorescence Microscopy Spectral Images." *Opt Express* 20, no. 12 (2012): 12729–41.

11. Bagatolli, L. A., E. Gratton, and G. D. Fidelio. "Water Dynamics in Glycosphingolipid Aggregates Studied by Laurdan Fluorescence." *Biophys J* 75, no. 1 (1998): 331–41.

12. Bagatolli, L. A., T. Parasassi, G. D. Fidelio, and E. Gratton. "A Model for the Interaction of 6-Lauroyl-2-(N,N-Dimethylamino)Naphthalene with Lipid Environments: Implications for Spectral Properties." *Photochem Photobiol* 70, no. 4 (1999): 557–64.

13. Golfetto, O., E. Hinde, and E. Gratton. "Laurdan Fluorescence Lifetime Discriminates Cholesterol Content from Changes in Fluidity in Living Cell Membranes." *Biophys J* 104, no. 6 (2013): 1238–47.

14. Los, D. A., K. S. Mironov, and S. I. Allakhverdiev. "Regulatory Role of Membrane Fluidity in Gene Expression and Physiological Functions." *Photosynth Res* 116, no. 2–3 (2013): 489–509.

15. Lin, C., L. H. Wang, T. Y. Fan, and F. W. Kuo. "Lipid Content and Composition During the Oocyte Development of Two Gorgonian Coral Species in Relation to Low Temperature Preservation." *PLoS One* 7, no. 7 (2012): e38689.

16. Marguet, D., P. F. Lenne, H. Rigneault, and H. T. He. "Dynamics in the Plasma Membrane: How to Combine Fluidity and Order." *EMBO J* 25, no. 15 (2006): 3446–57.

17. Nozawa, Y., R. Kasai, Y. Kameyama, and K. Ohki. "Age-Dependent Modifications in Membrane Lipids: Lipid Composition, Fluidity and Palmitoyl-CoA Desaturase in Tetrahymena Membranes." *Biochim Biophys Acta* 599, no. 1 (1980): 232–45.

18. Quinn, P. J., and D. Chapman. "The Dynamics of Membrane Structure." *CRC Crit Rev Biochem* 8, no. 1 (1980): 1–117.

19. Wang, T. Y., and J. R. Silvius. "Sphingolipid Partitioning into Ordered Domains in Cholesterol-Free and Cholesterol-Containing Lipid Bilayers." *Biophys J* 84, no. 1 (2003): 367–78.

20. Weeks, G., and F. G. Herring. "The Lipid Composition and Membrane Fluidity of Dictyostelium Discoideum Plasma Membranes at Various Stages During Differentiation." *J Lipid Res* 21, no. 6 (1980): 681–6.

21. Wisniewska, A., J. Draus, and W. K. Subczynski. "Is a Fluid-Mosaic Model of Biological Membranes Fully Relevant? Studies on Lipid Organization in Model and Biological Membranes." *Cell Mol Biol Lett* 8, no. 1 (2003): 147–59.

22. Hashimoto, M., S. Hossain, and S. Masumura. "Effect of Aging on Plasma Membrane Fluidity of Rat Aortic Endothelial Cells." *Exp Gerontol* 34, no. 5 (1999): 687–98.

23. Hitzemann, R. J., and D. A. Johnson. "Developmental Changes in Synaptic Membrane Lipid Composition and Fluidity." *Neurochem Res* 8, no. 2 (1983): 121–31.

24. Ayuyan, A. G., and F. S. Cohen. "Raft Composition at Physiological Temperature and pH in the Absence of Detergents." *Biophys J* 94, no. 7 (2008): 2654–66.

25. Bakht, O., P. Pathak, and E. London. "Effect of the Structure of Lipids Favoring Disordered Domain Formation on the Stability of Cholesterol-Containing Ordered Domains (Lipid Rafts): Identification of Multiple Raft-Stabilization Mechanisms." *Biophys J* 93, no. 12 (2007): 4307–18.

26. Fan, J., M. Sammalkorpi, and M. Haataja. "Lipid Microdomains: Structural Correlations, Fluctuations, and Formation Mechanisms." *Phys Rev Lett* 104, no. 11 (2010): 118101.

27. Gallegos, A. M., S. M. Storey, A. B. Kier, F. Schroeder, and J. M. Ball. "Structure and Cholesterol Dynamics of Caveolae/Raft and Nonraft Plasma Membrane Domains." *Biochemistry* 45, no. 39 (2006): 12100–16.

28. Martinez-Seara, H., T. Rog, M. Pasenkiewicz-Gierula et al. "Interplay of Unsaturated Phospholipids and Cholesterol in Membranes: Effect of the Double-Bond Position." *Biophys J* 95, no. 7 (2008): 3295–305.

29. Maurya, S. R., D. Chaturvedi, and R. Mahalakshmi. "Modulating Lipid Dynamics and Membrane Fluidity to Drive Rapid Folding of a Transmembrane Barrel." *Sci Rep* 3 (2013): 1989.

30. Niemela, P. S., S. Ollila, M. T. Hyvonen, M. Karttunen, and I. Vattulainen. "Assessing the Nature of Lipid Raft Membranes." *PLoS Comput Biol* 3, no. 2 (2007): e34.

31. Sengupta, P., B. Baird, and D. Holowka. "Lipid Rafts, Fluid/Fluid Phase Separation, and Their Relevance to Plasma Membrane Structure and Function." *Semin Cell Dev Biol* 18, no. 5 (2007): 583–90.

32. Wassall, S. R., M. R. Brzustowicz, S. R. Shaikh et al. "Order from Disorder, Corralling Cholesterol with Chaotic Lipids. The Role of Polyunsaturated Lipids in Membrane Raft Formation." *Chem Phys Lipids* 132, no. 1 (2004): 79–88.

33. Kusumi, A., and K. Suzuki. "Toward Understanding the Dynamics of Membrane-Raft-Based Molecular Interactions." *Biochim Biophys Acta* 1746, no. 3 (2005): 234–51.

34. Sanchez, S. A., M. A. Tricerri, and E. Gratton. "Laurdan Generalized Polarization Fluctuations Measures Membrane Packing Micro-Heterogeneity In Vivo." *Proc Natl Acad Sci U S A* 109, no. 19 (2012): 7314–9.

35. Bagatolli, L. A., S. A. Sanchez, T. Hazlett, and E. Gratton. "Giant Vesicles, Laurdan, and Two-Photon Fluorescence Microscopy: Evidence of Lipid Lateral Separation in Bilayers." *Methods Enzymol* 360 (2003): 481–500.

36. Parasassi, T., and E. Gratton. "Membrane Lipid Domains and Dynamics as Detected by Laurdan Fluorescence." *J Fluoresc* 5, no. 1 (1995): 59–69.

37. Parasassi, T., M. Di Stefano, M. Loiero, G. Ravagnan, and E. Gratton. "Cholesterol Modifies Water Concentration and Dynamics in Phospholipid Bilayers: A Fluorescence Study Using Laurdan Probe." *Biophys J* 66, no. 3 Pt 1 (1994): 763–8.

38. Kantar, A., P. L. Giorgi, E. Gratton, and R. Fiorini. "Probing the Interaction of Paf with Human Platelet Membrane Using the Fluorescent Probe Laurdan." *Platelets* 5, no. 3 (1994): 145–8.

39. Parasassi, T., M. Di Stefano, M. Loiero, G. Ravagnan, and E. Gratton. "Influence of Cholesterol on Phospholipid Bilayers Phase Domains as Detected by Laurdan Fluorescence." *Biophys J* 66, no. 1 (1994): 120–32.

40. Fiorini, R., G. Curatola, A. Kantar, P. L. Giorgi, and E. Gratton. "Use of Laurdan Fluorescence in Studying Plasma Membrane Organization of Polymorphonuclear Leukocytes During the Respiratory Burst." *Photochem Photobiol* 57, no. 3 (1993): 438–41.

41. Levi, M., P. V. Wilson, O. J. Cooper, and E. Gratton. "Lipid Phases in Renal Brush Border Membranes Revealed by Laurdan Fluorescence." *Photochem Photobiol* 57, no. 3 (1993): 420–5.

42. Parasassi, T., G. Ravagnan, R. M. Rusch, and E. Gratton. "Modulation and Dynamics of Phase Properties in Phospholipid Mixtures Detected by Laurdan Fluorescence." *Photochem Photobiol* 57, no. 3 (1993): 403–10.

43. Parasassi, T., M. Di Stefano, G. Ravagnan, O. Sapora, and E. Gratton. "Membrane Aging During Cell Growth Ascertained by Laurdan Generalized Polarization." *Exp Cell Res* 202, no. 2 (1992): 432–9.

44. Parasassi, T., and E. Gratton. "Packing of Phospholipid Vesicles Studied by Oxygen Quenching of Laurdan Fluorescence." *J Fluoresc* 2, no. 3 (1992): 167–74.

45. Parasassi, T., F. Conti, and E. Gratton. "Time-Resolved Fluorescence Emission Spectra of Laurdan in Phospholipid Vesicles by Multifrequency Phase and Modulation Fluorometry." *Cell Mol Biol* 32, no. 1 (1986): 103–8.

46. Ruan, Q., M.A. Cheng, M. Levi, E. Gratton, and W. Mantulin. "Spatial-temporal studies of membrane dynamics: Scanning fluorescence correlation spectroscopy (SFCS)." Biophys J 87, no. 2 (2004): pp. 1260–1267. doi: 10.1529/biophysj.103.036483 PMCID: PMC1304464.

14 Development of Optical Highlighter Fluorescent Proteins and Their Applications in Super-Resolution Fluorescence Microscopy

Yan Fu and George H. Patterson

CONTENTS

14.1 INTRODUCTION

Among the vast number of fluorescent proteins (FPs) engineered from molecules discovered in various marine organisms, a set of FPs have been developed with distinct optical properties in that they are capable of pronounced changes in their chromophore structure or conformation within the protein and consequently their spectral properties in response to irradiation with light of a specific wavelength and intensity. Here, a general term, *optical highlighter*, is used to broadly describe these proteins, which are initially nonfluorescent or can be made nonfluorescent at the excited fluorescent wavelength and increase in fluorescence with contrast over a darker background upon light irradiation. These optical highlighting properties have been discovered in wild-type proteins or have been introduced into FPs by mutating selected residues in or near their chromophores to change their spectral properties and responses to light irradiation. Optical highlighter FPs have proved to be excellent tools for the precise optical labeling and tracking of proteins in cellular systems. They offer an alternative to photobleaching approaches in the study of protein kinetics, gene expression, organelle dynamics, and even cellular dynamics within living specimen. Moreover, optical highlighter FPs have stimulated the development of super-resolution microscopy techniques to provide key information about cellular structure and function that is otherwise unattainable.

In addition to their various spectral characteristics, optical highlighter FPs can be classified according to whether their spectral changes are irreversible or reversible upon light irradiation, and these generally fall into three main categories, which are termed *photoactivatable*, *photoconvertible*, and *photoswitchable*. The literature may be confusing to some readers since these terms have often been used interchangeably. This is unfortunate but unavoidable and readers are cautioned to pay close attention to each optical highlighter's spectral characteristics. For this chapter, the optical highlighters are defined as follows. Irreversible dark-to-bright photoactivatable FPs (PA-FPs) have little or no fluorescence in the inactivated state but easily undergo irreversible photoactivation after ultraviolet (UV) or near-UV light irradiation to produce enhanced fluorescent emission. Photoconvertible FPs (PC-FPs) are capable of irreversible photoconversion from one fluorescent color to another and of generating a high fluorescence contrast in the new color. Photoswitchable FPs (PS-FPs) are able to reversibly switch from dark to bright upon light irradiation. Here, we discuss the optical properties of several of these proteins and briefly discuss the proposed mechanisms of their highlighting properties.

In addition, we describe some of the examples of the applications of these molecules as they relate to super-resolution imaging techniques, such as reversible saturable optical fluorescence transitions (RESOLFT) microscopy and single molecule localization microscopy. Single molecule localization microscopy techniques have helped take fluorescence microscopy into the 50–100 nm and sometimes even better super-resolution realm. Numerous versions of these techniques have been published, which rely on both organically synthesized and often referred to as conventional fluorophores as well as many of the optical highlighter FPs discussed here. We limit our discussion to the optical highlighter FPs and methods relying on these proteins.

Interested readers are referred to elsewhere[1-3] for discussion of the use of conventional fluorophores in localization microscopy.

14.2 IRREVERSIBLE DARK-TO-BRIGHT PA-FPs

These proteins initially have little or no fluorescence when excited at their photoactivated spectral wavelengths. These generally have major changes in absorption, excitation, and emission spectra upon photoactivation and the structural changes involve covalent modifications that render the reaction essentially irreversible. This category contains one of the first PA-FPs that was engineered specifically to be an optical highlighter (Table 14.1), but development in this area has lagged behind others in the volume of new discoveries or newly engineered molecules.

14.2.1 IRREVERSIBLE GREEN PA-FPs

This category includes PAGFP,[4] a variant of the *Aequorea victoria* green FP (GFP); PAmRFP1[5,6] and PAmCherry, both variants of DsRed; PATagRFP,[7] a variant developed from TagRFP;[8] and PAmKate,[9] a protein based on mKate.[10] The original wild-type GFP (wtGFP) from *A. victoria* can perhaps be considered the first PA-FP[11] since it produces an approximately threefold increase in 488 nm excited fluorescence after irradiation with UV light (Figure 14.1).

The mechanism behind this holds that the wtGFP chromophore normally exists as a mixed population of neutral phenols (protonated) and anionic phenolates (deprotonated) producing the major 397 nm and minor 475 nm absorbance peaks, respectively.[12,13] UV or near-UV light irradiation changes this ratio in favor of the anionic form by decarboxylation of Glu-222, which results in the rearrangement of hydrogen bond network and chromophore deprotonation (Figure 14.2a and b). This leads to an increase of green fluorescent emission upon excitation in the blue spectral region (~475 or 488 nm, for example). Evidence for this mechanism has been produced by comparing the crystal structures of the preactivated and photoactivated states.[14] On the basis of this mechanism, one of the first engineered PA-FPs was developed mainly as a result of a single-residue substitution of histidine to threonine at position 203 (Thr203His) in wtGFP.[4] Upon photoactivation with violet or UV light (usually in the spectral region of ~400 nm), the absorption maximum of PAGFP is shifted from 400 to 504 nm, and this is accompanied by a 100-fold increase in fluorescence when exciting at 488 nm (Figure 14.2c and d). Follow-up structural analysis of PAGFP photoactivation also resulted in Glu-222 decarboxylation.[15] In addition, subsequent addition of folding enhancement mutations has improved PAGFP for use in neuronal protein trafficking.[16]

14.2.2 IRREVERSIBLE RED PA-FPs

Red PA-FPs (Table 14.1) were first derived from the monomeric red fluorescent protein mRFP1 that had been previously derived from DsRed.[17] Several versions were engineered, PAmRFP1-1, PAmRFP1-2, and PAmRFP1-3,[5] having their most important substitutions at positions 148, 165, and 203 (numbering is based on *A. victoria*

TABLE 14.1
Irreversible Dark-to-Bright PA-FPs

Name		Abs Max (nm)[a]	Extinction Coefficient ($M^{-1} cm^{-1}$)	λ_{max} Em (nm)	Quantum Yield	Brightness (%)[b]	pK_a	Contrast (-fold)	Irradiation Light (nm)[c]	Oligomeric State[d]	Source Organism, Protein	Reference
Irreversible Dark-to-Green PA-FP												
PAGFP	N	400	20,700	515	0.13	8	4.5	100	↓405	M	A. victoria (jellyfish), wtGFP	4
	G	504	17,400	517	0.79	42						
Irreversible Dark-to-Red PA-FP												
PAmCherry	N	404	6500				6.3	4000	↓405	M	Discosoma sp. (coral), mCherry	6
	R	564	18,000	595	0.46	20						
PAmRFP1	N	564			<0.001		4.4	70	↓405	M	Discosoma sp. (coral), mRFP1	5
	R		10,000	605	0.08	3						
PATagRFP	N	N/A					5.3	540	↓405	M	Entacmaea quadricolor (anemone), TagRFP	7
	R	562	66,000	595	0.38	25						
PAmKate	N	442					5.6	100	↓405	M	E. quadricolor (anemone), mKate	9
	R	568	25,000	628	0.18	11						

[a] N, G, and R denote nonfluorescent (off or dark state), green, and red fluorescent state, respectively.

[b] Brightness is determined by the product of the extinction coefficient and quantum yield. It is expressed here as a percentage of EGFP brightness.

[c] The arrow direction indicates the direction of the spectral alteration resulting from irradiation with the indicated wavelength of light (e.g., [N] nonfluorescent to [G] green).

[d] M, monomer.

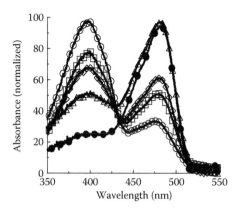

FIGURE 14.1 wtGFP from *A. victoria* undergoes a spectral shift in response to irradiation. Purified wtGFP protein was irradiated using 413 nm laser light in a cuvette and monitored by absorption spectroscopy at 0 min (open circles), 5 min (open squares), 10 min (open diamonds), 30 min (open triangles), and 60 min (filled circles). Over the course of the experiment, the major peak at ~400 nm decreases while the minor peak at ~475 nm increases.

GFP). The brightest, PAmRFP1-1, initially has weak fluorescence, but after its irreversible photoactivation at 380 nm, it results in an ~70-fold increase in red fluorescence with excitation and emission maxima at 578 nm and 605 nm, respectively.

Since PAmRFP1-1 lacks in brightness with a fluorescence quantum yield of only 0.08, this led to the development of PAmCherry.[6] PAmCherry1 was developed specifically for use in molecule localization experiments. It contains 10 amino acid residue substitutions compared with the parental mCherry sequence, and upon its irreversible photoactivation at 399 nm, it yields an ~4000-fold increase in red absorption with excitation and emission maxima at 564 and 594 nm, respectively (Figure 14.3a and b). On the basis of its crystal structure, the mechanism of PAmCherry photoactivation is thought to also require the decarboxylation of a glutamic acid (Glu-215) that is structurally equivalent to the *A. victoria* GFP Glu-222. UV light irradiation also results in the oxidation of the chromophore Tyr67 C_α–C_β bond, extending the π-conjugation of the chromophore to promote red fluorescence[18] (Figure 14.3c and d). Compared to PA-mRFP1-1, the PAmCherry features faster maturation, better pH stability, faster photoactivation, higher photoactivation contrast, and better photostability. These properties make PAmCherry a good red form for long-term visualization of the activated proteins and for dual-color super-resolution imaging.

Another development in the red part of the spectrum is PATagRFP,[7] which was engineered from monomeric TagRFP,[8] a bright red FP derived from Anthozoa species (corals and anemones). PATagRFP contains 12 substitutions compared with the parental TagRFP sequence, and after 405 nm light irradiation, PATagRFP results in an ~540-fold increase in red fluorescence with the excitation and emission maxima at 562 and 595 nm, respectively. In the activated state, PATagRFP has a threefold greater brightness than PAmCherry and also exhibits better pH stability and photostability. PATagRFP has slower photoactivation kinetics and red fluorescence photobleaching rate than found with PAmCherry. A crystal structure is currently

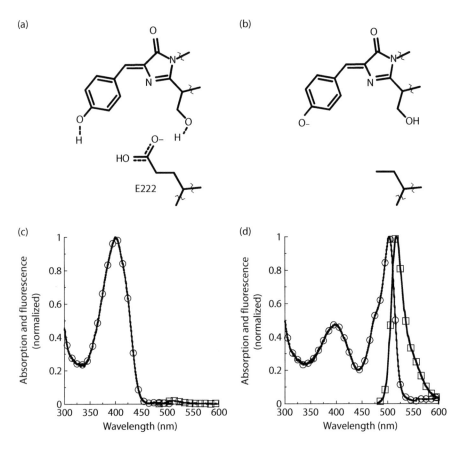

FIGURE 14.2 Photoactivation of green PA-FPs. (a) The chromophore of wtGFP and PAGFP is shown with the nearby Glu-222 (E222) amino acid side chain. The chromophore is protonated (neutral phenol) before photoactivation. (b) After photoactivation, the majority of the chromophore population is in an anionic form. A second important alteration is the decarboxylation of the Glu-222, which helps stabilize the anionic chromophore. (c) The absorption spectrum (open circles) and the fluorescence spectrum (open squares) of purified PAGFP in the pre-photoactivated form were measured before irradiation using 413 nm laser light. (d) The absorption spectrum (open circles) and the fluorescence spectrum (open squares) of purified PAGFP in the photoactivated form were measured after irradiation using 413 nm laser light. The fluorescence signal of the pre-photoactivated protein is normalized to the value of the post-photoactivated form.

unavailable, but it is hypothesized that the mechanism may be similar to PAGFP and PAmCherry at least with regard to a structurally equivalent glutamic acid (Glu-222). Spectroscopic analysis suggests that PATagRFP photoactivation is a two-step photochemical process involving sequential one-photon absorbance by two distinct chromophore forms.

Finally, in the constant pursuit of redder and better FPs, a photoactivatable version of the red-shifted protein mKate has been developed.[9] The protein was initially designed to mimic the crucial PAmCherry amino acid residues, subjected to random

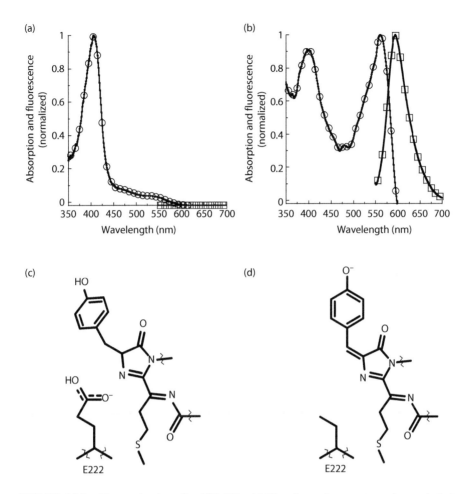

FIGURE 14.3 Photoactivation of red PA-FPs. (a) The absorption spectrum (open circles) and the fluorescence spectrum (open squares) of purified PAmCherry in the pre-photoactivated form were measured before irradiation using 405 nm laser light. (b) The absorption spectrum (open circles) and the fluorescence spectrum (open squares) of purified PAmCherry in the photoactivated form were measured after irradiation using 405 nm laser light. The fluorescence signal of the pre-photoactivated protein is normalized to the value of the post-photoactivated form. (c) Similar to PAGFP, the chromophore of PAmCherry is shown with the nearby Glu-222 (E222) amino acid side chain. The chromophore is protonated (neutral phenol) before photoactivation. However, after the cyclization reaction common to all FPs, the C_α and N bond of the methionine is the location of the first oxidation step instead of between the C_α and C_β of the tyrosine residue in the chromophore. A nonplanar chromophore, almost trans conformation is adopted. (d) Irradiation at ~400 nm results in glutamic acid decarboxylation, which is similar to PAGFP, but another difference is that the second oxidation reaction then occurs at the tyrosine position between C_α and C_β. After photoactivation, the majority of the chromophore population is in an anionic form, but in an uncommon trans configuration.

mutagenesis, and screened for 405 nm induced far-red emission. The final protein, PAmKate, has a major absorption peak at 442 nm before photoactivation and a 586 nm peak afterward. Excitation produces emission peaking at 628 nm, much shifted compared to PAmCherry or PATagRFP. In addition, PAmKate is more photostable and less pH sensitive than PAmCherry.

14.3   IRREVERSIBLE PC-FPs

The PC-FPs make up a large and diverse category, and these molecules have the defining characteristic of initially being produced as proteins emitting one color that can then be irreversibly photoconverted to the another fluorescent form upon near-UV light illumination (Table 14.2). These are described in Sections 14.3.1–14.3.3 in three major spectral range changes: cyan to green, green to red, and orange to far red.

14.3.1   IRREVERSIBLE CYAN-TO-GREEN PC-FP

Photoswitchable cyan fluorescent protein (PS-CFP)[19] was developed from a GFP-like protein aceGFP[20] (a fluorescent mutant of monomeric colorless jellyfish *Aequorea coerulescens* protein). It initially displays cyan fluorescence with an excitation peak at 402 nm and an emission peak at 468 nm. In response to intense 405 nm light irradiation, PS-CFP photoconverts into a green form with an excitation peak at 490 nm and a 300-fold increase in fluorescence emission at 511 nm (Figure 14.4a and b). The decrease in the cyan fluorescence is approximately fivefold and allows ratiometric analysis, an advantageous characteristic for PC-FPs. Readers should note that PS-CFP represents one of the examples that may be particularly confusing since it has the name "photoswitchable," but it displays the characteristics of a PC-FP under the definition given earlier. Moreover, the proposed mechanism of PS-CFP photoconversion is similar to PA-GFP, based on decarboxylation of the Glu-222 (the equivalent of the *A. victoria* Glu-222) residue, which results in the reorganization of hydrogen bond network and stabilization of a deprotonated chromophore (Figure 14.2a and b). An enhanced version, PS-CFP2, has been developed by Evrogen (Moscow, Russia) with faster maturation and brighter fluorescence both before and after photoconversion.

14.3.2   IRREVERSIBLE GREEN-TO-RED PC-FP

Often surprising to many is that a green-to-red photoconversion phenomenon was discovered very early after the advent of GFP. Several variants of the *A. victoria* GFP were found to undergo a spectral shift into a red form upon 488 nm irradiation with the stipulation that the environmental oxygen levels be low.[21,22] This phenomenon was found to be enhanced with the commonly used EGFP variant when riboflavin was added to the oxygen scavenged environment.[23] However, EGFP green-to-red photoconversion was eventually found to occur in the presence of oxygen with the addition of electron acceptors.[24] It was even found to occur in live mammalian cell lines. A proposed mechanism for this photoconversion is not well described, but

TABLE 14.2
Irreversible PC-FPs

Name		Abs Max (nm)[a]	Extinction Coefficient (M⁻¹ cm⁻¹)	λ_{max} Em (nm)	Quantum Yield	Brightness (%)[b]	pK_a	Contrast (-fold)	Irradiation Light (nm)[c]	Oligomeric State[d]	Source Organism, Protein	Reference
						Irreversible Cyan-to-Green PC-FP						
PS-CFP	C	402	34,000	468	0.16	16	4.0	1500 green/cyan	↓405	M	A. coerulescens (jellyfish), aceGFP	19
	G	490	27,000	511	0.19	15	6.0					
PS-CFP2	C	400	43,000	470	0.20	26	4.3	2000	↓405	M	A. coerulescens (jellyfish), PS-CFP	Evrogen
	G	490	47,000	511	0.23	33	6.1					
						Irreversible Green-to-Red PC-FP						
Kaede	G	508	98,800	518	0.80	264	5.6	2000 red/green	↓405	T	T. geoffroyi (coral)	25
	R	572	60,400	582	0.33	60	5.6					
KikGR	G	507	28,200	517	0.70	112	7.8	2000 red/green	↓405	T	Favia favus (coral)	26
	R	583	32,600	593	0.65	68	5.5					
mKikGR	G	505	49,000	515	0.69	101	6.6	2000	↓405	M	F. favus (coral), KikGR	27
	R	580	28,000	591	0.63	53	5.2					
EosFP	G	506	72,000	516	0.70	150		2000	↓405	T	L. hemprichii (coral)	28
	R	571	41,000	581	0.55	67						
mEosFP	G	505	67,200	516	0.64	128	5.5		↓405	M	L. hemprichii (coral), EosFP	28
	R	569	37,000	581	0.62	68	5.5					
tdEosFP	G	506	84,000	516	0.66	165	5.5	200	↓405	TD	L. hemprichii (coral), EosFP	29
	R	571	33,000	581	0.60	59	5.5					

(continued)

TABLE 14.2 (Continued)
Irreversible PC-FPs

Name		Abs Max (nm)[a]	Extinction Coefficient (M⁻¹ cm⁻¹)	λ_{max} Em (nm)	Quantum Yield	Brightness (%)[b]	pK_a	Contrast (-fold)	Irradiation Light (nm)[c]	Oligomeric State[d]	Source Organism, Protein	Reference
dEosFP	G	506	84,000	516	0.66	165			↓405	D	L. hemprichii (coral), EosFP	28
	R	569	33,000	581	0.60	59						
mEos2	G	506	56,000	519	0.84	140	5.6		↓405	M	L. hemprichii (coral), EosFP	30
	R	573	46,000	584	0.66	90	6.4					
mEos3.1	G	505	88,400	513	0.83	256	5.2		↓405	M	L. hemprichii (coral), mEos2	31
	R	570	33,500	580	0.62	63	6.0					
mEos3.2	G	507	63,400	516	0.84	158	5.4		↓405	M	L. hemprichii (coral), mEos2	31
	R	572	32,200	580	0.55	54	5.8					
Dendra	G	486	21,000	505	0.72	44	6.6	4500 red/green	↓405 or 488	M	Dendronephthya sp. (octocoral)	32
	R	558	20,000	575	0.70	43	6.9					
Dendra2	G	490	45,000	507	0.50	67	6.6	300	↓405 or 488	M	Dendronephthya sp. (octocoral), Dendra	Evrogen
	R	553	35,000	573	0.55	57	6.9					

mClavGR1	G	486	16,000	503	0.84	42	8.0		↓405	M	Clavularia sp. (coral), mTFP1	33
	R	565	21,000	582	0.56	36	7.4					
mClavGR2	G	488	19,000	504	0.77	45	8.0		↓405	M	Clavularia sp. (coral), mClavGR1	33
	R	566	32,000	583	0.53	51	7.3					
mMaple	G	489	15,000	505	0.74	33	8.2		↓405	M	Clavularia sp. (coral), mClavGR2	34
	R	566	30,000	583	0.56	51	7.3					
Irreversible Orange-to-Far-Red PC-FP												
PSmOrange	O	548	113,300	635	0.51	176	6.2	560	↓488	M	Discosoma sp. (coral), mOrange	35
	fR	565	32,700	662	0.28	28	5.6					

[a] C, G, R, O, and fR denote cyan, green, red, orange, and far-red fluorescent state, respectively.

[b] Brightness is determined by the product of the extinction coefficient and quantum yield. It is expressed here as a percentage of EGFP brightness.

[c] The arrow direction indicates the direction of the spectral alteration resulting from irradiation with the indicated wavelength of light (e.g., [G] green to [R] red).

[d] M, monomer; D, dimer; TD, tandem dimer; T, tetramer.

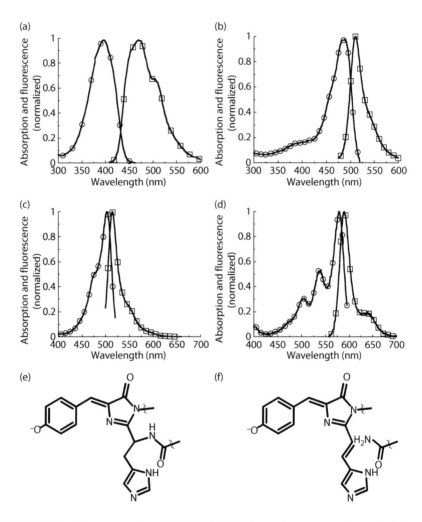

FIGURE 14.4 Photoconversion of PC-FPs. (a) The absorption spectrum (open circles) and the fluorescence spectrum (open squares) of purified PS-CFP in the pre-photoconverted form were measured before irradiation using 405 nm laser light. (b) The absorption spectrum (open circles) and the fluorescence spectrum (open squares) of purified PS-CFP in the photoconverted form were measured after irradiation using 405 nm laser light. The mechanism for PS-CFP photoconversion is hypothesized to be similar to PAGFP. (c) The absorption spectrum (open circles) and the fluorescence spectrum (open squares) of purified KikGR in the pre-photoconverted form were measured before irradiation using 405 nm laser light. (d) The absorption spectrum (open circles) and the fluorescence spectrum (open squares) of purified KikGR in the photoconverted form were measured after irradiation using 405 nm laser light. (e) The pre-photoconverted KikGR has a chromophore population made up of neutral phenol forms (not shown) and a majority anionic phenolate form similar to the photoactivated chromophore of PAGFP. (f) Irradiation at 405 nm results in extension of the π-conjugation at the histidine amino acid side-chain C_α–C_β bond, which leads to red-shifted absorption and fluorescence spectra as observed in (d).

it has been suggested that a tyrosine in the 66 position (*A. victoria* numbering) or equivalent is necessary.

More widely known are irreversible green-to-red PC-FPs (Table 14.2) that were discovered to be naturally photoconvertible, such as Kaede,[25] or were engineered to display this characteristic, such as KikGR[26] (Figure 14.4c and d). Kaede[25] was derived from a stony coral, *Trachyphyllia geoffroyi*. Kaede initially displays green fluorescence with excitation peaking at 508 nm and emission peaking at 518 nm. Serendipitously, Kaede was found to change to a red form after a purified protein sample was left on a laboratory bench in bright sunlight. Subsequent tests showed that upon irradiation with UV or near-UV light, Kaede undergoes photoconversion exhibiting red fluorescence with excitation peaking at 572 nm and emission peaking at 582 nm. This shift in both excitation and emission peaks results in a more than 2000-fold increase in the red-to-green fluorescence ratio. Unfortunately, Kaede forms tetramers, which limit its usefulness as a protein trafficking tool in the cell. Nevertheless, Kaede's large contrast with background after photoconversion makes it an excellent cell tracking marker in developing organisms.[36,37]

Kaede photoconversion is hypothesized to occur after excitation of the protonated form (Figure 14.4e) of the central chromophore by irradiation with UV or violet light. Structural studies show that this leads to a cleavage of a C_α–N bond[38] (Figure 14.4f). The C_α in this case is part of the histidine in the N terminal position of the three amino acids making up the chromophore. A second important modification is the formation of a double bond between the C_α and C_β of that histidine (Figure 14.4f), which extends the π-conjugation and ultimately red-shifts the excitation and emission spectra. This mechanism is thought to be common to several of the PC-FPs discussed below.

KikGR[26] was developed from the coral *Favia favus* protein, KikG, by engineering it based on the structure[38] of the previously discovered Kaede. KikGR initially displays green fluorescence with two principal peaks at 390 and 507 nm, and after irradiation with UV or violet light, it converts to red fluorescent form showing an emission peak at 593 nm and two absorption peaks at 360 and 583 nm (Figure 14.4c and d). Similar to Kaede, photoconversion of KikGR is highly dependent on irradiation wavelength (350–420 nm) and pH (efficient at lower pH); the photoconversion was hypothesized to initiate from excitation of the neutral chromophore form. From a comparative analysis with Kaede in a biological application, KikGR was found to show an approximately threefold faster photoconversion and higher red-to-green fluorescence ratio in cells than Kaede. KikGR was also found to be a tetramer. However, the monomeric version, mKikGR,[27] is now available, which expands the use of this highlighter in cell biology applications.

The green-to-red PC-FP, Dendra,[32] was cloned from octocoral *Dendronephthya* sp. It undergoes photoconversion from green fluorescence with excitation peaking at 486 nm and emission peaking at 505 nm to red fluorescence with excitation and emission maxima at 558 and 575 nm, respectively. Dendra yields a 4500-fold photoconversion from its green-to-red fluorescent forms. Dendra can be photoactivated with irradiation with an ~400 nm light, but in contrast to most of the proteins discussed here, it also allows the option of activation with a potentially less phototoxic wavelength (~488 nm). High intensity of 488 nm laser power is required to cause photoconversion, and even prolonged scanning with 488 nm light density below 50 mW/cm^2 did not result in green-to-red photoconversion. An improved version, Dendra2, is commercially available from Evrogen, providing an improvement in folding efficiency at 37°C.

The fluorescent protein EosFP[28] from the stony coral *Lobophyllia hemprichii* has led to the development of several PC-FP variations. It initially shows green fluorescence with excitation peaking at 506 nm and emission peaking at 516 nm. Upon activation at 400 nm, EosFP photoconverts to a red FP with the excitation peak at 571 nm and the emission peak at 581 nm. The original EosFP is a tetramer; however, it was engineered into two dimeric forms, d1EosFP and d2EosFP, and then a monomeric molecule, mEosFP. The emission maxima of these mutants remain constant, whereas the excitation maxima and brightness change slightly. mEosFP inefficiently forms a fluorescent molecule when expressed at 37°C, and its application is better suited for temperatures below 30°C. A tandem dimer[29] with two EosFP subunits connected by a flexible 12-amino-acid linker (tdEosFP) has also been engineered and has a good expression in cells at 37°C. Since having twice the size can affect the super-resolution imaging localization accuracy, efforts were made to further develop the mEosFP into an improved protein, mEos2.[30] At the time of its introduction, mEos2 was one of the brightest optical highlighter FPs. It has good photostability compared to other PA-FPs and PC-FPs and provides localization precisions in photoactivated localization microscopy (PALM) imaging on the order of ~10 nm. This version has been further developed into mEos3,[31] which has slightly better photon statistics and has less tendency to dimerize at high concentrations.

In a development similar to that of KikGR, a PC-FP named mMaple[34] was engineered from a conventional FP, monomeric teal FP1 (mTFP1). Positions of interest in the mTFP1 were converted to consensus residues, which were determined using sequence alignments of EosFP, Dendra2, KikGR, and Kaede. This simple step was enough to create a green protein, mClavGR1 (monomeric clavularia-derived green-to-red photoconvertible 1),[33] which could convert from green to red in the presence of white light. After being subjected to several rounds of mutagenesis, an improved variant, mClavGR2, was derived. This protein had good photostability compared to other PC-FPs, and its brightness in the photoconverted form was similar to that of Dendra2 and mKikGR, but it had very high pK_a (8.0 green and 7.3 red). The third generation, mMaple, still has a high pK_a but has the best green state photostability of the PC-FPs. This is an advantage when performing both structured illumination microscopy[39] and molecule localization on the same specimen, for which the mMaple was designed.

14.3.3 Irreversible Orange-to-Far-Red PC-FP

It has become clear that photoconversion in FPs is not such a rare characteristic. In fact, several common conventional green[21–24] and red FPs[40] have been found to undergo irradiation-induced spectral alterations. The findings with the red and orange molecules, Katushka, mKate, HcRed1, mOrange1, and mOrange2,[40] inspired development of PSmOrange (photoswitchable mOrange).[35] On the basis of the photoconversion of mOrange from an orange to a far-red emitting protein upon irradiation at 488 nm, the PSmOrange protein (Table 14.2) has an emission peak at 662 nm and currently represents the most red-shifted version of the optical highlighters. It has an excitation maximum in the photoconverted form at 635 nm, which fits well with a number of laser lines in this spectral range. The red shifts in the photoconversion, excitation, and emission wavelengths are particularly important since this readily allows use of blue lasers for photoconversion and red lasers for imaging in tissue where light scattering becomes limiting.

14.4   REVERSIBLE PS-FPs

Because of the covalent modifications such as glutamic acid decarboxylation or peptide backbone breakage, photoactivatable and photoconvertible reactions are generally considered irreversible and thus can occur only once. This is the major difference from PS-FPs since the proteins in this category display the capability of being reversibly switched "on" and switched "off" repeatedly by illumination at different wavelengths (Table 14.3). Thus, these allow repeated measurements with the same molecules.

Light-driven photoswitching in FPs was observed with *A. victoria* variants using single-molecule imaging by turning them on or off with 405 and 488 nm light, respectively.[41] Similarly, fluorescence correlation spectroscopy discovered rapid flickering events that were light driven to both on and off states.[42–44] However, photoswitching behavior was not well documented in bulk FP samples or widely utilized until the introduction of asFP595,[45] a protein isolated from the tentacle tips of sea anemone, *Anemonia sulcata*. Subsequent development of KFP1 from asFP595[46] and eventually the discovery of Dronpa from the stony coral, *Pectiniidae*,[47] proved to be major catalysts for an enormous amount of optical highlighter development, specifically in the PS-FP category.

14.4.1   REVERSIBLE DARK-TO-GREEN PS-FP

Dronpa was discovered in a cDNA screen of *Pectiniidae* and was found to be efficiently and repeatedly switched "off" and "on".[47] It initially displays green fluorescence with the absorbance maximum at 503 nm and emission maximum at 518 nm. With intense irradiation at 490 nm, the absorbance at 503 nm and the green fluorescence emission are decreased (Figure 14.5a). However, after weak irradiation at 400 nm, the 503 nm absorbance and the green fluorescence emission are rapidly restored (Figure 14.5b). Remarkably, the "off" state of Dronpa was found to be thermally stable with a $t_{1/2}$ of 840 min for returning to the on state in the absence of ~400 nm light. The "off" state structure of the chromophore has been proposed to be one of two slightly different configurations, a trans conformation with a protonated tyrosine form in the chromophore[48] (Figure 14.5c) or a nonplanar flexible chromophore with a protonated tyrosine along with a flexible portion of the β-barrel near the hydroxyl group of the tyrosines.[49,50] The disordered excited chromophore is considered to be more prone to nonradiative decay and therefore produces little to no fluorescence. Thus far, proposed structures for the "on" state suggest a deprotonated tyrosine in a chromophore in the cis isomerization (Figure 14.5d).[48–50]

TABLE 14.3
Reversible PS-FPs

Name		Abs Max (nm)[a]	Extinction Coefficient (M⁻¹ cm⁻¹)	λ_{max} Em (nm)	Quantum Yield	Brightness (%)[b]	pK_a	Contrast (-fold)	Irradiation Light (nm)[c]	Oligomeric State[d]	Source Organism, Protein	Reference
						Reversible Dark-to-Green PS-FP						
Dronpa	N	392						17	↓405	M	*Pectiniidae* (coral), 22G	47
	G	503	95,000	518	0.85	240	5.0		↑488			
Dronpa2	N								↓405	M	*Pectiniidae* (coral), Dronpa	51
	G	486	58,000	514	0.33	47			↑488			
Dronpa3	N								↓405	M	*Pectiniidae* (coral), Dronpa	51
	G	487	56,000	514	0.28	57			↑488			
rsFastLime	N	384						67	↓405	M	*Pectiniidae* (coral), Dronpa	52
	G	496	39,094	518	0.77	94			↑488			
bsDronpa	N	385						17	↓405	M	*Pectiniidae* (coral), Dronpa	53
	G	460	45,000	504	0.50	67			↑488			
Padron	N	505						143	↓488	M	*Pectiniidae* (coral), Dronpa	53
	G	503	43,000	522	0.64	82			↑405			
mGeos (a series)	N							20	↓405	M	*L. hemprichii* (coral), mEos2	54
	G	501–505	52,000–77,000	512–519	0.72–0.85		4.5–6.5		↑488			

Dreiklang	N	340							↓365	M	*A. victoria* (jellyfish), Citrine	55
	G	511	83,000	0.41	529	101	7.2	75	↑405			
rsEGFP	N	396							↓405	M	*A. victoria* (jellyfish), EGFP	56
	G	491	47,000	0.36	510	50	6.5		↑488			
rsEGFP2	N	408							↓405	M	*A. victoria* (jellyfish), EGFP	57
	G	478	61,300	0.3	503	44	5.8		↑488			
Reversible Dark-to-Red PS-FP												
asFP595	N	572	56,200	<0.001	595	<0.001			↓568	T	*A. sulcata* (anemone)	45
	R	572			595				↑450			
KFP1	N	580	123,000	<0.001	600	0.4		30	↓532	T	*A. sulcata* (anemone), asFP595	46
	R	580	59,000	0.07	600	13			↑458			
rsCherry	N	572							↓561	M	*Discosoma* sp. (coral), mCherry	58
	R	572	80,000	0.02	610	1.3	6.0	6.7	↑470			
rsCherryRev	N	572							↓470	M	*Discosoma* sp. (coral), mCherry	58
	R	572	84,000	0.005	608	5	5.5	20	↑546			
rsTagRFP	N	440	15,300	0.0013	585	0.5			↓470	M	*E. quadricolor* (anemone), TagRFP	59
	R	567	36,800	0.11	585	92	6.6	133	↑546			

a N, G, and R denote nonfluorescent (off or dark state), green, and red fluorescent state, respectively.

b Brightness is determined by the product of the extinction coefficient and quantum yield. It is expressed here as a percentage of EGFP brightness.

c The arrow direction indicates the direction of the spectral alteration resulting from irradiation with the indicated wavelength of light (e.g., [N] nonfluorescent to [G] green).

d M, monomer; T, tetramer.

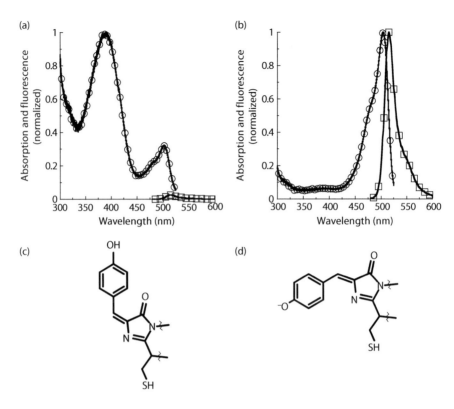

FIGURE 14.5 Photoswitching in PS-FPs. (a) The absorption spectrum (open circles) and the fluorescence spectrum (open squares) of purified Dronpa were measured after irradiation at 491 nm to push the chromophore population into the "off" state. (b) The absorption spectrum (open circles) and the fluorescence spectrum (open squares) of purified Dronpa in the photoswitched "on" form were measured after brief irradiation using 405 nm laser light. The fluorescence signal of the "off" state protein (a) is normalized to the value of the "on" state form (b). (c) Unlike PA-FPs and PC-FPs, structural alterations associated with PS-FPs are generally not covalent modifications. One mechanism for the Dronpa "off" state holds that the chromophore population consists mainly of the trans conformation, which is nonfluorescent. (d) The "on" state is predicted to have a deprotonated tyrosine in the chromophore in the cis conformation.

These changes allow Dronpa and similar PS-FPs to undergo the on–off cycling many times (Figure 14.6), albeit often with a limited number of cycles before photodestruction becomes limiting. In imaging experiments, the reversible nature of the fluorescence allows the same photoswitching experiment to be repeated multiple times within the same region of interest. Because it is monomeric and displays bright green fluorescence with high quantum yield, Dronpa has been used in a number of cell biology applications including super-resolution imaging as discussed later.

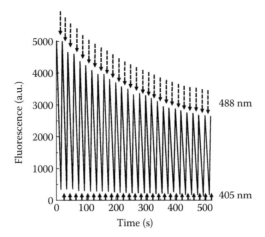

FIGURE 14.6 Dronpa photoswitching. Purified His_6-tagged Dronpa attached to an antibody (anti-His_6 tag)-coated coverslip was imaged with 488 nm excitation while alternately irradiating with higher levels of 488 nm to turn it "off" (dashed line arrows) or 405 nm light (solid line arrows) to turn it back "on".

Dronpa has also undergone numerous alterations (Table 14.3) to produce several variants. Dronpa2 and Dronpa3[51] were found to photoswitch off much more efficiently than the original by illumination at 490 nm. However, their off states were not thermally stable and Dronpa2 and Dronpa3 quickly returned to their emissive states with green fluorescence after an intense 490 nm light was turned off. Imaging experiments performed with a simultaneous scan using both 400 and 490 nm light was required to highlight the target subcellular structures with the FPs oscillating between their bright and dark states. The rsFastLime variant has a single point mutation (Val157Gly) compared with Dronpa,[52] which makes it more efficient in photoswitching to both its "on" and "off" states. The bsDronpa variant[53] has a broad on-state absorption spectrum that is blue-shifted ~44 nm compared with Dronpa and the other variants. Another mutant, Padron,[53] shows photoswitching under opposite irradiation protocols by being turned "on" by irradiation with 488 nm light and "off" by irradiation with 405 nm light. Padron maintains brightness of Dronpa but has the switching speed of rsFastLime. Moreover, it had a highest on-to-off fluorescence ratio of 150 among Dronpa variants (Dronpa, 17; rsFastLime, 67; and bsDronpa, 17). In addition to protein tracking, Dronpa and some of its derivatives, rsFastLime and Padron, have also shown their utility in super-resolution molecular localization experiments (see the molecule localization discussions later).

A series of PS-FPs named mGeos was derived from mutagenesis of EosFP at a single position in the chromophore.[54] Converting the histidine at position 62 of mEos2 to one of several amino acids eliminated the green-to-red photoconversion and introduced a photoswitching behavior while in the green state. These displayed a wide range of values in the characteristics important for a PS-FP. Initially, photoswitching "off" was slow, but an additional mutation, Phe173Ser, in the context of a cysteine, glutamic acid, phenylalanine, leucine, or methionine at position 62, increased the off-switching rates. The mutants displayed a wide range of photoswitching rates, brightnesses, and photostabilities, and while all are less bright than Dronpa, most photoswitch even faster than rsFastLime, a fast-switching derivative of Dronpa.

The protein Dreiklang[55] evolved from the yellow FP Citrine, a derivative of GFP. Dreiklang initially displays yellow-green fluorescence with the excitation maximum at 511 nm and the emission maximum at 529 nm. Irradiation at 405 nm light switches the protein to a nonfluorescent off state while illumination at 365 nm is required to switch it back into the on state. Unlike other PS-FPs, the wavelength used for generating the fluorescence emission is not identical to the wavelength used for switching the fluorescence on or off, which avoids a complex interlocking of switching and fluorescence readout during the imaging experiment. Mass spectrometry and high-resolution crystallographic analysis of the same protein crystal in the photoswitched on and off states demonstrate that switching is based on a reversible hydration/dehydration reaction that modifies the chromophore.[55] Dreiklang is a monomer and has been shown to achieve an average localization precision of ~15 nm in super-resolution imaging experiments.

This area of development has been advanced with the commonly used EGFP variant being converted into a PS-FP. The protein rsEGFP[56] can be reversibly switched "on" at 405 nm and "off" at 491 nm. It initially displays bright green fluorescence with a single absorption band peaking at 491 nm and an emission maximum peaking at 510 nm. Irradiation with 490 nm light decreases the rsEGFP fluorescence and results in an off state with a single absorption band at 396 nm, corresponding to the neutral state of the chromophore. Irradiation of the off-state rsEGFP with ~405 nm light switches the protein back to the on state. Compared to Dronpa, rsEGFP displays more than 10 times faster switchable rate and can undergo ~120× more cycles before reaching the same level of photodestruction. The mechanism of reversibly switching is believed to be associated with the ionization state of the chromophore, where on state corresponds to the ionized state of the phenolic hydroxyl of the chromophore and off state corresponds to the neutral state of the chromophore. The rsEGFP variant has been further developed into rsEGFP2, which has a photoswitching rate 25–250 times faster than rsEGFP.[57] Both have been instrumental in further development of super-resolution imaging techniques as discussed later.

14.4.2 Reversible Dark-to-Red PS-FP

The first phenomenon in a red form of reversible and switchable from "on" and "off" state (Table 14.3) was observed with asFP595.[45] The asFP595 protein initially displays red fluorescence with the absorbance maximum at 572 nm and emission maximum at 595 nm. The weak red fluorescence can be enhanced by exposure to green light and quenched by exposure to blue light. Because asFP595 is a tetramer, has a low fluorescence quantum yield, and matures slowly, it has been used sparingly as a marker. One asFP595 variant, KFP1,[46] was introduced as a PS-FP that has the capability to be reversibly or irreversibly photoswitched from dark to bright fluorescence. KFP1 initially exhibits little red fluorescence, but activation with 532 nm laser light increases its red fluorescence by approximately 30-fold with the excitation maximum at 580 nm and the emission maximum at 600 nm. The reversibility of KFP1 depends on the irradiation intensity and duration. For reversible photoswitching, a lower level (approximately 1 W/cm^2 for 2 min) of 532 nm laser irradiation produced red KFP1 fluorescence that relaxed to the nonfluorescent state with a half-time of approximately 50 s, whereas a high level (approximately 20 W/cm^2 for 20 min) of 532 nm laser irradiation irreversibly photoactivates approximately 50% of the population. However, KFP1 has tetrameric oligomerization, slow maturation, and an on-state quantum yield of 0.07, all of which limit its use as a marker.

Other red PS-FPs (Table 14.3) include two variants of mCherry, rsCherry and rsCherryRev,[58] which emit red fluorescence but display opposite switching modes. These molecules are switched back and forth between "on" and "off" states using red and green/yellow light. The rsCherry behaves similarly to Padron in that the more red-shifted irradiation (561 nm) turns it "on" whereas the more blue-shifted irradiation (470 nm) turns it "off". In the fluorescence-on state, rsCherry exhibits an absorption peak at 572 nm and emits at 610 nm. Irradiation with light of a wavelength (561 nm) that induces fluorescence converts the protein from the off to the on state, whereas irradiation with a shorter wavelength (450–470 nm) converts it from the on to the off state. However, follow-up analysis using Hg^{2+} arc lamp irradiation for switching found that rsCherry eventually switched its cycle dependence on wavelength of irradiation to a process similar to Dronpa or rsCherryRev. In the fluorescence-on state, rsCherryRev has an absorption peak at 572 nm and emission at 608 nm. Irradiation with 546 nm light switches rsCherryRev from "on" to "off," whereas irradiation with 470 nm light transfers rsCherryRev into on state. Because an ensemble of rsCherry molecules exhibits a residual fluorescence signal after switching off that corresponds to ~15% of its maximum signal, rsCherryRev, because of its more favorable dynamic range between the on and the off state, may be more suitable for most imaging applications that rely on photoswitching with good contrast.

Given its brightness, utility for imaging, and development into a photoactivatable form,[7] the TagRFP molecule[8] was another promising candidate for PS-FP development. The final result, rsTagRFP[59] (Table 14.3), is produced as a red FP with a major absorption peak at 567 nm and a minor peak at 440 nm. Excitation at either peak produces emission (brightness is wavelength dependent) peaking at 585 nm. Irradiation in the yellow region of the spectrum shifts the spectrum such that the major peak is 440 nm and the minor peak is 567 nm. Photoswitching "on" is accomplished by irradiation in the 440 nm region of the spectrum. A key feature of rsTagRFP is that the spectral changes during photoswitching are evident in the absorption spectra. This makes a photoswitchable version in the red region of the spectrum, a technique known as photoquenching fluorescence resonance energy transfer (PQ-FRET),[60] possible. In this technique, a more blue-shifted molecule, EYFP, has an emission spectrum that overlaps well with the absorption spectrum of the "on" rsTagRFP. FRET efficiency between fluorophores depends not only on their proximity but also on the overlap integral of the donor emission and acceptor absorption. Since the absorption spectrum of rsTagRFP changes depending on its "on" and "off" states, the overlap integral increases and decreases, respectively. Thus, a reversible, modulatable FRET acceptor results from the development of this PS-FP.

14.5 PHOTOCONVERTIBLE/PHOTOSWITCHABLE FLUORESCENT PROTEINS

Finally, we discuss a new class of unique green-to-red PC-FPs that display photoswitchable behavior in their native, nonphotoconverted green state as well as their photoconverted red state (Table 14.4). The first of these is IrisFP,[61] a derivative of the tetrameric form of EosFP. It can be irreversibly photoconverted just as EosFP upon irradiation with 405 nm light and also joins the photoswitchable category by having the capability to photoswitch between "off" and "on" states. Illumination of IrisFP by 488 nm light leads Iris to switch from "on" to "off" in the green form and recover to the "on" state slowly ($t_{1/2}$ = 5.5 h), which can be strongly accelerated by illuminating with 405 nm light. After photoconversion to the red form, Iris FP decreases in red fluorescence after illumination with 532 nm light and the dark form slowly reverts to the red state ($t_{1/2}$ = 3.2 h). Similar to many other red PS-FPs, the return is strongly accelerated by exposure to light in the 440 nm spectral range. Since IrisFP was developed from the tetrameric form of EosFP, its usefulness in protein trafficking and molecule localization experiments was deemed limited and spawned improvement into monomeric IrisFP (mIrisFP).[62] The mIrisFP was used in pulse chase experiments combined with molecule localization in which molecules could be tracked as a defined population in a specific cellular region and imaged at super-resolution detail, marked for trafficking studies by photoconversion into a red form and then imaged again at super-resolution detail.

This area of FP development was expanded to other PC-FPs with studies aimed at developing mEosFP and Dendra2 in PS-FPs.[63] Given the high structural similarity in the vicinity of the chromophore of many PC-FPs, such as Kaede, KikGR, EosFP, and Dendra (Figure 14.7), the development of IrisFP suggested that others might also be engineered to photoswitch in the green channel, remain photoconvertible, and photoswitch in the red channel. Targeting three amino acid positions, 157, 159, and 173, in single or combined mutagenesis efforts, several photoswitchable PC-FPs variants were produced. One in particular, Dendra2 Phe173Ser, which was named NijiFP, proved to be photochromic, although not as bright as many of the variants produced in these studies. The green molecules could be switched "on" with ~400 nm light and "off" with 488 nm light similar to Dronpa and many other green PS-FPs. The red molecules after photoconversion were switched "on" with ~440 nm light and "off" with 561 nm light. Further improving upon its utility, NijiFP was found to be monomeric in the 100–500 μm concentration range, whereas mEosFP and IrisFP were a population of monomers, dimers, and oligomers in this range.

TABLE 14.4

Irreversible PC-FPs/Reversible PS-FPs

Name		Abs Max (nm)[a]	Extinction Coefficient (M⁻¹ cm⁻¹)	λ_{max} Em (nm)	Quantum Yield	Brightness (%)[b]	pK_a	Irradiation Light (nm)[c]		Oligomeric State[d]	Source Organism, Protein	Reference
					Irreversibly PC-FPs and Reversible PS-FPs							
IrisFP	N									T	L. hemprichii (coral), EosFP	61
	G	487	52,200	516	0.43	83	6.4	↓405	↑488			
	R	551	35,400	580	0.47	40	7.2	↓532	↓405 ↑440			
	N											
mIrisFP	N	386	12,000							M	L. hemprichii (coral), IrisFP	62
	G	486	47,000	516	0.54	132	5.4	↓405	↑488			
	R	546	33,000	578	0.59	34	7.6	↓561	↓405 ↑440			
	N	446	21,000									
NijiFP	N	385								M	Dendronephthya sp. (octocoral), Dendra2	63
	G	469	41,100	507	0.64	78	7.0	↓405	↑488			
	R	526	42,000	569	0.65	81	7.3	↓561	↓405 ↑440			
	N	440										

[a] N, G, and R denote nonfluorescent (off or dark state), green, and red fluorescent state, respectively.

[b] Brightness is determined by the product of the extinction coefficient and quantum yield. It is expressed here as a percentage of EGFP brightness.

[c] The arrow direction indicates the direction of the spectral alteration resulting from irradiation with the indicated wavelength of light (e.g., [N] nonfluorescent to [G] green).

[d] M, monomer; T, tetramer.

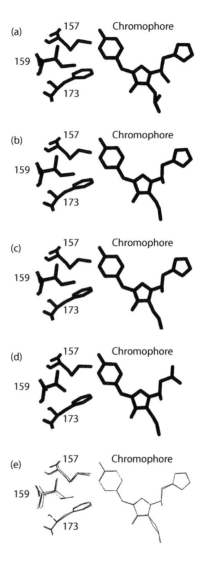

FIGURE 14.7 The chromophores and surrounding amino acids of the PC-FPs, Kaede, KikGR, EosFP, and Dendra are structurally similar. Crystal structures of (a) Dendra, (b) EosFP, (c) Kaede, and (d) KikGR chromophores and residues Phe-173, Met-159, and Ile-157 (Kaede, EosFP, and Dendra) or Val-157 (KikGR) show such a high degree of similarity. (e) Aligning and overlaying the chromophores show only slight differences in the structure of these key amino acids relative to the chromophores.

14.6 OPTICAL HIGHLIGHTER APPLICATIONS IN SUPER-RESOLUTION IMAGING

The wide range of optical highlighters has opened up several avenues of experimental approaches. Although our discussion of optical highlighter use is limited mainly to super-resolution imaging, most of the described necessities and desired characteristics are also applicable for diffraction-limited imaging. As discussed earlier, optical highlighting generally requires illumination with a wavelength separate from the excitation wavelength. After this step, imaging is similar to imaging conventional FPs and other probes. However, optical highlighters do have special considerations in imaging and since the range of the characteristics across the array of optical highlighters is quite broad, different proteins find usefulness in different experiments. For instance, an estimate of the signal after the highlighting step is needed in order to determine proper settings for the detector. In addition, the amount of light needed to "turn on" or "turn off" the proteins must be determined to minimize light exposure to the sample. An often-overlooked consideration is that some of the highlighters produce little or any signal prior to being photoactivated. This is problematic when trying to find positively expressing cells in a cell culture, tissue sample, or organism. Expression of a PC-FP is good option, but the PC-FP spectra (native and photoconverted) will use two major spectral emission bands and can thus be limiting in multicolor experiments. However, some approaches discussed in the following can circumvent this possible problem. An additional alternative is to use PS-FPs that can be switched "off" and then back "on" when needed. The examples discussed in the following are meant to provide readers with a template on which to base the protocols for imaging their favored proteins.

14.6.1 MOLECULE LOCALIZATION SUPER-RESOLUTION TECHNIQUES UTILIZING OPTICAL HIGHLIGHTERS

The majority of super-resolution techniques utilizing highlighter FPs are molecule localization techniques including PALM[64] and fluorescence PALM (FPALM).[65] In recent years, these types of imaging methods have gained in popularity and in number since more than a dozen variations have been reported,[66] including those relying on conventional organic fluorophores such as stochastic optical reconstruction microscopy (STORM).[67] Briefly, the techniques rely on being able to image single fluorescently tagged molecules among a much larger population of similar molecules. Given the limitations of diffraction, most single fluorescence molecules, which are 1–10 nm in size, are imaged as ~500 nm diameter spots. Since biological specimens can often have hundreds or thousands of molecules in a 500 nm spot, distinguishing individual molecules in such a pool of conventional fluorescent molecules is a daunting if not impossible task. Optical highlighters circumvent this problem by being able to be made dark in the spectral region to be imaged or they simply start with little or no fluorescence at those wavelengths. Subsequent photoactivation, photoconversion, or photoswitching "on" at very low levels maintains a sparse fluorescing population of single molecules that can be fitted with a function (usually a two-dimensional Gaussian) to define more precisely the coordinates of the molecules in the diffraction-limited spots. These molecule positions are plotted on a final image that offers higher resolution and more detail than an image of all of the molecules imaged at the same time. The data collection requirements of collecting hundreds of thousands of single-molecule signals while keeping the actively fluorescing molecule density low impose limitations on the potential experiments.

Nevertheless, investigators using PALM and other molecule localization techniques have devised approaches to perform live cell and multicolor experiments similar to those performed with conventional FPs.

14.6.2 STATIC LOCALIZATION MICROSCOPY IMAGING WITH OPTICAL HIGHLIGHTER FPS

Some of the first experiments relied heavily on cells fixed to maintain molecule positions over the long time course needed to collect localization data for all molecules in the sample. Experimentally, these are the equivalent of immunofluorescence imaging experiments that are widely used in cell and developmental biology. The major difference here is that the single localized molecules together can make an image with much more detail than an image collected while all molecules are fluorescent simultaneously.

Fixed cell imaging experiments were able to detect >10^5 molecules/μm^2 in some samples including detection of >5000 molecules in the matrix of a mitochondrion.[64] Furthermore, other densely populated cell structures that were imaged include focal adhesions, actin stress fibers, and plasma membrane proteins. In these examples, an array of optical highlighter FPs were utilized including mEosFP, dEosFP, tdEosFP, Kaede, KikGR, PAGFP, and Dronpa.

Imaging capabilities at subcellular organelle resolution have proved very useful for very small specimen, such as bacteria. For example, bacteria sensory cluster proteins, Tar receptor, CheY, and CheW, within *Escherichia coli* chemotaxis networks were imaged using mEosFP at ~15 nm resolution to show that they were formed by self-assembly without assistance from cytoskeletal elements or other protein trafficking machinery.[68] Both the dynamics (see below) and the structure of a ring involved in *Caulobacter crescentus*[69] and *E. coli*[70] cell division have been studied extensively using Dendra2 and mEos2 tags, respectively. The ring is located near the midpoint of the cell and is made up of a bacteria tubulin homolog, FtsZ, which shows an average thickness of 67 or 92 nm depending on the cell cycle stage in *C. crescentus*.[69] A similar thickness of ~110 nm was measured in *E. coli*.[70] Furthermore, the structure in the stalked cell stage of *C. crescentus* was noted to have ~650 nm outer diameter, consistent with the diameter of the cell and an ~150 nm opening in the center.[69] PALM studies were performed on the BfpB secretin protein tagged with PAmCherry to determine its localization in the cell envelope of enteropathogenic *E. coli*.[71] Here, BfpB proteins, which are part of the bundle forming pilus, were found to display various distributions depending on the cell, but the higher-resolution images showed a novel pattern of banding oriented obliquely relative to the long axis.

Membrane protein distributions on a subdiffraction scale have been further expanded in mammalian cell studies. For instance, the water channel, aquaporin-4, is known to form orthogonal arrays of particles, and tagging it with photoactivatable markers allowed the study of the size, shape, and composition of these arrays under various stimuli.[72] Another example is the fusion/fission cycle dependence on the location of oxidative phosphorylation complexes in the cristae of mitochondria.[73] These were imaged using photoactivatable tagged versions of complexes I, II, and

III and showed a much delayed mixing after fusion compared with outer membrane and matrix proteins. Membrane microdomains were studied using a linker for activation of T cells (LAT) transmembrane protein.[74] In fact, membrane proteins and associated molecules involved in T cell activation have been examined extensively by several groups using molecule localization techniques and found to show microclusters of many proteins[75–78] and nanoclusters of LAT[79] before activation. While the origin and physiological consequences of both types of clustering are being debated, it is clear that these molecule localization studies have yielded data concerning the sizes, shapes, and dynamics of protein domains that proved difficult to study with previous techniques.

The T cell activation studies highlight an additional capability of molecule localization techniques. Because the final displayed image represents single molecules localized precisely, this provides quantitative information on the number of molecules in specific domains and is readily subjected to cluster analysis. It is noteworthy that determining absolute numbers of molecules in molecule localization experiments is a daunting task. In fact, simply counting the molecules can be problematic owing to inefficient chromophore formation, inefficient photoactivation, blinking into dark states, or just simply low fluorescent signals. Typically, investigators have relied on PA-FPs, such as PAGFP and PAmCherry, or photoconvertible proteins, such as EosFP derivatives, because of the irreversible nature of their highlighting event. Despite the challenges, several good examples of these types of studies are discussed as follows. For instance, Gag stoichiometry in HIV virus-like particles (VLPs) was studied in cells expressing different Gag optical highlighter FPs.[80] This allowed characterization of intermediate stages of VLP formation and offered insight into protein packing and cluster morphological changes. Other molecule localization studies of HIV assembly concentrated on a host cell factor, tetherin, which incorporates into the viral membrane and acts to inhibit release of the virion. These studies showed several new features of the assembly sites and found four to seven tetherin dimers at each site.[81] Molecule counting was also applied to studies of endosome maturation as they moved from the plasma membrane into the cell and gained characteristics of other endosome classes.[82] These studies allowed determination of both the suborganelle location of numerous proteins and their stoichiometries. Bolder studies were aimed at the oligomeric state of molecules and their distributions. Using a combination of FRET and single-molecule counting, the two subunits of asialoglycoprotein receptor, RHL1 and RHL2, were found to exist in both homo- and hetero-oligomeric states.[83] While RHL1 formed higher-order homo-oligomers, RHL2 self-associated to form only dimers. The subunits formed higher-order hetero-oligomers at 2:1 stoichiometry. Each form was also found to display different ligand specificities. A similar quantitative PALM approach of protein kinase RAF localizations provided evidence of dimerization and multimerization to a lesser extent under various activating stimuli.[84]

As mentioned in the FP descriptions, many conventional FPs undergo similar photoswitching or photoconversion processes as optical highlighters. These are often less efficient but have the advantage that the conventional FP chimeras are often well characterized and lack the potential problems associated with making new chimeras specifically for molecule localization experiments. A great example of this is the EYFP derivative of the *A. victoria* GFP. Moerner and colleagues have made great use of EYFP by irradiating it until it goes into a dark state.[41,85,86] It can then relax stochastically or be driven by ~400 nm light irradiation back to the fluorescent state at a rate slow enough to image single molecules. A recent example of this is studies of the huntingtin protein exon 1 in which large inclusions were often observed; a smaller pool of monomers, oligomers, and fibrous aggregates ~100 nm in diameter and 1–2 μm long were prominent as well.[87] A similar phenomenon for EGFP as well as YFP has been utilized by Cremer and colleagues in their imaging of plasma membrane localized tyrosine kinases and histone H2B.[88] A different example of a conventional FP applied to molecule localization is the green-to-red photoconversion of the common EGFP variant of the *A. victoria* GFP. Here, the addition of reduced riboflavin was added to the imaging medium to increase the EGFP photoconversion efficiency. The resulting single molecules were reportedly as bright as the optical highlighter FPs and were used to study condensed chromosomes at 20 nm resolution and found ~70 nm filaments in *Drosophila* mitotic chromosomes labeled with H2AvD-EGFP, an H2A variant.[23]

An important but as yet underutilized advantage of static localization experiments is their combination with transmission electron microscopy (TEM). TEM provides much higher resolution images than PALM, and so on, but these are limited to contrasting structures, often sparsely populated antibody labels, or substrate precipitation experiments. As useful as these techniques are, the capability to localize thousands of molecules with high precision in an electron micrograph can propel the field further along. This correlative PALM/electron microscopy (EM) approach was first shown with a simple mitochondria matrix marker in which the dEosFP derivative was tagged to the signal sequence of cytochrome c oxidase.[64] Correlative PALM/EM of mitochondria has since been expanded to the study of mitochondria nucleoids using an mtDNA binding protein TFAM tagged with mEos2.[89] Other advances in this area include histone H2B, the mitochondria protein TOM20, and a presynaptic density protein, a-liprin.[90] The molecular tags in the latter examples included tdEosFP, Dendra, and a conventional FP, Citrine. As the fixation and embedding of the specimen often have detrimental consequences on an FP's fluorescence as well as the photoactivation, photoconversion, or photoswitching capabilities of the optical highlighters, much effort has been spent to optimize these methods.[91] Thus, while the protocol optimization has reaped rewards, future efforts in developing FPs with better tolerance for EM sample preparation would be very beneficial to the field.

14.6.3   LIVE CELL LOCALIZATION MICROSCOPY WITH OPTICAL HIGHLIGHTER FPS

Because of the unique data acquisition required for single molecule localization experiments, we discuss separately the movement of large macromolecular structures and the movement of individual molecules. While the distinction may seem arbitrary, the advantages and limitations encountered as well as the information derived from these experiments differ significantly. Studying movement of macromolecular structures is somewhat limited since positions for enough single molecules must be collected to make a useful image while simultaneously maintaining a low density of observed molecules per frame. For the examples discussed here, the typical super-resolution image collection time is ~30–60 s. This did prove rapid enough to image the movement of focal adhesions and the actin network of a crawling cell.[92] Moerner and colleagues imaged live *C. crescentus* cells and monitored the actin protein MreB tagged with EYFP to better understand the actin network in this organism[85] as well as the tubulin homolog FtsZ tagged with Dendra to monitor the doughnut-shaped Z-ring of the cell division machinery.[69] In similar studies to better characterize the Z-ring dynamics, FtsZ tagged with mEos2 was imaged in another bacteria, *E. coli.*[70] This approach was extended into neurobiology by Izeddin et al. using a low-affinity actin binding peptide tagged with tdEosFP.[93] This provided a readout of <1 min and was sufficient to monitor morphological changes in the spine in response to induced synaptic activity. This example brings up an important point for PALM imaging of macromolecular structures. Since enough molecules must be imaged to provide a sufficiently detailed structure, this signal can be rapidly depleted over a long time course. However, this can be circumvented if the probe is photoswitchable or exchanged with a pool of molecules not making up the structure of interest. A final example of macromolecular structure movement is the water channel aquaporin-4 that forms large orthogonal arrays of particles.[72] PALM studies show the arrays diffuse as a unit with slow diffusion coefficients on the order of 10^{-12} cm^2/s.

The second and perhaps more powerful use of optical highlighters in live cell molecule localization experiments is in single-particle tracking (SPT). SPT was used extensively long before the super-resolution techniques or optical highlighter FPs were introduced, but these generally required that the number of molecules studied in each cell be low enough to maintain sufficient average distance between single-molecule signals. The advantage with optical highlighters is that these allow single molecules to be tracking in a cell in the midst of thousands of other tagged molecules of interest. Second, as the imaged molecules photobleach, new molecules can be activated for further study. In doing so, data from thousands rather than tens or hundreds of molecules are gathered, and this produces molecule tracks, diffusion maps, and cluster analysis for an entire cell. One of the first studies of this kind was performed using FPALM on hemagglutinin-PAGFP located on the surface of fibroblasts to reveal clusters of various sizes and shapes from microns down to ~40 nm.[94] The technique and analyses were expanded in sptPALM (single-particle tracking PALM) to monitor and compare the dynamics of two dynamically different proteins, the vesicular stomatitis virus G protein and the HIV capsid protein Gag.[95] Optical highlighters have also provided useful in further studies of the actin network and behavior in dendritic spines. Tagging the actin monomers with PA-FP or PC-FP helped observe the flow of filaments into and out of the spine,[96] turnover of the molecules in individual filaments,[96] and polymerization rates in different regions of the dendritic spine. A final example is the study of DNA repair in live *E. coli.*[97] By imaging the polymerase or the ligase tagged with PAmCherry, the temporal characteristics of the DNA gap and nick searching and repairing processes were discerned. These studies found that the polymerase and ligase molecules spend ~80% in the search mode and require ~2.1 and 2.5 s, respectively, to complete a repair on a damaged site.

14.6.4   MULTICOLOR LOCALIZATION MICROSCOPY
WITH OPTICAL HIGHLIGHTER FPS

The capability to image multiple molecules at super-resolved detail was an important advance in localization microscopy. While it may seem trivial to simply expand to multiple colors, turning molecules "on" or "off" adds a new parameter that has different requirements for different FPs. For instance, Shroff et al.[92] had success when using green-to-red PC-FPs in conjunction with the green PS-FP Dronpa. In these experiments, the photoswitchable properties of Dronpa were advantaged because the protocol dictated photoconverting all of the PC-FP molecules from green to red upon collection of the red channel PALM image followed by photoswitching the Dronpa "off" and then back "on" upon collection of the green channel image. A Dronpa derivative, rsFastLime, was used in concert with a conventional organic fluorophore, cyanine 5, in which the photoswitching properties of both were used to generate dark images and monitor the single molecules as they returned from their respective dark states.[98] These were extended to just using PS-FPs with the introduction of bsDronpa and using it paired with Dronpa.[53] The switching half-times were markedly different, which was limiting for the experiment, but the blue-shifted spectra of bsDronpa proved sufficient to distinguish it from Dronpa and produce two-color subdiffraction-limited images. As an alternative solution, PAmCherry was developed specifically to be used as a red marker in PALM experiments.[6] The advantage with PAmCherry is that it has no signal prior to photoactivation and thus can be easily used with a green PA-FP or PS-FP since it does not produce overlap in these regions of the spectrum. Sherman et al.[79] relied on PAmCherry and Dronpa pairings to study the components of T cell antigen receptor complexes. In keeping with the approach to avoid signal overlap between molecule localization partners, the PATagRFP is a red PA-FP developed with the goal to provide a more photostable red molecule for two-color single-molecule tracking[7] as well as for other multicolor imaging experiments.[99] Alternatively, Gunewardene et al.[9] used an approach similar to one using organic fluorophores,[100] which relied on the ratio of signals in different channels to computationally overcome issues with spectral overlap. By doing so, they were able to image and separate the signals for three red FPs, Dendra, PAmCherry1, and PAmKate, tagged to plasma membrane proteins located in different membrane microdomains and to the actin cytoskeleton.[9]

14.6.5   RESOLFT MICROSCOPY

Finally, a technique that is still maturing but offers enormous promise because of its scalable super-resolution similar to stimulated emission depletion (STED) microscopy and the use of irradiation powers similar to those used in confocal microscopy. A recent implementation of the technique[56] is similar to STED microscopy in that a doughnut-shaped excitation pattern within a diffraction-limited spot is used to switch off the fluorescence. However, the population of molecules in the doughnut pattern is not turned "off" because they are driven from their singlet excited states back to the ground state without emitting fluorescence. Here, those molecules are switched into a dark state and hence do not produce fluorescence upon arrival of a second excitation pulse in the same diffraction-limited spot. The nature of this approach requires PS-FPs which can be switched numerous times. The first RESOLFT attempt[101] used the asFP595 protein discussed earlier, but its tetrameric characteristics, low brightness, and high tendency to undergo photodestruction limited further development of the method. The introduction of Dronpa and other PS-FPs offered molecules overcoming the tetramer and brightness problems, but the photostability remained a problem. This led to the development of the rsEGFP[56] and later the rsEGFP2[57] discussed earlier, which display better photostability than Dronpa and can undergo more on/off cycles. Demonstrations of RESOLFT capabilities included rewriteable data storage on subdiffraction limit scale.[56] In bacteria, the double-helical cytoskeletal network labeled by the actin protein, MreB, was imaged to show the improvement over the confocal microscopy. In mammalian cells, the keratin-19-rsEGFP-labeled intermediate filaments showed full width at half maximum of ~70 nm. Importantly, RESOLFT imaging was able to image lifeact-rsEGFP, an actin binding protein, over a 5 min period with a resolution comparable to STED but with approximately six orders of magnitude less irradiation.

14.7 FINAL COMMENTS AND OUTLOOK

Optical highlighter FPs and their uses have now matured into viable and routine options for imaging our favorite molecules. They provide more options for diffraction-limited imaging and extend imaging capabilities into the super-resolution realm. While they can often lack the brightness of their conventional counterparts; have less than desirable characteristics such as high photodestruction rates, low quantum yields in their optical highlighting reactions, and low contrast ratios of "on" and "off" states; and have aberrant behavior such as uncontrolled molecule blinking, investigators have devised clever workarounds until developments can optimize these characteristics.

With such a vast array of optical highlighters available, a major question that is often raised is "Which to use?" The answer unfortunately is not as simple as "Use this one or that one." As discussed throughout this chapter, each has strengths and weaknesses that must be assessed by each investigator for his or her specific purpose. For instance, if irradiation at ~400 nm is severely detrimental for your cells, perhaps Dendra or PSmOrange, which can be photoconverted using 488 nm, may work. If a reversible PS-FP is needed in the red spectral region, rsTagRFP or one of the reversible mCherry proteins may suffice. Finally, it is suggested that a few different proteins be tried since anecdotal evidence gathered through personal communication indicates that not all proteins work well with all proteins of interest. This is perhaps an unsatisfactory answer, but it may remain the situation until developments catch up to some of these problems.

Where are the developments going other than improving upon existing optical highlighters? While surprising characteristics are often found, the emphasis tends to be on redder and better, better meaning brighter and more photostable optical highlighters are sought, and since proteins are now being engineered on the basis of structural and mechanistic data from existing optical highlighters,[63] it is probable that development of conventional far-red FPs will shortly thereafter have optical highlighter counterparts.

ACKNOWLEDGMENTS

This work was supported by the Intramural Research Program of the National Institutes of Health including the National Institute of Biomedical Imaging and Bioengineering.

REFERENCES

1. Bates, M., S.A. Jones, and X. Zhuang. "Stochastic optical reconstruction microscopy (STORM): A method for superresolution fluorescence imaging." *Cold Spring Harb Protoc* 2013, no. 6 (2013): 498–520.
2. Dempsey, G.T. et al. "Evaluation of fluorophores for optimal performance in localization-based super-resolution imaging." *Nat Methods* 8, no. 12 (2011): 1027–36.
3. van de Linde, S. et al. "Direct stochastic optical reconstruction microscopy with standard fluorescent probes." *Nat Protoc* 6, no. 7 (2011): 991–1009.
4. Patterson, G.H. and J. Lippincott-Schwartz. "A photoactivatable GFP for selective photolabeling of proteins and cells." *Science* 297, no. 5588 (2002): 1873–7.
5. Verkhusha, V.V. and A. Sorkin. "Conversion of the monomeric red fluorescent protein into a photoactivatable probe." *Chem Biol* 12, no. 3 (2005): 279–85.
6. Subach, F.V. et al. "Photoactivatable mCherry for high-resolution two-color fluorescence microscopy." *Nat Methods* 6, no. 2 (2009): 153–9.
7. Subach, F.V. et al. "Bright monomeric photoactivatable red fluorescent protein for two-color super-resolution sptPALM of live cells." *J Am Chem Soc* 132, no. 18 (2010): 6481–91.
8. Merzlyak, E.M. et al. "Bright monomeric red fluorescent protein with an extended fluorescence lifetime." *Nat Methods* 4, no. 7 (2007): 555–7.
9. Gunewardene, M.S. et al. "Superresolution imaging of multiple fluorescent proteins with highly overlapping emission spectra in living cells." *Biophys J* 101, no. 6 (2011): 1522–8.
10. Shcherbo, D. et al. "Bright far-red fluorescent protein for whole-body imaging." *Nat Methods* 4, no. 9 (2007): 741–6.
11. Yokoe, H. and T. Meyer. "Spatial dynamics of GFP-tagged proteins investigated by local fluorescence enhancement." *Nat Biotechnol* 14 (1996): 1252–6.
12. Brejc, K. et al. "Structural basis for dual excitation and photoisomerization of the *Aequorea victoria* green fluorescent protein." *Proc Natl Acad Sci U S A* 94, no. 6 (1997): 2306–11.
13. Palm, G.J. et al. "The structural basis for spectral variations in green fluorescent protein." *Nat Struct Biol* 4, no. 5 (1997): 361–5.
14. van Thor, J.J. et al. "Phototransformation of green fluorescent protein with UV and visible light leads to decarboxylation of glutamate 222." *Nat Struct Biol* 9, no. 1 (2002): 37–41.
15. Henderson, J.N. et al. "Structure and mechanism of the photoactivatable green fluorescent protein." *J Am Chem Soc* 131, no. 12 (2009): 4176–7.
16. Ruta, V. et al. "A dimorphic pheromone circuit in *Drosophila* from sensory input to descending output." *Nature* 468, no. 7324 (2010): 686–90.
17. Matz, M.V. et al. "Fluorescent proteins from nonbioluminescent Anthozoa species." *Nat Biotechnol* 17, no. 10 (1999): 969–73.
18. Subach, F.V. et al. "Photoactivation mechanism of PAmCherry based on crystal structures of the protein in the dark and fluorescent states." *Proc Natl Acad Sci U S A* 106, no. 50 (2009): 21097–102.
19. Chudakov, D.M. et al. "Photoswitchable cyan fluorescent protein for protein tracking." *Nat Biotechnol* 22, no. 11 (2004): 1435–9.

20. Gurskaya, N.G. et al. "A colourless green fluorescent protein homologue from the non-fluorescent hydromedusa *Aequorea coerulescens* and its fluorescent mutants." *Biochem J* 373, no. Pt 2 (2003): 403–8.

21. Sawin, K.E. and P. Nurse. "Photoactivation of green fluorescent protein." *Curr Biol* 7, no. 10 (1997): R606–7.

22. Elowitz, M.B. et al. "Photoactivation turns green fluorescent protein red." *Curr Biol* 7, no. 10 (1997): 809–12.

23. Matsuda, A. et al. "Condensed mitotic chromosome structure at nanometer resolution using PALM and EGFP- histones." *PLoS One* 5, no. 9 (2010): e12768.

24. Bogdanov, A.M. et al. "Green fluorescent proteins are light-induced electron donors." *Nat Chem Biol* 5, no. 7 (2009): 459–61.

25. Ando, R. et al. "An optical marker based on the UV-induced green-to-red photoconversion of a fluorescent protein." *Proc Natl Acad Sci U S A* 99, no. 20 (2002): 12651–6.

26. Tsutsui, H. et al. "Semi-rational engineering of a coral fluorescent protein into an efficient highlighter." *EMBO Rep* 6, no. 3 (2005): 233–8.

27. Habuchi, S. et al. "mKikGR, a monomeric photoswitchable fluorescent protein." *PLoS One* 3, no. 12 (2008): e3944.

28. Wiedenmann, J. et al. "EosFP, a fluorescent marker protein with UV-inducible green-to-red fluorescence conversion." *Proc Natl Acad Sci U S A* 101, no. 45 (2004): 15905–10.

29. Nienhaus, G.U. et al. "Photoconvertible fluorescent protein EosFP: Biophysical properties and cell biology applications." *Photochem Photobiol* 82, no. 2 (2006): 351–8.

30. McKinney, S.A. et al. "A bright and photostable photoconvertible fluorescent protein." *Nat Methods* 6, no. 2 (2009): 131–3.

31. Zhang, M. et al. "Rational design of true monomeric and bright photoactivatable fluorescent proteins." *Nat Methods* 9, no. 7 (2012): 727–9.

32. Gurskaya, N.G. et al. "Engineering of a monomeric green-to-red photoactivatable fluorescent protein induced by blue light." *Nat Biotechnol* 24 (2006): 461–5.

33. Hoi, H. et al. "A monomeric photoconvertible fluorescent protein for imaging of dynamic protein localization." *J Mol Biol* 401, no. 5 (2010): 776–91.

34. McEvoy, A.L. et al. "mMaple: A photoconvertible fluorescent protein for use in multiple imaging modalities." *PLoS One* 7, no. 12 (2012): e51314.

35. Subach, O.M. et al. "A photoswitchable orange-to-far-red fluorescent protein, PSmOrange." *Nat Methods* 8, no. 9 (2011): 771–7.

36. Chen, C.C. et al. "Visualizing long-term memory formation in two neurons of the Drosophila brain." *Science* 335, no. 6069 (2012): 678–85.

37. Helker, C.S. et al. "The zebrafish common cardinal veins develop by a novel mechanism: Lumen ensheathment." *Development* 140, no. 13 (2013): 2776–86.

38. Mizuno, H. et al. "Photo-induced peptide cleavage in the green-to-red conversion of a fluorescent protein." *Mol Cell* 12, no. 4 (2003): 1051–8.

39. Gustafsson, M.G. "Surpassing the lateral resolution limit by a factor of two using structured illumination microscopy." *J Microsc* 198, no. Pt 2 (2000): 82–7.

40. Kremers, G.J. et al. "Photoconversion in orange and red fluorescent proteins." *Nat Methods* 6, no. 5 (2009): 355–8.

41. Dickson, R.M. et al. "On/off blinking and switching behaviour of single molecules of green fluorescent protein." *Nature* 388 (1997): 355–8.

42. Haupts, U. et al. "Dynamics of fluorescence fluctuations in green fluorescent protein observed by fluorescence correlation spectroscopy." *Proc Natl Acad Sci U S A* 95 (1998): 13573–8.

43. Schwille, P. et al. "Fluorescence correlation spectroscopy reveals fast optical excitation-driven intramolecular dynamics of yellow fluorescent proteins." *Proc Natl Acad Sci U S A* 97, no. 1 (2000): 151–6.

44. Heikal, A.A. et al. "Molecular spectroscopy and dynamics of intrinsically fluorescent proteins: Coral red (dsRed) and yellow (Citrine)." *Proc Natl Acad Sci U S A* 97, no. 22 (2000): 11996–2001.

45. Lukyanov, K.A. et al. "Natural animal coloration can be determined by a nonfluorescent green fluorescent protein homolog." *J Biol Chem* 275, no. 34 (2000): 25879–82.

46. Chudakov, D.M. et al. "Kindling fluorescent proteins for precise in vivo photolabeling." *Nat Biotechnol* 21, no. 2 (2003): 191–4.

47. Ando, R., H. Mizuno, and A. Miyawaki. "Regulated fast nucleocytoplasmic shuttling observed by reversible protein highlighting." *Science* 306, no. 5700 (2004): 1370–3.

48. Andresen, M. et al. "Structural basis for reversible photoswitching in Dronpa." *Proc Natl Acad Sci U S A* 104, no. 32 (2007): 13005–9.

49. Mizuno, H. et al. "Light-dependent regulation of structural flexibility in a photochromic fluorescent protein." *Proc Natl Acad Sci U S A* 105, no. 27 (2008): 9227–32.

50. Mizuno, H. et al. "Molecular basis of photochromism of a fluorescent protein revealed by direct 13C detection under laser illumination." *J Biomol NMR* 48, no. 4 (2010): 237–46.

51. Ando, R. et al. "Highlighted generation of fluorescence signals using simultaneous two-color irradiation on Dronpa mutants." *Biophys J* 92, no. 12 (2007): L97–9.

52. Stiel, A.C. et al. "1.8 A bright-state structure of the reversibly switchable fluorescent protein Dronpa guides the generation of fast switching variants." *Biochem J* 402, no. 1 (2007): 35–42.

53. Andresen, M. et al. "Photoswitchable fluorescent proteins enable monochromatic multi-label imaging and dual color fluorescence nanoscopy." *Nat Biotechnol* 26, no. 9 (2008): 1035–40.

54. Chang, H. et al. "A unique series of reversibly switchable fluorescent proteins with beneficial properties for various applications." *Proc Natl Acad Sci U S A* 109, no. 12 (2012): 4455–60.

55. Brakemann, T. et al. "A reversibly photoswitchable GFP-like protein with fluorescence excitation decoupled from switching." *Nat Biotechnol* 29, no. 10 (2011): 942–7.

56. Grotjohann, T. et al. "Diffraction-unlimited all-optical imaging and writing with a photochromic GFP." *Nature* 478, no. 7368 (2011): 204–8.

57. Grotjohann, T. et al. "rsEGFP2 enables fast RESOLFT nanoscopy of living cells." *Elife* 1 (2012): e00248.

58. Stiel, A.C. et al. "Generation of monomeric reversibly switchable red fluorescent proteins for far-field fluorescence nanoscopy." *Biophys J* 95, no. 6 (2008): 2989–97.

59. Subach, F.V. et al. "Red fluorescent protein with reversibly photoswitchable absorbance for photochromic FRET." *Chem Biol* 17, no. 7 (2010): 745–55.

60. Demarco, I.A. et al. "Monitoring dynamic protein interactions with photoquenching FRET." *Nat Methods* 3, no. 7 (2006): 519–24.

61. Adam, V. et al. "Structural characterization of IrisFP, an optical highlighter undergoing multiple photo-induced transformations." *Proc Natl Acad Sci U S A* 105, no. 47 (2008): 18343–8.

62. Fuchs, J. et al. "A photoactivatable marker protein for pulse-chase imaging with super-resolution." *Nat Methods* 7, no. 8 (2010): 627–30.

63. Adam, V. et al. "Rational design of photoconvertible and biphotochromic fluorescent proteins for advanced microscopy applications." *Chem Biol* 18, no. 10 (2011): 1241–51.

64. Betzig, E. et al. "Imaging intracellular fluorescent proteins at nanometer resolution." *Science* 313, no. 5793 (2006): 1642–5.

65. Hess, S.T., T.P. Girirajan, and M.D. Mason. "Ultra-high resolution imaging by fluorescence photoactivation localization microscopy." *Biophys J* 91, no. 11 (2006): 4258–72.

66. Patterson, G.H. "Fluorescence microscopy below the diffraction limit." *Semin Cell Dev Biol* 20, no. 8 (2009): 886–93.

67. Rust, M.J., M. Bates, and X. Zhuang. "Sub-diffraction-limit imaging by stochastic optical reconstruction microscopy (STORM)." *Nat Methods* 3, no. 10 (2006): 793–5.

68. Greenfield, D. et al. "Self-organization of the *Escherichia coli* chemotaxis network imaged with super-resolution light microscopy." *PLoS Biol* 7, no. 6 (2009): e1000137.

69. Biteen, J.S. et al. "Three-dimensional super-resolution imaging of the midplane protein FtsZ in live *Caulobacter crescentus* cells using astigmatism." *Chemphyschem* 13, no. 4 (2012): 1007–12.

70. Fu, G. et al. "In vivo structure of the E. coli FtsZ-ring revealed by photoactivated localization microscopy (PALM)." *PLoS One* 5, no. 9 (2010): e12682.

71. Lieberman, J.A. et al. "Outer membrane targeting, ultrastructure, and single molecule localization of the enteropathogenic *Escherichia coli* type IV pilus secretin BfpB." *J Bacteriol* 194, no. 7 (2012): 1646–58.

72. Rossi, A. et al. "Super-resolution imaging of aquaporin-4 orthogonal arrays of particles in cell membranes." *J Cell Sci* 125, no. Pt 18 (2012): 4405–12.

73. Wilkens, V., W. Kohl, and K. Busch. "Restricted diffusion of OXPHOS complexes in dynamic mitochondria delays their exchange between cristae and engenders a transitory mosaic distribution." *J Cell Sci* 126, no. Pt 1 (2013): 103–16.

74. Owen, D.M. et al. "Sub-resolution lipid domains exist in the plasma membrane and regulate protein diffusion and distribution." *Nat Commun* 3 (2012): 1256.

75. Lillemeier, B.F. et al. "TCR and Lat are expressed on separate protein islands on T cell membranes and concatenate during activation." *Nat Immunol* 11, no. 1 (2010): 90–6.

76. Williamson, D.J. et al. "Pre-existing clusters of the adaptor Lat do not participate in early T cell signaling events." *Nat Immunol* 12, no. 7 (2011): 655–62.

77. Rossy, J. et al. "Conformational states of the kinase Lck regulate clustering in early T cell signaling." *Nat Immunol* 14, no. 1 (2013): 82–9.

78. Hsu, C.J. and T. Baumgart. "Spatial association of signaling proteins and F-actin effects on cluster assembly analyzed via photoactivation localization microscopy in T cells." *PLoS One* 6, no. 8 (2011): e23586.

79. Sherman, E. et al. "Functional nanoscale organization of signaling molecules downstream of the T cell antigen receptor." *Immunity* 35, no. 5 (2011): 705–20.

80. Gunzenhauser, J. et al. "Quantitative super-resolution imaging reveals protein stoichiometry and nanoscale morphology of assembling HIV-Gag virions." *Nano Lett* 12, no. 9 (2012): 4705–10.

81. Lehmann, M. et al. "Quantitative multicolor super-resolution microscopy reveals tetherin HIV-1 interaction." *PLoS Pathog* 7, no. 12 (2011): e1002456.

82. Puchner, E.M. et al. "Counting molecules in single organelles with superresolution microscopy allows tracking of the endosome maturation trajectory." *Proc Natl Acad Sci U S A* 110, no. 40 (2013): 16015–20.

83. Renz, M. et al. "Plasticity of the asialoglycoprotein receptor deciphered by ensemble FRET imaging and single-molecule counting PALM imaging." *Proc Natl Acad Sci U S A* 109, no. 44 (2012): E2989–97.

84. Nan, X. et al. "Single-molecule superresolution imaging allows quantitative analysis of RAF multimer formation and signaling." *Proc Natl Acad Sci U S A* 110, no. 46 (2013): 18519–24.

85. Biteen, J.S. et al. "Super-resolution imaging in live *Caulobacter crescentus* cells using photoswitchable EYFP." *Nat Methods* 5, no. 11 (2008): 947–9.

86. Pavani, S.R. et al. "Three-dimensional, single-molecule fluorescence imaging beyond the diffraction limit by using a double-helix point spread function." *Proc Natl Acad Sci U S A* 106, no. 9 (2009): 2995–9.

87. Sahl, S.J. et al. "Cellular inclusion bodies of mutant huntingtin exon 1 obscure small fibrillar aggregate species." *Sci Rep* 2 (2012): 895.

88. Lemmer, P. et al. "Using conventional fluorescent markers for far-field fluorescence localization nanoscopy allows resolution in the 10-nm range." *J Microsc* 235, no. 2 (2009): 163–71.

89. Kopek, B.G. et al. "Correlative 3D superresolution fluorescence and electron microscopy reveal the relationship of mitochondrial nucleoids to membranes." *Proc Natl Acad Sci U S A* 109, no. 16 (2012): 6136–41.

90. Watanabe, S. et al. "Protein localization in electron micrographs using fluorescence nanoscopy." *Nat Methods* 8, no. 1 (2011): 80–4.

91. Watanabe, S. and E.M. Jorgensen. "Visualizing proteins in electron micrographs at nanometer resolution." In *Correlative Light and Electron Microscopy*, edited by Müller-Reichert, T. and Verkade, P. New York: Academic Press: 283–306 (2012).

92. Shroff, H. et al. "Dual-color superresolution imaging of genetically expressed probes within individual adhesion complexes." *Proc Natl Acad Sci U S A* 104, no. 51 (2007): 20308–13.

93. Izeddin, I. et al. "Super-resolution dynamic imaging of dendritic spines using a low-affinity photoconvertible actin probe." *PLoS One* 6, no. 1 (2011): e15611.

94. Hess, S.T. et al. "Dynamic clustered distribution of hemagglutinin resolved at 40 nm in living cell membranes discriminates between raft theories." *Proc Natl Acad Sci U S A* 104, no. 44 (2007): 17370–5.

95. Manley, S. et al. "High-density mapping of single-molecule trajectories with photoactivated localization microscopy." *Nat Methods* 5, no. 2 (2008): 155–7.

96. Tatavarty, V. et al. "Investigating sub-spine actin dynamics in rat hippocampal neurons with super-resolution optical imaging." *PLoS One* 4, no. 11 (2009): e7724.

97. Uphoff, S. et al. "Single-molecule DNA repair in live bacteria." *Proc Natl Acad Sci U S A* 110, no. 20 (2013): 8063–8.

98. Bock, H. et al. "Two-color far-field fluorescence nanoscopy based on photoswitchable emitters." *Appl Phys B* 88 (2007): 161–5.

99. Wilmes, S. et al. "Triple-color super-resolution imaging of live cells: Resolving submicroscopic receptor organization in the plasma membrane." *Angew Chem Int Ed Engl* 51, no. 20 (2012): 4868–71.

100. Bossi, M. et al. "Multicolor far-field fluorescence nanoscopy through isolated detection of distinct molecular species." *Nano Lett* 8, no. 8 (2008): 2463–8.

101. Hofmann, M. et al. "Breaking the diffraction barrier in fluorescence microscopy at low light intensities by using reversibly photoswitchable proteins." *Proc Natl Acad Sci U S A* 102, no. 49 (2005): 17565–9.

15 Targeting Dyes for Biology

Saumya Saurabh and Marcel P. Bruchez

CONTENTS

15.1 INTRODUCTION

Measurements of the structure, function, and interactions of proteins are crucial to our understanding of living systems. Biologists and chemists have developed a variety of methods to study these proteins both *in vitro* and *in vivo*. Among the methods to observe proteins, fluorescence spectroscopy has proven to be a unique tool in cell biology and biophysics, capable of revealing the dynamic nature of many processes. The prime requirement for observing a protein of interest (POI) using fluorescence spectroscopy is that the protein has to be labeled with a fluorescent probe. While *in vitro* labeling of biomolecules for biochemical methods is relatively straightforward as it relies on standard functional groups in purified proteins (typically cysteines) for covalent labeling, labeling POIs in living cells is a very formidable task. Labeling inside the cell requires balancing trade-offs between spatiotemporal control, specificity, selectivity, and modularity (e.g., the ability to swap one dye for another). Developments in fluorescent probes and microscopy techniques over the last two decades have given us tools that address all these challenges, thus making fluorescent labels the tool of choice for live cell imaging.

Cellular structures range from nanometers to microns in size, yet conventional optical microscopy is limited by the diffraction of light to resolve structures separated by ~200 nm. The emergence of superresolution microscopy and probes suited for it has made possible the resolution of cellular structures considerably beyond this limit and the localization of single molecules with a precision of 1 nm or better.[1,2] Protein interactions inside the cell occur across a wide range of time scales, anywhere from well under a second to hours or days. Typical fluorescent probes can emit up to 10^5–10^7 photons per second to allow for fast imaging of protein locations in real time.[3,4] However, most probes emit only ~10^5–10^6 photons, which limits the duration of such imaging. Finally, fluorescent probes come in a variety of colors, covering the spectrum from ultraviolet to infrared and enabling specific multicolor labeling (multiplexing).[5]

A protein inside a cell is surrounded by numerous other biomolecules with identical chemical building blocks (amino acids) and standard functional groups (SH, NH_2) in its microenvironment. This poses one of the most daunting challenges in labeling proteins. The ability to orthogonally label multiple POIs with different colors has been made possible through the development of organic dyes and genetically encoded fluorescent protein (FP) technology.[6–8] While organic dyes date back to over 150 years, and for specific fluorescence detection more than 60 years, tagging with FPs has become the most widely used technology since the discovery and development of the GFP (green fluorescent protein).[9,10] These genetically encoded proteins allow one to express an FP fusion with any POI without secondary labeling using standard molecular biology techniques. This approach has transformed fluorescence microscopy from a static method, applied to fixed cells, to a dynamic real-time approach to visualize changes within living cells and organisms. The FP family has been developed further to cover a large spectral range (from 440 to 720 nm) that allows the simultaneous tagging of multiple POIs with different colors.[11,12]

FPs are typically ~25–30 kDa in size and thus can perturb the function of the POI. Second, most FP chromophores mature posttranslationally, leading to a "lag time" before fluorescence can be observed from them. Finally, the photochemical properties of the FPs such as extinction coefficients (EC), quantum yields (QY), and photostability tend to be limiting factors in imaging, especially considering that many of the orange and red FPs show some photoconversion to alternate colors.[13] Organic dyes, on the other hand, are small molecules that can be targeted to POIs for fluorescence detection. Labeling with organic dyes is triggered by addition of dye to the cells, allowing controlled sequencing with biological treatments (e.g., labeling before or after drug addition) for detection of distinct biological processes. The synthetic chemistry involved in making organic dyes is well understood, allowing significant rational design of organic dyes with desirable properties, for example, photoactivation or photoconversion upon illumination with specific excitation wavelength or chemical sensing. This same synthetic control provides us with tunability of spectral and photochemical properties yielding a suite of organic fluorophores with a broader spectral range, higher molecular brightness (QY*EC), and higher photostability compared to FPs. Finally, different organic dyes can be tailored to bind specifically to functional groups or expressed tags on the POI through standard synthetic chemistry, providing the modularity that is needed to genetically target POIs in the cellular environment.

Traditionally, organic dyes have been targeted to POIs using antibodies. While this methodology has been useful in several *in vivo* and *in vitro* assays, it takes away the "small molecule" advantage from the dye. Covalent labeling approaches circumvent this disadvantage by employing specific functional groups on the proteins (NH_2, OH, SH) to target organic dyes with respective reactive functional groups. While the synthetic steps involved in this type of covalent labeling are well established, the nonspecific labeling poses a challenge to the widespread utility of simple, direct bioconjugation, especially in cellular systems, where all proteins have the same available functional groups. In another approach, various cell surface receptor ligands have been covalently tagged with fluorescent dyes. Following the work of Farinas and Verkman to target cell-permeable fluorescent ligands to receptors, several other ligands for cell surface receptors have been targeted successfully.[14] In particular, covalently labeled fluorescent conjugates of the epidermal growth factor (EGF) have been successfully employed in several studies of the epidermal growth factor receptor (EGFR).[15] While antibody labeling, bioconjugation, and affinity-directed labeling have several limitations as discussed above, they have, in some way, inspired chemists to develop hybrid chemical labeling approaches for targeting proteins.

An ideal fluorescent probe for labeling POIs for live cell imaging should have, of course, excellent spectroscopic and photochemical properties. It should have a small size so that it does not perturb protein function. It should also have the modularity with respect to binding partners and flexibility with respect to location of the probe on or inside the cell. The labeling reaction should complete in a specific and selective fashion in the shortest possible time and should not leave any background or nonspecific products. The labeling reagents should not be cytotoxic. Finally, the approach should be free of washing to allow for monitoring POIs in real time while the labeling reaction is going on (Figure 15.1a).

With the advent of bio-orthogonal chemistry, we have been able to incorporate chemical entities genetically or metabolically inside live cells. In the last 16 years, there has been a surge in the development of hybrid labeling approaches that utilize an organic molecule as a fluorescence reporter and a genetically encoded peptide tag as the bio-orthogonal targeting moiety. These approaches combine the synthetic control over the structure and function of the fluorescent reporter (dye) while maintaining the ease of labeling that is offered by genetic encoding. Since the discovery of the tetracysteine tags by Roger Tsien, the field has rapidly expanded and there are over two dozen tags that cover a wide range of bio-orthogonality and fluorescent properties.[16] Since many technologies are unique in their modalities, classifying them on the basis of the underlying chemistry is very useful for further discussions in this chapter (Figure 15.1b).

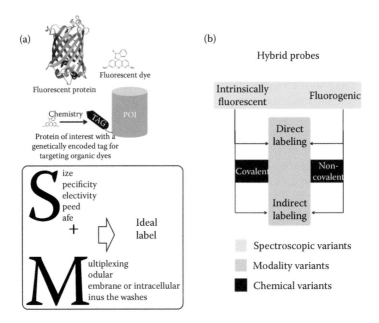

FIGURE 15.1 (a) A hybrid approach combining the properties of fluorescent dyes and genetically encoded proteins for labeling POIs. Also outlined are the qualities that are expected from an ideal label. (b) Categorization of probes in our discussion on the basis of spectroscopy, modality, and chemical variations.

15.2 INTRINSICALLY FLUORESCENT PROBES

Because of the availability of fluorescent dye conjugates of a wide range of antibodies, antibody-mediated labeling remains a very practical method to tag POIs on the surface of living cells as long as the bound antibodies do not perturb the protein's function. However, when the perturbation of protein function and structure is a concern, smaller tags need to be incorporated. Several approaches have been developed that utilize the chemistry of functional groups of a directly fused peptide tag to interact specifically and selectively with modified organic dye molecules. The final labeling can be as a result of a direct chemical reaction between the dye and the tag functional groups (direct labeling) as in the case of SNAP and CLIP tags or, alternatively, as a result of a reaction mediated by an enzyme such as PPTase or BirA, or any external means such as light, that leads to the dye binding the tag irreversibly. Finally, these interactions may be covalent or noncovalent depending on the chemistry used. Once a particular peptide tag has been engineered to perform a specific chemical reaction, any dye molecule with the cognate functional motif can be used to label the tagged POI, thus allowing for multiplexing as well as pulse chase measurements using the same tag with different dye molecules. Properties of the fluorescent probes discussed next are summarized in Table 15.1.

TABLE 15.1

Properties and Labeling Conditions for Fluorescent Hybrid Tags Discussed in This Study

Name (MW/kDa)	Steps	[Probe] (µM)/ Incubation Time (min)	Wash	Cell Permeability
SNAP[a] (20)	1	5/25	3×	Yes
CLIP (21)	1	5/20	3×	Yes
Halo (33)	1	5/15	3×	Yes
BL (29)	1	10/30–120	1×	Yes
A-TMP (18)	1	1/10	2×	Yes
Poly-His (1)	1	*0.1/5*	*1×*	*No*
DHFR–Mtx[a] (18)	1	*2/20 h*	*2×*	*Yes*
DHFR–TMP (18)	1	*0.1–10/5–120*	*3×*	*Yes*
Coiled coil (6)	1	*0.005/5*	*1×*	*No*
BirA–biotin[b] (2)	1	*<1/instantaneous*	*1×*	*No*
BirA–ketone-1[b] (2)	2	1000/60–120	2×	No
LipoicAl[b] (0.2)	2	100–400/20	3×	No
PPTase[b] (1)	1	1/20	5×	Yes
P-PALM[c] (27)	1	0.3–1/0–60	1×	Yes

Note: Noncovalent probes are italicized.

[a] Deficient cell lines needed.

[b] Enzyme mediated.

[c] Light mediated.

15.2.1 Direct Labeling

The selectivity that arises from a specific functional group binding to a specific tag makes the direct labeling approach a very versatile tool for targeting POIs. The absence of any enzymes or catalysts in the reaction circumvents the limitations of enzyme catalysis such as narrow substrate range, suboptimal efficiency of the reaction, compartment-specific labeling challenges, and the limited stability of enzymes under reaction conditions. Most reactions that result in the formation of a specific covalent bond employ weak electrophiles that liberate nonfluorescent and nonreactive side products that do not interfere with the measurements. Direct labeling techniques that utilize a noncovalent interaction between a targeting protein and its ligand produce a versatile and even exchangeable interaction without any leaving groups. In Sections 15.2.1.1 and 15.2.1.2, we will discuss some of the labels developed using this technology, where the dye binds in a covalent or noncovalent manner to a genetically encoded tag linked to the POI.

15.2.1.1 Covalent Labels

SNAP tag: SNAP tag is a classic example of a bio-inspired labeling approach. Human DNA repair protein O^6-alkylguanine-DNA alkyltransferase (hAGT) selectively and irreversibly transfers the alkyl residue from alkylated DNA or its substrate to a cysteine residue within the enzyme.[17] Kai Johnsson's laboratory used this technology to target O^6-benzylguanosine (BG) derivatives containing fluorescent probes to POIs (Figure 15.2a). This labeling approach has several attractive properties: the size of hAGT is small (207 amino acids); it can be fused to either the N- or the C-terminus of POI and retains its function; the ligated dye is covalently linked to

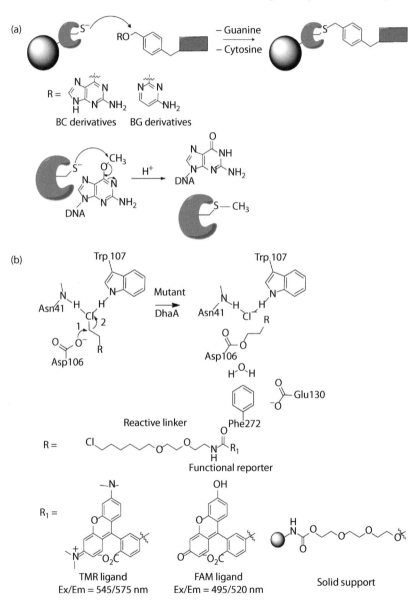

FIGURE 15.2 (a) SNAP and CLIP tag technologies and their mechanism of action. (b) The mechanism of action of the BL tag and some of the common fluorophores used in the BL tag technology.

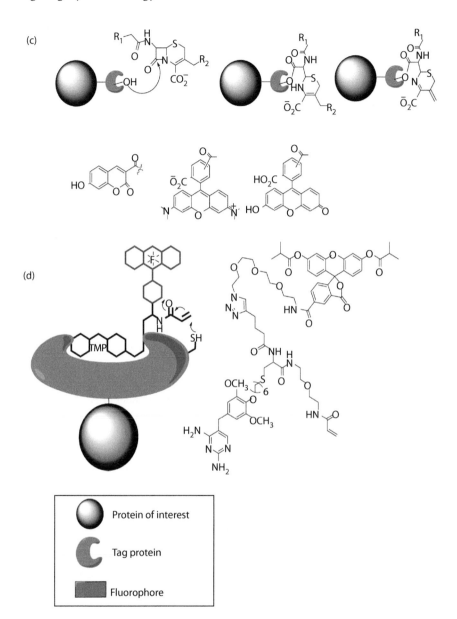

FIGURE 15.2 (Continued) (c) Mechanism of action of the HaloTag and some of the fluorophores optimized for this technology. (d) Mechanism of action of the covalent A-TMP tag and structure of the acrylamide trimethoprim probe.

the hAGT with a 1:1 stoichiometry; and the chemistry of BG-modification chemistry has been established very well in the literature. Several studies have successfully shown the applications of this tag *in vitro* and in living cells.[18–21] However, the inspiration from the DNA damage repair protein also has its disadvantages. Since alkylguanine-DNA alkyltransferase (AGT) is intrinsically present in cells for DNA repair, special cell lines that are deficient in AGT should be utilized in studies with SNAP tag. Cell lines that have endogenous AGT show a detectable labeling of AGT in the nucleus. This can be a major limitation for the general application of the SNAP tag technology, especially when the studies involve targeting proteins in the nucleus or studying proteins that may translocate to the nucleus. The second disadvantage to this technology comes from the high concentration of the substrate, typically ~10 μM for labeling cultured cells. Several dyes show nonspecific binding as well as dye–dye interactions at such high concentrations and thus may interfere with fluorescence observations. Finally, washing the unreacted BG derivatives may be cumbersome and needs optimization with each cell type and experimental condition.

CLIP tag: The CLIP tag is a logical extension of the SNAP tag technology where the molecular recognition consists of an AGT mutant that reacts specifically with an O²-benzylcytosine (BC) derivative (Figure 15.2a).[19] The discovery of the CLIP tag allowed for simultaneous and specific labeling of two different proteins with spectrally resolvable fluorescent probes. The CLIP tag can be used in conjunction with the SNAP tag owing to the marked differences between the molecular recognition mechanisms of AGT (SNAP) and its mutant (CLIP). The labeling achieved through the simultaneous use of the two probes can be attributed to the lack of interactions between AGT and BC because of the hydrogen bonding between Tyr114 and the N³ of guanine. Further, since cytosine is a less bulky group and has different hydrogen-binding interactions, the AGT mutants (CLIP) did not show any cross-reactivity toward the BG derivatives. One of the key breakthroughs that the CLIP tag achieves over the SNAP tag is in the labeling of cell lines that are not deficient in endogenous AGT. Since the CLIP tag uses a mutant of AGT, BC derivatives do not react with endogenous AGT in cell lines. The CLIP tag has been applied to studies involving pulse chase measurements, superresolution microscopy, and chromophore-assisted light inactivation of proteins.[22] Similar to the SNAP tag, the CLIP tag labeling requires high concentrations of the BC derivatives and extensive wash steps prior to imaging. Both SNAP tag and CLIP tag constructs, dyes, and targeting moieties (reactive versions of BG and BC) are available commercially from New England Biolabs.

HaloTag: The HaloTag is a commercially available, versatile probe from Promega that utilizes similar principles as the SNAP and CLIP tags. The tag uses a mutant of *Rhodococcus* dehalogenase (DhaA.H272F/K175M/C176G/Y273L) that reacts specifically and at a fast rate with haloalkanes.[23] The underlying chemistry involves the nucleophilic displacement of the terminal chloride with Asp¹⁰⁶, forming an alkyl-enzyme intermediate. The H272F mutation ensures that the hydrolysis of this intermediate is not catalyzed and hence trapped as the stable product (Figure 15.2b). The utility and versatility of the HaloTag arise primarily from the underlying linker chemistry. Since the ester bond formed with Asp¹⁰⁶ is seated deeply inside a hydrophobic pocket, it is stable under stringent conditions such as boiling with SDS, or even in the presence of formaldehyde. A direct application of this property is the use of HaloTag in fixed cell assays.[24] Second, alkyl dehalogenases are absent in *Escherichia coli* and eukaryotic cells, making this probe useful in a wide variety of cell types and organisms. Finally, the HaloTag technology has been used in a wide variety of assays owing to the generality of the approach and optimization of the chloroalkane linker that proves to be an excellent handle for performing cellular imaging, protein–protein and protein–DNA interaction studies, SDS-PAGE, Western blotting, and a variety of *in vivo* and *in vitro* assays. For live cell imaging, the probes are incubated at concentrations of 1–5 µM for 45 min and require extensive washing, limiting their applications in the imaging of real-time protein interactions during the labeling.

BL tag: Throughout the course of evolution, cells have developed a wide variety of electrophiles and nucleophiles to carry out chemical reactions required for biosynthesis and metabolism. The β-lactamase enzymes found in *E. coli* are similar to the hAGT proteins in that regard. They cleave β lactam moieties in several compounds very well and have been used widely as genetic reporters for colorimetric and fluorogenic assays. The Kukuchi laboratory utilized the underlying chemistry behind the β-lactamase in a mutant of the TEM-1-β-lactamase from *E. coli* to specifically covalently couple to substrates containing β-lactams (Figure 15.2c).[25] The BL tag is similar to the HaloTag in that it traps the reaction intermediate of the WT enzyme through a site-specific mutation. In the WT-TEM-1, Ser70 attacks the β-lactam ring to form an acyl intermediate. This is followed by the nucleophilic attack of Glu166 on the intermediate that releases the substrate and regenerates WT-TEM-1. In the BL tag, an E166N mutation uses an ineffective nucleophile (Asn) in the active site instead of Glu, trapping the acyl intermediate and covalently linking the dye to form a stable product. The TEM-1 mutant is not found endogenously in bacterial or eukaryotic cells, making the method widely applicable in intracellular and cell surface protein imaging.[26] However, background β-lactamase catalytic activity in cells may reduce the availability of the tag in the cellular context. The BL tag is orthogonal to SNAP tag and thus can be used in combination with it and with similar technologies. A potential disadvantage of the method is the high concentrations of probe that are incubated with the cells (typically 5 µM) that may lead to nonspecific binding on the basis of the cell type and dye used. Hence, optimization of incubation times and concentrations needs to be performed when using the BL tag for cell imaging. Additionally, for both HaloTag and BL tag, there are limited choices of probes for intracellular imaging.

Covalent A-TMP tag: The Cornish laboratory utilized rational design principles to synthesize an acrylamide conjugate of 2,4-diamino-5-(3,4,5-trimethoxy-benzyl)pyrimidine (acrylamide trimethoprim or A-TMP) that could specifically covalently link to a single engineered cysteine in an *E. coli*-derived dihydrofolate reductase mutant (eDHFR:L28C) (Figure 15.2d).[27] This tag could be used in wild-type mammalian cell lines with great success as TMP selectively binds to eDHFR (K_d = 1 nM) with over three orders of magnitude higher affinity compared to mammalian DHFR (K_d = 4 µM). Live cell imaging of proteins inside nuclear compartments could be performed using this tag owing to the excellent cell permeability of TMP. Moreover, only 1 µM of fluorescently labeled A-TMP is needed for live cell imaging. It is important to point out here that the reaction forming the eDHFR:A-TMP covalent bond takes ~2 h for >95% completion. This tag can be used for single-molecule imaging owing to the irreversible binding of the fluorophore to the target protein. This can also be used in conjunction with the noncovalent TMP tag as discussed later.

15.2.1.2   Noncovalent Labels

Polyhistidine tags: Polyhistidine tags have been widely used in affinity purification of proteins utilizing noncovalent binding with Ni^{2+}:nitrilotriacetic acid (Ni:NTA). The Ebright laboratory first demonstrated the successful targeting of Ni:NTA-conjugated cyanine dyes to proteins expressing a hexahistidine (His_6) tag.[28] They optimized the number of Ni:NTA per dye molecule such that, while mono Ni:NTA-conjugated cyanine dyes showed a K_d in excess of 10 μM, the Bis-Ni:NTA conjugates of the same dyes exhibited a K_d of 0.4–1 μM for binding a His_6 tag. The Piehler laboratory further improved on this technology by synthesizing tris-NTA conjugates of commercially available organic dyes that bound His_6 and His_{10} residues on POIs with high affinity and fast rates, ultimately achieving subnanomolar affinities with His_{10} and tris-Ni:NTA chelates (Figure 15.3a).[29] The poly-His:Ni:NTA binding is reversible in the presence of 20–100 mM imidazole; a method used very frequently in affinity purification of proteins and useful for reversal of labeling under moderate conditions at the cell surface. A critical drawback of poly-His tagging arises from the quenching of the fluorophores upon conjugation with the Ni:NTA owing to the electronic interactions with the empty d-orbitals of Ni^{2+}. There is typically further quenching of the fluorophore upon binding with the His-tagged protein. The combined quenching effect can sometimes lead to a loss of up to 80% in QY of the respective fluorophores. The Hamachi laboratory developed a complementary extension of this technology through the use of oligo-aspartate sequences and corresponding multinuclear Zn(II) complexes.[30] While moderate binding affinities weaken the signal because of incomplete labeling, there is no quenching of the fluorophore in this tag owing to the d10 configuration of Zn(II). One challenge with these metal coordination-based tags is that the poly-His and poly-Asp tags consist of clustered charges at the N-terminus or C-terminus of the protein and may interfere with protein solubility, interactions, and functions in cellular environments.

DHFR–Mtx: The Cornish laboratory utilized the noncovalent interaction between eDHFR and fluorescent conjugates of a small molecule, methotrexate (Mtx) (Figure 15.3b).[31] The equilibrium and kinetic properties of the DHFR–Mtx complex further make this approach very attractive. DHFR binds Mtx with subnanomolar affinities (K_d = 25 pM) with a sufficiently slow dissociation rate constant (k_{off}) of 10^{-4} s^{-1} in solution. Further, the formation of the DHFR–Mtx complex is thermodynamically favorable and it provides additional stability to DHFR particularly against proteolytic degradation. Finally, the chemical modification of Mtx is performed at the γ-carboxylate position that does not interfere with the receptor-binding moiety. Cell imaging using membrane and nuclear targeting DHFR in DHFR-deficient cell lines was performed using a Texas Red conjugate of Mtx (Mtx-TR) at a concentration of 2 μM (incubation with cells for 20 h), which is less than half of that used for the SNAP tag and HaloTag. Key disadvantages of the DHFR–Mtx labeling strategy arise from the fact that the interaction is noncovalent and hence reversible, and the Mtx-TR, for example, dissociates from DHFR-tagged proteins on the order of 1–2 h. Further, because Mtx binds to both human and bacterial DHFR, this approach has to be used in cell lines that are DHFR-deficient to reduce background that arises from the labeling of endogenous DHFR.

FIGURE 15.3   (a) Common tris-NTA probes and schematic showing the binding of Ni:NTA to His$_6$ motif on a POI. (b) Mechanism of action of an Mtx tag binding to DHFR. (c) Binding mechanism of the noncovalent TMP tag and some of the commonly used fluorophores for this technology.

DHFR-TMP tag: The TMP tag is a rationally designed tag that improves over the DHFR–Mtx tag and exploits the advantages of a noncovalent label. The Cornish labora-tory used it as a binding partner for the *E. coli* DHFR for imaging in wild-type mamma-lian cell lines, owing to the previously described 4000:1 selectivity of TMP for eDHFR compared to hDHFR (Figure 15.3c).[32] The conjugation of TMP to fluorescent dyes is

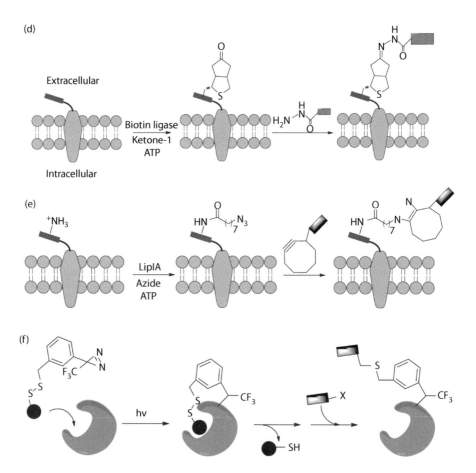

FIGURE 15.3 (Continued) (d) Mechanism of action of the BirA–ketone-1 tagging technology. (e) Mechanism of action of the LiplA-azide tagging technology. (f) Mechanism of labeling using P-PALM probes.

straightforward and does not interfere with the binding to eDHFR. Owing to the high affinity and excellent cell permeability, the dye-conjugated TMP tags can be used at low concentrations (10 nM) with 5–15 min incubation times. Therefore, TMP tags deliver low background imaging with fast binding kinetics for cell biology studies. Because TMP is recognized by both the mutant eDHFR and wt-eDHFR, these TMP-tagged dyes can be used with the covalent A-TMP-eDHFR tags for pulse chase experiments.

Coiled-coil tag: The coiled-coil (CC) tagging approach is unique from the previously discussed approach in that it uses complementary heptad-repeat peptide coil combinations for labeling cellular proteins.[33] Since it does not involve metal ions, a cleaner photochemistry of the probe is achieved that is advantageous for live cell imaging. Briefly, the approach uses four peptides K3 (KIAALKE)$_3$, K4 (KIAALKE)$_4$, E3 (EIAALEK)$_3$, and E4 (EIAALEK)$_4$. The K peptides are positively charged, whereas the E peptides are negatively charged (K#, E#, with # indicating the charge). K3 and E3 probes were expressed on the extracellular N-terminus of membrane proteins in mammalian cells, and TMR-labeled complementary probes (E3 and K3, respectively) were used for live cell imaging. Although this approach should be very modular, fluorescent labeling could only be achieved with the K probes and E3 peptide expressed on the POI at the cell surface. The labeling concentrations of the probes were low (<70 nM) and the incubation time was typically ~5 min. Finally, the probes were nontoxic even at concentrations of 10 μM in the media. Because the charged peptides do not cross the plasma membrane, the CC tag approach is presently limited to labeling membrane proteins.

15.2.2 Indirect Labeling

Indirect labeling approaches, for the purposes of discussion in this chapter, are defined as approaches where the formation of a covalent bond between a genetically encoded peptide sequence on the POI and a small molecule is mediated by enzymes or photochemically. Several of these methods are inspired by posttranslational modifications on proteins. Specific enzymes catalyze the formation of a covalent bond between many small molecules such as biotin, acetyl coenzyme A (CoA), and lipoic acid to specific short peptides in native proteins. These reactions can be exploited using the native enzymes or mutant and recombinant enzymes to form linkages between these peptides and dyes or other bio-orthogonal reactive groups.

15.2.2.1 Enzyme-Mediated Labeling

BirA labeling with biotin: The streptavidin–biotin complex has one of the highest known affinities among noncovalent complexes. The high affinity and the extremely slow off rates make this system very attractive for fluorescent labeling of proteins. Further, the systematic optimization of the bacterial biotin holoenzyme synthetase BirA has fueled the application of biotinylated proteins in pull-down assays, immunofluorescence, and single-molecule studies *in vitro* and in cells.[34–37] Of particular interest are the studies targeting streptavidin-conjugated Alexa Fluor dyes and streptavidin-conjugated QDots to enzymatically biotinylated proteins on the cell surface, such as the cystic fibrosis transmembrane conductance receptor, the EGFR, and α-amino-3-hydroxy-5-methyl-4-isoxazolepropionate receptor.[35,36]

BirA labeling with ketone-1: The Ting laboratory developed a cell surface protein labeling method derived from this approach to ligate an unnatural biotin analog (ketone-1) onto the AP (Figure 15.3d).[37] This required a combination of the unnatural biotin analog and a mutant BirA that could selectively ligate this new analog preferentially to native biotin. Because most biomolecules do not have a ketone group on them, this label can provide a very specific site for covalent labeling of POIs with ketone-1-modified APs using mild hydrazide chemistry. This approach was used to label AP-tagged EGFR and other transmembrane proteins with ketone-1 followed by covalent labeling with hydrazide conjugates of fluorescent dyes. The method is used to label surface proteins and cannot yet be applied inside cells because some intracellular molecules may be reactive toward hydrazides. This approach requires relatively long incubation times of the ketone-1–BirA complex followed by the fluorescent target incubation (20–120 min). The reaction between ketone-1 and the dye conjugated to a hydrazide is carried out at pH 6.2 (faster hydrazine formation), limiting the application in complex tissues or cells that may be pH sensitive. This method requires initial washing of the ketone prior to labeling with the dye, as well as washing of the unreacted fluorescent dye label.

Lipoic acid ligase: The reaction between an alkyne and an azide can be used to provide high specificity in cellular environments not only because they are generally not found in cells but also because they are not cytotoxic. The lipoic acid ligase (LiplA) tag exploits this principle and has been shown to label cell surface proteins with fluorescent dyes. The Ting laboratory discovered that an alkyl azide with a linker can bind selectively to the lysine side chain in the acceptor peptide sequence on the POI (Figure 15.3e).[38] Once this was achieved, a fluorescent probe conjugated with a cyclooctyne group could be covalently linked to the azide through the Staudinger ligation. This probe could be used as a complement to BirA labeling on the cell surface. The labeling protocol and wash steps for this approach are similar to the BirA approach. The labeling time is shorter than the BirA approach yet still requires more than an hour, and the lipoic acid and fluorophore cyclooctyne are added in two different steps. The approach can only be used on the cell membrane and requires washing out of the unreacted azide, LiplA, and unreacted fluorophores prior to imaging.

PPTase: Yin and coworkers discovered an enzymatic labeling method utilizing the phosphopantetheinyl transferase (PPTase) enzyme that could catalyze CoA ligation to the serine residue of an 11-amino-acid AP motif.[39] The underlying chemistry involves the transfer of the phosphopantetheinyl group from CoA to a specific serine moiety on a peptidyl carrier protein (PCP). Since the size of the PCP tag is slightly larger (80–100 amino acids), the Yin laboratory subsequently selected an 11-amino-acid residue through phage display and peptide synthesis, the ybbR AP. This compact tag can be inserted on the N- or the C-terminus of POIs, as well as on a flexible loop within the POI. Further, there were improvements made through the selection of two other AP tags (12 amino acids) through a phage display library selection, named the S6 and the A1 tag, which served as substrates of Sfp (catalytic efficiency of 442-fold for A1) and AcpS (catalytic efficiency of 30-fold for S6), respectively.[40] The methodology provided for two selective labels: one utilizing the Sfp pathway while the other utilizes an AcpS pathway. This methodology was successfully applied to image the EGFR (S6-EGFR) and the transferrin receptor 1 (A1-TfR1) on HeLa cells, labeled with small-molecule fluorophores. Although the cell impermeability aspect of the CoA enzyme conjugates has been touted as an advantage, the inability to label intracellular proteins is a key limitation of this method. Second, high labeling concentrations and stringent washing conditions further limit the applications of this method.

15.2.2.2 Light-Mediated Labeling

P-PALM: The Hamachi laboratory utilized local photochemical reactions in conjunction with electrophilic–nucleophilic substitution principles to obtain a post-photoaffinity labeling modification (P-PALM) method (Figure 15.3f).[41] They used concavalin A (ConA), a lectin, as the protein tag. The probe combined a high-affinity target ligand such as α-D-mannoside and α-D-glucoside, a diazirine group that is photoreactive, and a disulfide cleavage site that can generate a chemoselective nucleophilic thiol group upon reduction. After the saccharide moiety binds ConA, bringing the nucleophilic reduction site in proximity to the protein binding site, UV-irradiation of the probe resulted in the formation of a covalent bond between the diazirine groups of the probe and the ConA tag at the Tyr100 or Tyr12 residues close to the binding pocket. The Hamachi laboratory further applied this technique to synthesize, in a site-selective fashion, ConA with two fluorescent labels (coumarin and fluorescein). They showed that the fluorescence from fluorescein, which was closer to the protein–sugar binding pocket, was somewhat quenched, while that of coumarin was invariant to the changes in the microenvironment. They used this observation to build a ratiometric sensor for mannose-type saccharides on the surface of MCF-7 cells. When dual-labeled ConA was bound to the saccharide, the fluorescence from fluorescein was quenched relative to the free dual-labeled ConA in solution. Washing free ConA sensor away revealed cell surface signal related to mannose levels present. The probe could be chased away very easily by using 100 μM 1,6-mannotriose. Photochemical principles have not been exploited very well in protein labeling, and this technology may be a starting point in photo-mediated ligation of small molecules to POIs.

15.3 FLUOROGENIC PROBES

A key limitation of fluorescently labeled affinity tags is that washing steps are required to remove unbound and nonspecifically bound fluorescent labels. Further, incubation times are generally low only when the fluorescent probe is used at high concentrations, giving rise to nonspecific binding with intrinsic cellular proteins. A logical solution to these limitations would be the use of probes that light up only when bound to the specific target protein. A fluorogen is a small, nonfluorescent molecule that shows a fluorescent enhancement upon binding a partner protein. Fluorogens have been realized using three basic concepts: chemical cleavage produces an aromatic and fluorescent conjugated dye molecule, chemical cleavage removes a fluorescence quenching group, and binding results in enhancement of fluorescent properties of molecular rotor-like molecules. While one of the first attempts at protein labeling was fluorogenic (tetracysteine tags), only a handful of fluorogenic probes have since been discovered. Although the concept of fluorogenic detection is well established and highly effective in DNA detection, many of these molecules are unsuitable for fluorogenic protein labeling because of background from DNA and RNA activation. Fluorogenic labeling is a very attractive approach for both cell surface and intracellular labeling but is presently limited by a small selection of robust fluorogenic dyes with high brightness and low nonspecific activation with good cell-penetrating properties. Properties of the fluorogenic probes discussed next are summarized in Table 15.2.

15.3.1 COVALENT LABELS

BL tag: The BL tag, as discussed in the fluorescent dye labeling approach, employs the site-specific covalent labeling of small molecules conjugated to β-lactams and the TEM-1-β lactamase. In a related approach, the Kikuchi laboratory

TABLE 15.2

Properties and Labeling Conditions for Fluorogenic Hybrid Tags Discussed in This Study

Name (MW/kDa)	Mechanism	F_{bound}/F_{free}	[Probe] (µM)/ Incubation Time (min)	K_d (µM)/ k_{off} (s^{-1})	Cell Permeability
BL (29)	Chromophore quenching	142	10/30	—	No
SNAP (20)	Chromophore quenching	300	2/10–40	—	No
PYP (14)	Chromophore quenching	22	1/30	—	No
Tetra-Cys (0.6)	*Disruption of conjugation*	*1000*	*1/60*	—	*Yes*
Tetra-Ser (0.6)	*Disruption of conjugation*	*3*	*0.05/20*	*0.3/—*	*Yes*
FAP (26)	*Disruption of conjugation*	*18,000*	*0.1/5*	*6E−6/1E−5*	*Yes*

Note: Noncovalent probes are italicized.

synthesized a three-component fluorogenic probe that consisted of a single organic dye (7-hydroxycoumarin, fluorescein, or TAMRA), cephalosporin, and a collisional fluorescence quencher, DABCYL or azopyridine (Figure 15.4a).[42] The fluorescence of the respective organic dyes is quenched in the presence of the DABCYL or azopyridine until the cephalosporin β-lactam ring cleaves followed by the elimination of the 3′ bonded quencher. The remaining cephalosporin–dye adduct remained bound to the β-lactamase-labeled EGFR on HEK-293 cell surface. Although the probe is fluorogenic, high concentrations of the fluorogen (~10 µM) have to be used with cells for long incubation times (~2 h), achieving a fluorescence activation of 142-fold. Also, the fluorescence signal of the FCD reaches its maximum in over 200 min, limiting the application of this probe in experiments where fast labeling is not crucial.

SNAP tag: While the benzylguanine motif in SNAP tag probes is a fluorescence quencher for certain organic dyes, only a 30-fold fluorescence enhancement was achieved using this approach.[43] More recently, the Urano laboratory developed a SNAP tag BG probe that has a disperse red-1 quencher at the C8 position of the BG motif.[44] They synthesized a disperse red-BG-Fluorescein (DRBG-488) (Figure 15.4b) and a membrane-permeant version with a diacetyl protection (DRBFFL-DA) for labeling proteins. The fluorescence activation of these probes upon binding the SNAP tag was 300-fold, and they did not need any washing of the unreacted label owing to their negligible background fluorescence. SNAP-EGFR-expressing COS7 cells could be imaged using 2 µM of the DRBG-488 probe without washing within 40 min. These probes were successfully employed to study membrane trafficking in COS7 cells as well as cell migration of MDCK cells. This approach was used to study protein delivery on the HEK-293 cell surface in real time, as opposed to the

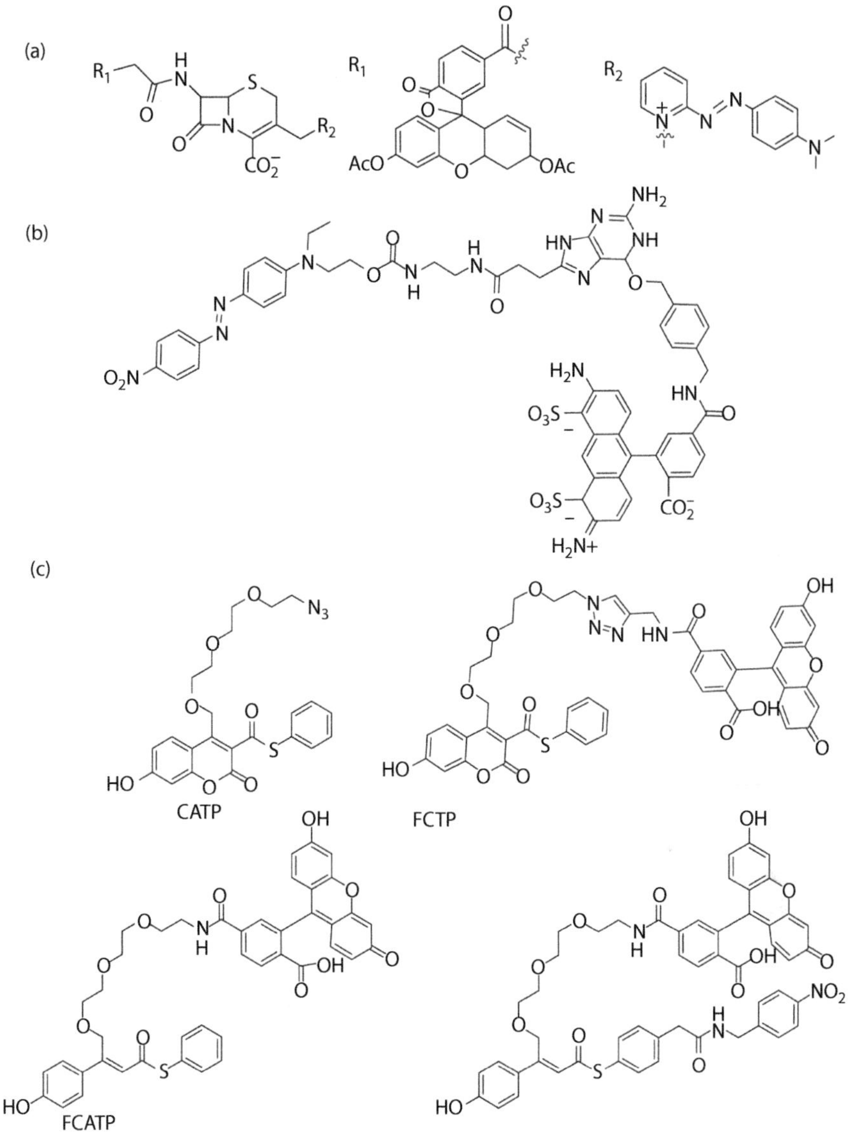

FIGURE 15.4 (a) Fluorogenic BL tag probes showing the structures of the fluorophore and the quencher. (b) Structure of the fluorogenic SNAP tag probe. (c) Structures of some commonly used PYP tag probes.

single time point measurements offered by pulse chase for probes where rigorous washing is needed.

PYP tag: PYP tag is based on a 125 kDa photoactive yellow protein found in bacteria. It can covalently bind to a variety of compounds containing a 7-hydroxy-coumarin-3-carboxylic acid thioester through transthioesterification with its Cys_{69}

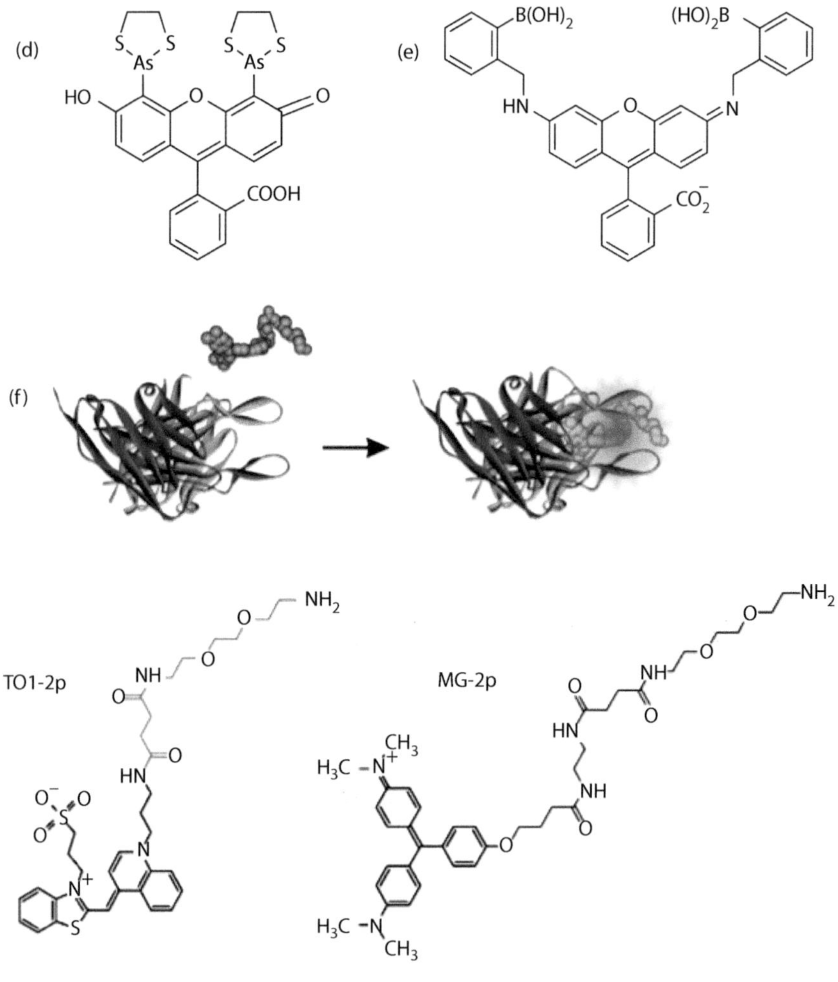

FIGURE 15.4 (Continued) (d) FlAsH. (e) RhoBo fluorogen. (f) Fluorogen-activating peptide technology and the structure of the commonly used fluorogens.

residue.[45-47] When the probe is in solution without the PYP tag, the fluorescence from fluorescein is quenched owing to intermolecular interactions between the coumarin thioester derivative and fluorescein. On covalently binding to the PYP tag, the location of coumarin in the protein binding pocket disrupts its interaction with fluorescein and fluorescence emission from fluorescein is observed. Common PYP probes are shown in Figure 15.4c. CATP is a cell-permeable dye while the other dyes can be only used on the cell surface. In another probe designated FCANB, nitrobenzene is used as a quencher for fluorescein. All but the environment-sensitive probes designated TMBDMA and CMBDMA need washing after incubation for ~30 min at several micromolar concentrations. They could be incubated at 1 μM concentration for 30 min to label mammalian cells. The key limitation of PYP tags is the use of fluorescein as the primary fluorophore. This limits the available colors when performing an experiment with PYP tags.

15.3.2 Noncovalent Labels

Tetracysteine: The tetracysteine tag is the first example of a hybrid tag and was systematically developed and reported by Roger Tsien's laboratory in 1998.[16] It utilizes 6–12 residues containing the sequence CCXBCC, where X and B can be any amino acids except cysteine and mostly proline and glycine. The four cysteines bind to biarsenical dyes such as FlAsH (Figure 15.4d), ReAsH, CrAsH, CHoXAsH, and AsCy3.[48–50] The tetracysteine motif has subpicomolar affinity for the FlAsH and ReAsH probes, and there is a 1000-fold fluorescence enhancement of the probes upon binding the tetracysteine motif. This combination of tight binding and high fluorogenicity results in a labeling system that does not require any washing prior to imaging the specifically labeled proteins. The biarsenical dyes are always administered with dithiols to minimize background labeling arising from their affinity for monothiols and to protect cells from arsenic toxicity. Typical labeling concentrations are 1 μM, and the incubation times are long, often up to 1 h. As the first hybrid tags that were developed and implemented in two colors, the biarsenicals have been used in a variety of applications, including affinity purification, pulse chase labeling, chromophore-assisted light inactivation, correlative light and electron microscopy, protein synthesis detection, and *in vivo* studies of protein folding to name just a few.[8]

Tetraserine tags: Tetraserine tags, developed by the Schepartz laboratory, to some extent solve the problems of cytotoxicity and background that are observed with TC tags. A rhodamine-derived bis-boronic acid dye (RhoBo) (Figure 15.4e) can bind specifically with submicromolar affinity to tetraserine motifs (SSPGSS) on POIs. RhoBo has higher QY (0.91) than FlAsH (0.5).[51] RhoBo is a cell-permeant dye and has been used at a concentration of 1 μM with 30 min of incubation time for the fluorescence imaging of intrinsic proteins inside HeLa cells. The relatively higher K_d (347 nM) and the abundance of proteins containing the SSPGSS motifs (particularly myosin) in human cell lines pose the main limitations to the use of this probe for live cell imaging.

Fluorogen-activating peptides: While noncovalent, fluorogenic labeling has several advantages, there is a constant trade-off between binding affinity, on rate, and brightness. Also, for some applications, having a reversible binding of the fluorescent complex can be very useful. Most importantly, the ability to target the probe to any location, on or inside the cell, is still an unmet need because of the limitations on the available tags and probes. Fluorogen-activating peptides are excellent hybrid labeling agents that address these limitations. They consist of a genetically encoded protein tag and a small-molecule fluorogen. The fluorogen in solution has rotational freedom around its pi-bond system that disrupts conjugation and fluorescence. However, when it is bound to a protein in a noncovalent fashion, the rotational freedom is restricted and fluorescence results from the formation of a planar, conjugated π-system. Derivatives of malachite green and thiazole orange were the first reported fluorogens with this technology (Figure 15.4f).[52] The last 5 years have seen a rapid increase in the number and type of fluorogens for this technology, covering the visible and far red spectrum as well as providing a variety of functionalities, such as resonance energy transfer, leading to signal amplification and pH sensing.[53–57] The fluorogens used with this technology show a fluorescence enhancement of up to 18,000-fold, the highest reported enhancement for any protein-based fluorogen. This ensures a completely wash-free system for cell imaging. Finally, since the interaction between the peptide and the fluorogen is noncovalent, it has been possible to obtain, through directed evolution, a vast variety of peptide–fluorogen pairs with varying affinities (6 pM to ~500 nM).[58] The protein–fluorogen binding is instantaneous, even at ~100 nM of the fluorogen. Directed evolution also allows for tunability of photochemical properties and has led to the discovery of fluorogens with enhanced photostability. This technology has been applied for single-molecule detection and superresolution microscopy on fixed and live cells.[52,59]

15.4   CONCLUSIONS AND FUTURE OUTLOOK

During the first wave of developing fluorophores, synthetic chemistry enabled us to provide the desired spectroscopic, photochemical, and targeting properties to a variety of fluorophores and fluorogens. The development of FP technology further fueled discovery through genetically encoded protein tagging techniques. The last 18 years, in what may be termed as a bio-inspired third wave of protein tagging, have seen some very smart systems that mimic natural enzymes and proteins to label POIs. During this period, most of the efforts have been toward the modification of the protein tag. Fluorogenic probes are catching up with other techniques and a surge in the number and variety of these probes has been observed in the last 4 years. While these wash-free labels will continue to be developed, in the future, we would finally like to have a "tag-less" tag system. For this to be achieved, the principles of fluorogenicity and bio-inspired specificity have to be utilized in sync. A recent example of that approach was the development of fluorescent saxitoxins by the Moerner laboratory.[60] These small-molecule probes directly bind to a POI and show a fluorogenic response. While it is hard to fathom that we would be able to find a selective fluorogen for every protein possible, it is definitely a good target for the design of the fourth-generation protein-labeling approaches. These may enable the direct detection of a specific native protein in the complex cellular environment.

ACKNOWLEDGMENTS

The authors thank Dr. Cheryl Telmer (Bruchez laboratory) for a critical reading of the manuscript. They also thank Joanna Burdyńska (Matyjaszewski laboratory) and Matharishwan Naganbabu (Bruchez laboratory) for help with the graphic content of the manuscript. This work was supported by grants from the National Institutes of Health (U54GM103529-MPB) and a McWilliams Fellowship (SS) from CMU.

REFERENCES

1. Fernández-Suárez, M., and A. Y. Ting. "Fluorescent Probes for Super-Resolution Imaging in Living Cells." *Nature Reviews Molecular Cell Biology* 9, no. 12 (2008): 929–43.
2. Yildiz, A., and P. R. Selvin. "Fluorescence Imaging with One Nanometer Accuracy: Application to Molecular Motors." *Accounts of Chemical Research* 38, no. 7 (2005): 574–82.

3. Xie, X. S., and J. K. Trautman. "Optical Studies of Single Molecules at Room Temperature." *Annual Review of Physical Chemistry* 49, no. 1 (1998): 441–80.

4. Eggeling, C., J. Widengren, R. Rigler, and C. A. M. Seidel. "Photostability of Fluorescent Dyes for Single-Molecule Spectroscopy: Mechanisms and Experimental Methods for Estimating Photobleaching in Aqueous Solution." In *Applied Fluorescence in Chemistry, Biology and Medicine*, edited by W. Rettig, B. Strehmel, S. Schrader, H. Seifert, 193–240. New York: Springer, 1999.

5. Depry, C., S. Mehta, and J. Zhang. "Multiplexed Visualization of Dynamic Signaling Networks Using Genetically Encoded Fluorescent Protein-Based Biosensors." *Pflügers Archiv—European Journal of Physiology* 465, no. 3 (2013): 373–81.

6. Wysocki, L. M., and L. D. Lavis. "Advances in the Chemistry of Small Molecule Fluorescent Probes." *Current Opinion in Chemical Biology* 15, no. 6 (2011): 752–9.

7. Remington, S. J. "Green Fluorescent Protein: A Perspective." *Protein Science* 20, no. 9 (2011): 1509–19.

8. Giepmans, B. N. G., S. R. Adams, M. H. Ellisman, and R. Y. Tsien. "The Fluorescent Toolbox for Assessing Protein Location and Function." *Science Signaling* 312, no. 5771 (2006): 217.

9. Coons, A. H., and M. H. Kaplan. "Localization of Antigen in Tissue Cells II. Improvements in a Method for the Detection of Antigen by Means of Fluorescent Antibody." *The Journal of Experimental Medicine* 91, no. 1 (1950): 1–13.

10. Tsien, R. Y. "The Green Fluorescent Protein." *Annual Review of Biochemistry* 67, no. 1 (1998): 509–44.

11. Day, R. N., and M. W. Davidson. "The Fluorescent Protein Palette: Tools for Cellular Imaging." *Chemical Society Reviews* 38, no. 10 (2009): 2887–921.

12. Shcherbo, D., C. Murphy, G. Ermakova et al. "Far-Red Fluorescent Tags for Protein Imaging in Living Tissues." *Biochemical Journal* 418 (2009): 567–74.

13. Kremers, G., K. L. Hazelwood, C. S. Murphy, M. W. Davidson, and D. W. Piston. "Photoconversion in Orange and Red Fluorescent Proteins." *Nature Methods* 6, no. 5 (2009): 355–8.

14. Farinas, J., and A. S. Verkman. "Receptor-Mediated Targeting of Fluorescent Probes in Living Cells." *Journal of Biological Chemistry* 274, no. 12 (1999): 7603–6.

15. Schlessinger, J., Y. Shechter, M. C. Willingham, and I. Pastan. "Direct Visualization of Binding, Aggregation, and Internalization of Insulin and Epidermal Growth Factor on Living Fibroblastic Cells." *Proceedings of the National Academy of Sciences* 75, no. 6 (1978): 2659–63.

16. Griffin, B. A., S. R. Adams, and R. Y. Tsien. "Specific Covalent Labeling of Recombinant Protein Molecules inside Live Cells." *Science* 281, no. 5374 (1998): 269–72.

17. Keppler, A., S. Gendreizig, T. Gronemeyer et al. "A General Method for the Covalent Labeling of Fusion Proteins with Small Molecules *In Vivo*." *Nature Biotechnology* 21, no. 1 (2002): 86–9.

18. Regoes, A., and A. B. Hehl. "SNAP-Tag-Mediated Live Cell Labeling as an Alternative to GFP in Anaerobic Organisms." *Biotechniques* 39, no. 6 (2005): 809–10.

19. Gautier, A., A. Juillerat, C. Heinis et al. "An Engineered Protein Tag for Multiprotein Labeling in Living Cells." *Chemistry & Biology* 15, no. 2 (2008): 128–36.

20. Srikun, D., A. E. Albers, C. I. Nam, A. T. Iavarone, and C. J. Chang. "Organelle-Targetable Fluorescent Probes for Imaging Hydrogen Peroxide in Living Cells Via Snap-Tag Protein Labeling." *Journal of the American Chemical Society* 132, no. 12 (2010): 4455–65.

21. Maurel, D., L. Comps-Agrar, C. Brock et al. "Cell-Surface Protein–Protein Interaction Analysis with Time-Resolved FRET and SNAP-Tag Technologies: Application to GPCR Oligomerization." *Nature Methods* 5, no. 6 (2008): 561–7.

22. Hinner, M. J., and K. Johnsson. "How to Obtain Labeled Proteins and What to Do with Them." *Current Opinion in Biotechnology* 21, no. 6 (2010): 766–76.

23. Los, G., A. Darzins, N. Karassina et al. "Halotag™ Interchangeable Labeling Technology for Cell Imaging and Protein Capture." *Cell Notes* 11 (2005): 2–6.

24. Schröder, J., H. Benink, M. Dyba, and G. V. Los. "*In Vivo* Labeling Method Using a Genetic Construct for Nanoscale Resolution Microscopy." *Biophysical Journal* 96, no. 1 (2009): L1–3.

25. Watanabe, S., S. Mizukami, Y. Hori, and K. Kikuchi. "Multicolor Protein Labeling in Living Cells Using Mutant B-Lactamase-Tag Technology." *Bioconjugate Chemistry* 21, no. 12 (2010): 2320–6.

26. Watanabe, S., S. Mizukami, Y. Akimoto, Y. Hori, and K. Kikuchi. "Intracellular Protein Labeling with Prodrug-Like Probes Using a Mutant B-Lactamase Tag." *Chemistry-A European Journal* 17, no. 30 (2011): 8342–9.

27. Gallagher, S. S., J. E. Sable, M. P. Sheetz, and V. W. Cornish. "An *In Vivo* Covalent TMP-Tag Based on Proximity-Induced Reactivity." *ACS Chemical Biology* 4, no. 7 (2009): 547–56.

28. Kapanidis, A. N., Y. W. Ebright, and R. H. Ebright. "Site-Specific Incorporation of Fluorescent Probes into Protein: Hexahistidine-Tag-Mediated Fluorescent Labeling with (Ni2+: Nitrilotriacetic Acid) N-Fluorochrome Conjugates." *Journal of the American Chemical Society* 123, no. 48 (2001): 12123–5.

29. Lata, S., M. Gavutis, R. Tampe, and J. Piehler. "Specific and Stable Fluorescence Labeling of Histidine-Tagged Proteins for Dissecting Multi-Protein Complex Formation." *Journal of the American Chemical Society* 128, no. 7 (2006): 2365–72.

30. Ojida, A., K. Honda, D. Shinmi et al. "Oligo-Asp Tag/Zn (II) Complex Probe as a New Pair for Labeling and Fluorescence Imaging of Proteins." *Journal of the American Chemical Society* 128, no. 32 (2006): 10452–9.

31. Miller, L. W., J. Sable, P. Goelet, M. P. Sheetz, and V. W. Cornish. "Methotrexate Conjugates: A Molecular *In Vivo* Protein Tag." *Angewandte Chemie* 116, no. 13 (2004): 1704–7.

32. Miller, L. W., Y. Cai, M. P. Sheetz, and V. W. Cornish. "*In Vivo* Protein Labeling with Trimethoprim Conjugates: A Flexible Chemical Tag." *Nature Methods* 2, no. 4 (2005): 255–7.

33. Yano, Y., A. Yano, S. Oishi et al. "Coiled-Coil Tag-Probe System for Quick Labeling of Membrane Receptors in Living Cells." *ACS Chemical Biology* 3, no. 6 (2008): 341–5.

34. Beckett, D., E. Kovaleva, and P. J. Schatz. "A Minimal Peptide Substrate in Biotin Holoenzyme Synthetase-Catalyzed Biotinylation." *Protein Science* 8, no. 04 (1999): 921–9.

35. Bates, I. R., B. Hébert, Y. Luo et al. "Membrane Lateral Diffusion and Capture of CFTR within Transient Confinement Zones." *Biophysical Journal* 91, no. 3 (2006): 1046–58.

36. Howarth, M., K. Takao, Y. Hayashi, and A. Y. Ting. "Targeting Quantum Dots to Surface Proteins in Living Cells with Biotin Ligase." *Proceedings of the National Academy of Sciences of the United States of America* 102, no. 21 (2005): 7583–8.

37. Chen, I., M. Howarth, W. Lin, and A. Y. Ting. "Site-Specific Labeling of Cell Surface Proteins with Biophysical Probes Using Biotin Ligase." *Nature Methods* 2, no. 2 (2005): 99–104.

38. Fernández-Suárez, M., H. Baruah, L. Martínez-Hernández et al. "Redirecting Lipoic Acid Ligase for Cell Surface Protein Labeling with Small-Molecule Probes." *Nature Biotechnology* 25, no. 12 (2007): 1483–7.

39. Yin, J., P. D. Straight, S. M. McLoughlin et al. "Genetically Encoded Short Peptide Tag for Versatile Protein Labeling by Sfp Phosphopantetheinyl Transferase." *Proceedings of the National Academy of Sciences of the United States of America* 102, no. 44 (2005): 15815–20.

40. Zhou, Z., P. Cironi, A. J. Lin et al. "Genetically Encoded Short Peptide Tags for Orthogonal Protein Labeling by Sfp and AcpS Phosphopantetheinyl Transferases." *ACS Chemical Biology* 2, no. 5 (2007): 337–46.

41. Hayashi, T., and I. Hamachi. "Traceless Affinity Labeling of Endogenous Proteins for Functional Analysis in Living Cells." *Accounts of Chemical Research* 45, no. 9 (2012): 1460–9.

42. Mizukami, S., S. Watanabe, Y. Akimoto, and K. Kikuchi. "No-Wash Protein Labeling with Designed Fluorogenic Probes and Application to Real-Time Pulse-Chase Analysis." *Journal of the American Chemical Society* 134, no. 3 (2012): 1623–9.

43. Stöhr, K., D. Siegberg, T. Ehrhard et al. "Quenched Substrates for Live-Cell Labeling of Snap-Tagged Fusion Proteins with Improved Fluorescent Background." *Analytical Chemistry* 82, no. 19 (2010): 8186–93.

44. Komatsu, T., K. Johnsson, H. Okuno et al. "Real-Time Measurements of Protein Dynamics Using Fluorescence Activation-Coupled Protein Labeling Method." *Journal of the American Chemical Society* 133, no. 17 (2011): 6745–51.

45. Hori, Y., K. Nakaki, M. Sato, S. Mizukami, and K. Kikuchi. "Development of Protein-Labeling Probes with a Redesigned Fluorogenic Switch Based on Intramolecular Association for No-Wash-Live-Cell Imaging." *Angewandte Chemie International Edition* 51, no. 23 (2012): 5611–4.

46. Hori, Y., H. Ueno, S. Mizukami, and K. Kikuchi. "Photoactive Yellow Protein-Based Protein Labeling System with Turn-on Fluorescence Intensity." *Journal of the American Chemical Society* 131, no. 46 (2009): 16610–1.

47. Sadhu, K. K., S. Mizukami, Y. Hori, and K. Kikuchi. "Switching Modulation for Protein Labeling with Activatable Fluorescent Probes." *ChemBioChem* 12, no. 9 (2011): 1299–308.

48. Uljana Mayer, M. "Crash: A Biarsenical Multi-Use Affinity Probe with Low Non-Specific Fluorescence." *Chemical Communications* no. 24 (2006): 2601–3.

49. Adams, S. R., R. E. Campbell, L. A. Gross et al. "New Biarsenical Ligands and Tetracysteine Motifs for Protein Labeling *In Vitro* and *In Vivo*: Synthesis and Biological Applications." *Journal of the American Chemical Society* 124, no. 21 (2002): 6063–76.

50. Cao, H., Y. Xiong, T. Wang et al. "A Red Cy3-Based Biarsenical Fluorescent Probe Targeted to a Complementary Binding Peptide." *Journal of the American Chemical Society* 129, no. 28 (2007): 8672–3.

51. Halo, T. L., J. Appelbaum, E. M. Hobert, D. M. Balkin, and A. Schepartz. "Selective Recognition of Protein Tetraserine Motifs with a Cell-Permeable, Pro-Fluorescent Bis-Boronic Acid." *Journal of the American Chemical Society* 131, no. 2 (2008): 438–9.

52. Szent-Gyorgyi, C., B. F. Schmidt, Y. Creeger et al. "Fluorogen-Activating Single-Chain Antibodies for Imaging Cell Surface Proteins." *Nature Biotechnology* 26, no. 2 (2007): 235–40.

53. Pow, C. L., S. A. Marks, L. D. Jesper et al. "A Rainbow of Fluoromodules: A Promiscuous ScFv Protein Binds to and Activates a Diverse Set of Fluorogenic Cyanine Dyes." *Journal of the American Chemical Society* 130, no. 38 (2008): 12620–1.

54. Shank, N. I., K. J. Zanotti, F. Lanni, P. B. Berget, and B. A. Armitage. "Enhanced Photostability of Genetically Encodable Fluoromodules Based on Fluorogenic Cyanine Dyes and a Promiscuous Protein Partner." *Journal of the American Chemical Society* 131, no. 36 (2009): 12960–9.

55. Shank, N. I., H. H. Pham, A. S. Waggoner, and B. A. Armitage. "Twisted Cyanines: A Non-Planar Fluorogenic Dye with Superior Photostability and Its Use in a Protein-Based Fluoromodule." *Journal of the American Chemical Society* 135, no. 1 (2012): 242–51.

56. Grover, A., B. F. Schmidt, R. D. Salter et al. "Genetically Encoded pH Sensor for Tracking Surface Proteins through Endocytosis." *Angewandte Chemie International Edition* 51, no. 20 (2012): 4838–42.

57. Szent-Gyorgyi, C., B. F. Schmidt, J. A. J. Fitzpatrick, and M. P. Bruchez. "Fluorogenic Dendrons with Multiple Donor Chromophores as Bright Genetically Targeted and Activated Probes." *Journal of the American Chemical Society* 132, no. 32 (2010): 11103–9.

58. Szent-Gyorgyi, C., R. L. Stanfield, S. Andreko et al. "Malachite Green Mediates Homodimerization of Antibody V_1 Domains to Form a Fluorescent Ternary Complex with Singular Symmetric Interfaces." *Journal of Molecular Biology* 425, no. 22 (2013): 4595–613.
59. Fitzpatrick, J. A., Q. Yan, J. J. Sieber et al. "STED Nanoscopy in Living Cells Using Fluorogen Activating Proteins." *Bioconjugate Chemistry* 20, no. 10 (2009): 1843–7.
60. Ondrus, A. E., H.-l. D. Lee, S. Iwanaga et al. "Fluorescent Saxitoxins for Live Cell Imaging of Single Voltage-Gated Sodium Ion Channels Beyond the Optical Diffraction Limit." *Chemistry & Biology* 19, no. 7 (2012): 902–12.

Section IV

Nanoscopy

16 Combined Topography, Recognition, and Fluorescence Measurements on Cells

Rong Zhu, Memed Duman, Josef Madl,
Gerhard J. Schütz, and Peter Hinterdorfer

CONTENTS

16.1   COMBINED OPTICAL AND ATOMIC FORCE MICROSCOPE

Conventional optical microscopy techniques, such as bright field, cross-polarized light, phase contrast, dark field, and differential interference contrast provide morphological and structural information of cells and cellular organelles, while fluorescence microscopy allows for imaging specific molecular components and for determining the localization of molecules in cells down to the single-molecule level,[1] making it possible to follow cellular processes and to monitor the dynamics of living cell components. The lateral and axial resolution of conventional optical microscopy is limited by diffraction, which is typically approximately 200–300 nm. Recently, optical super-resolution techniques have been developed, such as single-molecule optical microscopy,[2] saturated structured illumination microscopy,[3] stimulated emission depletion microscopy,[4] photoactivation localization microscopy,[5,6] and stochastic optical reconstruction microscopy,[7] which surpass the diffraction limit by applying concepts such as point-spread-function engineering or by utilizing the high accuracy of single-molecule localization. Thereby, a lateral resolution of 20–50 nm can be achieved and super-resolution in 3D is also feasible.

However, most of the optical techniques cannot provide information about the sample topography. Atomic force microscopy (AFM)[8] allows for obtaining 3D topographical images with subnanometer resolution. Compared with other high-resolution techniques (e.g., electron microscopy, etc.), the particular advantage of AFM is that the measurements can be carried out in aqueous and physiological environments. Recently, the imaging speed of AFM has been dramatically improved[9] from minutes to tens of milliseconds per frame, which makes it possible to film single biomolecules in action in real time.[10,11] This opens the possibility to study structure, dynamics, and function of biological samples in vivo. Since structure–function relationships play a key role in bioscience, their simultaneous detection is a promising approach to yield novel insights for the characterization of biological mechanisms.

In addition to high-resolution topographical imaging, AFM can also be used for force measurements, which provide insights into the mechanical properties of cells, for example, the stiffness.[12,13] Furthermore, the structural and energetic dynamics of biomolecules can be investigated by probing the interactions between a cell surface–bound molecule and a cantilever that carries a complementary binding partner, for example, another cell,[14] virus,[15,16] or single molecules.[17–19] Ligand binding to receptors is one of the most important functional elements because it is often the initiating step in reaction pathways and signaling cascades. The high resolution of AFM in both position and force is ideally suited to gain new insights into this field. Force spectroscopy experiments probe the molecular dynamics of ligand–receptor binding, which renders it possible for estimation of affinity, rate constants, and energy barriers, as well as the bond width of the binding pocket.[20–26] It also allows detection of association,[27] different functional and conformational states of proteins,[28] and sequential information of epigenetic modification of DNA.[29]

Besides studying ligand–receptor recognition processes, the localization of receptor binding sites by molecular recognition of a ligand is of particular interest. The information for topography and ligand–receptor interaction can be obtained by recognition imaging,[30] where receptor sites are localized with single-molecule accuracy. This opens new perspectives for nanometer-scale epitope mapping of bio-molecules and localizing receptor sites during biological processes. The recently developed simultaneous topography and recognition imaging technique (TREC)[31-33] yields a topographical image and a separate map of recognition sites from a single scan. When a ligand for a particular receptor is attached to an AFM tip, the AFM tip becomes a chemically selective nanosensor for the detection of specific receptor sites on the cell surface. The operating principle of TREC is based on the dynamic AFM mode. As shown in Figure 16.1, the functionalized tip is oscillated close to its resonance frequency and scanned across the surface. When the specific molecular binding occurs during the lateral scan, the upper part of the oscillation amplitude is consequently reduced. The electronic circuits in the PicoTREC box split the oscil-lation signal into lower and upper parts, the latter of which is used to construct the recognition image. Therefore, the corresponding recognition events appear as dark spots in the recognition image. Consequently, maps of binding sites across a variety of surfaces can be quickly and easily obtained. TREC imaging has been applied to detect isolated single molecules,[34-37] molecular complexes,[38] fabricated nanopatterns,[39,40] proteins in membranes,[41-44] cells,[45-50] and tissues,[51-53] with nano-meter resolution for isolated molecules in planar membranes and 5 nm resolution on cell surfaces.

The plasma membrane of cells has inherent complexity on various levels, which renders precise statements about the early signaling mechanisms still speculative. First of all, the formation of nanodomains, such as caveolae,[54] tetraspanin networks,[55] lipid rafts,[56] and so on, leads to association or segregation of plasma membrane con-stituents, with dramatic effects for ligand binding and signal transduction.[57-59] The intrinsic heterogeneity of nanodomains yields the presence of multiple platforms with distinct receptor occupancy. Second, receptors, adaptor proteins, and effectors are prone to posttranslational modifications (e.g., acylation and phosphorylation), which have dramatic effects not only on their affinity to plasma membrane domains but also on their ligand affinity and activity. Third, cellular signaling can be orga-nized in a highly redundant way, with multiple pathways capable of activating the same effect. The described complexity calls for a combined measurement strategy, by studying protein status and functions at the same time.

AFM has been successfully combined with some optical microscopy techniques to yield high-resolution images and more quantitative details that may not be possible to obtain using the individual techniques alone. The advantages and benefits of com-bined AFM and fluorescence microscopy allow more detailed characterization of cellular structures and processes.[60-62] With the help of the combined AFM/confocal laser scanning microscopy, the organization and distribution of intracellular proteins have been studied.[63] The cellular response of AFM-based manipulation was also detected using objective-type total internal reflection fluorescence microscopy.[64]

In our laboratory, we developed a versatile instrument that combines the topog-raphy, recognition, force spectroscopy, and optical imaging into a single system for cell investigations.[49,65] The combination of AFM and fluorescence microscopy is not merely a simple addition of two components. It rather provides a qualitatively new level in microscopic studies, giving unprecedented versatility in the detection and monitoring of cellular events, not only for the localization of individual molecules

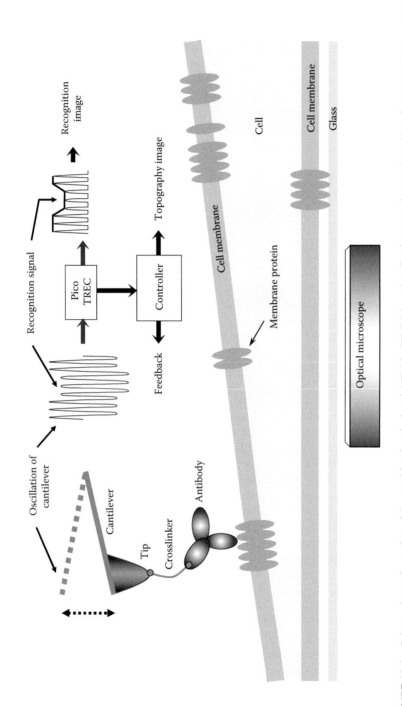

FIGURE 16.1 Schematic configuration of the combined optical and AFM for TREC imaging. During scanning on the cell surface, the AFM cantilever tip oscillates with constant amplitude. When the tip-tethered antibody binds with the cognate membrane protein on the cell surface, the upper part of the oscillation is reduced, which is detected by the electronic circuits of the PicoTREC box, shown as a dark spot in the recognition image.

and nanodomains but also for controlled substance delivery to the plasma membrane and for ligand-mediated stimulation of specific single receptor molecule. In Section 16.2, we will review the measurements of nanodomains of CD1d molecules on THP1 cells using a combination of AFM and fluorescence microscopy. In Section 16.3, we will introduce the fluorescence-guided force measurements, where the information obtained from fluorescence microscopy was used to position antibody-modified AFM tips above preselected sites on cells. With this approach, receptor-positive sites identified via fluorescence staining could be selectively addressed in molecular recognition force spectroscopy, thereby significantly increasing the binding probability. In Section 16.4, we will report on the T cell stimulation experiments, where Jurkat T cells loaded with Fura-2 were activated by AFM tips functionalized with anti-CD3 antibodies.

16.2 MULTIPLEX IMAGING OF THP1 CELLS EXPRESSING CD1d MOLECULES FUSED WITH YFP

CD1d molecules, nonpolymorphic major histocompatibility complex (MHC) class I-like molecules, are highly conserved antigen-presenting molecules expressed on several antigen-presenting cell types such as dendritic cells, monocytes, and B lymphocytes. Human invariant natural killer T (iNKT) cells express a semi-invariant T cell receptor (TCR) composed of an invariant TCR α chain (Vα24Jα18) that recognizes lipid antigens loaded onto the CD1d molecule. The presence of CD1d–lipid complexes on the cell surface allows the engagement of the iNKT TCR, leading to a rapid activation and secretion of Th1 (T helper type 1) and Th2 cytokines such as IFN-γ and IL-4.[66–69] Here, we used combined TREC and epifluorescence microscopy imaging to measure the density, distribution, and localization of yellow fluorescence protein (YFP)-labeled CD1d molecules loaded with α-galactosylceramide (αGalCer) on THP1 cells. Using an AFM tip tethered with the iNKT TCR, the recognition sites of cell receptors were detected in recognition images with domain sizes ranging from ~25 to ~160 nm, with the smallest domains corresponding to a single CD1d molecule.

16.2.1 MATERIALS AND METHODS

16.2.1.1 Instrumentation

For combined AFM and epifluorescence imaging, an Agilent 5500 AFM (Agilent Technologies, Arizona, USA) was placed on an iMIC 2000 fluorescence microscope (TILL Photonics, Germany). A specially designed quick-slide stage was used as the mechanical interface between the Agilent 5500 AFM and the iMIC 2000. The mechanical interface is very crucial for low-noise AFM measurements. All experiments with the combined setup were performed on a passive antivibration table (Newport GmbH, Darmstadt, Germany). The fluorescence images were recorded via an Olympus 40× objective (NA = 0.95) and a green fluorescent protein (GFP) filter set (excitation/bandwidth, 469/35 nm; emission/bandwith, 525/39 nm). AFM imaging was performed with top magnetic AC (top MAC, magnetic field excitation above the sample), bottom magnetic AC (bottom MAC, magnetic field excitation below the sample), and contact mode. The recognition data were recorded using a commercially available electronic unit (PicoTREC, Agilent Technologies). Magnetically coated Olympus cantilevers (with a nominal spring constant of 0.08 N m^{-1}) and magnetically coated applied nanostructure cantilevers (with a nominal spring constant of 0.28 N m^{-1}) were used for top MAC mode. A Veeco-C cantilever (with a nominal spring constant of 0.01 N m^{-1}) was used for contact mode imaging. All images were taken by closed-loop large-scan size scanner (100 μm × 100 μm). Integral and proportional gains were adjusted to optimize the sensitivity of the feedback loop. During TREC measurements, 5–10 nm free tip oscillation amplitude was chosen[70] at the optimum driving frequencies of each cantilever (~15 kHz for applied nanostructure and ~3 kHz for Olympus cantilevers).

16.2.1.2 Cell Culture and Sample Preparation

THP1 cells (American Type Culture Collection) transduced with a lentiviral vector encoding for YFP-labeled human CD1d[71] were grown in RPMI 1640 + 10% fetal bovine serum + 2 mM L-glutamine. Sodium pyruvate (1 mM), penicillin (100 U/ml), and streptomycin (100 μg/ml) were added to the medium to inhibit bacterial contamination. Cells were maintained between 2×10^5 and 9×10^5 cells/ml and grown at 37°C in 5% CO_2. Before immobilization of THP1 cells on a glass slide for TREC/fluorescence combined measurements, CD1d molecules on THP1 cells were loaded with 1 μg/ml αGalCer for 16 h at 37°C. Twenty-two-millimeter-diameter glass slides were coated with 0.01% poly-L-lysine aqueous solution and incubated for 15 min at room temperature. Afterward, they were washed with phosphate-buffered saline (PBS) and dried. THP1 cells loaded with αGalCer were immobilized on coated glass slides for 20 min. After 20 min fixation with 2% paraformaldehyde, glass slides were rinsed with PBS. To decrease autofluorescence, samples were treated with 1 mg/ml sodium borohydride ($NaBH_4$) in PBS buffer for 5 min to chemically reduce free aldehyde groups.[72] The sample was mounted in AFM and aligned according to the position of the AFM cantilever and illumination area of the epifluorescence microscope.

16.2.1.3 Functionalization of AFM Tips with iNKT-TCR

Tips (Si_3N_4) of the magnetically coated AFM cantilevers were functionalized with biotinylated iNKT-TCR.[73] First, the tips were treated with 3-aminopropyl-triethoxysilane (APTES) using a vapor phase deposition method described previously.[74] Subsequently, conjugation of aldehyde–PEG–NHS was performed by incubating the tips for 2 h in 0.5 ml of chloroform containing 3.3 mg of aldehyde–PEG–NHS and 30 μl of triethylamine.[75] Tips were rinsed with chloroform and dried with nitrogen. They were incubated with 10 μl of streptavidin solution (1.3 mg/ml) in 55 μl of PBS buffer plus 2 μl of 1 M $NaCNBH_3$ (freshly prepared by dissolving 32 mg of $NaCNBH_3$ in 50 μl of 100 mM NaOH and 450 μl Millipore water) for 1 h. Then, 5 μl of 1 M ethanolamine-hydrochloride aqueous solution (pH 9.6) was added to the solution in order to inactivate the remaining aldehyde groups. After 10 min, the tips were washed with PBS buffer (three times for 5 min) and stored in PBS buffer. As the last step, the streptavidin-modified tips were incubated with 20 μg/ml biotinylated iNKT-TCR in TRIS buffer overnight at 4°C. Tips were subsequently washed with the same buffer and stored (up to 3 days) at 4°C before measurement.

16.2.2 RESULTS AND DISCUSSION

The performance of the combined AFM/optical microscope system was first tested using a sample with fluorescein isothiocyanate (FITC) beads on a glass slide. Both the optical image and the AFM topographical image were measured at the same position. As shown in Figure 16.2, the optical image and the AFM topography could be accurately overlapped, which indicates that the closed-loop scanner has no distortion or nonlinearity. Thus, the image information from the two types of microscopes could be reliably compared and correlated.

In Figure 16.3, we show the measurements on THP1 cells expressing CD1d loaded with αGalCer[76] by using the combined AFM and optical microscope. From the standard bright-field imaging (Figure 16.3a), the AFM cantilever tip could be positioned above a proper cell. The expression level of CD1d molecules was shown by the fluorescence image (Figure 16.3b), which provided the distribution of αGalCer-CD1d on THP1 cells. Figure 16.3c shows the overlay of the AFM deflection and fluorescence images, with the cell plasma membrane and its underlying support resolved at nanometer resolution. TREC images of αGalCer-CD1d on THP1 cells were obtained with the AFM tip functionalized with iNKT-TCR. The oscillation amplitude of the cantilever (~8 nm) was set slightly smaller than the extended PEG tether length of ~10 nm. The suchlike selected imaging amplitude allows that the ligand molecule on the tip remains bound to the receptor molecule on the surface during scanning. For the control experiment, anti-CD1d antibodies were injected into the buffer solution, which resulted in an effective block of the CD1d molecules on the THP1 cell surface (data not shown). Recognition images were acquired on two different areas (Figure 16.3d). CD1d nanodomains were observed as dark spots on the recognition images, with a diameter ranging between 25 and 160 nm (Figure 16.3f). Since the diameter of the iNKT-TCR/CD1d complex is ~3.5 nm[77] and the free orientation of the PEG linker allows binding 10 nm before and 10 nm after the

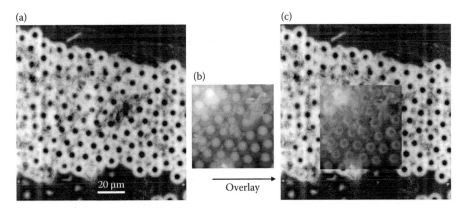

(a)

(b)

(c)

20 μm

Overlay →

FIGURE 16.2 The optical bright-field image (a) and the AFM topography (b) measured at the same position of the FITC bead sample on glass can be overlaid accurately (c).

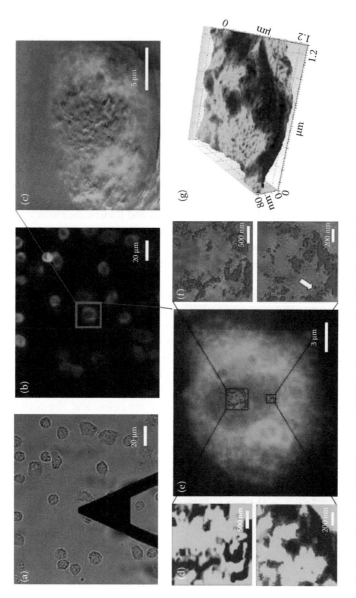

FIGURE 16.3 In situ optical and AFM images on THP1 cells expressing CD1d loaded with αGalCer. (a) Bright-field image, (b) fluorescence image, (c) overlay of fluorescence and deflection image, (d) recognition images, (e) superimposition of the recognition spots (from images [d], shown as red) on the fluorescence image, (f) higher magnification of the superimposition of the recognition and fluorescence images, (g) 3D overlay image of recognition and topography. (From Figure 5 of Ref. 49, with permission from IOP Publishing.)

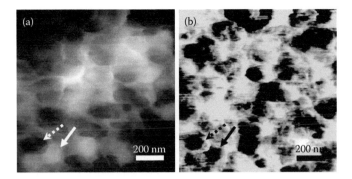

FIGURE 16.4 Simultaneous topography (a) and recognition (b) images on THP1 cells expressing CD1d loaded with αGalCer using a TCR-modified AFM tip. CD1d nanodomains are found not only in caveolae-like regions (e.g., indicated by dashed arrow) but also in protruding membrane regions (e.g., indicated by solid arrow). (From Figure 4 of Ref. 49, with permission from IOP Publishing.)

binding sites, the expected diameter of a single receptor recognition spot is 23.5 nm, which is approximately the minimal size of the recognition spots that we observed in the recognition images (see the arrow in Figure 16.3f). In Figure 16.3e, the recognition spots (red) were superimposed on the fluorescence image (green), revealing improved resolution as demonstrated further in Figure 16.3f. Recognition spots were also superimposed on the AFM topography image (Figure 16.3g) to investigate the correlation of αGalCer-CD1d molecules with membrane topographical features. Interestingly, some of the recognition spots are located in the caveolae-like regions (Figure 16.4, indicated by dashed arrows), whereas some other recognition spots are located in protruding membrane regions (Figure 16.4, indicated by solid arrows).

In summary, these measurements demonstrate the combination of topography, recognition, and fluorescence imaging for the localization of cellular membrane proteins with single-molecule resolution. While fluorescence imaging can be used to determine the overall expression level and the distribution of receptor sites on the cell surface, simultaneous topography and recognition imaging allows for exploring the distribution of specific membrane nanodomains and the cell topography in three dimensions. With TREC on the light microscope, single cellular receptor recognition sites can be detected at high signal-to-noise ratio with an apparent spot diameter of 25 nm. Therefore, epifluorescence microscopy becomes more powerful when combined with TREC imaging.

16.3   FLUORESCENCE-GUIDED FORCE SPECTROSCOPY

As shown in the last section, by applying two complementary techniques together, additional information on the nanodomains could be obtained. The synergic effect between fluorescence microscopy and AFM was further demonstrated here by probing fluorescence-labeled receptors in the cell membrane using force spectroscopy with AFM tips functionalized with specific antibodies. Two examples are shown in this section, for both of which AFM binding probability was found to be closely correlated with fluorescence intensity.

16.3.1   CHO Cells Expressing SRBI Fused with eGFP

Chinese hamster ovary (CHO) cells are widely used as expression systems for a number of proteins in cell biology. They have been used in our laboratory to study the uptake of high-density lipoprotein (HDL) particles into living cells.[78] The scavenger receptor class B type I (SRBI) plays an important role in mediating selective uptake of HDL-derived cholesterol and cholesteryl ester in liver and steroidogenic tissues. Here, we used information obtained from fluorescence microscopy to accurately position an antibody-modified tip above a preselected receptor domain in the cell membrane. With this approach, the binding probability of the molecular recognition force measurements could be significantly increased.

16.3.1.1   Materials and Methods

16.3.1.1.1   Instrumentation

A PicoPlus 5500 AFM (Molecular Imaging, Tempe, Arizona) was placed on an Axiovert 200 inverted optical microscope (Zeiss GmbH, Oberkochen, Germany) via a quick-slide stage (Molecular Imaging). This stage allows for convenient changing and positioning of samples, as the sample holder can be moved both relative to the optical axis of the objective and relative to the AFM cantilever. The whole setup was placed on a passive antivibration optical table (Newport GmbH) without any additional damping system. We used a 60× water objective (NA = 1.2, Olympus, Hamburg, Germany) for the fluorescence-guided force spectroscopy experiments. Fluorescence excitation was realized with a 488 nm laser (Sapphire 488-200; Coherent, Lübeck, Germany; approximately 100–500 W/cm^2 intensity). Fluorescence emission was acquired using an eGFP filter set (emission filter HQ535/50 M, 535,725 nm band pass, Chroma Tech) and a Cy3 filter set (emission filter HQ610/75M, 610,738 nm band pass, Chroma Tech) in addition. The fluorescence images were recorded using a CCD camera (Cascade 512B; Roper Scientific, Tucson, Arizona). For AFM force measurements, we used a PicoPlus multipurpose large scanner and contact mode cantilevers (10 pN/nm, silicon nitride) functionalized with antibodies as described in Section 16.3.1.1.3.

16.3.1.1.2   Cell Culture and Sample Preparation

CHO cells lacking the low-density lipoprotein receptor and expressing high levels of recombinant SRBI (ldlA7-SRBI cells) were used in this study. The receptor was fused with eGFP, which shows an absorption maximum at 488 nm and an emission maximum at 508 nm. Cells were grown in medium A (1:1 v/v mixture of Dulbecco's minimal essential medium and Ham's F-12 medium with 100 U/ml streptomycin sulfate) on 22 or 30 mm glass slides in conventional Petri dishes. The glass slides were mounted on the setup through a standard molecular imaging sample stage with a liquid cell. For AFM force spectroscopy, live CHO cells were fixed with 2% aqueous glutaraldehyde solution for 1 min and washed afterward carefully with PBS buffer. Fixation of the cells was necessary for preventing both endocytosis and diffusion of SRBI receptors, which was observed in living cells.[78] Shorter fixation times were used in order to minimize autofluorescence, arising mostly from glutaraldehyde fixation. In addition, we applied 1 mg/ml aqueous sodium borohydride (NaBH$_4$, in PBS buffer) for 2–5 min after the fixation process to further decrease autofluorescence by chemically reducing free aldehyde groups. Shorter fixation times also minimized degradation and inactiva-tion of the SRBI receptors in the cell membrane and preserved their ability to specifi-cally bind with antibodies.[79] Finally, the cells on the glass slide were aligned with the position of the AFM cantilever inside the illumination area of the inverted microscope.

16.3.1.1.3   Coupling of Antibodies to AFM Tips

Silicon nitride cantilevers (Veeco, Santa Barbara, California) were treated with ethanolamine-HCl (Sigma, Vienna, Austria) and subsequently coupled with het-erobifunctional tether (polyethylene glycol derivative, synthesized in our laboratory) as previously described in detail.[30,80] Affinity-purified polyclonal antibodies (anti-SRBI/II) were bound to the amino-reactive end of the tether in PBS buffer for an incu-bation time of 2 h. Tips were subsequently washed in PBS buffer and stored at 4°C.

16.3.1.2   Results and Discussion

At first, the fluorescence image of the sample was acquired using a GFP filter set. As shown in Figure 16.5a, clusters of eGFP-SRBI receptors were observed, one of

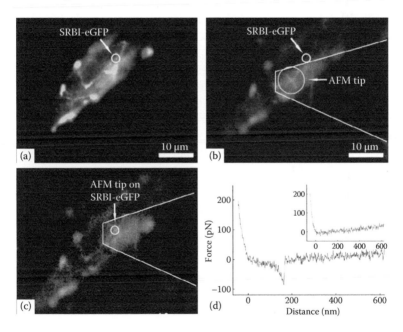

FIGURE 16.5 Fluorescence-guided force spectroscopy on CHO cells expressing SRBI-eGFP using an AFM tip functionalized with anti-SRBI/II antibody. (a) Fluorescence image of a fixed cell using the GFP filter set. An SRBI-eGFP-positive receptor site (white circle) was selected for force spectroscopy experiments, (b) switching to a Cy3 filter set (excitation still at 488 nm) revealing areas of autofluorescence. The AFM tip can be recognized by its typical X-shaped form resulting from its luminescence, (c) positioning of the AFM cantilever tip with the preselected SRBI-eGFP receptor cluster by overlapping the intersection of the X-shape with the center point of the small circle, (d) retrace curve recorded at an SRBI-eGFP-positive site, with a single unbinding event; the inset depicts a force curve without binding event on an SRBI-eGFP-negative site. (From Figures 4 and 5 of Ref. 65, with permission from Elsevier.)

which was marked with a white circle. Although autofluorescence of the fixed cells was reduced by applying NaBH$_4$, several areas still showed autofluorescence, which could be identified spectroscopically by switching to a Cy3 filter set, where the eGFP fluorescence was blocked.[81] Furthermore, this filter set allowed us to visualize the AFM tip position (Figure 16.5b), since an AFM tip made of silicon nitride shows some autoluminescence (in contrast to silicon cantilevers).[82] When the tip was illuminated with laser light (in our case, 488 nm), it emitted light at longer wavelengths up to 750 nm. After blocking the eGFP emission, the weak luminescence signal of the tip was sufficient to visualize its position on the cell (Figure 16.5b, X-shaped form), which enabled us to move the tip directly above the receptor cluster of interest, the position of which was known from the previously recorded fluorescence image using the GFP filter set (Figure 16.5a). Figure 16.5c shows the final position of the cantilever aligned on top of an SRBI-eGFP receptor cluster. Once the tip alignment had been accomplished, consecutive force–distance cycles were recorded. As shown in Figure 16.5d, a specific binding event between the tip-bound antibody and the cell membrane component was observed on an SRBI-eGFP-positive site. The inset in Figure 16.5d shows an example of a force–distance cycle without any binding event on an SRBI-eGFP-negative site. From several hundreds of cycles, the binding probability was determined (13.6% on eGFP-positive sites). The probability was much lower on either "blindly" probed plasma membrane without using guidance by fluorescence microscopy (3–4% binding probability) or deliberately selected eGFP-negative regions on the plasma membrane (2.5% binding probability). Therefore, guiding tip-bound proteins to their cognate binding partners on the cell surface via fluorescence microscopy showed the merits for force spectroscopy experiments of receptors with very low density on cells.

16.3.2   T24 CELLS EXPRESSING CD4-YFP AND LCK-CFP

CD4 is the major coreceptor in T cell activation, and Lck is the major Src family protein tyrosine kinase essential for early T cell signaling. T24 cells are a human bladder carcinoma cell line that does not contain endogenous CD4 and Lck.[83] Here, we measured force–distance curves on T24 cells transfected for expressing CD4-YFP and Lck-CFP using a cantilever tip functionalized with an anti-CD4 antibody and studied the correlation between the binding probability and the expression level of CD4-YFP and Lck-CFP.

16.3.2.1   Materials and Methods

16.3.2.1.1   Instrumentation

An Agilent 6000ILM AFM was mounted on a TILL Photonics more fluorescence microscope equipped with Oligochrome (TILL Photonics) as light source. For fluorescence imaging, single-band YFP and single-band CFP excitation filters in the Oligochrome were utilized sequentially. The setup was equipped with an image-splitter based on TILL Photonic's Dichrotome system (dichroic beamsplitter for CFP/YFP in combination with mirrors). Thereby, the image on the camera was split into two halves corresponding to the two color channels. The optical images were recorded with a CCD camera (Stingray F-145B) using the software Live Acquisition

(TILL Photonics). The combined AFM and optical microscope was placed on an active vibration control unit (Herzan). For AFM force–distance curve measurements, the scanning range is 3 µm and the sweep duration is 2 s/cycle.

16.3.2.1.2   Cell Culture and Sample Preparation

T24 cells expressing CD4-YFP and Lck-CFP were cultured in RPMI 1640 medium with 10% fetal calf serum (FCS), supplemented with penicillin–streptomycin (all cell culture media, buffers, and antibiotics were from PAA Laboratories, Pasching, Austria). Cells were passaged twice a week and were maintained under a humidified atmosphere with 5% CO_2 at 37°C. For AFM experiments, cells were seeded on glass bottom microwell dishes (MatTek, Ashland, Massachusetts) with three different dilutions to obtain an average of 40% confluence after 1 day. Before fixation, cells were rinsed in PBS to remove media components. Cells were then fixed with 4% formaldehyde in PBS at room temperature for 15 min and washed again in PBS. To quench the free aldehyde moieties, cells were incubated in 50 mM ethanolamine in PBS for 5 min followed by washing with PBS.

16.3.2.1.3   Coupling of Antibodies to AFM Tips

The antibodies specific for CD4 (MEM-241, EXBio) were covalently bound to Veeco MSCT cantilevers (nominal spring constant of 0.01 N m^{-1}) via NHS–PEG–acetal cross-linker.[84] The cantilevers were washed three times in chloroform, dried in air, washed with piranha solution (3 ml H_2O_2 with 7 ml H_2SO_4) for 30 min, rinsed three times in Millipore water, and finally dried at 160°C. The cleaned cantilevers were treated with APTES in gas phase.[85] Afterward, cantilevers were incubated for 1.5 h in 500 µl chloroform containing 1 mg NHS–PEG–acetal and 2.5 µl triethylamine. After being washed three times in chloroform and being air dried, cantilevers were treated with 1% citric acid (pH 2.2) for 10 min followed by washing in Millipore water three times and in ethanol once. The dried cantilever chips were put on a piece of clean parafilm in a small Petri dish. In parallel, the antibody solution was treated with dialysis to remove the sodium azide. Fifteen microliters of antibody solution was placed on the bottom of a dialysis tube (Slide-A-Lyzer MINI Dialysis Device, 10K MWCO, Pierce) and dialyzed against 1 L PBS two times (approximately 40 min and 19.5 h, respectively) in a 4°C room. The 25 µl antibody solution collected after dialysis was mixed with 2.5 µl of 200 mM $NaCNBH_3$ (32 mg $NaCNBH_3$ in 450 µl H_2O and 50 µl 100 mM NaOH, mixed with 2 ml buffer A [100 mM NaCl, 50 mM NaH_2PO_4, 1 mM EDTA, pH 7.5]). The antibody solution was then applied to the cantilevers and incubated for 1.5 h. Afterward, cantilevers were washed with buffer A three times and stored in buffer A treated with argon at 4°C before measurement.

16.3.2.2   Results and Discussion

According to the bright-field image and the fluorescence images at the same position using CFP and YFP filters, respectively (Figure 16.6), we found that the expression level of CD4-YFP and Lck-CFP varied significantly on different T24 cells, even in the same culture dish. For example, cells 4, 5, and 6 (Figure 16.6b) have high expression of Lck-CFP and low expression of CD4-YFP, while cells 7, 8, and 9

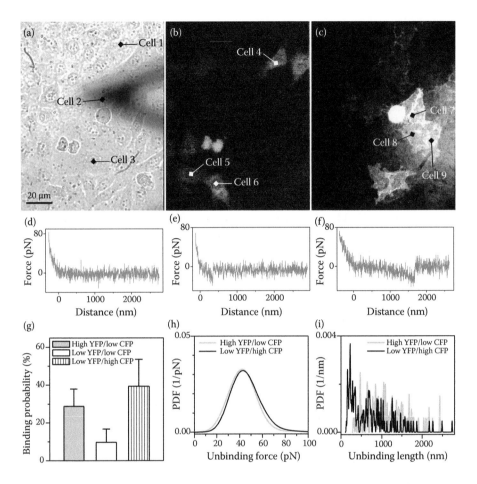

FIGURE 16.6 Fluorescence-guided force spectroscopy on T24 cells expressing CD4-YFP and Lck-CFP using an AFM tip functionalized with anti-CD4 antibody. (a) Bright-field, (b) CFP, and (c) YFP fluorescence images at the same position reveal that some cells (e.g., cells 4, 5, and 6) show high expression of Lck-CFP, while some cells (e.g., cells 7, 8, and 9) show high expression of CD4-YFP, whereas some other cells (e.g., cells 1, 2, and 3) show low expression for both. Every cell eventually shows force curves without binding (d) or with binding event (e and f), but the binding probability (g) is different. Cells with high expression of CD4-YFP and cells with high expression of Lck-CFP show a similar distribution of unbinding forces (h) but different distribution of unbinding lengths (i).

(Figure 16.6c) have low expression of Lck-CFP and high expression of CD4-YFP. In contrast, cells 1, 2, and 3 (Figure 16.6a) have low expression for both. We measured force–distance curves on each of the nine cells with the cantilever tip functionalized with the anti-CD4 antibody. On each cell, there were curves without binding event (e.g., Figure 16.6d) and curves with binding event (e.g., Figure 16.6e and f). The binding probability for each group of cells is shown in Figure 16.6g. On cells (7, 8, and 9) with high expression of CD4-YFP, the average binding probability was $28.8 \pm 9.1\%$, while on cells (1, 2, and 3) with low expression of both CD4-YFP and Lck-CFP, the binding probability was only 9.7 ± 7.1%. This result showed good correlation between the binding probability and the expression level of CD4-YFP. On cells (4, 5, and 6) that have high expression of Lck-CFP but low expression of CD4-YFP, the binding probability is 39.4 ± 14.2%. One possible interpretation for this high binding probability is that the overexpression of Lck might trigger the endogenous expression of CD4. The distributions of the unbinding force measured on cells (7, 8, and 9) with high expression of CD4-YFP and cells (4, 5, and 6) with high expression of Lck-CFP are shown in Figure 16.6h. The peak position (the most probable unbinding force) is 42.1 and 42.9 pN for the two groups of cells, respectively. The similar unbinding force measured on the two groups of cells supports the hypothesis that most of the binding events on cells (4, 5, and 6) with high expression of Lck-CFP might be contributed by the up-regulated endogenous CD4. The distributions of the unbinding length measured on cells with high expression of CD4-YFP (cells 7, 8, and 9) or Lck-CFP (cells 4, 5, and 6) are shown in Figure 16.6i. Both groups of cells have unbinding events with long lengths (>500 nm). However, the cells with high expression of Lck-CFP have a unique population of curves with an unbinding length shorter than 400 nm. Such shorter unbinding events might be attributed to the overexpressed Lck molecules, which could bind with CD4 molecules and associate with rafts, resulting in a more rigid plasma membrane.

16.4   ACTIVATION OF T CELL WITH SINGLE MOLECULE

For T cell activation, the initial key molecule is the TCR, which binds to the MHC molecule loaded with a specific peptide derived from an antigenic protein of the pathogen. Although the TCR is one of the best studied cell surface receptors, the mechanism involved in the early steps of T cell activation is still enigmatic.[86,87] Here, we explored the feasibility of using combined AFM and fluorescence microscopy to investigate the activation of a T cell with a single molecule. For this, a monoclonal antibody specific for the CD3 subunit of the TCR complex was conjugated onto the tip of the AFM cantilever, which was moved above individual Jurkat T cells for stimulation. The two Fab domains of the antibody can bind with the CD3 subunits of two TCR complexes, resulting in the formation of the TCR dimer, which could thus mimic the TCR triggering. By using the simultaneous fluorescence measurements, we examined whether such scenario was sufficient for signal initiation to induce a transient calcium release from the endoplasmic reticulum of the cell when touched by the AFM antibody tip.

16.4.1   Materials and Methods

16.4.1.1   Instrumentation

The Agilent 6000ILM AFM was mounted on the TILL Photonics *more* fluorescence microscope equipped with an Oligochrome (TILL Photonics) as light source. For the Fura-2 fluorescence imaging, the excitation light was filtered by the 340 and 380 nm excitation filters alternately in the Oligochrome. The optical images were recorded with a CCD camera (Stingray F-145B) using the software Live Acquisition (TILL Photonics). The combined AFM and optical microscope was placed on an active vibration control unit (Herzan) in an acoustic isolation chamber. For AFM force–distance curve measurements, the scanning range was 5 μm and the sweep duration was 1.5 s/cycle. A sample plate (Agilent) with temperature control was used, operated at 37°C.

16.4.1.2 Cell Culture and Sample Preparation

Wild-type Jurkat T cells (TIB152, Clone E6.1) were cultured in a medium of RPMI 1640 with 10% FCS in an incubator with 5% CO_2 at 37°C. They were passaged twice a week by giving 7 ml of fresh medium to 3 ml of cell solution from old passage. For the activation experiments, 1 ml of Jurkat T cells from the culture was washed by adding 9 ml of PBS with 2% FCS. The mixture was centrifuged at 1000 rpm for 5 min and the suspension was removed. One milliliter of culture medium was given to the cells and 10 μl of 1 mM Fura-2 (Molecular Probes) solution in DMSO was added. The cells were resuspended and incubated at 37°C with 5% CO_2 for approximately 45 min. Then, they were washed again as described above. Afterward, the cells were resuspended in 1 ml HBSS with Ca^{++} and Mg^{++} and with 10% FCS. A piece of glass slide with a diameter of 22 mm was mounted on the temperature-controlled sample plate. Five hundred microliters of HBSS with Ca^{++} and Mg^{++} and with 10% FCS was given on the glass. After the temperature reached 37°C, 50 μl of the above prepared cell suspension was added into the solution on the glass. The cells could settle down on the glass surface with slight movement.

16.4.1.3 Coupling of Antibodies to AFM Tips

The antibodies specific for CD3 (OKT3, EXBio) were covalently bound to the silicon tips of the Bruker MSNL cantilevers via NHS–PEG–acetal cross-linker.[84] The cantilevers were washed three times in chloroform, dried in air, washed with piranha solution (3 ml H_2O_2 with 7 ml H_2SO_4) for 30 min, rinsed three times in Millipore water, and finally dried at 160°C. The cleaned cantilevers were treated with APTES in gas phase.[85] Afterward, the cantilevers were incubated for 1.5 h in 500 μl of chloroform containing 1 mg NHS–PEG–acetal and 2.5 μl of triethylamine. After being washed three times in chloroform and being air dried, the cantilevers were treated with 1% citric acid (pH 2.2) for 10 min followed by washing in Millipore water three times and in ethanol once. The dried cantilever chips were put on a piece of clean parafilm in a small Petri dish. In parallel, the antibody solution was treated with dialysis to remove the sodium azide. Twenty microliters of antibody solution was placed on the bottom of a dialysis tube (Slide-A-Lyzer MINI Dialysis Device, 10K MWCO, Pierce) and dialyzed against 1 L PBS two times (approximately 2 and 19 h, respectively) in a 4°C room. The 60 μl antibody solution collected after dialysis was mixed with 2 μl of 200 mM $NaCNBH_3$ (32 mg $NaCNBH_3$ in 450 μl H_2O and 50 μl 100 mM NaOH, mixed with 2 ml buffer A [100 mM NaCl, 50 mM NaH_2PO_4, 1 mM EDTA, pH 7.5]). The antibody solution was then applied to the cantilevers and incubated for 3 h. Subsequently, cantilevers were washed with buffer A three times and stored in buffer A treated with argon at 4°C before measurement.

16.4.2 RESULTS AND DISCUSSION

The experimental configuration for the T cell activation is shown in Figure 16.7. During the experiment, the cantilever tip tethered with the anti-CD3 antibody was used to stimulate a randomly selected living Jurkat cell loaded with Fura-2. Meanwhile, the fluorescence images were continuously recorded at two excitation wavelengths: 340 and 380 nm. The ratio of the fluorescence signal from the two channels was calculated, for sensitive monitoring of the change of the calcium concentration in the cytosol of the cell. First, the measurements were performed at room temperature and the cells were washed and measured in PBS. With this condition, the efficiency of T cell activation was low. From 10 cells, only one cell could be activated. Therefore, the temperature was increased to 37°C and the HBSS with Ca^{++} and Mg^{++} and with 10% FCS was used as solution for the measurement. With this condition, the efficiency of the activation was improved. From randomly selected 15 cells, 12 were activated by the functionalized cantilever tips. One example of the measurement result is shown in Figure 16.8. As shown by the bright-field image in Figure 16.8a, the functionalized cantilever tip (approximately 8.5 μm from the end of the dark rectangle cantilever that had a width of approximately 23 μm) was moved above a Jurkat T cell (shown as a bright ball with a diameter of approximately 8.5 μm, indicated by a white arrow). Before force–distance curve measurement, the calcium concentration in the cytosol of this cell was as low as that of most other cells, which was shown by the fluorescence ratio image in Figure 16.8b. The fluorescence ratio

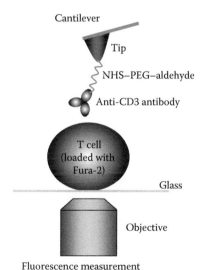

Fluorescence measurement

FIGURE 16.7   Schematic configuration of the T cell activation experiment. The AFM cantilever tip is functionalized with the anti-CD3 antibody via the NHS–PEG–aldehyde crosslinker. Jurkat T cells loaded with Ca^{++} indicator Fura-2 are placed on the glass surface. The AFM tip brings the antibody to the cell surface for engagement; meanwhile, fluorescence images at two excitation wavelengths (340 and 380 nm) are continuously recorded for the detection of the change of the Ca^{++} concentration in the cytosol of the cell.

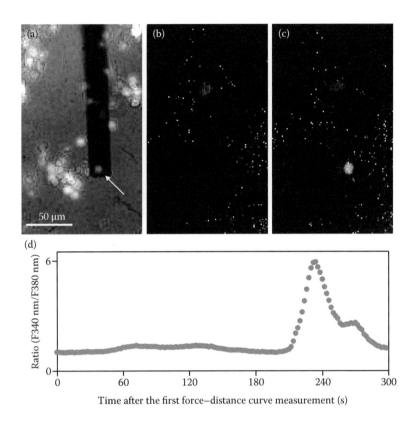

FIGURE 16.8 Activation of a Jurkat T cell using an AFM tip functionalized with anti-CD3 antibody. (a) Using bright-field imaging, the AFM tip was positioned above a Jurkat T cell (marked with the arrow). The image was taken with both light sources for bright field and fluorescence on, so that the cantilever and the cell under the cantilever can be shown simultaneously. (b) The fluorescence ratio image indicated that before the AFM tip touched the cell, the Ca^{++} concentration in the cytosol of this cell is similar to that of most other cells. (c) The fluorescence ratio image measured at 228 s after the first force–distance curve measurement indicated that the Ca^{++} concentration in the cell touched by the antibody tip became significantly higher than that in other cells. (d) The time course of the fluorescence ratio signal within the cell stimulated by the antibody tip.

signal within this cell was recorded every 2 s as shown in Figure 16.8d. After the force–distance curve measurements were performed for approximately 3.5 min, the calcium concentration in the cytosol of this cell started to increase (Figure 16.8d). A fluorescence ratio image measured at 228 s after the start of force–distance curve measurement is shown in Figure 16.8c; the calcium concentration in this cell was much higher than that in other cells. From Figure 16.8d, it was found that it took approximately 20 s for the calcium concentration to reach the maximum after cell activation, and the concentration decreased subsequently for approximately 1 min before it restored to the normal value.

As control experiment, the cantilever tip was functionalized with nonspecific goat IgG and the measurement was performed under the same conditions. With this kind of cantilever tip, nine Jurkat T cells were measured and none was activated.

In summary, the combined AFM and fluorescence microscopy was shown not only to be capable of mapping specific nanodomains on cell surface and providing additional information from correlation between fluorescence and force spectroscopy but also to be feasible for delicate experiments on manipulation of single cells via precise delivery of single molecules to the cell membrane for signal transduction. The cantilever tips can also be functionalized with MHC molecules loaded with the cognate peptide[88] or various mutants with neutral, agonistic, or antagonistic effect for activation experiments on other types of T cells. Moreover, by varying the force loading rate, the combined instrument allows for systematic investigations of the interaction kinetics for antigen recognition. This will altogether help for the comprehensive understanding of mechanisms involved in the early steps of T cell activation.

ACKNOWLEDGMENTS

The authors would like to thank Dr. Julian Weghuber for providing the T24 cell lines and Anna-Maria Lipp for Jurkat T cells; Doris Vater, Dr. Mariolina Salio, Dawn Shepherd, Paolo Polzella, and Dr. Sebastian Rhode for technical assistance; Dr. Christian Rankl, Dr. Ferry Kienberger, and Dr. Gerald Kada for software and hardware support; Prof. Dr. Rainer Uhl, Prof. Dr. Hermann Gruber, Prof. Dr. Vincenzo Cerundolo, Prof. Dr. Andreas Ebner, Dr. Mario Brameshuber, Dr. Birgit Plochberger, Dr. Barbara Unterauer, Dr. Bianca Bozna, Dr. Barbara Lackner, Prof. Dr. Herbert Stangl, and Prof. Dr. Hannes Stockinger for helpful discussions; and Agilent Technologies and TILL Photonics for the support of instruments. This work was supported by the Christian Doppler Society, the EC grant SMW ("Single Molecule Workstation," grant no. 213717), the EC grant Immunanomap (grant no. 35946), and the Austrian Science Foundation (FWF project SFB-F35).

REFERENCES

1. Hinterdorfer, P., G. Schütz, F. Kienberger, and H. Schindler. "Detection and Characterization of Single Biomolecules at Surfaces." *Rev Mol Biotechnol* 82, no. 1 (2001): 25–35.
2. Schmidt, T., G. J. Schütz, W. Baumgartner, H. J. Gruber, and H. Schindler. "Imaging of Single Molecule Diffusion." *Proc Natl Acad Sci USA* 93, no. 7 (1996): 2926–9.
3. Gustafsson, M. G. L. "Nonlinear Structured-Illumination Microscopy: Wide-Field Fluorescence Imaging with Theoretically Unlimited Resolution." *Proc Natl Acad Sci USA* 102, no. 37 (2005): 13081–6.
4. Willig, K. I., S. O. Rizzoli, V. Westphal, R. Jahn, and S. W. Hell. "STED Microscopy Reveals That Synaptotagmin Remains Clustered after Synaptic Vesicle Exocytosis." *Nature* 440, no. 7086 (2006): 935–9.
5. Betzig, E., G. H. Patterson, R. Sougrat et al. "Imaging Intracellular Fluorescent Proteins at Nanometer Resolution." *Science* 313, no. 5793 (2006): 1642–5.
6. Hess, S. T., T. P. K. Girirajan, and M. D. Mason. "Ultra-High Resolution Imaging by Fluorescence Photoactivation Localization Microscopy." *Biophys J* 91, no. 11 (2006): 4258–72.

7. Rust, M. J., M. Bates, and X. Zhuang. "Sub-Diffraction-Limit Imaging by Stochastic Optical Reconstruction Microscopy (STORM)." *Nat Methods* 3, no. 10 (2006): 793–6.

8. Binnig, G., C. F. Quate, and C. Gerber. "Atomic Force Microscope." *Phys Rev Lett* 56, no. 9 (1986): 930–3.

9. Ando, T., N. Kodera, E. Takai et al. "A High-Speed Atomic Force Microscope for Studying Biological Macromolecules." *Proc Natl Acad Sci USA* 98, no. 22 (2001): 12468–72.

10. Kodera, N., D. Yamamoto, R. Ishikawa, and T. Ando. "Video Imaging of Walking Myosin V by High-Speed Atomic Force Microscopy." *Nature* 468, no. 7320 (2010): 72–6.

11. Uchihashi, T., R. Iino, T. Ando, and H. Noji. "High-Speed Atomic Force Microscopy Reveals Rotary Catalysis of Rotorless F1-ATPase." *Science* 333, no. 6043 (2011): 755–8.

12. Oberleithner, H., C. Riethmüller, H. Schillers et al. "Plasma Sodium Stiffens Vascular Endothelium and Reduces Nitric Oxide Release." *Proc Natl Acad Sci USA* 104, no. 41 (2007): 16281–6.

13. Lekka, M., D. Gil, K. Pogoda et al. "Cancer Cell Detection in Tissue Sections Using AFM." *Arch Biochem Biophys* 518, no. 2 (2012): 151–6.

14. Benoit, M., D. Gabriel, G. Gerisch, and H. E. Gaub. "Discrete Interactions in Cell Adhesion Measured by Single-Molecule Force Spectroscopy." *Nat Cell Biol* 2, no. 6 (2000): 313–7.

15. Rankl, C., F. Kienberger, L. Wildling et al. "Multiple Receptors Involved in Human Rhinovirus Attachment to Live Cells." *Proc Natl Acad Sci USA* 105, no. 46 (2008): 17778–83.

16. Sieben, C., C. Kappel, R. Zhu et al. "Influenza Virus Binds Its Host Cell Using Multiple Dynamic Interactions." *Proc Natl Acad Sci USA* 109, no. 34 (2012): 13626–31.

17. Puntheeranurak, T., L. Wildling, H. J. Gruber, R. K. H. Kinne, and P. Hinterdorfer. "Ligands on the String: Single-Molecule AFM Studies on the Interaction of Antibodies and Substrates with the Na+-Glucose Co-Transporter SGLT1 in Living Cells." *J Cell Sci* 119, no. 14 (2006): 2960–7.

18. Bozna, B. L., P. Polzella, C. Rankl et al. "Binding Strength and Dynamics of Invariant Natural Killer Cell T Cell Receptor/Cd1d-Glycosphingolipid Interaction on Living Cells by Single Molecule Force Spectroscopy." *J Biol Chem* 286, no. 18 (2011): 15973–9.

19. Wildling, L., C. Rankl, T. Haselgrübler et al. "Probing Binding Pocket of Serotonin Transporter by Single Molecular Force Spectroscopy on Living Cells." *J Biol Chem* 287, no. 1 (2012): 105–13.

20. Lee, G. U., L. A. Chrisey, and R. J. Colton. "Direct Measurement of the Forces between Complementary Strands of DNA." *Science* 266, no. 5186 (1994): 771–3.

21. Florin, E., V. T. Moy, and H. E. Gaub. "Adhesion Forces between Individual Ligand–Receptor Pairs." *Science* 264, no. 5157 (1994): 415–7.

22. Hinterdorfer, P., W. Baumgartner, H. J. Gruber, K. Schilcher, and H. Schindler. "Detection and Localization of Individual Antibody-Antigen Recognition Events by Atomic Force Microscopy." *Proc Natl Acad Sci USA* 93, no. 8 (1996): 3477–81.

23. Evans, E., and K. Ritchie. "Dynamic Strength of Molecular Adhesion Bonds." *Biophys J* 72, no. 4 (1997): 1541–55.

24. Merkel, R., P. Nassoy, A. Leung, K. Ritchie, and E. Evans. "Energy Landscapes of Receptor-Ligand Bonds Explored with Dynamic Force Spectroscopy." *Nature* 397, no. 6714 (1999): 50–3.

25. Schwesinger, F., R. Ros, T. Strunz et al. "Unbinding Forces of Single Antibody-Antigen Complexes Correlate with Their Thermal Dissociation Rates." *Proc Natl Acad Sci USA* 97, no. 18 (2000): 9972–7.

26. Strunz, T., K. Oroszlan, R. Schafer, and H. J. Guntherodt. "Dynamic Force Spectroscopy of Single DNA Molecules." *Proc Natl Acad Sci USA* 96, no. 20 (1999): 11277–82.

27. Baumgartner, W., P. Hinterdorfer, W. Ness et al. "Cadherin Interaction Probed by Atomic Force Microscopy." *Proc Natl Acad Sci USA* 97, no. 8 (2000): 4005–10.
28. Nevo, R., C. Stroh, F. Kienberger et al. "A Molecular Switch between Alternative Conformational States in the Complex of Ran and Importin beta1." *Nat Struct Mol Biol* 10, no. 7 (2003): 553–7.
29. Zhu, R., S. Howorka, J. Pröll et al. "Nanomechanical Recognition Measurements of Individual DNA Molecules Reveal Epigenetic Methylation Patterns." *Nat Nanotechnol* 5, no. 11 (2010): 788–91.
30. Raab, A., W. Han, D. Badt et al. "Antibody Recognition Imaging by Force Microscopy." *Nat Biotechnol* 17, no. 9 (1999): 901–5.
31. Stroh, C. M., A. Ebner, M. Geretschläger et al. "Simultaneous Topography and Recognition Imaging Using Force Microscopy." *Biophys J* 87, no. 3 (2004): 1981–90.
32. Stroh, C., H. Wang, R. Bash et al. "Single-Molecule Recognition Imaging Microscopy." *Proc Natl Acad Sci USA* 101, no. 34 (2004): 12503–7.
33. Ebner, A., F. Kienberger, G. Kada et al. "Localization of Single Avidin-Biotin Interactions Using Simultaneous Topography and Molecular Recognition Imaging." *ChemPhysChem* 6, no. 5 (2005): 897–900.
34. Lin, L., H. Wang, Y. Liu, H. Yan, and S. Lindsay. "Recognition Imaging with a DNA Aptamer." *Biophys J* 90, no. 11 (2006): 4236–8.
35. Lin, L., D. Hom, S. M Lindsay, and J. C. Chaput. "In Vitro Selection of Histone H4 Aptamers for Recognition Imaging Microscopy." *J Am Chem Soc* 129, no. 47 (2007): 14568–9.
36. Wang, H., L. Obenauer-Kutner, M. Lin et al. "Imaging Glycosylation." *J Am Chem Soc* 130, no. 26 (2008): 8154–5.
37. Leitner, M., N. Mitchell, M. Kastner et al. "Single-Molecule AFM Characterization of Individual Chemically Tagged DNA Tetrahedra." *ACS Nano* 5, no. 9 (2011): 7048–54.
38. Wang, H., R. Bash, and D. Lohr. "Two-Component Atomic Force Microscopy Recognition Imaging of Complex Samples." *Anal Biochem* 361, no. 2 (2007): 273–9.
39. Preiner, J., N. S. Losilla, A. Ebner et al. "Imaging and Detection of Single Molecule Recognition Events on Organic Semiconductor Surfaces." *Nano Lett* 9, no. 2 (2008): 571–5.
40. Zhu, R., A. Ebner, M. Kastner et al. "Topography and Recognition Imaging of Protein-Patterned Surfaces Generated by AFM Nanolithography." *ChemPhysChem* 10, no. 9–10 (2009): 1478–81.
41. Ebner, A., D. Nikova, T. Lange et al. "Determination of CFTR Densities in Erythrocyte Plasma Membranes Using Recognition Imaging." *Nanotechnology* 19, no. 38 (2008): 384017.
42. Tang, J., A. Ebner, H. Badelt-Lichtblau et al. "Recognition Imaging and Highly Ordered Molecular Templating of Bacterial S-Layer Nanoarrays Containing Affinity-Tags." *Nano Lett* 8, no. 12 (2008): 4312–9.
43. Jiang, J., X. Hao, M. Cai et al. "Localization of Na+-K+ ATPases in Quasi-Native Cell Membranes." *Nano Lett* 9, no. 12 (2009): 4489–93.
44. Zhu, R., A. Rupprecht, A. Ebner et al. "Mapping the Nucleotide Binding Site of Uncoupling Protein 1 Using Atomic Force Microscopy." *J Am Chem Soc* 135, no. 9 (2013): 3640–6.
45. Chtcheglova, L. A., J. Waschke, L. Wildling, D. Drenckhahn, and P. Hinterdorfer. "Nano-Scale Dynamic Recognition Imaging on Vascular Endothelial Cells." *Biophys J* 93, no. 2 (2007): L11–3.
46. Chtcheglova, L. A., F. Atalar, U. Ozbek et al. "Localization of the Ergtoxin-1 Receptors on the Voltage Sensing Domain of hERG K+ Channel by AFM Recognition Imaging." *Pflügers Arch* 456, no. 1 (2008): 247–54.
47. Chtcheglova, L. A., L. Wildling, J. Waschke, D. Drenckhahn, and P. Hinterdorfer. "AFM Functional Imaging on Vascular Endothelial Cells." *J Mol Recognit* 23, no. 6 (2010): 589–96.

48. Lee, S., J. Mandic, and K. J. Van Vliet. "Chemomechanical Mapping of Ligand-Receptor Binding Kinetics on Cells." *Proc Natl Acad Sci USA* 104, no. 23 (2007): 9609–14.

49. Duman, M., M. Pfleger, R. Zhu et al. "Improved Localization of Cellular Membrane Receptors Using Combined Fluorescence Microscopy and Simultaneous Topography and Recognition Imaging." *Nanotechnology* 21, no. 11 (2010): 115504.

50. Duman, M., L. A. Chtcheglova, R. Zhu et al. "Nanomapping of CD1d-Glycolipid Complexes on THP1 Cells by Using Simultaneous Topography and Recognition Imaging." *J Mol Recognit* 26, no. 9 (2013): 408–14.

51. Rankl, C., R. Zhu, G. S. Luengo et al. "Detection of Corneodesmosin on the Surface of Stratum Corneum Using Atomic Force Microscopy." *Exp Dermatol* 19, no. 11 (2010): 1014–9.

52. Creasey, R., S. Sharma, J. E. Craig et al. "Detecting Protein Aggregates on Untreated Human Tissue Samples by Atomic Force Microscopy Recognition Imaging." *Biophys J* 99, no. 5 (2010): 1660–7.

53. Creasey, R., S. Sharma, C. T. Gibson et al. "Atomic Force Microscopy-Based Antibody Recognition Imaging of Proteins in the Pathological Deposits in Pseudoexfoliation Syndrome." *Ultramicroscopy* 111, no. 8 (2011): 1055–61.

54. Parton, R. G. "Caveolae: From Ultrastructure to Molecular Mechanisms." *Nat Rev Mol Cell Biol* 4, no. 2 (2003): 162–7.

55. Yunta, M., and P. A. Lazo. "Tetraspanin Proteins as Organisers of Membrane Microdomains and Signalling Complexes." *Cell Signal* 15, no. 6 (2003): 559–64.

56. Jacobson, K., O. G. Mouritsen, and R. G. W. Anderson. "Lipid Rafts: At a Crossroad between Cell Biology and Physics." *Nat Cell Biol* 9, no. 1 (2007): 7–14.

57. Engelman, D. M. "Membranes Are More Mosaic Than Fluid." *Nature* 438, no. 7068 (2005): 578–80.

58. McIntosh, T. J., and S. A. Simon. "Roles of Bilayer Material Properties in Function and Distribution of Membrane Proteins." *Annu Rev Biophys Biomol Struct* 35 (2006): 177–98.

59. Vereb, G., J. Szöllosi, J. Matko et al. "Dynamic, yet Structured: The Cell Membrane Three Decades after the Singer-Nicolson Model." *Proc Natl Acad Sci USA* 100, no. 14 (2003): 8053–8.

60. Dvorak, J. A. "The Application of Atomic Force Microscopy to the Study of Living Vertebrate Cells in Culture." *Methods* 29, no. 1 (2003): 86–96.

61. Wallace, M., J. Molloy, and D. Trentham. "Combined Single-Molecule Force and Fluorescence Measurements for Biology." *J Biol* 2, no. 1 (2003): 4.

62. Hards, A., C. Zhou, M. Seitz, C. Bräuchle, and A. Zumbusch. "Simultaneous AFM Manipulation and Fluorescence Imaging of Single DNA Strands." *ChemPhysChem* 6, no. 3 (2005): 534–40.

63. Meller, K., and C. Theiss. "Atomic Force Microscopy and Confocal Laser Scanning Microscopy on the Cytoskeleton of Permeabilised and Embedded Cells." *Ultramicroscopy* 106, no. 4 (2006): 320–5.

64. Nishida, S., Y. Funabashi, and A. Ikai. "Combination of AFM with an Objective-Type Total Internal Reflection Fluorescence Microscope (TIRFM) for Nanomanipulation of Single Cells." *Ultramicroscopy* 91, no. 1 (2002): 269–74.

65. Madl, J., S. Rhode, H. Stangl et al. "A Combined Optical and Atomic Force Microscope for Live Cell Investigations." *Ultramicroscopy* 106, no. 8 (2006): 645–51.

66. Kawano, T., J. Cui, Y. Koezuka et al. "CD1d-Restricted and TCR-Mediated Activation of V-Alpha-14 NKT Cells by Glycosylceramides." *Science* 278, no. 5343 (1997): 1626–9.

67. Spada, F. M., Y. Koezuka, and S. A. Porcelli. "CD1d-Restricted Recognition of Synthetic Glycolipid Antigens by Human Natural Killer T Cells." *J Exp Med* 188, no. 8 (1998): 1529–34.

68. Hermans, I. F., J. D. Silk, U. Gileadi et al. "NKT Cells Enhance CD4+ and CD8+ T Cell Responses to Soluble Antigen In Vivo through Direct Interaction with Dendritic Cells." *J Immunol* 171, no. 10 (2003): 5140–7.

69. Fujii, S., K. Shimizu, C. Smith, L. Bonifaz, and R. M. Steinman. "Activation of Natural Killer T Cells by α-Galactosylceramide Rapidly Induces the Full Maturation of Dendritic Cells in vivo and Thereby Acts as an Adjuvant for Combined CD4 and CD8 T Cell Immunity to a Coadministered Protein." *J Exp Med* 198, no. 2 (2003): 267–79.

70. Preiner, J., A. Ebner, L. Chtcheglova, R. Zhu, and P. Hinterdorfer. "Simultaneous Topography and Recognition Imaging: Physical Aspects and Optimal Imaging Conditions." *Nanotechnology* 20, no. 21 (2009): 215103.

71. Salio, M., A. O. Speak, D. Shepherd et al. "Modulation of Human Natural Killer T Cell Ligands on TLR-Mediated Antigen-Presenting Cell Activation." *Proc Natl Acad Sci USA* 104, no. 51 (2007): 20490–5.

72. Beisker, W., F. Dolbeare, and J. W. Gray. "An Improved Immunocytochemical Procedure for High-Sensitivity Detection of Incorporated Bromodeoxyuridine." *Cytometry* 8, no. 2 (1987): 235–9.

73. McCarthy, C., D. Shepherd, S. Fleire et al. "The Length of Lipids Bound to Human CD1d Molecules Modulates the Affinity of NKT Cell TCR and the Threshold of NKT Cell Activation." *J Exp Med* 204, no. 5 (2007): 1131–44.

74. Ebner, A., P. Hinterdorfer, and H. J. Gruber. "Comparison of Different Amino-functionalization Strategies for Attachment of Single Antibodies to AFM Cantilevers." *Ultramicroscopy* 107, no. 10 (2007): 922–7.

75. Ebner, A., L. Wildling, A.S.M. Kamruzzahan et al. "A New, Simple Method for Linking of Antibodies to Atomic Force Microscopy Tips." *Bioconjugate Chem* 18, no. 4 (2007): 1176–84.

76. Cerundolo, V., J. D. Silk, S. H. Masri, and M. Salio. "Harnessing Invariant NKT Cells in Vaccination Strategies." *Nat Rev Immunol* 9, no. 1 (2009): 28–38.

77. Borg, N. A., K. S. Wun, L. Kjer-Nielsen et al. "CD1d–Lipid–Antigen Recognition by the Semi-Invariant NKT T-Cell Receptor." *Nature* 448, no. 7149 (2007): 44–9.

78. Rhode, S., A. Breuer, J. Hesse et al. "Visualization of the Uptake of Individual HDL Particles in Living Cells Via the Scavenger Receptor Class B Type I." *Cell Biochem Biophys* 41, no. 3 (2004): 343–56.

79. Mleczko, J., L. L. Litke, H. S. Larsen, and W. L. Chaffin. "Effect of Glutaraldehyde Fixation on Cell Surface Binding Capacity of Candida Albicans." *Infect Immun* 57, no. 10 (1989): 3247–9.

80. Bonanni, B., A. S. Kamruzzahan, A. R. Bizzarri et al. "Single Molecule Recognition between Cytochrome C 551 and Gold-Immobilized Azurin by Force Spectroscopy." *Biophys J* 89, no. 4 (2005): 2783–91.

81. Mörtelmaier, M., E. J. Kögler, J. Hesse et al. "Single Molecule Microscopy in Living Cells: Subtraction of Autofluorescence Based on Two Color Recording." *Single Mol* 3, no. 4 (2002): 225–31.

82. Gaiduk, A., R. Kühnemuth, M. Antonik, and C. A. M. Seidel. "Optical Characteristics of Atomic Force Microscopy Tips for Single-Molecule Fluorescence Applications." *ChemPhysChem* 6, no. 5 (2005): 976–83.

83. Schwarzenbacher, M., M. Kaltenbrunner, M. Brameshuber et al. "Micropatterning for Quantitative Analysis of Protein–Protein Interactions in Living Cells." *Nat Methods* 5, no. 12 (2008): 1053–60.

84. Wildling, L., B. Unterauer, R. Zhu et al. "Linking of Sensor Molecules with Amino Groups to Amino-Functionalized AFM Tips." *Bioconjugate Chem* 22, no. 6 (2011): 1239–48.

85. Riener, C. K., C. M. Stroh, A. Ebner et al. "Simple Test System for Single Molecule Recognition Force Microscopy." *Analytica Chimica Acta* 479, no. 1 (2003): 59–75.

86. Choudhuri, K., and P. A. van der Merwe. "Molecular Mechanisms Involved in T Cell Receptor Triggering." *Seminars in Immunology* 19, no. 4 (2007): 255–61.

87. Xu, C., E. Gagnon, M. E. Call et al. "Regulation of T Cell Receptor Activation by Dynamic Membrane Binding of the CD3ε Cytoplasmic Tyrosine-Based Motif." *Cell* 135, no. 4 (2008): 702–13.

88. Huppa, J. B., M. Axmann, M. A. Mörtelmaier et al. "TCR-Peptide-MHC Interactions In Situ Show Accelerated Kinetics and Increased Affinity." *Nature* 463, no. 7283 (2010): 963–7.

17 Super-Resolution Imaging with Single-Molecule Localization

Anna Oddone, Ione Verdeny Vilanova,
Johnny Tam, Štefan Bálint, and Melike Lakadamyali

CONTENTS

17.1 INTRODUCTION

Over the years, fluorescence microscopy has become the workhorse of almost every biology laboratory around the world. Far-field imaging with visible light provides several advantages over methods such as electron microscopy. The immense toolbox of fluorescence probes, in particular the revolution that has led to the development of a large palette of fluorescent proteins, has given us the ability to label almost anything inside cells with high molecular specificity and in many colors. The non-invasive quality of visible light allows us to study dynamic biological processes in real time inside living cells or even living animals. Key technological developments have extended the capabilities of fluorescence microscopes and have provided us with several different imaging modalities from total internal reflection fluorescence (TIRF) to confocal and two-photon microscopy. These methods have overcome barriers such as reduction of background fluorescence and deep tissue imaging. However, one major barrier has remained impenetrable until recently—the diffraction limit. It has been known since the time of Ernst Abbe that structures smaller than the wavelength of light become blurred when imaged with a light microscope. As a result, two objects that are closer in distance than the wavelength of light cannot be resolved as two separate objects. The resolving power of an optical microscope can be approximated by $\lambda/(2NA)$ in the lateral (x–y) and $(2\lambda n)/NA^2$ in the axial (z) direction, where NA is the numerical aperture of the microscope objective, λ is the wavelength of light, and n is the refractive index of the medium. For visible light and high-NA objectives, the resolution of conventional optical microscopes is limited to ~200 and ~500 nm in the lateral and axial directions, respectively. This limitation is highly problematic in biology because many structures of interest are below the diffraction limit (e.g., protein complexes, DNA, cytoskeletal filaments, and viruses), and these structures are densely packed inside the crowded environment of the cell.

The diffraction limit has finally been broken through the development of truly innovative methods. With the experimental demonstration of stimulated emission depletion (STED) in 1999,[1] followed by the demonstration of saturated structured-illumination microscopy (SSIM),[2] stochastic optical reconstruction microscopy (STORM),[3] and (fluorescence) photoactivated localization microscopy (PALM[4] and fPALM[5]), we have entered the era of "nanoscopy." All these methods have improved the spatial resolution of fluorescence microscopy by one order of magnitude (~20 nm in the lateral and ~50 nm in the axial dimensions). This chapter will describe the sub-class of nanoscopy methods based on stochastic detection and localization of single molecules (STORM, PALM, fPALM, GSDIM, dSTORM, PAINT, etc.) with a special focus on STORM. We will refer to these methods in general as single-molecule localization microscopy (SMLM) and use the appropriate acronym when referring to a specific method in particular. For recent reviews on this topic, the reader is directed to Refs. 6 through 9.

17.2 SMLM: GENERAL CONCEPTS AND TECHNICAL DEVELOPMENTS

17.2.1 SINGLE-MOLECULE DETECTION AND LOCALIZATION

When imaged by an optical microscope, the image of a single fluorescence emitter will have a size that is determined by diffraction. This image is often referred to as the point spread function (PSF) of the microscope. Even though the PSF is much larger than the emitter itself, its position can nevertheless be determined with high precision.[10] The concept of high-precision, single-molecule localization is very powerful. For example, Yildiz et al. used this concept (fluorescence imaging with one-nanometer accuracy or FIONA) to determine the step size of a motor protein.[11] However, the resolving power of an optical microscope is related to the ability to discriminate two single emitters in proximity. This ability is still limited by diffraction, since the PSFs of these emitters will overlap when they are closer than $\lambda/2NA$. Therefore, the concept of single-molecule localization alone is not enough to break the diffraction limit when imaging densely labeled samples, where the PSFs of single emitters overlap significantly.

17.2.2 SMLM CONCEPT

The breakthrough that allowed the extension of the single-molecule localization concept to super-resolution microscopy came with the discovery of photoswitchable fluorophores.[12–14] These fluorophores can be cycled between bright and dark states (or between two different spectral colors). In particular, the majority of fluorophores in a sample can be put into a dark state with only a very small fraction of them activated into the bright state. Even in a densely labeled sample, the PSFs of this sparse subset of activated fluorophores will no longer overlap and therefore their positions can be localized with high precision. Through iterative cycles of activation and deactivation, the positions of all the fluorescent probes can be precisely determined, and these positions can then be used to reconstruct a high-resolution image of the underlying structure, which is no longer limited by diffraction (Figure 17.1). This concept was initially demonstrated with the use of a fluorophore pair (Cy3–Cy5)[13,14] as an optical switch (STORM) as well as with the use of a photoactivatable GFP (PA-GFP)[12] (PALM and fPALM) but since then has been extended to a large number of other photoswitchable probes.

17.2.3 PHOTOSWITCHABLE PROBES

A wide range of probes such as fluorescent proteins, small fluorescent dyes, and quantum dots have been proposed for SMLM. The common feature to all probes is their ability to exist in distinct fluorescent states—either an "on" (bright) and an "off" (dark) state, or two states with different spectral properties (e.g., different emission colors).

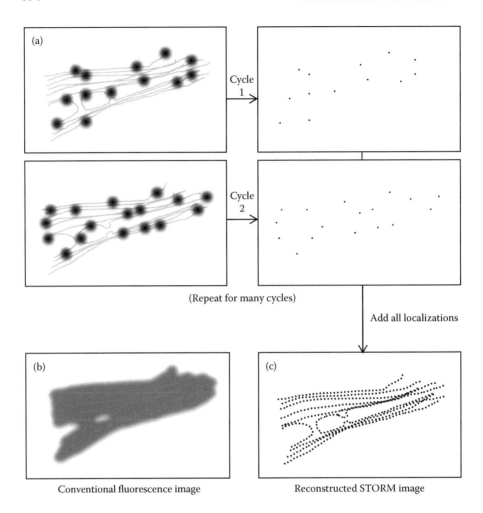

FIGURE 17.1 Schematic showing the basic strategy for SMLM: (a) Using photoswitchable fluorophores, it is possible to turn "on" and image only a sparse subset of fluorophores. These fluorophores are localized with nanometer precision and then turned "off" (by photobleaching or by switching to a dark state). A second subset is then turned "on," imaged, and localized. This process is repeated until all fluorophores are localized. By combining all the localizations, the diffraction-limited image (b) can thus be resolved at much higher resolution (c).

17.2.3.1 Fluorescent Proteins

Fluorescent proteins that are suitable for SMLM are proteins that can be either photoactivated (from a dark to a bright state) or photoconverted (from one state to another state with different spectral properties) by light. The first type includes irreversibly photoactivatable fluorescent proteins such as PA-GFP and PA-mCherry[12,15] and reversibly photoactivatable proteins such as EYFP, rsEGFP, Dronpa, and

Dreiklang,[16–20] all undergoing a dark-to-bright transition upon illumination with ultraviolet (UV) light. The second type includes the commonly used photoconvertible proteins Dendra2 and mEos2 (and its monomeric derivatives mEos3.1 and mEos3.2), which change from green to red emission upon illumination with UV light.[21–24]

17.2.3.2   Organic Dyes

Organic dyes are also popular probes for SMLM. Most organic dyes can switch many times between a dark and a bright state. Examples include cyanines (Cy5, Cy5.5, Cy7, Alexa Fluor 647 [A647], etc.), rhodamines (Alexa Fluor 488 [A488], Alexa Fluor 532 [A532], Alexa Fluor 568 [A568], ATTO488, ATTO532, ATTO565, tetramethylrhodamine, etc.), and oxazines (ATTO655, ATTO680, etc.).[25,26] In STORM, fluorescent dyes such as A647, Cy5.5, and Cy7 are often combined with a second fluorophore such as Alexa Fluor 405 (A405), Cy2, A488, or Cy3 in an activator–reporter pair configuration to increase the photoswitching efficiency and to facilitate multicolor imaging[27,28] (see Section 17.2.6). In this case, the fluorescent state of the reporter (the red or near-infrared dye) can be effectively recovered upon illumination of the activator dye with the corresponding wavelength laser.

In addition, some fluorophores that can directly bind to the structure of interest have been shown to be photoswitchable. These include DNA-binding dyes such as Picogreen[29] or YOYO-1,[30] and membrane-binding dyes such as Nile Red, DiI, DiD, DiR, MitoTracker Orange/Red/Deep Red, ER-Tracker Red, and LysoTracker Red.[31,32]

Organic fluorophores with quencher moieties have also been demonstrated as photoswitchable probes.[33–36]

It is important to note that in the case of fluorescent dyes, the photoswitching is often made possible or enhanced by the use of specific buffers. The most important component of the buffer is a reducing agent such as a primary thiol (β-mercaptoethanol [BME] or cysteamine [MEA]),[13,37,38] ascorbic acid,[29] or a phosphine.[39] For the photoswitching mechanisms, the reader is redirected to reviews on the topic.[25]

17.2.3.3   Quantum Dots

Inorganic nanoparticles such as quantum dots have also been proposed as SMLM probes.[40,41] Currently, the main limitation of quantum dots is their short "off" times (or high duty cycle, as discussed in Section 17.2.4.2), but future advances such as chemical caging and nanocrystal modifications can be expected to boost the use of quantum dots in SMLM imaging.[41,42]

Different SMLM techniques have been historically associated to different types of probes, essentially based on the type of fluorophores that had been used in the original publication. PALM and fPALM are hence associated with photoswitchable fluorescent proteins. STORM, dSTORM, and GSDIM are associated with fluorescent organic dyes. Nevertheless, all SMLM imaging techniques rely on the same concept: single-molecule localization combined with an active control of the density of fluorophores that are in the "on" state.

17.2.4 Probe Characteristics

The choice of the probe is critical for the quality of the final super-resolution image. Indeed, despite the large variety of probe types demonstrated for SMLM, to date only a few probes have been consistently used for imaging.

First, general considerations that apply to all fluorescent probes are also important for the photoswitchable probes. For example, spectral overlap (for multicolor imaging) and photostability must be taken into account when choosing a probe. The labeling strategy is also an important consideration. For intracellular labeling in living cells, fluorescent proteins outperform organic dyes since they can be genetically encoded. However, because fluorescent proteins are typically introduced via transfection, one needs to be careful about overexpression-induced artifacts. Organic dyes are often targeted to the structure of interest via immunostaining and therefore label the endogenous protein in the cell. However, they rely on the performance of the available antibodies and are more challenging to use for live-cell intracellular labeling. In the latter case, hybrid systems can be used that combine genetically encoded tags such as SNAP, CLIP, and HALO tags together with a fluorophore-labeled synthetic component that binds to the tag.[26,43–45] Nevertheless, most fluorophores are membrane impermeable, limiting these hybrid systems to a small number of cell-permeable fluorophores or to labeling of cell surface proteins. Structures such as DNA/RNA can also be labeled with small fluorophores using click chemistry, by modifying the nucleic acids with a terminal alkyne group that reacts with a modified fluorophore containing an azide group.[46]

In particular, three considerations are crucial when choosing a good probe for SMLM.

17.2.4.1 Brightness

Although bright probes are desirable for fluorescence microscopy in general, this is particularly true for SMLM, because the precision with which a single fluorescent molecule can be localized largely depends on the number of photons that it emits.[10] As a result, probes with higher photon yield allow a more accurate determination of the probe position and a subsequent higher resolution of the final image. Fluorophores such as Cy5 or A647 are generally much brighter than other fluorophores and most fluorescent proteins. mEos2 and its derivatives are among fluorescent proteins with the highest photon output.

17.2.4.2 On/Off Duty Cycle

To achieve single-molecule detection and localization, only a low number of fluorescent molecules should be "on" at any given time, to ensure that their PSFs do not overlap. This is most easily achieved if the probes have a low on/off duty cycle, meaning that they spend a long time in their "off" (dark) state and only a relatively short time in their "on" (bright) state.[38] A fluorophore with a high duty cycle, which spends a long time in the bright state, will lead to a high fraction of fluorophores that are "on" at any time, therefore causing the PSFs of the fluorophores to overlap. To avoid this problem, one could keep the labeling density low, but this would lead to low spatial resolution (see Section 17.2.5). Fluorophores with low duty cycle, such as A647 and Cy5, and irreversible fluorescent proteins are therefore preferred.

17.2.4.3 Switching Kinetics

The time that it takes for the fluorophore to switch off is important as it sets the acquisition time. In general, the camera frame rate is set such that most probes switch "off" within one camera frame. Therefore, probes with faster switching rates allow faster data acquisition rates and shorten the time needed to acquire the super-resolution image.[38,43] This is particularly important in live-cell imaging, which requires high temporal resolution to avoid motion blur (see Section 17.2.8). The off rate of certain fluorophores such as A647 is proportional to the laser power used to image them: at high powers, they switch "off" faster but still emit similar number of photons. Fluorescent proteins, on the other hand, switch with slower rates and their photon output usually decreases with increasing laser illumination intensities.[43]

To summarize, high photon yield and low on/off duty cycle are essential characteristics for SMLM probes in order to achieve high-resolution images. Fast switching times are desirable whenever fast data acquisition is needed.

These and other characteristics have been analyzed in depth for a number of currently available SMLM probes,[38,47] and the different probe types have been discussed in recent reviews.[25,26,48]

17.2.5 SPATIAL RESOLUTION IN SMLM

Spatial resolution in SMLM is limited not only by the accuracy in localizing each molecule but also by additional factors that are sample specific, such as labeling density or probe size. In the following, we summarize the contribution from these different factors.

17.2.5.1 Localization Precision

The location of a single fluorescent molecule can be precisely determined by finding the centroid position of its PSF as long as the molecule is isolated and spatial overlap is avoided. In this case, localization precision depends largely on the number of photons collected from the single emitter. Considering only the error generated from photon counting and assuming the PSF to be of Gaussian shape, the localization precision (σ) would be given by $\sigma = s/\sqrt{N}$, where s is the standard deviation of the Gaussian fit of the PSF and N is the number of photons detected. However, additional sources of error such as pixelation noise and background noise generated by CCD (charge-coupled device) readout, dark current, or cellular autofluorescence must also be taken into account. Several papers have discussed the fundamental limits to localization uncertainty and proposed different expressions for it.[10,49,50] Additionally, different computational methods for determining the centroid position, such as nonlinear least squares fitting to a Gaussian PSF or the maximum likelihood estimation (MLE) using a Gaussian PSF model, have been investigated and compared.[49,51–53] It has been shown that, in general, the MLE method is able to determine position with higher accuracy. The latest analytical approximation for localization precision was proposed in 2012 by Stallinga and Rieger:[50]

$$\sigma^2_{\text{Localization precision}} = \frac{s^2 + a^2/12}{N}\left(1 + 4\tau + \sqrt{\frac{2\tau}{1+4\tau}}\right),$$

(17.1)

where s is the width of the Gaussian that is used to fit the PSF, a is the pixel size, N is the number of collected photons, and τ is a normalized dimensionless background parameter defined as $\tau = 2\pi b(s^2 + a^2/12)/(Na^2)$, with b being the number of background photons per pixel.

In practice, localization precision can be experimentally determined by measuring the standard deviation or the full width at half maximum of a cluster of multiple localizations originating from a single fluorophore.[3,54] For bright organic dyes such as A647, a localization precision of 8–9 nm is common. Fluorescent proteins, which have lower photon output, give rise to lower localization precision (~20 nm).

17.2.5.2 Labeling Density and the Nyquist Criterion

Labeling density also affects the final spatial resolution. Low labeling densities (not all target molecules labeled) typically cause continuous structures to appear discontinuous, resulting in a loss of detail (Figure 17.2).

The effects of the labeling density on the effective spatial resolution can be quantified by the Nyquist criterion (see Ref. 55 for further details), which states that structural features smaller than twice the fluorophore-to-fluorophore distance cannot be reliably discerned:

$$\sigma_{\text{Nyquist}} = \frac{2}{\rho^{1/D}}. \tag{17.2}$$

Here, ρ is the labeling density calculated as the number of localizations per unit area or volume and D is the dimension of the structure to be imaged (2 for two-dimensional and 3 for three-dimensional [3D] STORM imaging). To determine the effective resolution, a common approach is to convolute the contribution due to localization precision and to the labeling density:

$$\sigma_{\text{Effective}} = \sqrt{\sigma^2_{\text{Localization precision}} + \sigma^2_{\text{Nyquist}}}. \tag{17.3}$$

For high spatial resolution, it is essential to obtain optimal labeling density. Antibody labeling may lead to low labeling efficiency owing to steric hindrance,

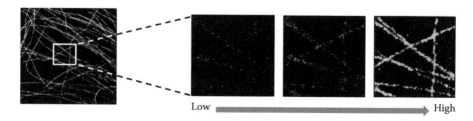

Low ➞ High

FIGURE 17.2 Effects of labeling density on effective spatial resolution for the specific case of a microtubule network. As the labeling density increases, a significant improvement in resolution can be appreciated.

low affinity of antibodies, or low accessibility of epitopes. Fluorescent proteins are typically introduced via transfection, and several factors can affect the final labeling density, including the presence of unlabeled endogenous proteins and the incomplete maturation or photoactivation of fluorescent proteins.[56] The specific probe that should be used to achieve optimal labeling depends on the target and the availability of high-quality antibodies or fluorescent protein fusion constructs.

17.2.5.3 Probe Size

The physical size of the probe also has an effect on how accurately the final super-resolution image resembles the actual structure. This is particularly important for super-resolution methods as the probe dimensions have the same order of magnitude as the achievable spatial resolution. Fluorescent proteins (3–4 nm) are among the smallest probes, although the low photon budget lowers the localization precision and effective resolution. While organic dyes are very small (1 nm), they are often linked to the target by indirect immunostaining with primary and secondary antibodies (10–15 nm) creating a rather large probe. The probe size can be substantially decreased via the use of Fab fragments (~5–6 nm) or camelid antibodies (nanobodies, ~4 nm).[57] Alternatively, organic dyes can be introduced into the cell via SNAP, CLIP, or HALO tag technology, resulting in a probe size similar to that of fluorescent proteins. Direct labeling (e.g., with membrane- or organelle-specific markers, DNA-binding dyes, or via click chemistry) will further reduce the probe size.

17.2.6 Multicolor Imaging

In many biological systems, it is not sufficient to examine a single protein. An important capability of fluorescence microscopy is the ability to detect different proteins or structures within the same region of interest. Typically, distinct fluorophores are used to label distinct objects of interest. In the case of SMLM imaging, the implementation requires a few additional considerations, but the end result is similar.

One way to extend SMLM imaging to multiple colors is to use fluorophores with different emission spectra. For example, combinations of photoconvertible, photoswitchable, and photoactivatable fluorescent proteins with different emission spectra, such as PA-GFP/PA-mCherry, PA-mCherry1/PS-CFP2, Dronpa/EosFP, and PS-CFP2/EosFP, have been used for multicolor PALM imaging.[58–60] It is also possible to use photoswitchable organic dyes with different emission spectra. However, since organic dyes require specific buffers for photoswitching, different dyes may not photoswitch with the same efficiency in the same buffer and may require different buffer components. In addition, when using photoswitchable dyes or fluorescent proteins with different spectral properties, it is important to consider chromatic aberrations and the possibility that the sensitivity of the detector is wavelength dependent.

To avoid this problem, a common approach to extend STORM imaging to multiple colors is to label each protein of interest with a different activator–reporter dye pair.[27] It is simplest to vary only the activator dye while keeping the reporter dye constant. As an example, suppose one wants to image both mitochondria and microtubules. The strategy would be to perform immunostaining using antibodies labeled with different activator–reporter pairs, resulting, for example, in mitochondria labeled with

A405–A647 and microtubules labeled with Cy3–A647. STORM data acquisition is composed of cycles that alternate "activation" (during which the corresponding activator–reporter pair is activated) and "imaging" (during which the signals arising from the reporter, in this case A647, are recorded). By alternating activation with 405 nm light (which activates the A405–A647 pairs) and activation with 561 nm light (which activates the Cy3–A647 pairs) and recording the A647 signal after each activation, mitochondria and microtubules are easily distinguished. An example of a multicolor STORM image acquired under these conditions is shown in Figure 17.3a.

One problem in using different activators but the same reporter is the possibility that a detected fluorophore is assigned to the wrong color (referred to as cross talk).[28] For example, cross talk can occur when fluorophores undergo spontaneous activation independently of the activation laser or if the activation laser activates the wrong activator–reporter pair. Although it is difficult to eliminate cross talk during image acquisition, there are effective ways to remove it using postprocessing based on statistical modeling.[27,61] An example of cross talk and cross talk removal is shown in Figure 17.3b through e.

This strategy can be extended to additional colors by selecting as many unique activator–reporter dye pairs as possible. Currently, there are nine spectral pairs that have been experimentally optimized for STORM, which combine A405, Cy2 (or A488), and Cy3 (or A555) as the activator and Cy5 (or A647), Cy5.5 (or A680), and Cy7 (or A750) as the reporter,[27,28] although additional potential fluorophores have also been suggested.[38] It is important to note that not all activator–reporter pairs will perform equally well, which can result in nonuniform image quality with respect to each of the different colors.

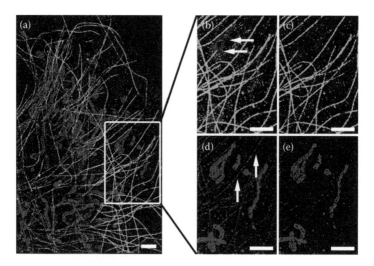

FIGURE 17.3 Multicolor imaging. (a) STORM image of microtubules and mitochondria. Microtubules (b and c) and mitochondria (d and e) are shown before (b and d) and after (c and e) cross talk removal. Arrows in (b) and (d) are examples of false color assignments that are corrected by the cross talk removal procedure. All scale bars represent 2 μm.

To summarize, although it is relatively straightforward to image in multiple colors using SMLM, it is important to consider that as the number of colors increases, it can become harder to achieve the same level of high resolution for all colors.

17.2.7   3D IMAGING

Most biological structures are 3D. Although there are now several methods for extending SMLM to three dimensions, one of the simplest approaches is to use a cylindrical lens to introduce astigmatism (3D STORM). This method can yield an axial resolution of 50–60 nm over a range of ~800 nm (~400 nm above and below the focal plane).[54] With this method, molecules that are exactly in the focal plane appear circular, whereas molecules above or below the focal plane appear elongated either horizontally or vertically, depending on the orientation of the astigmatic lens (Figure 17.4). With proper calibration, the ellipticity of each PSF can be converted into an amount of displacement above or below the focal plane. Calibration can be performed using a piezoelectric stage and a glass coverslip with fluorescent beads prepared in such a way that the beads are not clustered on the glass. By acquiring a series of images at fixed z-steps, a calibration curve relating z to the width (in either x or y) of the PSFs can be generated. This calibration curve can then be used to calculate the z position of subsequent single-molecule localizations acquired using the same system (see Figure 17.4). For additional details, the reader is referred to Ref. 54. It is also possible to combine astigmatism with a dual-objective geometry in order to capture more photons and improve the z-resolution to approximately ~20 nm at the expense of imaging depth.[62]

In general, the main requirement for 3D SMLM is a method to distinguish between fluorophores that are in different focal planes. Astigmatism, described above, is one of a class of 3D methods referred to as "point spread function engineering." In the case of astigmatism, the PSF is engineered to appear elliptical when the molecule

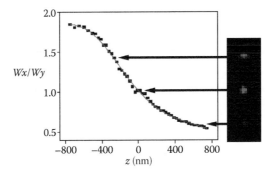

FIGURE 17.4   3D STORM imaging using the astigmatic lens approach. The z position of each raw data point is calculated by measuring the width in the x and y directions (Wx and Wy) and then by comparing the measured values to the calibration data. Representative molecules for various z positions are shown, which appear elongated because of the presence of an astigmatic lens placed before the camera.

is not in the focal plane.[54] An alternative approach is to engineer a PSF in the shape of a double helix with two maxima.[63] In this case, the midpoint between the two maxima reports the $x–y$ position, whereas the pitch of the double helix, which rotates depending on the molecule's axial position, reports the z position. In addition to PSF engineering, other methods also exist. An example is bifocal imaging in which two focal planes are captured simultaneously using one objective, by splitting the image into two paths with different focal lengths.[64] Finally, dual-objective geometry can be used to generate depth-dependent interferometric patterns (iPALM)[65] producing 3D images with an impressive 10 nm axial resolution but at the expense of imaging depth.

17.2.8   LIVE-CELL IMAGING

There is no fundamental restriction that prevents the concept of SMLM from being applied to live cells. The main requirement is that the temporal resolution is faster than the dynamics of the process to be imaged. The temporal resolution depends on how much time is allocated to construct a high-quality SMLM image. In order to accumulate a sufficient number of fluorophore localizations to satisfy the Nyquist criterion (see Figures 17.1 and 17.2), a long acquisition time is needed (STORM imaging in a fixed cell often proceeds for 10 to 60 min, yielding up to tens of millions of single-molecule localizations). Shortening the acquisition time results in a decrease in spatial resolution. Typically, there is a trade-off between maximizing spatial and temporal resolution. The rate-limiting step is that fluorophores require a relatively long time to undergo a complete switching cycle (off–on–off, on the range of tens of milliseconds, depending on the fluorophore and the experimental conditions).

Despite the trade-offs, live-cell super-resolution imaging has been achieved with a range of fluorescent probes. While fluorescent proteins provide straightforward intracellular labeling, their low photon output and slow switching kinetics lead to limited spatial and temporal resolution (60–70 nm and tens of seconds).[55] Organic dyes are typically brighter and photoswitch with faster kinetics. For example, an impressive 30 nm lateral and 50 nm axial spatial resolution at a temporal resolution of 1–2 s has been achieved by using A647.[43]

Typically, to achieve single-molecule localization, the density of fluorophores in each frame needs to be kept relatively low, which in turn limits the achievable temporal resolution. This constraint has recently been overcome with the development of new data analysis methods that can determine the position of fluorophores with high precision even when their PSFs are highly overlapping (see Section 17.3.3). These approaches allow for acquisition of SMLM images in a shorter amount of time, permitting even higher temporal resolution. For example, using this approach in combination with very fast scientific complementary metal-oxide semiconductor (sCMOS) cameras, Huang et al. have demonstrated high spatial resolution imaging with very fast (millisecond) temporal resolution.[66]

To summarize, live-cell SMLM imaging implies finding a balance between spatial and temporal resolution requirements. Thanks to recent developments, it is now possible to significantly increase temporal resolution in SMLM by relaxing the requirement for sparse single-molecule images in each frame. These and future strategies will help expand the capabilities of live-cell SMLM imaging. For a recent review on the topic, the reader is directed to Ref. 67.

17.2.9   CORRELATIVE LIVE-CELL AND SUPER-RESOLUTION IMAGING

As illustrated above, currently available live-cell super-resolution techniques must still deal with the trade-offs between spatial and temporal resolution, as well as other factors such as the size of the field of view, photobleaching, and phototoxicity. Achieving nanoscale image resolution with millisecond temporal resolution is still challenging. Many biological processes, such as microtubule-dependent cargo transport, are often faster than the typical temporal resolution that can be achieved with live-cell super-resolution microscopy, obscuring their observation in living cells. One approach to circumvent this problem is to combine live-cell imaging with SMLM in a correlative way, in which the same cell is imaged under two different modalities.[68]

In general terms, the target of interest is first labeled with a fluorescent marker and a time-lapse movie of the dynamics of the process is recorded with high temporal resolution (millisecond scale). The sample is subsequently fixed in situ at a time point of interest. Fixation is typically fast and structures are generally preserved as they appear in the final frame of the movie. Then, the structure to be imaged at high resolution is labeled using appropriate labeling methods and a super-resolution image of the target structure is acquired. Using a single-particle tracking routine, the trajectories of the target objects are obtained from the time-lapse movie. The trajectories can then be mapped onto the super-resolution image using fiduciary markers (fluorescent beads). A precise alignment with a final error of 9–10 nm can be easily achieved.

Figure 17.5 shows the application of this technique to study intracellular cargo transport. The trajectory of a cargo can be mapped onto the individual microtubule

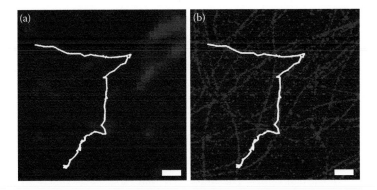

FIGURE 17.5   Full trajectory (white line) of a lysosome (not displayed) mapped on top of the endpoint image of microtubules, either with conventional fluorescence microscopy (a) or with the correlative live-cell and super-resolution imaging approach (b). The scale bar represents 1 μm.

tracks with high precision. Many biological questions, such as how cargo overcomes roadblocks for efficient transport, can be studied with this approach.

17.3   SMLM: PRACTICAL CONSIDERATIONS

This section summarizes some practical considerations for SMLM.

17.3.1   MICROSCOPE COMPONENTS

- TIRF or inclined illumination geometries are often used to minimize unwanted background.
- Laser intensities around 0.5–5 kW/cm^2 are typical for both fluorescent proteins and organic dyes (with somewhat higher powers for the latter).
- SMLM requires a very sensitive detector. The most commonly used detectors are EMCCDs (electron multiplying charge-coupled devices). Alternatively, sCMOS cameras can be used.[66]

17.3.2   SAMPLE PREPARATION

Since SMLM has much higher spatial resolution than conventional microscopy, additional care must be taken to not introduce sample preparation artifacts that might otherwise be unnoticeable at lower resolution. Accurate preservation of the structure of interest, high labeling density, and low background are key to the final quality of the reconstructed image.

Specific imaging buffers are needed in order to keep most molecules in the dark state when using organic dyes. Common buffers contain a reducing agent (e.g., BME, MEA, ascorbic acid). An overview of fluorophores and buffers for SMLM can be found in Ref. 38.

17.3.3   DATA ANALYSIS

SMLM data analysis involves three major steps: peak detection, position determination, and final rendering into a super-resolution image. There are many software options for SMLM analysis including publicly available software such as QuickPALM,[69] RapidSTORM,[70] and GraspJ.[71] Open source software that can localize single molecules in densely activated samples include DAOSTORM,[72] compressed sensing,[73] and Bayesian analysis.[74]

17.4   CONCLUSIONS AND OUTLOOK

Despite their short history, super-resolution methods have already made a high impact in biological imaging. The impressive and rapid development in this field has already started to transform these methods from complex tools available only for specialists into commercially available products that can be readily installed in any laboratory. The combination of high spatial resolution, molecular specificity, multiple colors, and live-cell imaging capability holds great promise for making important discoveries in biology, where being able to observe protein nanoclusters, DNA fibers, cytoskeletal filaments, vesicles, viruses, and other biological structures with high resolution in space and in time is critical for understanding their function. In the future, super-resolution microscopes will likely become a new workhorse of the biology laboratory. However, before that can happen, new developments, especially in the field of photoswitchable fluorescent probes, are needed. Bright fluorescent probes with high photostability, low duty cycle, and fast switching kinetics will allow us to push both spatial and temporal resolution limits to unprecedented levels and open the door for exciting biological discoveries at the nanoscale.

REFERENCES

1. Klar, T. A., and S. W. Hell. "Subdiffraction Resolution in Far-Field Fluorescence Microscopy." *Opt Lett* 24, no. 14 (1999): 954–6.
2. Gustafsson, M. G. "Nonlinear Structured-Illumination Microscopy: Wide-Field Fluorescence Imaging with Theoretically Unlimited Resolution." *Proc Natl Acad Sci USA* 102, no. 37 (2005): 13081–6.
3. Rust, M. J., M. Bates, and X. Zhuang. "Sub-Diffraction-Limit Imaging by Stochastic Optical Reconstruction Microscopy (STORM)." *Nat Methods* 3, no. 10 (2006): 793–5.
4. Betzig, E., G. H. Patterson, R. Sougrat et al. "Imaging Intracellular Fluorescent Proteins at Nanometer Resolution." *Science* 313, no. 5793 (2006): 1642–5.
5. Hess, S. T., T. P. Girirajan, and M. D. Mason. "Ultra-High Resolution Imaging by Fluorescence Photoactivation Localization Microscopy." *Biophys J* 91, no. 11 (2006): 4258–72.
6. Sahl, S. J., and W. Moerner. "Super-Resolution Fluorescence Imaging with Single Molecules." *Curr Opin Struct Biol* 23, no. 5 (2013): 778–87.
7. Kamiyama, D., and B. Huang. "Development in the STORM." *Dev Cell* 23, no. 6 (2012): 1103–10.
8. Sengupta, P., S. van Engelenburg, and J. Lippincott-Schwartz. "Visualizing Cell Structure and Function with Point-Localization Superresolution Imaging." *Dev Cell* 23, no. 6 (2012): 1092–102.
9. Bates, M., S. A. Jones, and X. Zhuang. "Stochastic Optical Reconstruction Microscopy (STORM): A Method for Superresolution Fluorescence Imaging." *Cold Spring Harb Protoc* 2013, no. 6 (2013): 498–520.
10. Thompson, R. E., D. R. Larson, and W. W. Webb. "Precise Nanometer Localization Analysis for Individual Fluorescent Probes." *Biophys J* 82, no. 5 (2002): 2775–83.
11. Yildiz, A., H. Park, D. Safer et al. "Myosin VI Steps via a Hand-Over-Hand Mechanism with Its Lever Arm Undergoing Fluctuations When Attached to Actin." *J Biol Chem* 279, no. 36 (2004): 37223–6.
12. Patterson, G. H., and J. Lippincott-Schwartz. "A Photoactivatable GFP for Selective Photolabeling of Proteins and Cells." *Science* 297, no. 5588 (2002): 1873–7.
13. Bates, M., T. R. Blosser, and X. Zhuang. "Short-Range Spectroscopic Ruler Based on a Single-Molecule Optical Switch." *Phys Rev Lett* 94, no. 10 (2005): 108101.
14. Heilemann, M., E. Margeat, R. Kasper, M. Sauer, and P. Tinnefeld. "Carbocyanine Dyes as Efficient Reversible Single-Molecule Optical Switch." *J Am Chem Soc* 127, no. 11 (2005): 3801–6.
15. Subach, F. V., G. H. Patterson, S. Manley et al. "Photoactivatable mCherry for High-Resolution Two-Color Fluorescence Microscopy." *Nat Methods* 6, no. 2 (2009): 153–9.
16. Dickson, R. M., A. B. Cubitt, R. Y. Tsien, and W. E. Moerner. "On/Off Blinking and Switching Behaviour of Single Molecules of Green Fluorescent Protein." *Nature* 388, no. 6640 (1997): 355–8.

17. Biteen, J. S., M. A. Thompson, N. K. Tselentis et al. "Super-Resolution Imaging in Live Caulobacter Crescentus Cells Using Photoswitchable EYFP." *Nat Methods* 5, no. 11 (2008): 947–9.

18. Habuchi, S., R. Ando, P. Dedecker et al. "Reversible Single-Molecule Photoswitching in the GFP-Like Fluorescent Protein Dronpa." *Proc Natl Acad Sci USA* 102, no. 27 (2005): 9511–6.

19. Brakemann, T., A. C. Stiel, G. Weber et al. "A Reversibly Photoswitchable GFP-Like Protein with Fluorescence Excitation Decoupled from Switching." *Nat Biotechnol* 29, no. 10 (2011): 942–7.

20. Grotjohann, T., I. Testa, M. Leutenegger et al. "Diffraction-Unlimited All-Optical Imaging and Writing with a Photochromic GFP." *Nature* 478, no. 7368 (2011): 204–8.

21. Wiedenmann, J., S. Ivanchenko, F. Oswald et al. "EosFP, a Fluorescent Marker Protein with UV-Inducible Green-to-Red Fluorescence Conversion." *Proc Natl Acad Sci USA* 101, no. 45 (2004): 15905–10.

22. McKinney, S. A., C. S. Murphy, K. L. Hazelwood, M. W. Davidson, and L. L. Looger. "A Bright and Photostable Photoconvertible Fluorescent Protein." *Nat Methods* 6, no. 2 (2009): 131–3.

23. Gurskaya, N. G., V. V. Verkhusha, A. S. Shcheglov et al. "Engineering of a Monomeric Green-to-Red Photoactivatable Fluorescent Protein Induced by Blue Light." *Nat Biotechnol* 24, no. 4 (2006): 461–5.

24. Zhang, M., H. Chang, Y. Zhang et al. "Rational Design of True Monomeric and Bright Photoactivatable Fluorescent Proteins." *Nat Methods* 9, no. 7 (2012): 727–9.

25. Furstenberg, A., and M. Heilemann. "Single-Molecule Localization Microscopy—Near-Molecular Spatial Resolution in Light Microscopy with Photoswitchable Fluorophores." *Phys Chem Chem Phys* 15, no. 36 (2013): 14919–30.

26. van de Linde, S., M. Heilemann, and M. Sauer. "Live-Cell Super-Resolution Imaging with Synthetic Fluorophores." *Annu Rev Phys Chem* 63 (2012): 519–40.

27. Bates, M., B. Huang, G. T. Dempsey, and X. Zhuang. "Multicolor Super-Resolution Imaging with Photo-Switchable Fluorescent Probes." *Science* 317, no. 5845 (2007): 1749–53.

28. Bates, M., G. T. Dempsey, K. H. Chen, and X. Zhuang. "Multicolor Super-Resolution Fluorescence Imaging via Multi-Parameter Fluorophore Detection." *ChemPhysChem* 13, no. 1 (2012): 99–107.

29. Benke, A., and S. Manley. "Live-Cell dSTORM of Cellular DNA Based on Direct DNA Labeling." *ChemBioChem* 13, no. 2 (2012): 298–301.

30. Flors, C. "Photoswitching of Monomeric and Dimeric DNA-Intercalating Cyanine Dyes for Super-Resolution Microscopy Applications." *Photochem Photobiol Sci* 9, no. 5 (2010): 643–8.

31. Shim, S. H., C. Xia, G. Zhong et al. "Super-Resolution Fluorescence Imaging of Organelles in Live Cells with Photoswitchable Membrane Probes." *Proc Natl Acad Sci USA* 109, no. 35 (2012): 13978–83.

32. Sharonov, A., and R. M. Hochstrasser. "Wide-Field Subdiffraction Imaging by Accumulated Binding of Diffusing Probes." *Proc Natl Acad Sci USA* 103, no. 50 (2006): 18911–6.

33. Maurel, D., S. Banala, T. Laroche, and K. Johnsson. "Photoactivatable and Photoconvertible Fluorescent Probes for Protein Labeling." *ACS Chem Biol* 5, no. 5 (2010): 507–16.

34. Gee, K. R., E. S. Weinberg, and D. J. Kozlowski. "Caged Q-Rhodamine Dextran: A New Photoactivated Fluorescent Tracer." *Bioorg Med Chem Lett* 11, no. 16 (2001): 2181–3.

35. Belov, V. N., C. A. Wurm, V. P. Boyarskiy, S. Jakobs, and S. W. Hell. "Rhodamines NN: A Novel Class of Caged Fluorescent Dyes." *Angew Chem Int Ed Engl* 49, no. 20 (2010): 3520–3.

36. Lord, S. J., H. L. Lee, R. Samuel et al. "Azido Push-Pull Fluorogens Photoactivate to Produce Bright Fluorescent Labels." *J Phys Chem B* 114, no. 45 (2010): 14157–67.

37. Heilemann, M., S. van de Linde, A. Mukherjee, and M. Sauer. "Super-Resolution Imaging with Small Organic Fluorophores." *Angew Chem Int Ed Engl* 48, no. 37 (2009): 6903–8.

38. Dempsey, G. T., J. C. Vaughan, K. H. Chen, M. Bates, and X. Zhuang. "Evaluation of Fluorophores for Optimal Performance in Localization-Based Super-Resolution Imaging." *Nat Methods* 8, no. 12 (2011): 1027–36.

39. Vaughan, J. C., G. T. Dempsey, E. Sun, and X. Zhuang. "Phosphine Quenching of Cyanine Dyes as a Versatile Tool for Fluorescence Microscopy." *J Am Chem Soc* 135, no. 4 (2013): 1197–200.

40. Dertinger, T., R. Colyer, G. Iyer, S. Weiss, and J. Enderlein. "Fast, Background-Free, 3D Super-Resolution Optical Fluctuation Imaging (SOFI)." *Proc Natl Acad Sci USA* 106, no. 52 (2009): 22287–92.

41. Hoyer, P., T. Staudt, J. Engelhardt, and S. W. Hell. "Quantum Dot Blueing and Blinking Enables Fluorescence Nanoscopy." *Nano Lett* 11, no. 1 (2011): 245–50.

42. Han, G., T. Mokari, C. Ajo-Franklin, and B. E. Cohen. "Caged Quantum Dots." *J Am Chem Soc* 130, no. 47 (2008): 15811–3.

43. Jones, S. A., S. H. Shim, J. He, and X. Zhuang. "Fast, Three-Dimensional Super-Resolution Imaging of Live Cells." *Nat Methods* 8, no. 6 (2011): 499–508.

44. Klein, T., A. Loschberger, S. Proppert et al. "Live-Cell dSTORM with SNAP-Tag Fusion Proteins." *Nat Methods* 8, no. 1 (2011): 7–9.

45. Lee, H. L., S. J. Lord, S. Iwanaga et al. "Superresolution Imaging of Targeted Proteins in Fixed and Living Cells Using Photoactivatable Organic Fluorophores." *J Am Chem Soc* 132, no. 43 (2010): 15099–101.

46. Zessin, P. J., K. Finan, and M. Heilemann. "Super-Resolution Fluorescence Imaging of Chromosomal DNA." *J Struct Biol* 177, no. 2 (2012): 344–8.

47. Lippincott-Schwartz, J., and G. H. Patterson. "Photoactivatable Fluorescent Proteins for Diffraction-Limited and Super-Resolution Imaging." *Trends Cell Biol* 19, no. 11 (2009): 555–65.

48. Dempsey, G. T. "A User's Guide to Localization-Based Super-Resolution Fluorescence Imaging." *Methods Cell Biol* 114 (2013): 561–92.

49. Mortensen, K. I., L. S. Churchman, J. A. Spudich, and H. Flyvbjerg. "Optimized Localization Analysis for Single-Molecule Tracking and Super-Resolution Microscopy." *Nat Methods* 7, no. 5 (2010): 377–81.

50. Stallinga, S., and B. Rieger. "The Effect of Background on Localization Uncertainty in Single Emitter Imaging." *IEEE Int Symp Biomedical Imaging* (2012): 988–91.

51. Ober, R. J., S. Ram, and E. S. Ward. "Localization Accuracy in Single-Molecule Microscopy." *Biophys J* 86, no. 2 (2004): 1185–200.

52. Abraham, A. V., S. Ram, J. Chao, E. S. Ward, and R. J. Ober. "Quantitative Study of Single Molecule Location Estimation Techniques." *Opt Express* 17, no. 26 (2009): 23352–73.

53. Smith, C. S., N. Joseph, B. Rieger, and K. A. Lidke. "Fast, Single-Molecule Localization That Achieves Theoretically Minimum Uncertainty." *Nat Methods* 7, no. 5 (2010): 373–5.

54. Huang, B., W. Wang, M. Bates, and X. Zhuang. "Three-Dimensional Super-Resolution Imaging by Stochastic Optical Reconstruction Microscopy." *Science* 319, no. 5864 (2008): 810–3.

55. Shroff, H., C. G. Galbraith, J. A. Galbraith, and E. Betzig. "Live-Cell Photoactivated Localization Microscopy of Nanoscale Adhesion Dynamics." *Nat Methods* 5, no. 5 (2008): 417–23.

56. Durisic, N., L. Laparra-Cuervo, A. Sandoval-Alvarez, J. S. Borbely, and M. Lakadamyali. "Single-Molecule Evaluation of Fluorescent Protein Photoactivation Efficiency Using an In Vivo Nanotemplate." *Nat Methods* 11, no. 2 (2014): 156–62.

57. Ries, J., C. Kaplan, E. Platonova, H. Eghlidi, and H. Ewers. "A Simple, Versatile Method for GFP-Based Super-Resolution Microscopy via Nanobodies." *Nat Methods* 9, no. 6 (2012): 582–4.

58. Renz, M., B. R. Daniels, G. Vamosi, I. M. Arias, and J. Lippincott-Schwartz. "Plasticity of the Asialoglycoprotein Receptor Deciphered by Ensemble FRET Imaging and Single-Molecule Counting Palm Imaging." *Proc Natl Acad Sci USA* 109, no. 44 (2012): E2989–97.

59. Shroff, H., C. G. Galbraith, J. A. Galbraith et al. "Dual-Color Superresolution Imaging of Genetically Expressed Probes within Individual Adhesion Complexes." *Proc Natl Acad Sci USA* 104, no. 51 (2007): 20308–13.

60. Annibale, P., M. Scarselli, M. Greco, and A. Radenovic. "Identification of the Factors Affecting Co-Localization Precision for Quantitative Multicolor Localization Microscopy." *Opt Nanoscopy* 1, no. 1 (2012): 1–13.

61. Dani, A., B. Huang, J. Bergan, C. Dulac, and X. Zhuang. "Superresolution Imaging of Chemical Synapses in the Brain." *Neuron* 68, no. 5 (2010): 843–56.

62. Xu, K., H. P. Babcock, and X. Zhuang. "Dual-Objective STORM Reveals Three-Dimensional Filament Organization in the Actin Cytoskeleton." *Nat Methods* 9, no. 2 (2012): 185–8.

63. Pavani, S. R., M. A. Thompson, J. S. Biteen et al. "Three-Dimensional, Single-Molecule Fluorescence Imaging Beyond the Diffraction Limit by Using a Double-Helix Point Spread Function." *Proc Natl Acad Sci USA* 106, no. 9 (2009): 2995–9.

64. Juette, M. F., T. J. Gould, M. D. Lessard et al. "Three-Dimensional Sub-100 Nm Resolution Fluorescence Microscopy of Thick Samples." *Nat Methods* 5, no. 6 (2008): 527–9.

65. Shtengel, G., J. A. Galbraith, C. G. Galbraith et al. "Interferometric Fluorescent Super-Resolution Microscopy Resolves 3D Cellular Ultrastructure." *Proc Natl Acad Sci USA* 106, no. 9 (2009): 3125–30.

66. Huang, F., T. M. Hartwich, F. E. Rivera-Molina et al. "Video-Rate Nanoscopy Using Scmos Camera-Specific Single-Molecule Localization Algorithms." *Nat Methods* 10, no. 7 (2013): 653–8.

67. Lakadamyali, M. "Super-Resolution Microscopy: Going Live and Going Fast." *ChemPhysChem* 15, no. 4 (2014): 630–6.

68. Balint, S., I. Verdeny Vilanova, A. Sandoval Alvarez, and M. Lakadamyali. "Correlative Live-Cell and Superresolution Microscopy Reveals Cargo Transport Dynamics at Microtubule Intersections." *Proc Natl Acad Sci USA* 110, no. 9 (2013): 3375–80.

69. Henriques, R., M. Lelek, E. F. Fornasiero et al. "QuickPALM: 3D Real-Time Photoactivation Nanoscopy Image Processing in ImageJ." *Nat Methods* 7, no. 5 (2010): 339–40.

70. Wolter, S., A. Loschberger, T. Holm et al. "rapidSTORM: Accurate, Fast Open-Source Software for Localization Microscopy." *Nat Methods* 9, no. 11 (2012): 1040–1.

71. Brede, N., and M. Lakadamyali. "GraspJ—An Open Source, Real-Time Analysis Package for Super-Resolution Imaging." *Opt Nanoscopy* 1 (2012): 11.

72. Holden, S. J., S. Uphoff, and A. N. Kapanidis. "DAOSTORM: An Algorithm for High-Density Super-Resolution Microscopy." *Nat Methods* 8, no. 4 (2011): 279–80.

73. Zhu, L., W. Zhang, D. Elnatan, and B. Huang. "Faster STORM Using Compressed Sensing." *Nat Methods* 9, no. 7 (2012): 721–3.

74. Cox, S., E. Rosten, J. Monypenny et al. "Bayesian Localization Microscopy Reveals Nanoscale Podosome Dynamics." *Nat Methods* 9, no. 2 (2012): 195–200.

18 Visualization and Resolution in Localization Microscopy

Robert P.J. Nieuwenhuizen,
Sjoerd Stallinga, and Bernd Rieger

CONTENTS

18.1 INTRODUCTION

Imaging beyond the diffraction limit via a set of techniques nowadays termed *localization microscopy* has seen a sharp rise after the initial works around 2006; the most notable methods introduced were (fluorescence) photoactivated localization microscopy (PALM)[1,2] and stochastic optical reconstruction microscopy.[3] The common idea to achieve imaging below the diffraction limit in the optical far field is to localize single stochastically activated fluorescent molecules. These molecules are switched between a fluorescent on-state and a nonfluorescent off-state. The on-state molecules form a sparse subset of all molecules such that only one is active in a region the size on the order of the diffraction limit. The positions of these emitting molecules are estimated, after which they return to the off-state and other molecules are activated and localized until all molecules have been imaged. Essential to this process is the *localization* of single fluorescent molecules, hence the common name for the techniques. The high-resolution capability of these techniques follows from the precision with which the positions of the molecules can be estimated, which is much better than the diffraction limit.[4,5] This precision is on the order of $\sigma_{psf}/\sqrt{n}$, where n is the number of recorded emission photons and σ_{psf} is the width of the point spread function (PSF).[6,7] Typically, hundreds or thousands of photons can be recorded and with $\sigma_{psf} \approx 250$ nm, this results in commonly achieved localization precisions on the order of tens of nanometers, although smaller values in the range of nanometers have been reported.[8–10] In comparison, Abbe's diffraction limit is given by $\lambda/(2NA) \approx 200$ nm, where λ is the wavelength of light and NA is the numerical aperture of the imaging system. This superior precision is what makes localization microscopy images crisper and sharper than widefield images and explains the widespread use of the technique nowadays. Even now, more and more flavors of localization-based microscopy techniques are introduced; we give by no means an exhaustive list.[11–18]

18.2 RESOLUTION

As the family of localization microscopy techniques came of age and sharper and sharper images were recorded, the question "what is the resolution for these types of images?" arose. In other techniques for super-resolution imaging, such as stimulated emission depletion (STED) microscopy,[19,20] structured illumination microscopy (SIM),[21,22] or image scanning microscopy (ISM),[23,24] the system can be identified as having a smaller effective PSF. Once the width of this PSF is measured or calculated, the resolution in the Abbe sense can be given. Where Abbe and Nyquist defined resolution as the inverse of the spatial bandwidth of the imaging system,[25,26] Rayleigh and Sparrow captured resolution empirically. Rayleigh found a limit of 0.61λ/NA and Sparrow found a limit of 0.47λ/NA, which is very similar to Abbe's diffraction limit of 0.5λ/NA for incoherent light. For localization microscopy, there is no natural extension of the PSF methodology as the position estimation of a single emitter from a PSF image is the key concept.

18.2.1 RESOLUTION MEASURES

Which factors then play a role in the resolution of a localization-based image and how can the resolution easily be assessed for experimental data? Already in one of the first key publications by Betzig et al.,[1] it was noted that "both parameters, localization precision and the density of rendered molecules, are key to defining performance." However, it took a few years before this realization was developed further. Initially, researchers simply equated resolution with the average localization uncertainty of the recordings or the average density of localizations. Others showed full width at half maximum (FWHM) values of cross sections of line-like structures. These concepts will be discussed in the following.

18.2.1.1 Localization Uncertainty

The localization uncertainty indicates the expected standard deviation of the error that was made in estimating a single emitter's position. The localization uncertainty of a single fit to a PSF is only returned by some localization algorithms, mostly those based on maximum-likelihood estimation (MLE) fitting. The uncertainty is then computed using the inverse Fisher matrix,[5,27–31] which gives the theoretically best localization precision that could be achieved. It was shown that fitting with a simple Gaussian PSF model to the data is actually sufficient to achieve the best possible fit in 2D.[32,33] As MLE fitting is in many cases slower than nonlinear least mean squares (LMS) fitting, the latter is very popular and actually quite accurate for a few hundred signal photon counts.

As many algorithms lack the explicit computation of the uncertainty, a very concise and practical formula by Thompson et al. is often used for computing the average localization uncertainty Δx for LMS fitting[34]

$$\left\langle (\Delta x)^2 \right\rangle = \frac{\sigma_a^2}{n}\left(1 + \frac{8\pi\sigma^2 b}{na^2} \right), \tag{18.1}$$

with $\sigma_a^2 = \sigma_{psf}^2 + a^2/12$. Here, σ_{psf} is the width of the Gaussian that is used to fit the PSF, a is the pixel size, n is the number of signal photons, and b is the number of background photons per pixel. This formula is very widely used in the field as only easily accessible experimental parameters are required to evaluate it. It turned out, however, that it is also unduly optimistic for all cases where the background intensity b is nonzero.[6,7,28] Mortensen et al. presented a formula for the localization uncertainty for MLE fitting:[6]

$$\left\langle (\Delta x)^2 \right\rangle = \frac{\sigma_a^2}{n}\left(1 + \int_0^1 dt \, \frac{\ln t}{1 + t/\tau} \right)^{-1}, \tag{18.2}$$

where τ is a normalized dimensionless back ground parameter, $\tau = 2\pi\sigma_a^2 b/(na^2)$. This formula can be approximated within a few percent by an analytical expression derived by us earlier:[7]

$$\left\langle (\Delta x)^2 \right\rangle = \frac{\sigma_a^2}{n}\left(1 + 4\tau + \sqrt{\frac{2\tau}{1 + 4\tau}} \right). \tag{18.3}$$

None of these equations consider the excess noise of the electron multiplication process that is present in the EMCCD (electron-multiplying charge-coupled device) cameras that are normally used for single-molecule imaging.[30] Theoretically, this deteriorates the performance by a factor of $\sqrt{2}$ compared to Equations 18.2 and 18.3.[30] Recently, Huang et al.[35] showed that for this reason, sCMOS (scientific complementary metal oxide semiconductor) cameras outperform EMCCD cameras for localization microscopy, except in cases with fewer than ~100–200 signal photons per emitter and little background. If only a few photons are detected per pixel on average, EMCCD cameras can be used to achieve the best localization precision.[36]

Even though the Thompson formula is too optimistic for nonzero background intensities, it is still used because of its simplicity. We would recommend using Equation 18.3 instead, as it requires the same input parameters, is simple, and is correct for all cases to within a few percent.

18.2.1.2 Full Width at Half Maximum

Directly related to the localization uncertainty is the FWHM. For a line-like structure with a Gaussian cross section, the relation between its standard deviation σ and the FWHM is $2\sqrt{2\ln 2}\sigma \approx 2.35\sigma$. For a Gaussian distribution of localization errors, the FWHM represents the effective width of the system's PSF. In that sense, stating the FWHM instead of the localization uncertainty provides a fairer comparison to the widefield resolution. A related approach used in all publications by Hell et al. is to indicate the performance of the imaging by extracting line profiles across narrow line-like structures such as tubulin filaments. Also, in localization microscopy, this is a useful measure as it incorporates experimental effects such as the wider appearance of structures owing to the size of the linker plus fluorescent label.[16] The downside of this experimental procedure is that the user must handpick one or more cross sections. This is susceptible to bias toward selecting the best lines instead of representative lines.

18.2.1.3 Two-Point Resolution

The so-called two-point resolution has been defined in the context of localization microscopy by Ram et al.,[37] thus extending the Rayleigh criterion to this imaging modality. Their definition of two-point resolution was the minimal standard deviation with which the distance between two emitters can be estimated. This measure, however, was not used by practitioners in the field as it is not easy to assess this resolution measure by experimentally accessible parameters.

18.2.1.4 Density of Localizations

Another commonly stated quantity intended to indicate the resolution is the density of localizations ρ, which is easily computed directly from the data. It can also be used to compute the two-dimensional (2D) Nyquist random sampling resolution as $2/\sqrt{\rho}$ in 2D or $2\rho^{-1/3}$ in 3D. The Nyquist sampling theorem, however, does not strictly apply since localizations do not constitute samples of a bandwidth-limited function. In addition, a problem that has not received much attention is that individual fluorophores are typically activated and localized several times during an acquisition. The number of times an emitter is reactivated can be quite substantial depending on the imaging and buffer conditions (~5–50 times). Even for imaging with fluorescent proteins, repeated activations have been reported where emitters should have become permanently disabled because of photobleaching.[38,39] If this is the case, then the sampling density is artificially overestimated and, in turn, also the resolution based on the Nyquist density. Nevertheless, the density of localizations is used in the field and describes an additional quality besides the localization uncertainty.

As mentioned above, it has been already realized in 2006 that localization density and uncertainty must both play a role in the resolution;[1] these effects have since been investigated experimentally.[40,41] In the following, we review methods that combine both quantities into one resolution assessment.

18.2.1.5 Kernel Density Estimation

One approach for quantifying the resolution in localization microscopy that takes into account both localization precision and labeling density was proposed by Rees et al.[42] These authors draw on the literature on density estimation and consider filter kernels that provide the best estimation of the fluorophore density of the underlying imaged object. The authors argue that the filtered images show this object blurred first by the localization error and second by the smoothing kernel. The resolution is then defined as the minimal distance for which an intensity minimum can still be seen between two emitters in the filtered image (i.e., the Sparrow resolution criterion). Unfortunately, the determination of the optimal filter kernel size is rather difficult in practice. First, this requires knowledge about the stage drift in the acquisition and the size of the fluorescent labels. Second, the proposed scheme for dealing with variations in the density of localizations is based on statistics of the nearest neighbors of each localization. Since fluorophores are localized an unknown number of times, it is unclear which fluorophores are typically represented by these nearest neighbors. Therefore, rules for determining the kernel size will be susceptible to inconsistent outcomes depending on the statistics of the localizations per fluorophore.

18.2.1.6 Information Transfer Function

The information transfer function[43,44] is a conceptual approach for quantifying resolution that considers the filtering of localization microscopy images in the spatial frequency domain. It describes the theoretically minimal error that can be attained by any linear or nonlinear filtering procedure in estimating the spatial frequency content of the underlying imaged object. The maximum spatial frequency at which this relative error is larger than a certain threshold then defines the resolution of the image. Unfortunately, determining the resolution using this framework requires knowledge of the spatial frequency content of the underlying image structure. It has been suggested that such knowledge may be obtained by using a databank of electron microscopy (EM) images or that the spatial frequency content of the underlying structure can be iteratively estimated.[43] Nevertheless, this requirement severely hinders the practical application of this resolution concept on experimental data.

The above approaches consider the localization uncertainty and density but are not usable in practice and omit the fact that, additionally, the resolution depends on many more factors such as the link between the label and the structure, the underlying spatial structure of the sample itself, and the extensive data processing and visualization required to produce a final super-resolution image. Moreover, these approaches neglect the problems that arise owing to repeated localizations of the same emitter from different activation cycles. This will bias the resolution estimation substantially if not properly taken into account. Therefore, only an integral, image-based resolution measure not depending on a priori information is suitable for determining what level of detail can be reliably discerned in a specific image.

18.2.2   FOURIER RING CORRELATION

We proposed Fourier ring correlation (FRC) or, equivalently, the spectral signal-to-noise ratio as a practical approach for defining and quantifying resolution in localization microscopy.[45] The FRC is the standard for resolution assessment in the field of cryo-EM single-particle reconstructions of macromolecular complexes.[46–49] In cryo-EM, the resolution is much worse than the diffraction limit given by the electron wavelength and the opening angle, attributed to aberrations in the optical systems. Furthermore, the signal-to-noise ratio is so low (≤ 1) that the actual image content has to be considered. FRC provides an image-resolution measure that does not require any prior knowledge and is sensitive to the effects of both localization precision and labeling density. Moreover, it is also sensitive to the other factors that influence the resolution mentioned above.

To compute the FRC resolution, the full set of estimated fluorophore positions is divided into two independent subsets. This yields two subimages $f_1(\vec{r})$ and $f_2(\vec{r})$, where $\vec{r}$ denotes the spatial coordinates. Statistical correlation of their Fourier transforms $\hat{f}_1(\vec{q})$ and $\hat{f}_2(\vec{q})$ over the pixels on the perimeter of circles of constant spatial frequency magnitude $q = |\vec{q}|$ then gives the FRC:[47]

$$\text{FRC}(q) = \frac{\sum_{\vec{q} \in \text{circle}} \hat{f}_1(\vec{q}) \hat{f}_2(\vec{q})^*}{\sqrt{\sum_{\vec{q} \in \text{circle}} \hat{f}_1(\vec{q})^2} \sqrt{\sum_{\vec{q} \in \text{circle}} \hat{f}_2(\vec{q})^2}}. \tag{18.4}$$

The Fourier transformation of $f(\vec{r})$ is given by $\hat{f}(\vec{q}) = \int d\vec{r} f(\vec{r}) e^{-i2\pi \vec{q} \cdot \vec{r}}$. For low spatial frequencies, the FRC curve is close to unity, and for high spatial frequencies, noise dominates the data and the FRC decays to zero. The image resolution is defined as the inverse of the spatial frequency $R = 1/q_R$ for which the FRC curve drops below a given threshold. See Figure 18.1 for an illustration of the steps needed to compute the FRC resolution. Currently, there is no consensus on what threshold should be used in the field of single-particle EM. Lately, the field does appear to converge on the use of a fixed threshold of 1/7 though.[49,50] We investigated the various threshold criteria empirically[46,50–52] and concluded that the fixed threshold of $1/7 \approx 0.143$ is also the most appropriate one for localization microscopy; that is, $FRC(q_R) = 1/7$.

The expectation of the FRC is given by[45]

$$\langle \text{FRC}(q) \rangle = \frac{\sum_{\vec{q} \in \text{circle}} \left(Q + N |\hat{\psi}(\vec{q})|^2 \right) \exp\left(-4\pi^2 \sigma^2 q^2 \right)}{\sum_{\vec{q} \in \text{circle}} \left[2 + \left(Q + N |\hat{\psi}(\vec{q})|^2 \right) \exp\left(-4\pi^2 \sigma^2 q^2 \right) \right]}, \tag{18.5}$$

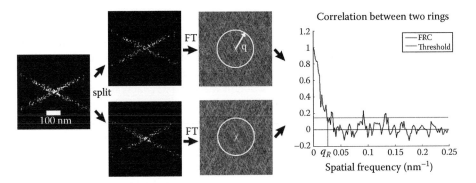

FIGURE 18.1 Schematic illustration of FRC resolution computation. All localizations are divided into two halves, and the correlation of their Fourier transforms over the perimeter of circles in Fourier space of radius q is calculated. This results in an FRC curve indicating the decay of the correlation with spatial frequency. The image resolution is the inverse of the spatial frequency q_R or which the FRC curve drops below the threshold $1/7 \approx 0.143$; thus, for example, $q_R = 0.04$ nm^{-1} is equivalent to 25 nm resolution.

where N is the total number of localized emitters, σ is the average localization uncertainty, and $\hat{\psi}(\vec{q})$ is the Fourier spectrum of the object. The parameter Q takes into account the repeated activation of the same emitter. Each emitter contributing to the image is localized once for $Q = 0$ and in general $Q/(1 - e^{-Q})$ times on average, provided the emitter activation follows Poisson statistics. The term with Q in the numerator of Equation 18.5 is a measure for spurious correlations at high frequencies and can result in overestimation of the resolution. However, this can be corrected for by estimating the parameter Q from the data as explained in Ref. 45. If done so, we have shown that more frequent localization of the same emitter is always beneficial to the final resolution.[53]

For a sample consisting of two parallel lines with a sinusoidal cross section, Equation 18.5 can be solved analytically for $Q = 0$. This results in a resolution $R = 2\pi\sigma/\sqrt{W(6\pi\rho\sigma^2)}$,[45] where $W(x)$ is the Lambert W-function.[54] This also shows that the localization precision σ and the density of localizations ρ are combined into the FRC resolution estimation in a natural way. More generally, Equation 18.5 shows that the FRC resolution also takes into account the frequency contents of the underlying object without it being known explicitly.

The FRC resolution measure reduces to common resolution measures in limiting cases. In the limit of perfect localization precision, that is, $\sigma \to 0$, the resolution for the two-line sample becomes $R = \sqrt{\pi/6} \, R_{\text{Nyquist}} \approx R_{\text{Nyquist}}$. When the FRC is applied to widefield acquisitions, the resolution reduces to the Abbe resolution in the limit of infinite SNR.[45]

In Section 18.3, the FRC-based resolution approach will be used to evaluate the image resolution attained with various visualization methods for localization microscopy data.

18.2.3 LOCAL AND ANISOTROPIC (2D AND 3D) RESOLUTION

For experimental images, the apparent resolution is often not homogeneous across the sample, for example, owing to differences in labeling density. In such cases, the FRC resolution and most of the other resolution measures listed above only provide a single number to indicate the smallest details that can be reliably interpreted on average. However, by computing the FRC resolution locally for smaller image patches, it is possible to obtain an indication of the local resolution across the image. This local resolution can be visualized using a false color overlay on the super-resolution image, where the color indicates the local resolution.

Experimental images also often exhibit anisotropy owing to inherent anisotropy in the imaged structure or imaging method. In 2D imaging, this can occur for example if the underlying imaged structure consists of filaments with the same orientation. In three-dimensional imaging, resolution anisotropy often results from anisotropy in the localization precision, which is typically two to three times worse in the axial direction than in the lateral direction.[55–57] For these situations, one would expect that the resolution is also anisotropic, that is, not the same for all directions. Anisotropic image resolution can be described similar to FRC by correlating two images of half the data set in Fourier space over a line in 2D (Fourier line correlation [FLC]) or a plane in 3D (Fourier plane correlation [FPC]) perpendicular to spatial frequency vectors $\vec{q}$. This results in an image with a value for the FLC or FPC for all directions and every spatial frequency magnitude $\left\| \vec{q} \right\|$. The resolution can then be assessed by identifying the spatial frequencies where the FLC/FPC is above the threshold.

18.3 VISUALIZATION

Localization microscopy has no natural way to display the recordings. It does not sample the image at pixel locations as in standard widefield microscopy. In widefield microscopy, images are typically recorded on a CCD (charge-coupled device) camera. The pixels of the camera together with the magnification of the objective lens naturally define the way how an image is sampled. The back-projected pixel size is chosen such that it fulfills Nyquist sampling, that is, a pixel should be smaller than half the diffraction limit $d \leq \lambda/(4NA)$, where λ is the wavelength of light and NA is the numerical aperture of the imaging system. The emission photons recorded per CCD pixel bin are translated into analog-to-digital units (ADU) with a linear amplification factor (gain). These ADU are typically discretized into 8-, 12-, or 16-bit integers and they represent the intensity or count values. The recorded sample is therefore visualized as a pixelated image where the discrete intensity scale is about linearly proportional to the recorded number of photons and thus the density of fluorescent molecules. The same natural visualization is shared by confocal microscopy, where the CCD pixel is replaced by a point detection device such as a photomultiplier tube or an avalanche photodiode. The stepping of the scan mirror naturally defines the pixel size. Please note that it is common to have a regular (square) sampling grid of pixels or scan positions, but that is not strictly necessary. To avoid phototoxicity, adaptive schemes of illuminating and recording have been proposed.[58,59]

As localization microscopy lacks any of the above natural ways of visualization, it is an important issue how data should be visualized. Basically, the positions of single fluorescent emitters are estimated from the asynchronous recordings of blinking emitters. To this end, different localization schemes are employed that estimate the positions (i.e., a list of 2D or 3D coordinates), as well as the estimated fluorophore intensities, background intensities, localization precisions, and possibly other parameters depending on the localization method.[5,28,29,31] Thus, localization microscopy produces data sets but no images initially. To make these data comprehensible, these localization data need to be translated into a visual representation in the form of an image. Subsequently, this image needs to be translated into brightness values of the pixels in the display device. Reconstruction (in the Nyquist sense) of the fluorophore distribution of the underlying imaged object from the set of localizations is not considered to be a part of the visualization process.

This section is concerned with the choice of the visualization method for translating localization data into an image. Several methods have been proposed in the literature that will be discussed here: scattergram plots,[3] histogram binning,[13] Gaussian rendering,[1] jittered histogram binning,[60] Delaunay triangulation,[61] and quad-tree visualization.[61]

18.3.1   DESCRIPTION OF VISUALIZATION METHODS

In this subsection, the various visualization methods are first illustrated and described, before moving on to discussing the merits and implications of using the methods in Section 18.3.2. See Figure 18.2 for an illustration of the different visualization methods, except the scattergram method.

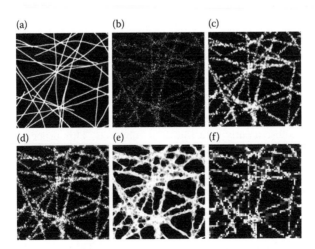

FIGURE 18.2 Illustration of different visualization methods. The images show the different visualization methods applied to simulated localization data of filaments for a density of localizations $\rho = 2.0 \times 10^3$ μm^{-2} and localization precision $\sigma = 10$ nm. (a) The ground truth structure, (b) histogram binning, (c) Gaussian rendering, (d) jittering, (e) Delaunay triangulation, and (f) quad-tree visualization. Images are individually 95th percentile stretched for better visibility on paper.

Scattergram: Each coordinate is plotted as a symbol, typically a cross or plus, in a Cartesian coordinate system.[3]

Histogram binning: The field of view is divided into a complete set of square pixel bins and the number of localizations that fall in each bin is counted and used to assign intensity values to bins.[13] The size of the pixel bins should generally not exceed one quarter of the image resolution in order not to deteriorate the resolution.[45] Histogram images often appear rather noisy because of the low signal-to-noise ratio per pixel, which can be resolved by postblurring the histogram images. This blurring also prevents problems with aliasing if the sampling density of the display device is too low. If a radially symmetric kernel is used for blurring, then the image resolution remains unchanged for reasonably isotropic structures.[45]

Gaussian rendering: An image is rendered where localizations are represented with Gaussian blobs with a width proportional to the estimated localization precision in the respective axial and lateral dimensions.[1] Thus, the resulting image conveys information on the localization precision of each localization. It should be noted that effects such as imperfect correction for stage drift effectively lead to an additional localization error that is not taken into account in the estimated localization precision. Therefore, the rendered Gaussian blobs cannot always be interpreted to be likelihood functions for the positions of the fluorophores.

Jittered histogram binning: Each localization gives rise to a fixed number of offspring points (typically 10 or 20) that are randomly displaced (i.e., jittered) with a zero-mean normal distribution whose standard deviation is equal to the estimated localization precision.[60] Thus, for very large numbers of offspring points, this visualization method gives the same result as Gaussian rendering.

Delaunay triangulation: A tiling is created in the image plane using triangles whose vertices correspond to the estimated emitter locations.[61] The triangles are rendered with a grayscale intensity inversely proportional to the area of the triangle such that higher local densities of emitters result in higher intensities. The size of the triangles emphasizes the local density of localizations.

Quad-tree visualization: An image is formed using square pixels whose size depends on the local density of localizations.[61] Initially, the image plane is divided into four pixels. Each pixel that contains more than a fixed threshold number of localizations is subsequently split into four subpixels. This process is repeated for the subpixels, until each pixel contains fewer localizations than the threshold value.

18.3.2 Comparison of Visualization Methods

With the multitude of available visualization methods, the question as to which method is best for representing experimental data arises. A number of relevant considerations in choosing a visualization method were discussed by Baddeley et al.[61] Here, we will focus on the most important of those: the extent to which images produced with a visualization method can be intuitively interpreted and the resolution of these images.

Intuitive interpretation of localization microscopy images requires that the images conform to users' expectations based on other fluorescence microscopy methods, such as widefield or confocal imaging. In these microscopy techniques, the local intensity in the image can be described by a convolution of the fluorophore density in the sample with the effective PSF. Hence, the image intensity values are linear in the density of imaged molecules and typically vary smoothly owing to the effective blurring by the PSF. This linearity is also inherent in super-resolution imaging techniques such as STED,[19,20] SIM,[21,22] and ISM.[23,24]

The expected linearity of intensity values argues against the use of the scattergram visualization method: at a high localization density, the symbols in the scattergram overlap and lead to a saturated image. The Delaunay triangulation and quad-tree methods are also not linear in the density of localized molecules, but these do not provide saturated images.

Linearity is more generally an issue for localization microscopy because the acquisitions are nonlinear in the density of labeled molecules. Some molecules are not localized in an experiment and do not contribute to the final image. Additionally, fluorophore activation events are sometimes not recognized or rejected by the localization software. This could happen, for example, if fluorophores are too dim to be picked up by the algorithm that selects candidates for fitting or too dim to pass the threshold for the allowed localization precision. Also, if nearby fluorophores are simultaneously active such that their emissions overlap in the image plane, then the localization algorithm results in a position intermediate between the two simultaneously active molecules. Although, currently, methods toward multifluorophore fitting[62–64] are proposed, the application of these methods to nonideal acquisitions outside TIRF (total internal reflection fluorescence) imaging remains a challenge. In the worst case, overlapping emissions may result in unnoticed missing structures. Hence, the final images are always nonlinear in the density of labeled molecules. None of the above visualization methods, however, shows activation events missed by the preprocessing software for candidate selection.

The smooth, blurry appearance of images produced with conventional fluorescence microscopy methods normally conveys a sense of the resolution of the imaging system. Therefore, the Gaussian rendering and jittered binning methods vary the apparent width of localizations in images to indicate how well the corresponding fluorophores can be distinguished from nearby molecules. The ability, however, to resolve structures in localization microscopy depends not only on the localization precision but also, for example, on the labeling density.[45] Therefore, the apparent size of localizations in Gaussian rendering and jittered binning methods does not indicate the actual image resolution. Delaunay triangulation and quad-tree visualization emphasize local variations in the image resolution by adjusting the triangle sizes or subpixel sizes to the labeling density. Unfortunately, these sizes do not correspond to the image resolution that would be determined with the FRC method.

18.3.2.1   Simulations

The second consideration for choosing a visualization method that merits attention, next to intuitive interpretation, is the actual image resolution in the image that is produced. This issue will be addressed by studying the resolution of images produced with different visualization methods for simulation data. By using simulation data where the underlying imaged structure is known, it is possible to identify if the FRC between images of two halves of the simulated data is biased. Such a bias could result in inaccurate resolution determination for experimental data.

18.3.2.2 Setup

Localization microscopy acquisitions of filaments were simulated where both the chosen average localization precision σ and density of localizations ρ were varied. For these simulations, the ground truth structure consisted of 100 filaments generated with a worm-like chain model[65–67] for a persistence length of 15 μm (i.e., approximately the persistence length of F-actin[68]). Each filament had a random starting position and starting orientation inside the field of view of 5.12 μm by 5.12 μm. All filaments were then Gaussian blurred with a standard deviation of 5 nm to provide the filaments with a finite width. Subsequently, they were rendered in an image with a pixel size of 2.5 nm.

For this ground truth structure, 100 acquisitions were simulated for each combination of densities ρ and localization uncertainties σ. For each acquisition, a Poisson-distributed number of points was generated with a density proportional to the ground truth structure and average density equal to ρ. These points were then randomly displaced with a Gaussian probability density with variance $d^2 + \sigma_0^2 / n_{photons}$ to simulate the finite label size and localization error. Here, d represents the finite size of fluorescent labels and had a value $d = 5$ nm. For each point, σ_0 was randomly drawn from a normal distribution with a mean specified by $\langle\sigma_0\rangle = 450$ nm and standard deviation of $0.1 \langle\sigma_0\rangle$. The parameter $n_{photons}$ was randomly drawn from a geometric distribution, which is the distribution for the photon counts of a photon source whose duration has an exponential distribution. These values give a localization uncertainty of 10 nm at 2000 photons.

The simulated localization data were used to compute the resolutions of the images generated by the various visualization methods. For each acquisition, the localizations were split into two half sets to obtain two images per visualization methods. All images had pixel sizes of 5 nm, except the images obtained with Delaunay triangulation, which were rendered using the PALM-siever software[69] with a pixel size of 2.5 nm. For the quad-tree visualization, the threshold number of localization per pixel for splitting into subpixels was 6. Subsequently, the resolution was obtained with these images by computing the FRC and finding the spatial frequency for which the FRC dropped below the threshold of 1/7. To investigate potential biases in the computed FRC curves, additional images were made with all localizations of each acquisition. These were then used to compute the FRC between those images and the ground truth structure. The spatial frequency at which this full data FRC crosses a threshold of 1/2 should give the same result as before for unbiased resolution estimation.[50]

18.3.2.3 Results

The results of the simulations are summarized in Figures 18.3 and 18.4. Figure 18.3 shows the resolution between the full data images and the ground truth structure for the various visualization methods. From this figure, it becomes clear that generally histogram binning, jittering, and Gaussian rendering result in more or less the same resolution. Gaussian rendering provides the best resolution, especially when the mean localization error σ is large and strongly affects the image resolution. This result will be discussed in more detail in the next paragraph. Delaunay triangulation and quad-tree visualization result in substantially deteriorated resolutions when the density ρ is not very high. For Delaunay triangulation, this deterioration is attributed to the hard edges that are introduced. For the quad-tree method, the deterioration is attributed to the lack of shift invariance of the pixel splitting.

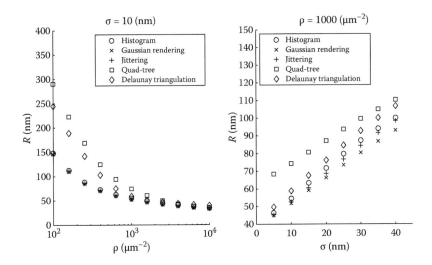

FIGURE 18.3 Resolution for the different visualization methods as a function of the density of localizations ρ and localization precision σ. The resolution is computed from the FRC between images of the full data sets and the ground truth structure. The standard error of the mean is smaller than the marker sizes in this plot.

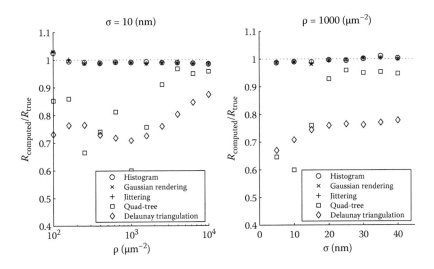

FIGURE 18.4 Bias in resolution estimation for the different visualization methods as a function of the density of localizations ρ and localization precision σ. R_{true} is the resolution obtained from the FRC between images of the full data sets and the ground truth structure, whereas R_{computed} is the resolution obtained from the FRC between two images of half data sets. The standard error of the mean is smaller than the marker sizes in this plot.

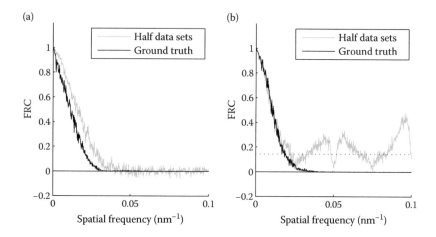

FIGURE 18.5 FRC curves for (a) Delaunay triangulation and (b) quad-tree visualization. The FRC between two images of half data sets is compared here with the curve that would be expected based on the FRC between images of the full data sets and the ground truth structure.

Figure 18.4 shows that Delaunay triangulation and quad-tree visualization bias the resolution estimation with two half data sets for small ρ and small σ. The bias is also evident in Figure 18.5 where the FRC curves between two half data sets are compared with the expected FRC curves based on the FRC between the full data and the ground truth images for these visualization methods. The irregular bias in the quad-tree FRC curve for two half data sets also explains the irregularity in the resolution bias as a function of ρ and σ for that method. All this implies that these visualization methods should not be used to compute and assess the resolution for experimental data.

18.3.2.4 Theoretical Considerations

This section provides a theoretical explanation for why Gaussian rendering performs better than histogram binning. To this end, the expected FRC will be derived for the case where the localization precision σ is not constant for both the Gaussian rendering method and the histogram binning method. Consistent with the simulations above, it will be assumed for simplicity that all fluorophores on the structure at hand are localized exactly once.

Before deriving the expected FRCs, we provide a few definitions. First, the ground truth object for this derivation is given by

$$\psi(\vec{r}) = \sum_{j=1}^{N} \delta\left(\vec{r} - \vec{r}_j^{\,\mathrm{em}}\right), \tag{18.6}$$

where δ is the Dirac delta function. The object depends on the set of positions $\left\{\vec{r}_j^{\,\mathrm{em}} \mid j = 1,\ldots,N\right\}$ of the N fluorophores or labels. These labels are localized at positions $\left\{\vec{r}_j \mid j = 1,\ldots N\right\}$ with probability $P\left(\vec{r}_j\right) = \left(2\pi\sigma_j^2\right)^{-1} \exp\left(-\left\|\vec{r}_j - \vec{r}_j^{\,\mathrm{em}}\right\|^2 \big/ 2\sigma_j^2\right)$. In the following, we assume no specific dimensionality, but typically $\vec{r}_j \in \mathbb{R}^2$ or $\vec{r}_j \in \mathbb{R}^3$. For the 3D case, the localization uncertainty is typically two to three times worse in the axial direction than in the lateral direction,[55–57] except for very specific experimental setups.[70,71] For the sake of compactness, 2D acquisitions with isotropic localization uncertainties will be assumed, although the conclusions derived here are also valid for anisotropic localization uncertainties.

The set of localizations is split into two subsets of size N_1 and N_2 to produce two images $f_1(\vec{r})$ and $f_2(\vec{r})$, with $N_1 + N_2 = N$ and $N_1 \approx N_2$. The FRC between such images is defined as given by Equation 18.4. The expected value of the numerator of the FRC when emitters are localized is

$$\left\langle \sum_{\vec{q} \in \text{circle}} \hat{f}_1(\vec{q}) \hat{f}_2(\vec{q})^* \right\rangle = \sum_{\vec{q} \in \text{circle}} \left\langle \hat{f}_1(\vec{q}) \right\rangle \left\langle \hat{f}_2(\vec{q})^* \right\rangle, \tag{18.7}$$

where $\left\langle f(\vec{r}) \right\rangle \equiv \int d\vec{r}_1 \ldots d\vec{r}_N f(\vec{r}) P(\{\vec{r}_j\})$. For Gaussian rendering, the images are denoted by $g_m(\vec{r})$ with $m = \{1, 2\}$, and equal to

$$g_m(\vec{r}) = \sum_{j=1}^{N_m} \frac{1}{2\pi\sigma_j^2} e^{-|\vec{r}-\vec{r}_j|^2/2\sigma_j^2}, \tag{18.8}$$

with Fourier transformation

$$\hat{g}_m(\vec{g}) = \sum_{j=1}^{N_m} e^{-2\pi^2 q^2 \sigma_j^2} e^{-i2\pi\vec{q}\cdot\vec{r}j}. \tag{18.9}$$

For the case of constant $\sigma_j \equiv \sigma \forall j$, this expression simply describes a convolution of the found positions r_j with a Gaussian kernel of size σ. Assuming that σ_j is given (i.e., not a stochastic variable), the expected value of $f_m(\vec{q})$ becomes

$$\left\langle \hat{g}_m(\vec{q}) \right\rangle = \int d\vec{r}_j \sum_{j=1}^{N_m} e^{-2\pi^2 q^2 \sigma_j^2} e^{-i2\pi\vec{q}\cdot\vec{r}_j} P(\{\vec{r}_j\}) \tag{18.10}$$

$$= \sum_{j=1}^{N_m} e^{-2\pi^2 q^2 \sigma_j^2} \int d\vec{r}_j e^{-i2\pi\vec{q}\cdot\vec{r}_j} P(\{\vec{r}_j\}) \tag{18.11}$$

$$= \sum_{j=1}^{N_m} e^{-4\pi^2 q^2 \sigma_j^2} e^{-i2\pi\vec{q}\cdot\vec{r}_j^{\text{em}}} \approx \frac{1}{N} \hat{\psi}(\vec{q}) \sum_{j=1}^{N_m} e^{-4\pi^2 q^2 \sigma_j^2}. \tag{18.12}$$

If the effect of low-pass filtering attributed to finite pixel size is neglected, $f_m(\vec{r})$ for histogram binning is equal to

$$f_m(\vec{r}) = \sum_{j=1}^{N_m} \delta(\vec{r} - \vec{r}_j),$$

(18.13)

which leads to

$$\left\langle \hat{f}_m(\vec{q}) \mid \sigma_j \right\rangle \approx \frac{1}{N} \hat{\psi}(\vec{q}) \sum_{j=1}^{N_m} e^{-2\pi^2 q^2 \sigma_j^2}.$$

(18.14)

The difference between the two visualization methods already becomes apparent here. Comparing Equations 18.12 and 18.14 show that an extra factor, 2, appears in the exponent because of the extra blurring of the Gaussian rendering. For the expected value of the denominator of the FRC, the expected value of $\left| f_m(\vec{q}) \right|^2$ needs to be evaluated. For Gaussian rendering, this goes as follows:

$$\left\langle \left| \hat{g}_m(\vec{q}) \right|^2 \right\rangle = \left\langle \sum_{j=1}^{N_m} \sum_{k=1}^{N_m} e^{-2\pi^2 q^2 \sigma_j^2} e^{-2\pi^2 q^2 \sigma_k^2} e^{-i2\pi \vec{q} \cdot (\vec{r}_k - \vec{r}_j)} \right\rangle$$

(18.15)

$$= \left\langle \sum_{j=1}^{N_m} \sum_{k \neq j} e^{-2\pi^2 q^2 \sigma_j^2} e^{-2\pi^2 q^2 \sigma_k^2} e^{-i2\pi \vec{q} \cdot (\vec{r}_k - \vec{r}_j)} \right\rangle + \left\langle \sum_{j=1}^{N_m} e^{-4\pi^2 q^2 \sigma_j^2} \right\rangle$$

(18.16)

$$\approx \left| \left\langle \sum_{j=1}^{N_m} e^{-2\pi^2 q^2 \sigma_j^2} e^{-i2\pi \vec{q} \cdot \vec{r}_j} \right\rangle \right|^2 + \left\langle \sum_{j=1}^{N_m} e^{-4\pi^2 q^2 \sigma_j^2} \right\rangle$$

(18.17)

$$= \left| \left\langle \hat{g}_m(\vec{q}) \right\rangle \right|^2 + \left\langle \sum_{j=1}^{N_m} e^{-4\pi^2 q^2 \sigma_j^2} \right\rangle.$$

(18.18)

Thus, if the average spectrum of the object over rings of constant spatial frequency is defined as $S(q) = \dfrac{1}{N^2} \int d^2 q' \dfrac{\delta(|\vec{q}'| - q)}{2\pi q} \left| \hat{\psi}(\vec{q}') \right|^2$, the expected FRC becomes

$$\left\langle \text{FRC} \right\rangle = \frac{NS(q) \left\langle \exp\left(-4\pi^2 \sigma^2 q^2\right) \right\rangle^2}{2 \left\langle \exp\left(-4\pi^2 \sigma^2 q^2\right) \right\rangle + NS(q) \left\langle \exp\left(-4\pi^2 \sigma^2 q^2\right) \right\rangle^2}$$

(18.19)

$$= \frac{NS(q)\langle\exp(-4\pi^2\sigma^2 q^2)\rangle}{2 + NS(q)\langle\exp(-4\pi^2\sigma^2 q^2)\rangle}. \tag{18.20}$$

Similarly, for histogram binning, the expected value of $|f_m(\vec{q})|^2$ is

$$\langle|\hat{f}_m(\vec{q})|^2\rangle = \left\langle\sum_{j=1}^{N_m}\sum_{k=1}^{N_m}e^{-i2\pi\vec{q}\cdot(\vec{r}_k-\vec{r}_j)}\right\rangle \approx |\langle\hat{f}_m(\vec{q})\rangle|^2 + N_m, \tag{18.21}$$

which leads to the following expected FRC:

$$\langle\text{FRC}\rangle = \frac{NS(q)\langle\exp(-2\pi^2\sigma^2 q^2)\rangle^2}{2 + NS(q)\langle\exp(-2\pi^2\sigma^2 q^2)\rangle^2}. \tag{18.22}$$

The superiority of the Gaussian rendering over histogram binning now follows from comparing Equations 18.20 and 18.22 and observing that

$$\langle e^{-4\pi^2\sigma^2 q^2}\rangle - \langle e^{-2\pi^2\sigma^2 q^2}\rangle^2 = \left\langle\left(e^{-2\pi^2\sigma^2 q^2} - \langle e^{-2\pi^2\sigma^2 q^2}\rangle\right)^2\right\rangle \geq 0. \tag{18.23}$$

The explanation for this general superiority on the basis of the equations above is that Gaussian rendering effectively weights the contribution of localizations to spatial frequency components depending on their localization precision. This weighting was already obvious from the comparison of Equations 18.12 and 18.14, which showed that Gaussian rendering introduces an extra factor, 2, in the exponent. This causes the exponentials corresponding to imprecise localizations to decrease faster, and therefore, those localizations contribute less to high-frequency components. This leads to higher correlations at those frequencies. For a constant localization uncertainty for all localizations, that is, $\sigma_j \equiv \sigma \forall j$, both visualization methods are equivalent as the difference in Equation 18.23 is then equal to zero.

This derivation did not include the effects of finite pixel size and multiple localizations per emitter. Low-pass filtering attributed to finite pixel sizes introduces an extra damping of $S(q)$, which is the same for histogram binning and Gaussian rendering. For very large pixel sizes, the damping owing to finite pixel size will be stronger than damping owing to the localization error, thus negating the benefits of Gaussian rendering. For multiple localizations per emitter, the impact of Gaussian rendering on the FRC is more subtle and dependent on the statistics of the localization uncertainties σ_j.

18.4   DISCUSSION AND CONCLUSION

The above results lead to the conclusion that the Gaussian rendering method provides the best resolution of the evaluated visualization methods. Please note that this is only true if the Gaussian blobs reflect the localization uncertainty of each single fluorophore and not if one applies one global Gaussian kernel to all localizations. Since this method is also linear in the density of localizations and conveys information about the localization precision, it seems to be the visualization method of choice. However, the histogram binning method provides a similar resolution in a shorter computation time and is therefore a good alternative method. In particular, the reduced computation time makes histogram binning the preferred method for fast and unbiased resolution determination. When this method is used for visualization, it is recommended to postblur the image, for example, with a Gaussian kernel with a standard deviation equal to the average localization precision. This reduces the noise in the image without reducing the resolution. The jittering method provides a compromise between the histogram binning and Gaussian rendering methods, with a better resolution than histogram binning and typically a shorter computation time than Gaussian rendering. Quad-tree visualization and Delaunay triangulation lead to resolution deterioration and biased resolution estimation and are therefore not recommended.

A significant limitation of this simulation study is that the ground truth structure and the Delaunay triangulation results had to be pixelated to compute their Fourier transforms, even though they contain infinitely high spatial frequency components. In principle, this could lead to changes in frequency contents caused by aliasing and the effective low-pass filtering attributed to the finite pixel size. The resolutions, however, in these simulations were typically more than 20 times the pixel size of these images. Therefore, these problems should not play a role at the spatial frequencies where the FRC drops below the threshold and should not affect the computed resolution.

REFERENCES

1. Betzig, E., G. Patterson, R. Sougrat, O. Lindwasser, S. Olenych, J. Bonifacino, M. Davidson, J. Lippincott-Schwartz, and H. Hess. "Imaging intracellular fluorescent proteins at nanometer resolution." *Science 313* (2006): 1643–5.
2. Hess, S., T. Girirajan, and M. Mason. "Ultra-high resolution imaging by fluorescence photoactivation localization microscopy." *Biophysical Journal 91* no. 11 (2006): 4258–72.
3. Rust, M., M. Bates, and X. Zhuang. "Sub-diffraction-limit imaging by stochastic optical reconstruction microscopy (STORM)." *Nature Methods 3* no. 10 (2006): 793–5.
4. Ober, R., Z. Lin, and Q. Zou. "Calculations of the fisher information matrix for multidimensional data sets." *IEEE Transactions on Signal Processing 51* no. 10 (2003): 2679–91.
5. Ober, R., S. Ram, and S. Ward. "Localization accuracy in single-molecule microscopy." *Biophysical Journal 86* no. 2 (2004): 1185–200.
6. Mortensen, K., L. Churchman, J. Spudich, and H. Flyvbjerg. "Optimized localization analysis for single-molecule tracking and super-resolution microscopy." *Nature Methods 7* no. 5 (2010): 377–84.

7. Stallinga, S. and B. Rieger (2012). "The effect of background on localization uncertainty in single emitter imaging." In *IEEE International Symposium on Biomedical Imaging*, Barcelona, Spain, pp. 988–91.

8. Pertsinidis, A., Y. Zhang, and S. Chu. "Subnanometre single-molecule localization, registration and distance measurements." *Nature 466* (2010): 647–51.

9. Vaughan, J., S. Jia, and X. Zhuang. "Ultrabright photoactivatable fluorophores created by reductive caging." *Nature Methods 9* no. 12 (2012): 1181–4.

10. Xu, K., G. Zhong, and X. Zhuang. "Actin, spectrin, and associated proteins form a periodic cytoskeletal structure in axons." *Science 339* (2013): 452–6.

11. Hofmann, M., C. Eggeling, S. Jakobs, and S. Hell. "Breaking the diffraction barrier in fluorescence microscopy at low light intensities by using reversibly photoswitchable proteins." *Proceedings of the National Academy of Sciences USA 102* no. 49 (2005): 17565–9.

12. Bock, H., C. Geisler, C. A. Wurm, C. V. Middendorff, S. Jakobs, A. Schönle, A. Egner, S. W. Hell, and C. Eggeling. "Two-color far-field fluorescence nanoscopy based on photoswitchable emitters." *Applied Physics B—Lasers and Optics 88* no. 2 (2007): 161–5.

13. Egner, A., C. Geisler, C. V. Middendorff, H. Bock, D. Wenzel, R. Medda, M. Andresen, A. Stiel, S. Jakobs, C. Eggeling, A. Schönle, and S. Hell. "Fluorescence nanoscopy in whole cells by asynchronous localization of photoswitching emitters." *Biophysical Journal 93* no. 9 (2007): 3285–90.

14. Bates, M., B. Huang, G. T. Dempsey, and X. Zhuang. "Multicolor super-resolution imaging with photo-switchable fluorescent probes." *Science 317* no. 5845 (2007): 1749–53.

15. Heilemann, M., S. V. d. Linde, M. Schüttpelz, R. Kasper, B. Seefeldt, A. Mukherjee, P. Tinnefeld, and M. Sauer. "Subdiffraction-resolution fluorescence imaging with conventional fluorescent probes." *Angewandte Chemie 47* no. 33 (2008): 6172–76.

16. Ries, J., C. Kaplan, E. Platonova, H. Eghlidi, and H. Ewers. "A simple, versatile method for GFP-based super-resolution microscopy via nanobodies." *Nature Methods 9* no. 6 (2012): 582–7.

17. Fölling, J., M. Bossi, H. Bock, R. Medda, C. Wurm, B. Hein, S. Jacobs, C. Eggeling, and S. Hell. "Fluorescence nanoscopy by ground-state depletion and single-molecule return." *Nature Methods 5* (2008): 943–5.

18. Grotjohann, T., T. Testa, M. Leutenegger, H. Bock, N. Urban, F. Lavoie-Cardinal, K. Willig, C. Eggeling, and S. Hell. "Diffraction-unlimited all-optical imaging and writing with a photochromic GFP." *Nature 478* (2011): 204–8.

19. Hell, S. and J. Wichmann. "Breaking the diffraction limit resolution by stimulated emission: Stimulated-emission-depletion microscopy." *Optics Letters 19* no. 11 (1994): 780–3.

20. Hell, S. "Far-field optical nanoscopy." *Science 316* (2007): 1153–8.

21. Gustafsson, M. "Surpassing the lateral resolution limit by a factor of two using structured illumination microscopy." *Journal of Microscopy 198* no. 2 (2000): 82–7.

22. Heintzmann, R. and M. Gustafsson. "Subdiffraction resolution in continuous samples." *Nature Photonics 3* (2009): 362–4.

23. Sheppard, C. "Super-resolution in confocal microscopy." *Optik 80* no. 2 (1988): 53–4.

24. Müller, C. and J. Enderlein. "Image scanning microscopy." *Physical Review Letters 104* (2010): 198101.

25. Abbe, E. "Beiträge zur Theorie des Mikroskopes und der mikroskopischen Wahrnehmung." *Archiv für Mikroskopische Anatomie 9* (1873): 413–68.

26. Nyquist, H. "Certain topics in telegraph transmission theory." *Transactions of the AIEE 90* (1928): 617–44. (reprinted in: *Proceedings of the IEEE 90* no. 2 [2002]: 280–305).

27. Aguet, F., D. V. D. Ville, and M. Unser. "Dynamic multiple-target tracing to probe spatiotemporal cartography of cell membranes." *Optics Express 13* no. 26 (2005): 10503–22.

28. Smith, C., N. Joseph, B. Rieger, and K. Lidke. "Fast, single-molecule localization that achieves theoretically minimum uncertainty." *Nature Methods 7* no. 5 (2010): 373–5.

29. Abraham, A., S. Ram, J. Chao, E. Ward, and R. Ober. "Quantitative study of single molecule location estimation techniques." *Optics Express 17* no. 26 (2009): 23352–73.

30. Chao, J., E. Ward, and R. Ober. "Fisher information matrix for branching processes with application to electron-multiplying charge-coupled devices." *Multidimensional System and Signal Processing 23* (2012): 349–79.

31. Wolter, S., A. Löschberger, T. Holm, S. Aufmkolk, M.-C. Dabauvalle, S. V. D. Linde, and M. Sauer. "rapidSTORM: Accurate, fast open-source software for localization microscopy." *Nature Methods 9* no. 11 (2012): 1040–1.

32. Zhang, B., J. Zerubia, and J.-C. Olivio-Marin. "Gaussian approximations of fluorescence microscope point-spread function models." *Applied Optics 46* no. 10 (2007): 1819–29.

33. Stallinga, S. and B. Rieger. "Accuracy of the Gaussian point spread function model in 2D localization microscopy." *Optics Express 18* no. 24 (2010): 24461–76.

34. Thompson, R., D. Larson, and W. Webb. "Precise nanometer localization analysis for individual fluorescent probes." *Biophysical Journal 82* (2002): 2775–83.

35. Huang, F., T. Hartwich, F. Rivera-Molina, Y. Lin, C. Whitney, J. Long, P. Uchil, J. Myers, M. Baird, W. Mothes, M. Davidson, D. Toomre, and J. Bewersdorf. "Video-rate nanoscopy using sCMOS camera-specific single-molecule localization algorithms." *Nature Methods 10* no. 7 (2013): 653–8.

36. Chao, J., S. Ram, E. Ward, and R. Ober. "Ultrahigh accuracy imaging modality for super-localization microscopy." *Nature Methods 10* (2013): 335–8.

37. Ram, S., E. Ward, and R. Ober. "Beyond Rayleighs criterion: A resolution measure with application to single-molecule microscopy." *Proceedings of the National Academy of Sciences USA 103* no. 12 (2006): 4457–62.

38. Annibale, P., S. Vanni, M. Scarselli, U. Rothlisberger, and A. Radenovic. "Quantitative photo activated localization microscopy: Unraveling the effects of photoblinking." *PLoS ONE 6* no. 7 (2011): e22678.

39. Annibale, P., S. Vanni, M. Scarelli, U. Rothlisberger, and A. Radenovic. "Identification of clustering artifacts in photoactivated localization microscopy." *Nature Methods 8* no. 7 (2011): 527–8.

40. Linde, S. V. D., S. Wolter, M. Heilemann, and M. Sauer. "The effect of photoswitching kinetics and labeling densities on super-resolution fluorescence imaging." *Journal of Biotechnology 149* (2010): 260–6.

41. Cordes, T., J. Vogelsang, M. Anaya, C. Spaguolo, A. Gietl, W. Summerer, A. Herrmann, K. Müllen, and P. Tinnefeld. "Single-molecule redox blinking of perylene diimide derivatives in water." *Journal of the American Chemical Society 132* no. 7 (2010): 2404–9.

42. Rees, E., M. Erdelyi, D. Pinotsi, A. Knight, D. Metcalf, and C. Kaminski. "Blind assessment of localization microscope image resolution." *Optical Nanoscopy 1* (2012): 12.

43. Fitzgerald, J., J. Lu, and M. Schnitzer. "Estimation theoretic measure of resolution for stochastic localization microscopy." *Physical Review Letters 109* (2012): 048102.

44. Mukamel, E. and M. Schnitzer. "Unified resolution bounds for conventional and stochastic localization fluorescence microscopy." *Physical Review Letters 109* (2012): 168102.

45. Nieuwenhuizen, R., K. Lidke, M. Bates, D. Leyton Puig, D. Grünwald, S. Stallinga, and B. Rieger. "Measuring image resolution in optical nanoscopy." *Nature Methods 10* (2013): 557–62.

46. Saxton, W. and W. Baumeister. "The correlation averaging of a regularly arranged bacterial cell envelope protein." *Journal of Microscopy 127* no. 2 (1982): 127–38.

47. Heel, M. V. "Similarity measures between images." *Ultramicroscopy 21* (1987): 95–100.

48. Unser, M., B. Trus, and A. Steven. "A new resolution criterion based on spectral signal-to-noise ratio." *Ultramicroscopy 23* (1987): 39–52.

49. Scheres, S. and S. Chen. "Prevention of overfitting in cryo-em structure determination." *Nature Methods 9* no. 9 (2012): 853–4.

50. Rosenthal, P. and R. Henderson. "Optimal determination of particle orientation, absolute hand, and contrast loss in single-particle electron cryomicroscopy." *Journal of Molecular Biology 333* no. 4 (2003): 721–45.

51. Beckmann, R., D. Bubeck, R. Grassucci, P. Penczek, A. Verschoor, G. Blobel, and J. Frank. "Alignment of conduits for the nascent polypeptide chain in the ribosome–sec61 complex." *Science 278* no. 5346 (1997): 213–6.

52. Böttcher, B., S. Wynne, and R. Crowther. "Determination of the fold of the core protein of hepatitis B virus by electron cryomicroscopy." *Nature 386* no. 6620 (1997): 88–91.

53. Nieuwenhuizen, R., S. Stallinga, and B. Rieger (2013, August 26–30). "Image resolution in optical nanoscopy." In P. Verma and A. Egner (Eds.), *Nanoimaging and Nanospectroscopy*, SPIE Conference vol. 8815, San Diego, USA, p. 881508.

54. Barry, D., J.-Y. Parlange, L. Li, H. Prommer, C. Cunningham, and F. Stagnitti. "Analytical approximations for real values of the Lambert W-function." *Mathematics and Computers in Simulation 53* no. 1–2 (2000): 95–103.

55. Holtzer, L., T. Meckel, and T. Schmidt. "Nanometric three-dimensional tracking of individual quantum dots in cells." *Applied Physics Letters 90* (2007): 053902.

56. Pavani, S. and R. Piestun. "Three dimensional tracking of fluorescent microparticles using a photon-limited double-helix response system." *Optics Express 16* no. 26 (2008): 22048–57.

57. Toprak, E., J. Enderlein, S. Syed, S. McKinney, R. Petschek, T. Ha, Y. Goldman, and P. Selvin. "Defocused orientation and position imaging (DOPI) of myosin V." *Proceedings of the National Academy of Sciences USA 103* no. 17 (2006): 6495–9.

58. Hoebe, R., C. V. Oven, T. J. Gadella, P. Dhonukshe, C. V. Noorden, and E. Manders. "Controlled light-exposure microscopy reduces photobleaching and phototoxicity in fluorescence live-cell imaging." *Nature Biotechnology 25* no. 2 (2007): 249–53.

59. Caarls, W., B. Rieger, A. D. Vries, D. Arndt-Jovin, and T. Jovin. "Minimizing light exposure with the programmable array microscope." *Journal of Microscopy 241* no. 1 (2011): 101–10.

60. Krizek, P., I. Raska, and G. Hagen. "Minimizing detection errors in single molecule localization microscopy." *Optics Express 19* no. 4 (2011): 3226–35.

61. Baddeley, D., M. Cannell, and C. Soeller. "Visualization of localization microscopy data." *Microscopy and Microanalysis 16* (2010): 64–72.

62. Holden, S., S. Uphoff, and A. Kapanidis. "DAOSTORM: An algorithm for high-density super-resolution microscopy." *Nature Methods 8* no. 4 (2011) 279–80.

63. Huang, F., S. Schwartz, J. Byars, and K. Lidke. "Simultaneous multiple-emitter fitting for single molecule super-resolution imaging." *Biomedical Optics Express 2* no. 5 (2011): 1377–93.

64. Zhu, L., W. Zhang, D. Elnatan, and B. Huang. "Faster STORM using compressed sensing." *Nature Methods 9* no. 7 (2012): 721–6.

65. Kratky, O. and G. Porod. "Röntgenuntersuchungen gelöster Fadenmoleküle." *Recueil des Travaux Chimies des Pays-Bas 68* (1949): 1106–24.

66. Landau, L. and E. Lifshitz (1969). *Statistical Physics, Part 1*, second ed. Oxford: Pergamon Press.

67. Faas, F., B. Rieger, L. V. Vliet, and D. Cherny. "DNA deformations near charged surfaces: Electron and atomic force microscopy views." *Biophysical Journal 97* no. 4 (2009): 1148–57.

68. Gittes, F., J. Mickey, B. Nettleton, and J. Howard. "Flexural rigidity of microtubules and actin filaments measured from thermal fluctuations in shape." *Journal of Cell Biology 120* no. 4 (1993): 923–34.

69. Pengo, T. (2013). "PALM-siever: Visualization and analysis platform for single-molecule localization microscopy." Available at http://www.code.google.com/p/palm-siever (accessed September 12, 2013).

70. Middendorff, C. V., A. Egner, C. Geisler, S. Hell, and A. Schönle. "Isotropic 3D nanoscopy based on single emitter switching." *Optics Express 16* no. 25 (2008): 20774–88.

71. Shtengel, G., J. Galbraith, C. Galbraith, J. Lippincott-Schwartz, J. Gillette, S. Manely, R. Sougrat, C. Waterman, P. Knachanawong, M. Davidson, R. Fetter, and H. Hess. "Interferometric fluorescent super-resolution microscopy resolves 3D cellular ultrastructure." *Proceeding of the National Academy of Science USA 106* no. 9 (2009): 3125–30.

19 Molecular Plasma Membrane Dynamics Dissected by STED Nanoscopy and Fluorescence Correlation Spectroscopy (STED-FCS)

Christian Eggeling and Alf Honigmann

CONTENTS

19.1 INTRODUCTION

19.1.1 MOLECULAR INTERACTIONS AND DIFFUSION DYNAMICS IN THE CELLULAR PLASMA MEMBRANE

The cellular plasma membrane is built up by a lipid bilayer and contains a multitude of different lipids and proteins, which among other things play a central role in cellular signaling (Figure 19.1). It is well acknowledged that the different membrane molecules are highly dynamic but do not just simply diffuse freely as introduced in 1972 by the "fluid mosaic model."[1] Rather, molecular membrane diffusion is usually restricted and hindered; that is, it shows highly anomalous diffusion patterns and

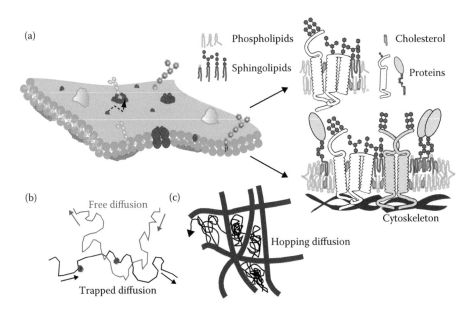

FIGURE 19.1 Plasma membrane heterogeneity. (a) Sources of membrane heterogeneity may be lipid–protein interactions, asymmetric molecular distribution to the leaflets, the underlying cytoskeleton (membrane anchored via proteins), and membrane curvature and pits. These heterogeneities result in hindered diffusion of lipids and proteins and may be the basis for the coalescence of transient signaling platforms—often denoted membrane domains or lipid rafts, spatially confined molecular assemblies of different lipids and proteins that are essential for a cellular signaling event. (Adapted from Lingwood, D., and K. Simons, *Science* 327 [2010]: 46–50.[2]) Hindered diffusion may be caused by (b) transient molecular interactions or incorporations into domains, which leads to an interruption or slowdown of diffusion, or (c) compartmentalization of the membrane, which causes a hopping diffusion.

only for a few molecules appears free, following free Brownian motion (e.g., Refs. 2 through 7) (Figure 19.1). For example, interactions with immobilized or slow-moving proteins lead to the local trapping of molecules, and the time to get from one point of the membrane to another is prolonged, especially on small spatial scales (e.g., Refs. 4 and 8). Similarly, the incorporation into putative domains of high molecular order leads to a local, transient slowdown (e.g., Refs. 2, 4 through 7, 9, and 10). Such slowdown may also stem from molecular crowding, since the mobility of molecules may already be retarded by the proximity to immobilized or relatively slow-moving molecules without direct interaction.[11] On the other hand, the influence of the cellular cytoskeleton, underlying the plasma membrane such as cortical actin, can be manifold. Proteins may transiently be arrested to the filament, thereby hindering their own mobility or, through interactions, the diffusion path of other molecules. Further, proteins that are anchored along the filament may be an obstacle for other diffusing molecules, acting like a picket or fence, and dividing the plasma membrane into compartments, whose boundaries may be hard to cross. As a consequence of this picket-fence model, molecules may show a kind of hopping diffusion with fast diffusion inside the compartments and hindered diffusion from one compartment to the next (see, for example, Refs. 3, 12, and 13). Therefore, diffusion may be fast on small spatial scales,[14] but extremely slowed down on long spatial scales.[4,10] Further, hindrances of molecular membrane motility may stem from obstacles such as membrane curvature or pits, induced by the cortical actin or proteins such as clathrin or caveolin (e.g., Refs. 15 through 17).

19.1.2 PLASMA MEMBRANE LIPIDS

Plasma membrane lipids have been acknowledged as a fundamental part of the functionality and regulation of integral or associated membrane proteins (e.g., Refs. 2, 7, and 18). This follows from novel experimental techniques and the recognition that membrane functionality is governed by the extremely high structural and chemical diversity of lipids and their highly heterogeneous spatiotemporal distribution.[19,20] It has been shown that specific lipid–protein interactions may induce conformational changes of proteins, thereby influencing the proteins' activity (e.g., Refs. 21 through 25). Lipids may, on the other hand, also be direct molecular receptors of, for example, viral particles or toxins, paving their way into or out of cells (for a review, see Refs. 2 and 7).

19.1.3 LIPID-INDUCED NANODOMAINS

An important feature of plasma membrane lipids is believed to be their ability to transiently bring together different proteins, thereby compartmentalizing cellular signaling events. Such signaling platforms are spatially localized and involve the tight packing of several proteins and lipids, and they are often referred to as membrane nanodomains or "rafts" (e.g., Refs. 2, 5 through 7, and 9) (Figure 19.1). The stabilization of such platforms may occur spontaneously or be triggered by extra- or intracellular events. While such nanodomains were initially believed to be stable,[6] they have recently be recognized as being of transient nature (e.g., Refs. 2 and 7). The higher local concentration of lipids and proteins may induce an increased molecular order, thereby resulting in changes of the involved proteins' structure and functionality. Prominent examples of such platform-triggered processes include the modulation of cell growth,[26,27] the activation of lymphocytes such as T-cells,[28,29] viral uptake and budding such as of HIV,[19,30,31] or cellular internalization of molecules during endocytosis[32–37] (for an overview, see Refs. 2 and 7). In a lot of these cases, cellular signaling is governed by distinct lipid–protein interactions. For example, cellular uptake and thus toxicity of the cholera toxin is triggered by its binding to the ganglioside lipid GM1 (e.g., Refs. 33 and 37); similarly, GM1 acts as a receptor and thus initiator of internalization of the VP1 protein of the simian virus 40 (e.g., Ref. 36). Here, the binding affinity and, thus, the efficiency of the cellular uptake are influenced by both the multivalency of the binding (i.e., the necessity to simultaneously bind several GM1 lipids) and the lipid structure. It has been shown that the incorporation of these virus or toxins is most effective for saturated and long-chained GM1 analogues, while short unsaturated GM1 analogues hardly facilitate this process.[36] This observation supports the assumption that such processes are realized by domains of tight molecular packing (such as rafts), since long saturated lipids prefer areas of higher molecular order (e.g., Refs. 38 though 41).

Specifically, sphingolipids and membrane-associated cholesterol seem to play a central role in the formation of aforementioned signaling platforms. It has been shown several times that a lowering of the level of sphingolipids and cholesterol resulted in an interruption or disorder of cellular signaling processes (e.g., Refs. 2, 7, and 42 through 45).

Further, lipids are asymmetrically distributed to the inner and outer leaflet of the plasma membrane, thereby adding another cause for membrane heterogeneity. For example, certain phospholipids are rather found in the inner leaflet while sphingolipids such as gangliosides rather prefer the outer leaflet (e.g., see Ref. 46).

19.1.4 Cortical Cytoskeleton

Cytoskeleton structures such as microtubule, actin, or spectrin underlying the cellular plasma membrane play another central role in the membrane's bioactivity (Figure 19.1). Aforementioned hindrance of molecular mobility by proteins anchored to the cortical cytoskeleton (e.g., Refs. 3, 12, 47, and 48) may, on one hand, stabilize the lipid nanodomains or molecular clusters (e.g., Refs. 47 and 49) and, on the other hand, increase the interaction probability of less abundant molecules (e.g., Refs. 50 and 51). Another implication of the anchoring to the cortical cytoskeleton is that the plasma membrane cannot be considered as a planar layer.[17] The resulting membrane curvatures (e.g., at a local invagination such as clathrin-coated pits or caveolae) may be another cause of heterogeneous membrane organization and dynamics (e.g., Refs. 15, 17, and 52 through 55).

19.2 DETECTION OF MEMBRANE HETEROGENEITY BY OPTICAL MICROSCOPY—LIMITATIONS

Optical far-field microscopy has proven valuable for live-cell studies, since the use of focused light has proven to be minimally invasive (e.g., Ref. 56). Often, far-field microscopy is combined with the fluorescence readout, where the studied molecule (e.g., a membrane protein or a lipid) is labeled with a fluorophore, and its fluorescence emission is excited, for example, by a laser and registered by a light detector. As a consequence, the position of a labeled molecule can be followed over space and time. In a confocal fluorescence microscope, a laser beam is focused to a small spot by an objective lens, which as well collects the emitted fluorescence and guides it onto a point detector. Scanning of the focused laser spot over the sample then allows reconstructing the spatial distribution of the fluorescently tagged molecules. Similarly, in wide-field microscopy, a larger area of the sample is illuminated at once and the spatial distribution of the fluorescence signal observed at once on a camera.

Molecular assemblies may be detected by spectroscopic techniques such as Förster resonance energy transfer (e.g., Refs. 18, 47, and 57) or by the use of fluorescent dyes that specifically label certain areas of the plasma membrane (e.g., Refs. 58 and 59). However, such experiments may be biased once they require an overexpression, that is, a very large concentration of the investigated molecules or membrane incorporation of the dyes, both of which may induce changes of the membrane.

19.2.1 IMAGING—TEMPORAL RESOLUTION

A challenge is that most of the mentioned membrane heterogeneities are highly dynamic (such as the diffusing molecules), which makes the direct imaging of the heterogeneous distribution of fluorescently labeled molecules difficult.[57,60–64] On one hand, imaging techniques such as scanning confocal microscopy are usually too slow to follow these dynamics, such as the formation of transient domains. On the other hand, molecules have to be unevenly distributed between their free and bound state to be able to visualize molecular assemblies.[65] Many experiments, therefore, fix the cells and observe the state of a cell at a certain point of time. Unfortunately, fixation may result in artifacts or some membrane molecules might still be mobile after fixation.[66]

19.2.2 SINGLE-MOLECULE TRACKING

The direct observation of hindered diffusion of labeled molecules (instead of acquiring an instantaneous image) realizes a much better way of exploring membrane heterogeneity (e.g., see Refs. 3, 12, and 67). A prominent method is the spatiotemporal tracking of single isolated fluorescent molecules (single-molecule or single-particle tracking [SPT]): the emitted fluorescence signal is detected on a spatial sensitive detector such as a camera or several point detectors, and the molecule's position is determined over time with nanometer precision (e.g., Refs. 3, 12, 50, 51, and 67 through 70). Unfortunately, an accurate assignment of a diffusion mode, such as trapping versus hopping diffusion, is often not feasible.[71] Furthermore, SPT is a stochastic method, and either very long trajectories or a large number of short trajectories are required for a statistically relevant analysis, which usually entails long and extensive measurement times. On the other hand, the recording of especially long trajectories as well as a high spatiotemporal resolution demands extremely bright and photostable fluorescent labels.[72] Therefore, SPT often employs large and bulky markers such as 20–40 nm large gold beads or 10 nm large quantum dots, which may themselves influence and thus bias the diffusion of the marked molecule.[73]

19.2.3 FLUORESCENCE CORRELATION SPECTROSCOPY

Methods such as fluorescence recovery after photobleaching (FRAP)[74,75] or fluorescence correlation spectroscopy (FCS)[4,76–79] usually require much shorter measurement times and small labels to acquire statistically relevant conclusions about the diffusion behavior of the investigated molecules. This follows from the fact that both techniques simultaneously observe the diffusion characteristics of a multitude of single molecules, which in SPT is only approximated by a large field of view or the use of photoswitchable fluorophores (e.g., Ref. 80). In FRAP, all fluorescent molecules within a micrometer-large area are photobleached (i.e., turned nonemissive) and the recovery of the fluorescence from this area is detected as nonphotobleached molecules diffuse into the area. The recovery curve allows the determination of diffusion coefficients and fractions of immobile species. Instead of photobleaching, one may also institute photoswitchable fluorescent labels.[81] In FCS, the temporal fluctuations of the observed fluorescence signal is monitored over time as molecules diffuse in and out of the observation area or volume (e.g., given by the micrometer-large focal laser spot of a confocal microscope[82]), and the correlation function of these fluctuations is calculated. The decay time of this correlation function usually renders the average transit time of the molecules through the observation area. Hindrances or anomalies in diffusion therefore result in a shift of the correlation curve toward larger times and the stretching of the decay.

19.2.4 OPTICAL MICROSCOPY—THE SPATIAL RESOLUTION LIMIT

The imaging or spectroscopic probing of molecular assemblies, or the probing of diffusion dynamics through FCS or FRAP on a far-field microscope, introduces a major limitation. Far-field optics introduce the diffraction of light, which limits the spatial resolution of such a lens-based microscope to approximately 200 nm for visible light.[83] As a consequence, a far-field microscope cannot distinguish alike molecules that are closer together than 200 nm and the structures below this size will appear blurred in the final image. In SPT, this issue is solved by detecting only single isolated (>200 nm apart) molecules and determining the central position of their blurred image spots. Because of the diffraction limit, FRAP and FCS experiments on a far-field microscope will average over nanoscopic hindrances in the diffusion characteristics.[8,65] A remedy to this issue has been suggested by spot-variation FCS (svFCS[4,8,84,85]), where correlation data are recorded for different sizes of the observation area above the diffraction limit. The resulting dependency of the average transit time through the observation spot allows more detailed information of diffusion modes (free, trapping, or hopping diffusion). Using svFCS in 200 nm to >1 μm large observation areas, the diffusion characteristics of several different membrane lipids and proteins could be assigned to these modes.[10] Unfortunately, this assignment was only realized by an extrapolation to even smaller areas, and further details of the molecular dynamics such as a trapping period or area could only be estimated. Further, it cannot be ruled out that the extrapolation might be biased because of changes in the dependencies for observation areas smaller than the 200 nm diffraction limit. A remedy to all these limitations would be precise FCS measurements on the relevant scales, that is, with observation areas <200 nm. This has been facilitated by recording FCS data near nanometer-sized apertures, as for example realized by placing the membrane sample in zero-mode waveguides[86] or on a pattern of isolated nanoapertures milled in a metallic film,[87] or by placing a small tip with a nanometer-sized aperture near the sample (near-field microscopy).[88] Unfortunately, the collateral nanometer proximity of the sample to a surface might introduce unforeseeable bias. A more noninvasive way is the combination of FCS with subdiffraction far-field nanoscopy such as stimulated emission depletion (STED) nanoscopy (STED-FCS).[89,90]

19.2.5 FAR-FIELD OPTICAL NANOSCOPY

Starting in the 1990s,[91] developments in optical microscopy have opened up the possibility to distinguish structures below the 200 nm diffraction limit with far-field optics (e.g., see Ref. 92). The key idea is to reversibly transfer the fluorescence markers between states of different emission properties, such as a dark and a bright state, thereby allowing the modulation or, reversibly, inhibition of fluorescence emission in space and time.[93–95] The first of such an optical nanoscope (or super-resolution microscope) was based on stimulated emission (STED) microscopy.[91,96] In a preferred implementation of STED nanoscopy, a laser is added to a conventional scanning (confocal) far-field microscope, which forces the fluorescent labels to their dark ground state, that is, inhibits fluorescence emission everywhere but at the center of the exciting laser focus (Figure 19.2). The wavelength of this second laser is tuned to the red edge of the fluorophore's emission spectrum and induces the stimulated de-excitation of the fluorophore's excited (and fluorescent) electronic (ON) to its ground (dark OFF) state. By detecting only the spontaneous (and not the stimulated) emission, the registered signal is efficiently decreased and completely switched off when increasing the intensity of the STED laser above a certain threshold (Figure 19.2). The introduction of a phase plate into the STED beam distorts its wave front and, once focused by the microscope objective, creates an intensity distribution that features one or several local zeros, such as a doughnut-shaped intensity distribution (Figure 19.2). However, while this intensity pattern is still ruled by diffraction, only an enhancement of the intensity of the STED laser drives the area in which fluorescence emission is still allowed to smaller and smaller subdiffraction scales. The spatial resolution of the STED microscope is therefore tuned by the intensity of the STED laser (Figure 19.2).

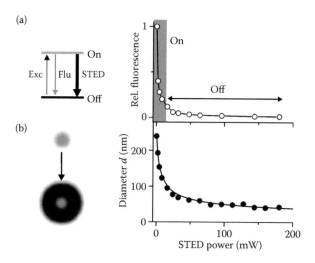

FIGURE 19.2 STED nanoscopy. (a) Optical nanoscopy relies on the transition between states of the fluorescent label with different emission characteristics. In the case of STED, these are the excited ON state, which is populated by the excitation laser (Exc) and which spontaneously depopulates by fluorescence emission (Flu), and the ground OFF state, to which the label is driven by (nondetected) stimulated emission using the additional STED laser. As a consequence, the STED laser inhibits spontaneous fluorescence emission. The efficiency of inhibition increases with the power of the STED laser, and the spontaneous fluorescence is efficiently switched off above a certain power threshold (right). (b) In a STED nanoscope, the diffraction-limited excitation (and thus fluorescence spot, gray) is overlaid with the STED laser, whose focal intensity distribution features at least one intensity-zero (black) (left). As a consequence, spontaneous fluorescence is inhibited everywhere but at the zero-intensity point, leaving a subdiffraction-sized area where emission is still allowed: the new observation spot, whose diameter d scales with the power of the STED laser (right).

19.3 STED-FCS

19.3.1 REDUCED OBSERVATION SPOT: THE CONCENTRATION ISSUE

In conventional (confocal) FCS measurements, the average number of fluorescent molecules in the observation volume has to be kept rather low (<100–1000 depending on the signal-to-noise level), meaning that the concentration of fluorescently labeled molecules has to be kept low as well (<1 μM). This is however a concentration range that is often far below that of endogenous (biological) conditions. In contrast to measuring in zero-mode waveguides[86] or to photobleach[97] or switching off[98] large parts of the ensemble, the most obvious way to handle larger, endogenous concentrations would be lowering the observation spot's length scale.[99,100] Figure 19.3 shows FCS measurements of a fluorescent lipid analogue freely diffusing in a membrane on glass support. Switching from confocal (240 nm diameter of the observation spot) to STED recordings (60 nm diameter) clearly results in two effects:[89,90] (1) The average transit time through the observation spot, t_D, which correlates with the decay time of the FCS curve, decreases, as expected for a molecule following free Brownian

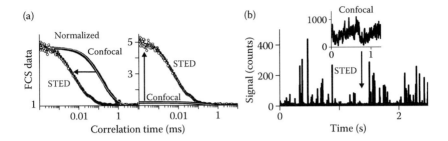

FIGURE 19.3 STED-FCS—reducing the observation spot. (a) STED-FCS analysis of free two-dimensional diffusion of a fluorescent lipid analogue in a multilamellar membrane. Representative correlation data (left, normalized amplitudes; right, original data) for confocal (black) and STED (60 nm) recordings (open dots). The confinement of the observation spot by STED reduces both the transit time and the average number of fluorescent molecules, leading to a shift of the correlation data to shorter correlation times (left) and an increase of the amplitude (right), respectively. (b) STED allows FCS-based single-molecule observations at high concentrations: fluorescence signal over time for the same concentration of a fluorescent lipid analogue diffusing in a multilamellar membrane indicates diffusion of single molecules only for the STED (right) but not for the confocal (left) recordings. (Adapted from Ringemann, C. et al., *New Journal of Physics* 11, 103054, 2009.)

diffusion; and (2) the average number, N, of fluorescent molecules in the observation volume, V, which changes inversely to the FCS curve's amplitude, decreases as well, as expected when lowering the observation volume but keeping the concentration ($c = N/V$) constant. As a consequence, much larger concentrations of fluorescently marked molecules can be used in measurements. For example, when moving from 240 nm large diffraction-limited to <50 nm large observation spots of the STED nanoscope, >25-fold concentrations (i.e., >20 µM) can in principle be employed for FCS measurements, as exemplified in Figure 19.3b, where clear fluctuations in the fluorescence signal caused by single-molecule transits (i.e., fluorescent bursts) can only be observed in the STED but not in the confocal recordings.

Similar to the aforementioned two-dimensional diffusion in a membrane, a shortening of the average transit time is equally well observed for three-dimensional diffusion when moving from diffraction-limited confocal to STED recordings.[89,90] While this makes STED-FCS measurements in solution or inside the cellular cytosol in principle feasible, these measurements are challenged by a lowered signal-to-background ratio owing to noninhibited out-of-focus fluorescence signal.[89,90]

19.3.2 TUNING OF THE OBSERVATION SPOT: STUDYING MOLECULAR INTERACTIONS

An important feature of the STED nanoscope for FCS is that the size of its observation spot can be tuned by the intensity of the added STED laser (Figure 19.2). One can use the principle of svFCS (compare previous discussions in Section 19.2.4[4,84,85]) and record and analyze FCS data at different sizes of the observation spot to determine the details of the hindrances in molecular diffusion. In contrast to the diffraction-limited svFCS data, STED-FCS can now directly study these molecular diffusion dynamics at the relevant scales.[8,65,90,101,102] For this, FCS data are recorded and average transit times, t_D, were determined for different STED intensities, I_{STED}. Since the dependency of the observation spot's diameter, d, on the intensity, I_{STED}, can straightforwardly be obtained from calibration measurements,[8,101,102] the dependency of the apparent diffusion coefficient D ($\sim d^2/t_D$) on d discloses different diffusion modes (Figure 19.4):[101,102] (1) Normal diffusion: A constant value $D(d)$ for free Brownian diffusion. (2) Transient trapping: An ongoing decrease of D toward small d for a transient interaction with immobilized or slow-moving binding partners (slow relative to the interaction period). (3) Transient domain incorporation: A decrease of D toward small d but with a leveling off and even increase in values of D for spot diameters d smaller than the diameter of the domains.[103] (4) Hopping diffusion: An increase of D toward small d for the aforementioned cytoskeleton meshwork-based diffusion.[104] Even more, analysis of the STED-FCS data for $d < 80$–100 nm allows the determination of kinetic parameters, such as on and off rates of molecular complexes[8,65,90,101,102] or meshwork sizes and hopping probabilities.[105]

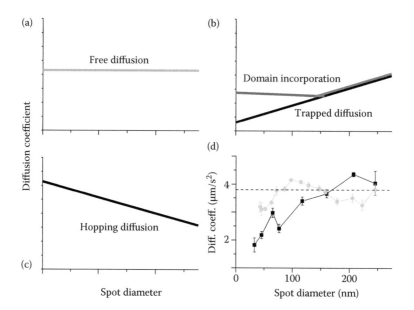

FIGURE 19.4 STED-FCS—observing diffusion modes by tuning the observation spot diameter. (a) Changing the STED power allows the determination of values of the apparent diffusion coefficient D for different diameters d of the observation spot. Sketched dependencies $D(d)$ for (a) free Brownian diffusion, (b) transient interaction with immobilized or slow-moving binding partners (transient trapping, black line) or transient domain incorporation (gray line), and (c) cytoskeleton meshwork-based hopping diffusion. (d) $D(d)$ dependency of the two-dimensional diffusion of a fluorescent lipid analogue in a fluid membrane bilayer on plasma-cleaned (gray circles) and non-plasma-cleaned (black squares) glass. Irregularities of the membrane bilayer by surface roughness and impurities may lead to a hindered diffusion in the case of the noncleaned glass substrate.

As an example, Figure 19.4b shows dependencies $D(d)$ recorded for a fluorescent lipid analogue diffusing in a fluid membrane bilayer on plasma-cleaned and noncleaned cover glass. While diffusion on the plasma-cleaned support was clearly free Brownian, diffusion on the noncleaned glass showed hindered diffusion, most probably attributed to transient trapping of the lipid analogues following irregularities of the membrane bilayer by surface roughness and impurities. Unfortunately, the transient trapping, that is, the deviation from normal diffusion, was too small to determine any kinetic parameters.

19.4 STUDYING LIPID–MEMBRANE DYNAMICS USING STED-FCS

19.4.1 LIVE-CELL LIPID PLASMA MEMBRANE DYNAMICS: PHOSPHOLIPID VERSUS SPHINGOLIPID DIFFUSION

Figure 19.5 shows the dependency of the apparent diffusion coefficient $D(d)$ on the diameter d of the observation area ($d = 30–240$ nm) as determined from STED-FCS data recorded for two fluorescent lipid analogues in the plasma membrane of live mammalian cells: phosphoethanolamine (PE) and sphingomyelin (SM) labeled with

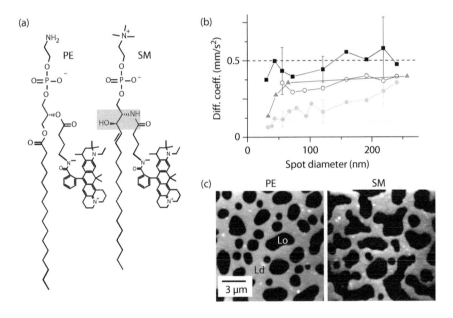

FIGURE 19.5 STED-FCS—lipid plasma membrane dynamics. (a) Structures of the fluorescent lipid analogues PE and SM both tagged with the organic dye Atto647N. Gray-shaded area: Ceramide or sphingosine group of the SM lipid. (b) Dependency of the apparent diffusion coefficient $D(d)$ on the diameter d of the observation spot for the diffusion of PE (black squares), SM (light gray circles), SM after cholesterol depletion (open circles), and SM after actin depolymerization (gray triangles) in the plasma membrane of live mammalian cells, indicating trapped cholesterol- and cytoskeleton-dependent diffusion of SM. (c) Comparison to phase separation in model membranes: both PE and SM hardly enter the liquid-ordered (Lo) domain, but rather prefer the liquid-disordered (Ld) domain of a model membrane bilayer composed of a ternary mixture[106] (confocal scanning fluorescence image; black, low signal; white, high signal).

the organic dye Atto647N.[8,65,90,101,102] These dependencies reveal an almost free diffusion of PE and a trapped diffusion of SM. A closer analysis of the FCS data for $d < 80$ nm revealed transient trapping of the lipids with on and off rates in the range of 190 s^{-1} and 800 s^{-1} for PE and of 80 s^{-1} and 80 s^{-1} for SM. While the fast on and off rates (equilibrium constant < 0.25) result in an almost normal diffusion of PE with a diffusion coefficient of ≈0.5 μm^2/s, the SM lipids are transiently arrested for approximately 10 ms on average every 10 ms (with a diffusion coefficient of ≈0.5 μm^2/s every 200–300 nm).[90,101] The fact that the SM lipids hardly move during trapping indicates that they interact with other molecules such as membrane proteins, which are either relatively slow moving or even immobilized. It has to be pointed out that an accurate appointment of these on/off rates was impossible for diffraction-limited or even >60 nm large observation areas, even when interpolating to smaller scales.[90] Furthermore, the values of the on and off rates rendered an equilibrium constant of approximately 1 for SM; that is, at a certain point of time, 50% of all SM lipids were bound (and immobilized) and 50% were freely diffusing. As a consequence, there was no contrast between bound and unbound SM, and it is impossible to image this heterogeneous distribution of lipids, even with a STED nanoscope.[8,65]

19.4.2 LIVE-CELL LIPID PLASMA MEMBRANE DYNAMICS: POSSIBLE ARTIFACTS

Aforementioned STED-FCS experiments on lipid plasma membrane dynamics are prone to many artifacts. Most importantly, the relatively large organic dye label might influence the dynamics of the lipid, thus not reflecting the true lipid dynamics. While one never can fully exclude such bias, extensive control experiments indicated that, apart from a label-induced change in the lipids' affinity for molecular ordered phases (as highlighted further in Section 19.4.4), the molecular dynamics of the fluorescent lipid analogues hardly depended on the properties and position of the dye label but instead depended on the chemical structure of the lipid.[8,101,102,107] Only the introduction of a very polar dye by acyl-chain replacement introduced biased diffusion, namely, faster mobility and negligible trapping (most probably from the polar label avoiding the hydrophobic membrane environment).[8] Further controls could rule out improper or nonspecific incorporation of the lipid analogues into the cellular plasma membrane[8,102] and influence by the laser light attributed to photobleaching, phototoxicity, heating, or trapping.[8] For example, it could be shown that—as expected from theory—the decrease of the average transit time t_D with increasing STED intensity coincided well with the decrease of the average number N of fluorescent molecules in the observation area, a correlation that could only be explained by the optically controlled decrease of the observation spot's length scale.[8] In the meantime, parts of the STED-FCS experiments could be confirmed by fast single-molecule tracking experiments,[70] as well as near-field microscopy observations.[88]

19.4.3 LIVE-CELL LIPID PLASMA MEMBRANE DYNAMICS: MOLECULAR DEPENDENCIES

It could be shown that the molecular interactions of SM decreased upon treatment for cholesterol depletion (diffusion was almost free afterward, similar to PE), for depolymerization of the underlying cellular cytoskeleton, and for lowering the level of endogenous SM (Figure 19.5). This indicated that either the binding interaction or the immobilization of the binding partner was assisted by cholesterol and SM and that most probably the binding partner was linked to the cytoskeleton.[8,101] Measurements at temperatures between 22°C and 37°C on the other hand revealed an Arrhenius-like dependency of the free diffusion coefficients but hardly any variation in trapping strength of SM.[101,102] The comparison of several different fluorescent lipid analogues, differing in their head group as well fatty acid chains, revealed lipid-specific dependencies of the lipids' molecular dynamics. Mainly, the ceramide (i.e., the NH and OH-) unit of the lipid backbone (gray in Figure 19.5a) was responsible for cholesterol- and cytoskeleton-dependent interactions, probably via hydrogen bonds. However, the polar head groups of, for example, ganglioside lipids such as GM1 induced transient binding as well, but less efficient and independent of cholesterol and the cytoskeleton.[101] In general, the interaction strength, frequency, and duration seemed very lipid specific, which points to specific and functional lipid–protein bindings.

19.4.4 LIVE-CELL LIPID PLASMA MEMBRANE DYNAMICS: RELATION TO LIPID RAFTS

Summarizing aforementioned results, the observed cholesterol- and cytoskeleton-dependent interactions of the fluorescent SM sphingolipid are well described by transient (~10 ms long) binding to relatively immobile binding partners and only uncovered by STED-FCS. The >200 nm large diffraction-limited observation areas average over details on the nanoscale. The binding partners are most probably membrane proteins, whose mobility is restricted by the cytoskeleton. We can exclude that the lipids move during trapping; that is, it does not wander around inside a domain (or raft), where diffusion is slowed down. However, because the only dynamics of single molecules was observed, one cannot rule out the possibility that additional lipids or proteins molecules were (temporarily) included in this complex. However, the complex was not of very high molecular order, which was shown by a comparison with experiments on model membranes.[101,106,107] A model bilayer membrane of a ternary mixture of unlabeled saturated SM, unlabeled and unsaturated phosphoglycerolipids, and cholesterol separates into two different phases: a fluid liquid-disordered phase (Ld), which mainly includes the unsaturated lipids, and a liquid-ordered (Lo) phase and less fluid Lo phase of higher molecular order, which mainly includes the saturated lipid and cholesterol (e.g., see Refs. 38, 40, and 41). The Lo phase is often considered as a physical model system for membrane domains or rafts in the plasma membrane of living cells. The labeled SM analogue, however, did not partition into the Lo phase of this model system but favored the Ld phase (Figure 19.5b). Consequently, the lipid analogue was also not able to stain areas (or domains) of high molecular order in the plasma membrane, which were therefore missed by the previously mentioned STED-FCS experiments. Still, we can conclude that the observed strong interactions of the SM analogue were not driven by differences in molecular order; that is, the results of STED-FCS and phase separation experiments were not correlated.[101,107] This is also exemplified by the fact that the fluorescent PE analogue partitioned similarly to the SM analogue but interacted much weaker with other constituents (Figure 19.5). Further, an elaborate study on a multitude of different lipid analogues using STED-FCS has shown that the partitioning characteristics of the analogue did not influence the transient trapping.[101,107]

It is possible that the interactions exposed by the STED-FCS experiments are those lipid–protein affinities that are the physicochemical basis of the coalescence of several molecules to the previously mentioned signaling platforms (or membrane rafts). However, it is unlikely that the investigation of this coalescence is possible with the presented fluorescent lipid analogues, since in comparison to the lipid, the rather large and often charged dye restricted the accessibility to highly ordered molecular assemblies such as the Lo phase or putative membrane rafts.[107] Nevertheless, it has been shown that the order of the Lo phase generated in cellular plasma membranes (which were treated by swelling procedures generating vesicular bilayers composed of native membranes such as giant plasma membrane vesicles[108] or plasma membrane spheres[109]) is much lower compared to model systems[110] and that more ordered phases of the plasma membrane are thus much more efficiently penetrated by the fluorescent lipid analogues.[107]

19.5   CONCLUSIONS

To investigate the discussed coalescence of potential signaling forms and existence of liquid-ordered nanodomains (or rafts) in the plasma membrane of living cells, it will be very important to study a functional fluorescent lipid analogue that does not alter phase partitioning and is compatible with STED-FCS, such as introduced recently.[103] First experiments using an Lo-partitioning fluorescent cholesterol analogue recently revealed fast and free diffusion of this probe, once again opposing a strong separation of model-membrane Lo-like domains in the plasma membrane of resting living cell.[111] It will therefore be very important to investigate lipid membrane dynamics after triggering of cellular functions including activation of different receptors.[2] Here, the development of two-color STED-FCS will allow relating lipid dynamics to changes in protein reorganization.[101] Scanning STED-FCS[112] or STED-RICS (raster image correlation spectroscopy),[113] as well as similar fluorescence fluctuation-based methods,[114] will highlight spatial heterogeneities in lipid diffusion.

At first, STED microscopy was realized with both the excitation and STED laser in a pulsed mode.[96,115] By letting the STED pulse swiftly follow the excitation laser, the fluorescence inhibition process is optimized, since the STED laser approaches the dye at the right point in time: in its excited state. STED microscopy, however, has also been realized with continuous-wave lasers,[116] an approach that has recently been significantly improved by the use of a gated detection scheme.[117,118] In this gated STED modality, the size of the observation spot (and thus the spatial resolution) can be tuned by both the power of the STED laser and the position of the gated detection window.[118,119] Gated STED-FCS has the potential to investigate temporal changes in lipid diffusion.[118]

STED-FCS is a sensitive and unique tool for studying nanoscale membrane organization and determining the cellular functions and molecular interdependencies of membrane components. More generally, STED-FCS expands currently available optical microscopy and spectroscopy techniques to the nanoscale and opens up exceptional possibilities to characterize and disclose complex cellular signaling events and therefore new approaches for drug screening and development.[120]

ACKNOWLEDGMENTS

This work could not have been realized without the work of the people from the Department of NanoBiophotonics: Christian Ringemann, Veronika Mueller, Rebecca Medda, Vladimir Belov, Svetlana Polyakova, Birka Llaken, Class von Middendorf, and Andreas Schönle, especially by the extraordinary support and interaction with Stefan Hell, as well as by the lipid syntheses and discussions with Günter Schwarzmann (University Bonn). Further fruitful discussions with Herve Rigneault (Marseille), the Simons group (MPI Dresden), and the Schwille group (Bioquant Dresden) are greatly acknowledged.

REFERENCES

1. Singer, S., and G. L. Nicolson. "The Fluid Mosaic Model of the Structure of Cell Membranes." *Science* 175 (1972): 720–31.
2. Lingwood, D., and K. Simons. "Lipid Rafts as a Membrane-Organizing Principle." *Science* 327 (2010): 46–50.
3. Kusumi, A., C. Nakada, K. Ritchie et al. "Paradigm Shift of the Plasmamembrane Concept from the Two-Dimensional Continuum Fluid to the Partitioned Fluid: High-Speed Single-Molecule Tracking of Membrane Molecules." *Annual Review of Biophysics and Bioengineering* 34 (2005): 351–78.
4. Wawrezinieck, L., H. Rigneault, D. Marguet, and P. F. Lenne. "Fluorescence Correlation Spectroscopy Diffusion Laws to Probe the Submicron Cell Membrane Organization." *Biophysical Journal* 89 (2005): 4029–42.
5. Jacobson, K., O. G. Mouritsen, and G. W. Anderson. "Lipid Rafts: At a Crossroad between Cell Biology and Physics." *Nature Cell Biology* 9, no. 1 (2007): 7–14.
6. Simons, K., and E. Ikonen. "Functional Rafts in Cell Membranes." *Nature* 387 (1997): 569–72.
7. Simons, K., and M. J. Gerl. "Revitalizing Membrane Rafts: New Tools and Insights." *Nature Reviews Molecular Cell Biology* 11 (2010): 688–99.
8. Eggeling, C., C. Ringemann, R. Medda et al. "Direct Observation of the Nanoscale Dynamics of Membrane Lipids in a Living Cell." *Nature* 457 (2009): 1159–62.
9. Joly, E. "Hypothesis: Could the Signalling Function of Membrane Microdomains Involve a Localized Transition of Lipids from Liquid to Solid State?" *BMC Cell Biology* 5, no. 5 (2004): 3.
10. Lenne, P. F., L. Wawrezinieck, F. Conchonaud et al. "Dynamic Molecular Confinement in the Plasma Membrane by Microdomains and the Cytoskeleton Meshwork." *EMBO Journal* 25 (2006): 3245–56.
11. Niemela, P. S., M. S. Miettinen, L. Monticelli et al. "Membrane Proteins Diffuse as Dynamic Complexes with Lipids." *Journal of the American Chemical Society* 132 (2010): 7574–5.
12. Kusumi, A., Y. M. Shirai, I. Koyama-Honda, K. G. N. Suzuki, and T. K. Fujiwara. "Hierarchical Organization of the Plasma Membrane: Investigations by Single-Molecule Tracking vs. Fluorescence Correlation Spectroscopy." *FEBS Letters* 584 (2010): 1814–23.

13. Destainville, N., F. Dumas, and L. Salome. "What do Diffusion Measurements Tell us about Membrane Compartmentalisation? Emergence of the Role of Interprotein Interactions." *Journal of Chemical Biology* 1 (2011): 37–48.

14. Fujiwara, T., K. Ritchie, H. Murakoshi, K. Jacobson, and A. Kusumi. "Phospholipids undergo Hop Diffusion in Compartmentalized Cell Membrane." *Journal of Cell Biology* 157, no. 6 (2002): 1071–81.

15. Parton, R. G. "Caveolae—from Ultrastructure to Molecular Mechanism." *Nature Reviews Molecular Cell Biology* 4 (2003): 162–7.

16. Baumgart, T., B. R. Caparo, C. Zhu, and S. L. Das. "Thermodynamics and Mechanics of Membrane Curvature Generation and Sensing by Proteins and Lipids." *Annual Review of Physical Chemistry* 62 (2011): 483–506.

17. Adler, J., I. S. Andrew, P. Novak, Y. E. Korchev, and I. Parmryd. "Plasma Membrane Topography and Interpretation of Single-Particle Tracks." *Nature Methods* 7, no. 3 (2010): 170–1.

18. van Meer, G., D. R. Voelker, and G. W. Feigenson. "Membrane Lipids: Where They Are and How They Behave." *Nature Reviews Molecular Cell Biology* 9 (2008): 112–24.

19. Brügger, B., B. Glass, P. Haberkant et al. "The HIV Lipidome: A Raft with an Unusual Composition." *Proceedings of the National Academy of Sciences of the United States of America* 103, no. 8 (2006): 2641–6.

20. Shevchenko, A., and K. Simons. "Lipidomics: Coming to Grips with Lipid Diversity." *National Reviews Molecular Cell Biology* 11 (2010): 593–8.

21. Bhushan, A., and M. G. McNamee. "Correlation of Phospholipid Structure with Functional Effects on the Nicotinic Acetylcholine Receptor." *Biophysical Journal* 64 (1993): 716–23.

22. Mantipragada, S. B., L. I. Horvath, H. R. Arias et al. "Lipid–Protein Interactions and Effect of Local Anesthetics in Acetylcholine Receptor-Rich Membranes from Torpedo Marmorata Electric Organ." *Biochemitry* 42, no. 30 (2003): 9167–75.

23. Fantini, J. "How Sphingolipids Bind and Shape Proteins: Molecular Basis of Lipid–Protein Interactions in Lipid Shells, Rafts and Related Biomembrane Domains." *Cellular and Molecular Life Sciences* 60 (2003): 1027–32.

24. Coskun, Ü., M. Grzybek, D. Drechsler, and K. Simons. "Regulation of Human EGF Receptor by Lipids." *Proceedings of the National Academy of Sciences of the United States of America* 108, no. 22 (2011): 9044–8.

25. Contreras, F.-X., A. M. Ernst, P. Haberkant et al. "Molecular Recognition of a Single Sphingolipid Species by a Protein's Transmembrane Domain." *Nature* 481 (2012): 525–9.

26. Bremer, E. G., J. Schlessinger, and S. Hakomori. "Ganglioside-Mediated Modulation of Cell Growth." *Journal of Biological Chemistry* 261, no. 5 (1986): 2434–40.

27. Kawashima, N., S.-J. Yoon, K. Itoh, and K. Nakayama. "Tyrosine Kinase Activity of Epidermal Growth Factor Receptor Is Regulated by GM3 Binding through Carbohydrate to Carbohydrate Interactions." *Journal of Biological Chemistry* 284, no. 10 (2009): 6147–55.

28. Zech, T., C. S. Ejsing, K. Gaus et al. "Accumulation of Raft Lipids in T-Cell Plasma Membrane Domains Engaged in TCR Signalling." *EMBO Journal* 28 (2009): 466–76.

29. Mahammad, S., J. Dinic, J. Adler, and I. Parmryd. "Limited Cholesterol Depletion Causes Aggregation of Plasma Membrane Lipid Rafts Inducing T Cell Activation." *Biochimica et Biophysica Acta (BBA)—Biomembranes* 1801 (2010): 625–34.

30. Chan, R., P. D. Uchil, J. Jin et al. "Retroviruses Human Immunodeficiency Virus and Murine Leukemia Virus Are Enriched in Phosphoinositides." *Journal of Virology* 82, no. 22 (2008): 11228–38.

31. Waheed, A. A., and E. O. Freed. "Lipids and Membrane Microdomains in HIV-1 Replication." *Virus Research* 143 (2009): 162–76.

32. Tsai, B., J. M. Gilbert, T. Stehle et al. "Gangliosides Are Receptors for Murine Polyoma Virus and SV40." *EMBO Journal* 22, no. 17 (2003): 4346–55.

33. Chinnapen, D. J. F., H. Chinnapen, D. Saslowsky, and W. Lencer. "Rafting with Cholera Toxin: Endocytosis and Tracking from Plasma Membrane to ER." *FEMS Microbiology Letters* 266 (2007): 129–37.

34. Römer, W., L. Berland, V. Chambon et al. "Shiga Toxin Induces Tubular Membrane Invaginations for Its Uptake into Cells." *Nature* 450 (2007): 670–5.

35. Hebbar, S., E. Lee, M. Manna et al. "A Fluorescent Sphingolipid Binding Domain Peptide Probe Interacts with Sphingolipids and Cholesterol-Dependent Raft Domains." *Journal of Lipid Research* 49, no. 5 (2008): 1077–89.

36. Ewers, H., W. Römer, A. E. Smith et al. "GM1 Structure Determines SV40-Induced Membrane Invagination and Infection." *Nature Cell Biology* 12 (2009): 11–8.

37. Wernick, N. L. B., D. J. F. Chinnapen, J. A. Cho, and W. Lencer. "Cholera Toxin: An Intracellular Journey into the Cytosol by Way of the Endoplasmic Reticulum." *Toxins* 2, no. 3 (2010): 310–25.

38. Bacia, K., D. Scherfeld, N. Kahya, and P. Schwille. "Fluorescence Correlation Spectroscopy Relates Rafts in Model and Native Membranes." *Biophysical Journal* 87 (2004): 1034–43.

39. Bagatolli, L. A. "To See or Not to See: Lateral Organization of Biological Membranes and Fluorescence Microscopy." *Biochimica et Biophysica Acta* 1758, no. 10 (2006): 1541–56.

40. Baumgart, T., G. Hunt, E. R. Farkas, W. W. Webb, and G. W. Feigenson. "Fluorescence Probe Partitioning between Lo/Ld Phases in Lipid Membranes." *Biochimica et Biophysica Acta* 1768, no. 9 (2007): 2182–94.

41. Marsh, D. "Cholesterol-Induced Fluid Membrane Domains: A Compendium of Lipid-Raft Ternary Phase Diagrams." *Biochimica et Biophysica Acta* 1788, no. 10 (2009): 2114–23.

42. Brown, D. A., and E. London. "Structure and Function of Sphingolipid- and Cholesterol-Rich Membrane Rafts." *Journal of Biological Chemistry* 275, no. 23 (2000): 17221–4.

43. Hao, M. M., S. Mukherjee, and F. R. Maxfield. "Cholesterol Depletion Induces Large Scale Domain Segregation in Living Cell Membranes." *Proceedings of the National Academy of Sciences of the United States of America* 98, no. 23 (2001): 13072–7.

44. Pike, L. J. "Rafts Defined: A Report on the Keystone Symposium on Lipid Rafts and Cell Function." *Journal of Lipid Research* 47 (2006): 1597–8.

45. Wüstner, D., L. Solanko, E. Sokol et al. "Quantitative Assessment of Sterol Traffic in Living Cells by Dual Labeling with Dehydroergosterol and Bodipy-Cholesterol." *Chemistry and Physics of Lipids* 164 (2011): 221–35.

46. Mondal, M., B. Mesmin, S. Mukherjee, and F. R. Maxfield. "Sterols Are Mainly in the Cytoplasmic Leaflet of the Plasma Membrane and the Endocytic Recycling Compartment in Cho Cells." *Molecular Biology of the Cell* 20, no. 2 (2009): 581–8.

47. Goswami, D., K. Gowrishankar, S. Bilgrami et al. "Nanoclusters of GPI-Anchored Proteins Are Formed by Cortical Actin-Driven Activity." *Cell* 135, no. 6 (2008): 1085–97.

48. Chichili, G. R., and W. Rodgers. "Cytoskeleton–Membrane Interactions in Membrane Raft Structure." *Cellular and Molecular Life Sciences* 66 (2009): 2319–28.

49. Machta, B. B., S. Papanikolaou, J. P. Sethna, and S. L. Veatch. "Minimal Model of Plasma Membrane Heterogeneity Requires Coupling Cortical Actin to Criticality." *Biophysical Journal* 100 (2011): 1668–77.

50. Andrews, N. L., K. A. Lidke, J. R. Pfeiffer et al. "Actin Restricts FcεRI Diffusion and Facilitates Antigen-Induced Receptor Immobilization." *Nature Cell Biology* 10, no. 8 (2008): 955–63.

51. Jaqaman, K., H. Kuwata, N. Touret et al. "Cytoskeletal Control of CD36 Diffusion Promotes Its Receptor and Signaling Function." *Cell* 146 (2011): 593–606.

52. Anderson, R. G. W., and K. Jacobson. "A Role for Lipid Shells in Targeting Proteins to Caveolae, Rafts, and Other Lipid Domains." *Science* 296 (2002): 1821–5.

53. Cheng, Z.-J., R. D. Singh, D. L. Marks, and R. E. Pagano. "Membrane Microdomains, Caveolae, and Caveolar Endocytosis of Sphingolipids (Review)." *Molecular Membrane Biology* 23, no. 1 (2006): 101–10.

54. Reynwar, B. J., G. Illya, V. A. Harmandaris et al. "Aggregation and Vesiculation of Membrane Proteins by Curvature-Mediated Interactions." *Nature* 447 (2007): 461–4.

55. Hatzakis, N. S., V. K. Bhatia, J. Larsen et al. "How Curved Membranes Recruit Amphipathic Helices and Protein Anchoring Motifs." *Nature Chemical Biology* 5 (2009): 835–41.

56. Pawley, J. B. *Handbook of Biological Confocal Microscopy*, 2nd ed. New York: Springer, 2006.

57. Hancock, J. F. "Lipid Rafts: Contentious Only from Simplistic Standpoints." *Nature Reviews. Molecular Cell Biology* 7 (2006): 457–62.

58. Parasassi, T., E. K. Krasnowska, L. Bagatolli, and E. Gratton. "Laurdan and Prodan as Polarity-Sensitive Fluorescent Membrane Probes." *Journal of Fluorescence* 8, no. 4 (1998): 365–73.

59. Kucherak, O. A., S. Oncul, Z. Darwich et al. "Switchable Nile Red-Based Probe for Cholesterol and Lipid Order at the Outer Leaflet of Biomembranes." *Journal of the American Chemical Society* 132 (2010): 4907–16.

60. Munro, S. "Lipid Rafts: Elusive or Illusive?" *Cell* 115 (2003): 377–88.

61. Lommerse, P. H. M., H. P. Spaink, and T. Schmidt. "In Vivo Plasma Membrane Organization: Results of Biophysical Approaches." *Biochimica et Biophysica Acta* 1664 (2004): 119–31.

62. Shaw, A. S. "Lipid Rafts: Now You See Them, Now You Don't." *Nature Immunology* 7, no. 11 (2006): 1139–42.

63. Groves, J. T., R. Parthasarathy, and M. B. Forstner. "Fluorescence Imaging of Membrane Dynamics." *Annual Review of Biomedical Engineering* 10 (2008): 311–38.

64. Pike, L. J. "The Challenge of Lipid Rafts." *Journal of Lipid Research* 50 (2009): S323–8.

65. Eggeling, C. "Sted-Fcs Nanoscopy of Membrane Dynamics." In *Fluorescent Methods to Study Biological Membranes*, edited by Y. Mely and G. Duportail, 291–309. Berlin: Springer-Verlag, 2012.

66. Tanaka, K. A. K., K. G. N. Suzuki, Y. M. Shirai et al. "Membrane Molecules Mobile Even after Chemical Fixation." *Nature Methods* 7 (2010): 865–6.

67. Lagerholm, B. C., G. E. Weinreb, K. Jacobson, and N. L. Thompson. "Detecting Microdomains in Intact Cells Membranes." *Annual Reviews Physical Chemistry* 56 (2005): 309–36.

68. Schutz, G. J., H. Schindler, and T. Schmidt. "Single-Molecule Microscopy on Model Membranes Reveals Anomalous Diffusion." *Biophysical Journal* 73 (1997): 1073–80.

69. Nishimura, S. Y., M. Vrljic, L. O. Klein, H. M. McConnell, and W. E. Moerner. "Cholesterol Depletion Induces Solid-Like Regions in the Plasma Membrane." *Biophysical Journal* 90 (2006): 927–38.

70. Sahl, S. J., M. Leutenegger, M. Hilbert, S. W. Hell, and C. Eggeling. "Fast Molecular Tracking Maps Nanoscale Dynamics of Plasma Membrane Lipids." *Proceedings of the National Academy of Sciences of the United States of America* 107, no. 15 (2010): 6829–34.

71. Wieser, S., M. Moertelmaier, E. Fuertbauer, H. Stockinger, and G. Schutz. "(Un) Confined Diffusion of CD59 in the Plasma Membrane Determined by High-Resolution Single Molecule Microscopy." *Biophysical Journal* 92 (2007): 3719–28.

72. Thompson, R. E., D. R. Larson, and W. W. Webb. "Precise Nanometer Localization Analysis for Individual Fluorescent Probes." *Biophysical Journal* 82 (2002): 2775–83.

73. Clausen, M., and B. C. Lagerholm. "The Probe Rules in Single Particle Tracking." *Current Protein and Peptide Science* 12 (2011): 699–713.

74. Yechiel, E., and M. Edidin. "Micrometer-Scale Domains in Fibroblast Plasma-Membranes." *Journal of Cell Biology* 105, no. 2 (1987): 755–60.

75. Feder, T. J., I. Brust-Mascher, J. P. Slattery, B. A. Baird, and W. W. Webb. "Constrainted Diffusion or Immobile Fraction on Cell Surfaces: A New Interpretation." *Biophysical Journal* 70 (1996): 2767–73.

76. Magde, D., W. W. Webb, and E. Elson. "Thermodynamic Fluctuations in a Reacting System—Measurement by Fluorescence Correlation Spectroscopy." *Physical Review Letters* 29, no. 11 (1972): 705–8.

77. Ehrenberg, M., and R. Rigler. "Rotational Brownian Motion and Fluorescence Intensity Fluctuations." *Chemical Physics* 4, no. 3 (1974): 390–401.

78. Fahey, P. F., D. E. Koppel, L. S. Barak et al. "Lateral Diffusion in Planar Lipid Bilayers." *Science* 195, no. 4275 (1977): 305–6.

79. Schwille, P., J. Korlach, and W. W. Webb. "Fluorescence Correlation Spectroscopy with Single-Molecule Sensitivity on Cell and Model Membranes." *Cytometry* 36 (1999): 176–82.

80. Manley, S., J. M. Gillette, G. H. Patterson et al. "High-Density Mapping of Single-Molecule Trajectories with Photoactivated Localization Microscopy." *Nature Methods* 5, no. 2 (2008): 155–7.

81. Lippincott-Schwartz, J., N. Altan-Bonnet, and G. H. Patterson. "Photobleaching and Photoactivation: Following Protein Dynamics in Living Cells." *Nature Cell Biology* 5 (2003): S7–14.

82. Widengren, J., and R. Rigler. "Ultrasensitive Detection of Single Molecules Using Fluorescence Correlation Spectroscopy." In *Bioscience*, edited by B. Klinge and C. Owman, 180–3. Lund: Lund University Press, 1990.

83. Abbe, E. "Beiträge zur Theorie des mikroskops und der mikroskopischen Wahrnehmung." *Archiv für Mikroskopische Anatomie* 9 (1873): 413–68.

84. Humpolickova, J., E. Gielen, A. Benda et al. "Probing Diffusion Laws within Cellular Membranes by Z-Scan Fluorescence Correlation Spectroscopy." *Biophysical Journal* 91, no. 3 (2006): L23–5.

85. He, H. T., and D. Marguet. "Detecting Nanodomains in Living Cell Membrane by Fluorescence Correlation Spectroscopy." *Annual Review of Physical Chemistry* 62 (2011): 417–36.

86. Levene, M. J., J. Korlach, S. W. Turner et al. "Zero-Mode Waveguides for Single-Molecule Analysis at High Concentrations." *Science* 299 (2003): 682–6.

87. Wenger, J., F. Conchonaud, J. Dintinger et al. "Diffusion Analysis within Single Nanometric Apertures Reveals the Ultrafine Cell Membrane Organization." *Biophysical Journal* 92, no. 3 (2007): 913–9.

88. Manzo, C., T. S. van Zanten, and M. F. Garcia-Parajo. "Nanoscale Fluorescence Correlation Spectroscopy on Intact Living Cell Membranes with NSOM Probes." *Biophysical Journal* 100 (2011): L08–10.

89. Kastrup, L., H. Blom, C. Eggeling, and S. W. Hell. "Fluorescence Fluctuation Spectroscopy in Subdiffraction Focal Volumes." *Physical Review Letters* 94 (2005): 178104.

90. Ringemann, C., B. Harke, C. V. Middendorff et al. "Exploring Single-Molecule Dynamics with Fluorescence Nanoscopy." *New Journal of Physics* 11 (2009): 103054.

91. Hell, S. W., and J. Wichmann. "Breaking the Diffraction Resolution Limit by Stimulated-Emission—Stimulated-Emission-Depletion Fluorescence Microscopy." *Optics Letters* 19, no. 11 (1994): 780–2.

92. Hell, S. W. "Far-Field Optical Nanoscopy." *Science* 316, no. 5828 (2007): 1153–8.

93. Hell, S. W., S. Jakobs, and L. Kastrup. "Imaging and Writing at the Nanoscale with Focused Visible Light through Saturable Optical Transitions." *Applied Physics A: Materials Science & Processing* 77 (2003): 859–60.

94. Hell, S. W. "Strategy for Far-Field Optical Imaging and Writing without Diffraction Limit." *Physics Letters. Section A: General, Atomic and Solid State Physics* 326, no. 1–2 (2004): 140–5.

95. Hell, S. W. "Microscopy and Its Focal Switch." *Nature Methods* 6, no. 1 (2009): 24–32.

96. Klar, T. A., S. Jakobs, M. Dyba, A. Egner, and S. W. Hell. "Fluorescence Microscopy with Diffraction Resolution Barrier Broken by Stimulated Emission." *Proceedings of the National Academy of Sciences of the United States of America* 97 (2000): 8206–10.

97. Moertelmaier, M., M. Brameshuber, M. Linimeier, G. J. Schutz, and H. Stockinger. "Thinning out Clusters While Conserving Stoichiometry of Labeling." *Applied Physics Letters* 87 (2005): 263903.

98. Eggeling, C., M. Hilbert, H. Bock et al. "Reversible Photoswitching Enables Single-Molecule Fluorescence Fluctuation Spectroscopy at High Molecular Concentration." *Microscopy Research and Technique* 70, no. 12 (2007): 1003–9.

99. Weiss, S. "Shattering the Diffraction Limit of Light: A Revolution in Fluorescence Microscopy?" *Proceedings of the National Academy of Sciences of the United States of America* 97, no. 16 (2000): 8747–9.

100. Blom, H., L. Kastrup, and C. Eggeling. "Fluorescence Fluctuation Spectroscopy in Reduced Detection Volumes." *Current Pharmaceutical Biotechnology* 7, no. 1 (2006): 51–66.

101. Mueller, V., C. Ringemann, A. Honigmann et al. "STED Nanoscopy Reveals Molecular Details of Cholesterol- and Cytoskeleton-Modulated Lipid Interactions in Living Cells." *Biophysical Journal* 101 (2011): 1651–60.

102. Mueller, V., A. Honigmann, C. Ringemann et al. "FCS in STED Microscopy: Studying the Nanoscale of Lipid Membrane Dynamics." In *Methods in Enzymology*, edited by S. Y. Tetin, 1–38. Burlington: Academic Press, Elsevier, 2013.

103. Honigmann, A., V. Mueller, S. W. Hell, and C. Eggeling. "STED Microscopy Detects and Quantifies Liquid Phase Separation in Lipid Membranes Using a New Far-Red Emitting Fluorescent Phosphoglycerolipid Analogue." *Faraday Discussion* 161 (2013): 77–89.

104. Mueller, V., PhD thesis, University Heidelberg, 2012.

105. Andrade, D. M., M. P. Clausen, J. Keller et al. "Lipids Are Compartmentalized at the Plasma Membrane by the ARP2/3-Dependent Cortical Actin Cytoskeleton." *Nature Structural Biology* (2014): submitted.

106. Honigmann, A., C. Walter, F. Erdmann, C. Eggeling, and R. Wagner. "Characterization of Horizontal Lipid Bilayers as a Model System to Study Lipid Phase Separation." *Biophysical Journal* 98, no. 12 (2010): 2886–94.

107. Sezgin, E., I. Levental, M. Grzybek et al. "Partitioning, Diffusion, and Ligand Binding of Raft Lipid Analogs in Model and Cellular Plasma Membranes." *Biochimica et Biophysica Acta (BBA)—Biomembranes* 1818 (2012): 1777–84.

108. Baumgart, T., A. T. Hammond, P. Sengupta et al. "Large-Scale Fluid/Fluid Phase Separation of Proteins and Lipids in Giant Plasma Membrane Vesicles." *Proceedings of the National Academy of Sciences of the United States of America* 104, no. 9 (2007): 3165–70.

109. Lingwood, D., J. Ries, P. Schwille, and K. Simons. "Plasma Membranes Are Poised for Activation of Raft Phase Coalescence at Physiological Temperature." *Proceedings of the National Academy of Sciences of the United States of America* 105, no. 29 (2008): 10005–10.

110. Kaiser, H.-J., D. Lingwood, I. Levental et al. "Order of Lipid Phases in Model and Plasma Membranes." *Proceedings of the National Academy of Sciences of the United States of America* 106, no. 39 (2009): 16645–50.

111. Solanko, M. L., A. Honigmann, H. S. Midtiby et al. "Membrane Orientation and Lateral Diffusion of BODIPY-Cholesterol as a Function of Probe Structure." *Biophysical Journal* 105 (2013): 2082–92.

112. Mueller, V., A. Honigmann, H. Ta et al. "Scanning STED-FCS Reveals Spatiotemporal Heterogeneity of Lipid Diffusion in the Plasma Membrane of Living Cells." *Proceedings of the National Academy of Sciences of the United States of America* (2013): submitted.

113. Hedde, P. N., R. M. Dorlich, R. Blomley et al. "Stimulated Emission Depletion-Based Raster Image Correlation Spectroscopy Reveals Biomolecular Dynamics in Live Cells." *Nature Communications* 4 (2013): 2093.

114. Digman, M. A., and E. Gratton. "Lessons in Fluctuation Correlation Spectroscopy." *Annual Review of Physical Chemistry* 62 (2011): 645–68.

115. Donnert, G., J. Keller, R. Medda et al. "Macromolecular-Scale Resolution in Biological Fluorescence Microscopy." *Proceedings of the National Academy of Sciences of the United States of America* 103, no. 31 (2006): 11440–5.

116. Willig, K. I., B. Harke, R. Medda, and S. W. Hell. "STED Microscopy with Continuous Wave Beams." *Nature Methods* 4, no. 11 (2007): 915–8.

117. Moffitt, J. R., C. Osseforth, and J. Michaelis. "Time-Gating Improves the Spatial Resolution of STED Microscopy." *Optics Express* 19, no. 5 (2011): 4242–54.

118. Vicidomini, G., G. Moneron, K. Y. Han et al. "Sharper Low-Power STED Nanoscopy by Time Gating." *Nature Methods* 8, no. 7 (2011): 571–3.

119. Vicidomini, G., A. Schoenle, H. Ta et al. "STED Nanoscopy with Time-Gated Detection: Theoretical and Experimental Aspects." *PLoS One* 8, no. 1 (2013): e54421.

120. Eggeling, C., L. Brand, D. Ullmann, and S. Jaeger. "Highly Sensitive Fluorescence Detection Technology Currently Available for HTS." *Drug Discovery Today* 8, no. 14 (2003): 632–41.

20 Nanophotonic Approaches for Nanoscale Imaging and Single-Molecule Detection at Ultrahigh Concentrations

Mathieu Mivelle, Thomas S. van Zanten,
Carlo Manzo, and Maria F. Garcia-Parajo

CONTENTS

20.1 INTRODUCTION

One of the ultimate goals in biology is to understand the relationship between structure, function, and dynamics of biomolecules in their natural environment: the living cell. Although modern molecular biology has made enormous progress in identifying a full repertoire of proteins, lipids, and other molecular components both inside the cell and at the cell membrane, direct visualization of molecular interactions in living cells remains a major challenge.

Take for example the cell membrane, which is highly crowded and heterogeneous in terms of structure, composition, and dynamics. In recent years, it has become evident that membrane components do not operate separately but are part of well-organized

453

multimolecular aggregates. Indeed, many membrane receptors exhibit clear but distinct spatial patterns, which might arise from protein–lipid interactions,[1,2] interactions with the cortical cytoskeleton,[3,4] or with other local organizers of the cell membrane, such as tetraspanins[5,6] or galectins.[7] Evidence for this persistent aggregation at multiple spatial scales has led to the concept that in addition to receptor expression, spatiotemporal organization on the cell surface is tightly controlled and crucial for function. Moreover, recent research is providing evidence that receptors might also exist in preassembled nanoclusters prior to ligand activation, in the absence of interactions with other molecular components.[8–11] As such, the overall result is that most plasma membrane receptors distribute heterogeneously in small domains that are diverse in terms of size, composition, and stability. This complex, heterogeneous arrangement has been shown to be critical to various physiological processes.[8,12–14] Yet, very little is known about the molecular mechanisms leading to the nonrandom organization of the cell membrane, in particular, prior to cell activation, since this compartmentalization occurs at the nanometer scale,[1,3,4,10] which is a size regime not accessible by standard microscopy techniques as they suffer from diffraction.

In recent years, the emergence of far-field optical techniques able to surpass the diffraction limit of light is advancing our understanding of the cell surface organization at the nanometer scale. These techniques make use of specific photophysical properties of fluorescence probes in conjunction with tailored ways of illumination. For instance, stimulated emission depletion (STED) based on reversible saturable transitions on a fluorescent dye can achieve ~30 nm resolution on fixed cells.[9,15] Alternatively, the "apparent" resolution (more correctly localization accuracy) can, in principle, reach the molecular scale by allowing only a subset of fluorescent molecules (autofluorescent proteins or organic dyes) to be photoactive at a given time and ensuring that their separation distance is larger than the diffraction limit. These techniques known in general as single-molecule localization methods[16–18] allow for the reconstruction of an image on a molecule-by-molecule basis using computational algorithms. Although these emerging techniques are already providing highly detailed information at the nanometer scale, they are still slow, preventing the visualization of dynamic events in living cells at these small spatial scales.

Given the importance of measuring single-molecule dynamic processes in living cells, techniques such as single-particle tracking (SPT)[19,20] and fluorescence correlation spectroscopy (FCS)[21,22] have been gaining increasing interest within the biological community. SPT allows the diffusion of individual microscopic particles (either fluorescent molecules, quantum dots, or fluorescent beads) attached to relevant biomolecules to be tracked with high precision. Normally, the sample is illuminated in wide field, either using epi- or total internal reflection excitation, and the fluorescence emission from multiple individual particles is recorded using a CCD (charge-couple device) camera. The temporal resolution is essentially given by the camera speed, while the number of photons collected in each fluorescent spot mainly determines the spatial localization precision. The information garnered from measurement of particle trajectories provides useful information about the mechanisms and forces that drive and constrain the particle's motion. Because of its simplicity and versatility, the number of SPT applications has grown significantly in the last decade based mainly on advances in microscopy and labeling techniques (for reviews in the field, see

Refs. 19 and 20). An alternative technique able to provide dynamic information with higher temporal resolution than SPT is FCS. In FCS, fluorescence fluctuations arising from the diffusion of molecules through a small excitation volume are recorded and correlated in time to provide information on the diffusion properties of molecules. Normally, excitation is performed in a confocal fashion by focusing the light using a high-numerical aperture (NA) objective and the fluorescent photons are collected using single photon counting avalanche photodiode (APD) detectors. Unfortunately, although both SPT and FCS are extremely powerful, the diffraction limit of light imposes a restriction on the number of molecules that can be labeled, and as such, both techniques work best at sublabeling conditions, which essentially means that only a small fraction of the total population of the molecules is accessible during experiments. This is obviously a main drawback given the crowded nature of the living cell. Moreover, although constrained diffusion arising from nanoscale hetero-geneities are in principle resolvable by SPT, standard FCS approaches tend to average out these details and more sophisticated approaches are needed to infer information on the diffusion of molecules at length scales smaller than the diffraction limit.[22]

Although, in principle, single-molecule dynamic events on in vitro conditions can be studied in a much easier way using several optical approaches, most tran-sient interactions between proteins and nucleic acids, and between enzymes and their ligands, occur at micromolar ligand concentrations.[23] Currently, single-molecule detection by fluorescence is commonly performed by confocal microscopy and far-field optics, in combination with FCS approaches. Because of the diffraction limit of light, the focal illumination volume in confocal corresponds to approximately 1 fl, which implies that for detection of individual molecules, concentrations in the order of picomolar to a few nanomolar should be used. As a consequence, at higher sample concentrations, more than one molecule resides in the observation volume, prevent-ing the detection of individual interactions at the relevant concentrations.

Different experimental strategies have been implemented in recent years to allow for in vitro single-molecule detection at high concentrations (for a recent review in the field, see Ref. 23). One of the most obvious ways to guarantee that only one molecule is pres-ent in the excitation volume is by reducing the size of the illumination volume. This has been successfully accomplished by making use of subwavelength apertures surrounded by an opaque metal film, also known as zero-mode waveguides (ZMWs).[24] By combin-ing the evanescent character of the axial field emanating from these structures (less than 100 nm) together with the reduced lateral dimensions of the nanoapertures (between 50 and 200 nm in size), effective illumination volumes orders of magnitude smaller than that in confocal can be achieved (a few tens of zeptoliters, i.e., 10^{-21} L), allowing the detection of individual molecules at high sample concentrations.[24] Unfortunately, as the dimensions of these nanostructures are reduced, very small transmitted light is obtained. This low light throughput together with the finite skin depth of the metal used (normally aluminum) restricts the practical size of the nanoapertures to approximately 50–70 nm.

In this chapter, we focus on recent advancements in the field of nanophotonics toward nanometric optical resolution as well as single-molecule detection at ultrahigh sample concentrations. These novel approaches, denoted as nanoantennas or optical antennas, might become key players in modern biology by providing tools to study processes both in vitro and in vivo at relevant spatial scales and physiological concentrations.

20.2 NEAR-FIELD OPTICS FOR SUPER-RESOLUTION IMAGING

In far-field optical microscopy, the diffraction limit implies that the minimum distance Δx required to resolve independently two distinct objects is dependent on the wavelength λ of the light used to observe the specimen, and by the condenser and objective lens system, through their refractive indices n and angle of acceptance α, such that $\Delta x = \lambda/2n \sin\alpha$. This implies that Δx typically exceeds 300 nm in the case of visible light. When an object, such as a microscopic specimen, is illuminated with a monochromatic plane wave, the transmitted or reflected light is collected by a lens and projected onto a detector to form the image. Usually, for convenience and practicality, the detector is placed in the far field, so that the far-field component of the light, which propagates in an unconfined way, is the only component used to generate the image. On the other hand, the interaction between the imaging light and the specimen also generates a near-field component, which consists of a nonpropagating (evanescent) field existing only near the object at distances less than the wavelength of the light. Because the near field decays exponentially within a distance less than the wavelength, usually it cannot be collected by the lens; thus, it is not detected. This effect leads to the well-known Abbé's diffraction limit.

By detecting the near-field component before it undergoes diffraction, near-field scanning optical microscopy (NSOM) allows non-diffraction-limited high-resolution optical imaging. This is commonly achieved by illuminating the sample using a subwavelength aperture probe placed in proximity to the sample. The spatial resolution Δx no longer depends on λ but instead on the diameter of the aperture (typically between 50 and 100 nm).

In its most commonly implemented mode, a subwavelength aperture probe is scanned in proximity (<10 nm) to the specimen under study (Figure 20.1) to generate an image. Using the probe as a near-field excitation source, the interaction with the sample surface induces changes in the far-field radiation, which is collected in the far field by conventional optics and directed to highly sensitive detectors to provide an optical image.[25–27] An independent mechanism is used to control the separation distance between the tip and the sample and to simultaneously generate a topographic image.[25,27] In this way, a singular feature pertaining to NSOM is produced: correlative optical and topographical imaging with a spatial resolution determined by the probe configuration. Another unique characteristic of near-field excitation is given by the finite size of the probe itself: decreasing the area of illumination obviously reduces the interaction volume and background scatter, which is of major importance in enhancing the sensitivity for spectroscopic applications (fluorescence, Raman, etc.).

For biological applications, the most widely used configuration is an aperture-type NSOM, incorporated into an inverted optical microscope, with near-field excitation and far-field detection (Figure 20.1). This scheme preserves most of the conventional imaging modes (confocal microscopy for instance), which remain available in combination with the near-field approach. In fluorescence applications, the near-field light excites fluorophores on the sample. The fluorescence is collected in the far field using a high-NA objective and sent to sensitive detectors, such as APDs or photomultiplier tubes, via suitable dichroic mirrors for spectral splitting or through a polarizing beam splitter cube for polarization detection.[26,27]

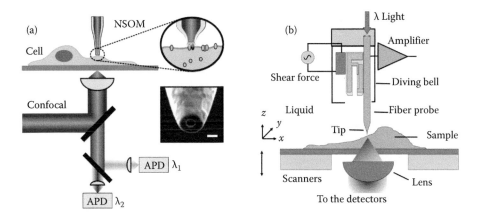

FIGURE 20.1 Schematics of a combined confocal/NSOM for biological applications. (a) General scheme of the setup. The sample can be illuminated either in confocal fashion using a high-NA objective or by the NSOM probe. In NSOM, only fluorophores close to the aperture are excited. The emitted fluorescence is collected with the objective and sent to the detectors after appropriate filtering. The inset shows a scanning electron microscopy (SEM) image of a typical NSOM probe of 70 nm in diameter. (b) Close-up detail of the NSOM head. The probe is mounted on one of the legs of a tuning fork, which works as a sensing element to control the distance separation between the tip and the sample. The tuning fork is laterally oscillated above the sample and a shear force feedback system maintains the tip above the sample with an accuracy of 1 nm. For live-cell applications, the tuning fork is encapsulated in a diving bell system that keeps the fork oscillating in air while the tip is immersed in solution.[28] The tip is aligned with respect to the objective and the sample is scanned with respect to the tip using an x,y,z scanner to provide the image.

As a surface-sensitive technique, NSOM has been extensively applied to study the organization of different lipids and receptors on the cell membrane. In the lipid context, single-molecule NSOM has been recently used to visualize the nano-landscape of ganglioside GM1 after tightening by its ligand cholera toxin (CTxB) on intact fixed monocytes and dendritic cells (DCs).[29] CTxB tightening of GM1 was sufficient to initiate a minimal raft coalescence unit, resulting in the formation of cholesterol-dependent GM1 nanodomains smaller than 120 nm in size (Figure 20.2a). These CTxB-GM1 nanodomains were further capable of recruiting certain types of transmembrane and lipid-anchored proteins without physical intermixing (Figure 20.2b), but not the transferring receptor CD71, a classical nonraft marker. These results demonstrated the existence of raft-based compositional connectivity at the nanometer scale crucially mediated by cholesterol. The data further suggested that such connective condition on resting membranes constitute an obligatory step toward the hierarchical evolution of large-scale raft coalescence upon cell activation.

The recruitment of specific receptors to lipid raft regions has been also studied using near-field nanoscopy. For instance, single-molecule NSOM has been exploited to capture the spatio-functional relationship between the integrin receptor LFA-1 involved in leukocyte adhesion and raft components (GPI-anchored proteins).[10] While LFA-1 formed nanoclusters of ~85 nm in size on resting monocytes, ~70% of the GPIs organized as monomers and the remaining 30% formed small oligomers

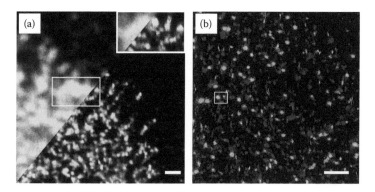

FIGURE 20.2 Application of single-molecule dual-color NSOM to study lipid nanoscale organization on intact cell membranes. (a) Combined confocal (left part) and NSOM (right part) of CTxB-labeled GM1 lipids on the membrane of fixed monocytes. The increased resolution of NSOM is apparent when comparing both parts of the image. Nanodomains of GM1 are clearly resolved on the NSOM part of the image. The optical resolution is 70 nm. (b) Dual-color NSOM of the GPI-AP protein CD55 (green) and CTxB-GM1 nanodomains (red). The absence of colocalization at the nanometer scale indicates that GM1 nanodomains and CD55 do not intermix at the nanoscale despite the fact that both components are raftophilic.[29]

containing two to four molecules. Surprisingly, whereas GPI monomers distributed randomly on the cell surface, GPI oligomers resided in regions proximal to each other (within ~250 nm). Moreover, the distribution of GPIs with respect to LFA-1 nanoclusters significantly deviated from randomness. In the resting state, that is, prior to LFA-1 activation, ~50% of the GPI oligomers were found close to LFA-1 nanoclusters, whereas GPI monomers exhibited no particular spatial correlation with respect to LFA-1. Interestingly, ligand-mediated LFA-1 activation not only resulted in a spatial interlocking of the integrin and GPIs generating nascent adhesion sites but importantly resulted in an interconversion from monomers to nanodomains of GPI-anchored proteins. These data demonstrated the existence of nanoplatforms composed of integrins and rafts as essential intermediates in nascent cell adhesion.

Dual-color NSOM has also been used to investigate the association of β-adrenergic receptors (β-ARs) and caveolae on the surface of cardiac myocytes.[30] The study showed that ~15–20% β_2AR clusters colocalized in caveolae, while the remaining nanoclusters were proximal to it. Additional work showed that increasing the β_2AR expression level increased the number of clusters and density on the membrane but not their size. Hence, β_2AR molecules preferentially reside in specific membrane compartments restricted in size, in line with a recent view on membrane rafts as having an upper limit on resting cells.

In addition to lipid rafts, other mechanisms are responsible for orchestrating the organization of the cell surface at different spatial scales. In particular, homophilic protein–protein interactions could also lead to the formation of protein nanoclusters. One example is the receptor DC-SIGN, a transmembrane tetrameric protein expressed on antigen-presenting cells and involved in the recognition of several pathogens.[8] Single-molecule NSOM showed that ~80% of the receptors form clusters of 185 nm in size on the membrane of immature DCs.[31] Interestingly, these nanoclusters showed a remarkable heterogeneity in their packing density, suggesting that this particular arrangement might serve to maximize binding strength to a large variety of viruses and pathogens having different binding affinities to DC-SIGN. More recently, using a mutagenesis approach combined with super-resolution imaging, we demonstrated that the neck region of the receptor is crucial not only for tetramer formation but also for DC-SIGN nanoclustering and binding capacity to virus-size pathogens.[11]

At a different level of hierarchical organization, interactions between clusters of different proteins have been also predicted and resolved using simultaneous dual-color excitation/detection NSOM.[32] As single receptors, IL2R and IL15R (two members of the interleukin family expressed in human T lymphoma cells) did not spatially colocalize and randomly scattered on the cell membrane. However, in their clustered form, both receptors significantly colocalized in the same nanocompartments. Interestingly, IL2R and IL15R clusters exhibited constant packing density albeit forming clusters of different sizes, suggesting a general "building block" type of assembly of these receptors as opposed to the heterogeneous packing density exhibited by DC-SIGN.

These successful applications not only demonstrate the powerfulness of NSOM as a super-resolution multicolor surface imaging technique but also highlight some of its drawbacks. Typical optical resolutions are in the order of 70 to 100 nm, mainly determined by the size of the aperture. Although, in principle, smaller apertures can be fabricated nowadays by taking advantage of focus ion beam (FIB) technology, the light throughput from the probe considerably decreases as the size of the aperture is reduced. This low light throughput limits in practice the attainable resolution to approximately 50 nm at best. Current developments using optical antennas to concentrate and enhance the excitation light hold great promise for generation of new nanoscale sources for nanoimaging applications.[33]

20.3   THE CONCEPT OF OPTICAL ANTENNAS

Optical antennas represent a class of optical components that couple electromagnetic radiation in the visible wavelengths in the same way as radioelectric antennas do at the corresponding wavelengths. As such, optical antennas represent the counterparts of conventional radio and microwave antennas for frequencies in the visible regime (hundreds of terahertz). In the broader sense, optical antennas can be defined as optical elements that efficiently convert localized energy (in the near field) into propagating radiation (in the far field), and vice versa (Figure 20.3). In the context of microscopy, an optical antenna effectively replaces a conventional focusing lens or objective, concentrating external laser radiation to dimensions smaller than the diffraction limit.[33,34]

As example, the working principle of an optical dipole antenna is shown in Figure 20.4. The modal field of the antenna is localized in a volume with dimensions smaller than the wavelength of the light used, and it is concentrated at the antenna ends. Moreover, the antenna can be also seen as a resonator. A bound wave traveling along the elongated metal antenna will be reflected at the antenna ends so that resonant cavity modes are formed. These resonant modes occur when the antenna length is approximately close to a multiple of half the bound wave wavelength. In this way, two main features pertaining to optical antennas are produced: a large field enhancement attributed to resonance as well as strong confinement of this field to the dimensions of the antenna ends (Figure 20.4).

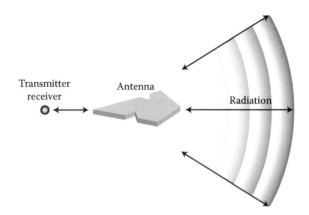

FIGURE 20.3 Working principle of an optical antenna. In the receiver mode, radiation from the far field is collected by the antenna and coupled to the receiver in the near field. In transmission mode, the antenna couples to the transmitter in the near field and radiates in the far field. (Reprinted from Novotny, L., and van Hulst, N.F., *Nat. Photonics* 5, 83–90, 2011. With permission.)

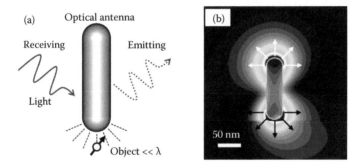

FIGURE 20.4 Optical dipole antenna and field localization. (a) Schematics of a dipole antenna. The antenna receives far-field radiation and concentrates near field at the antenna ends. If a dipole emitter (a single molecule for instance) is located in proximity to the near field of the antenna, it will interact with it. (b) Simulations of the near field localized and amplified at the antenna ends. (Figures were kindly provided by N.F. van Hulst.)

If a single molecule, or single emitter in general, is accurately positioned close to this enhanced and localized antenna near-field, it will interact with the antenna affecting in turn the emitter photophysical properties. Indeed, the antenna modifies both the electric field formed at the emitter position under external illumination and the electric field radiated by the emitter.[34] As a result, the total transition rates of the emitter can be enhanced, both in emission and in excitation. In excitation, the locally enhanced field at the antenna increases the excitation rate of an emitter by external illumination. In emission, optical antennas can enhance the total radiative transition rate.[34–36] Therefore, if the antenna–emitter system is properly designed, one can enhance the total amount of photons absorbed and emitted. In addition, it has also been shown that in both excitation and emission, the spectral dependence, polarization dependence, and angular dependence can be controlled.[36]

One of the essential requirements for optical antennas to operate in the visible and near-infrared wavelength range is that they need to have characteristic dimensions of the order of the wavelength of light, demanding fabrication accuracies better than 10 nm. The advent of nanoscience and nanotechnology provides access to this length scale with the use of novel top-down nanofabrication tools (e.g., FIB milling and electron beam lithography) and bottom-up self-assembly schemes. Nowadays, a large variety of optical antenna designs can be found in the literature that include different materials and shapes.[34,36] Depending on the application, the antenna can be directly carved or engineered at the end of standing probes (Figure 20.5a) or

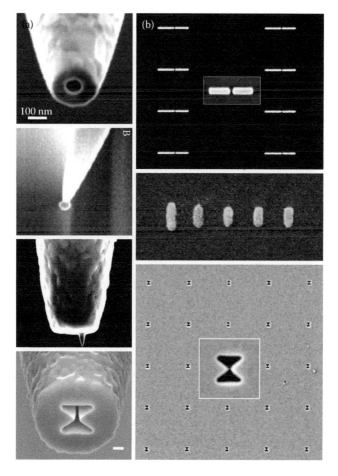

FIGURE 20.5   Different antenna geometries. (a) Fabricated at the apex of probes and used in combination with scanning probe techniques, such as NSOM. From top to bottom: subwavelength aperture, gold nanoparticle on a probe, monopole on a metal-coated NSOM probe, bowtie aperture on NSOM probe. (b) Fabricated as arrays on 2D substrates. From top to bottom: dimer antenna arrays, Yagi–Uda antenna, bowtie antenna arrays. (Reprinted from Novotny, L., and van Hulst, N.F., *Nat. Photonics* 5, 83–90, 2011. With permission; Mivelle, M. et al., *Nano Lett.* 12, 5972–5978, 2012.)

fabricated on two-dimensional (2D) substrates (Figure 20.5b). In the following, we highlight specific examples on how antennas (either on probes or 2D) are starting to be applied to biology for imaging and sensing applications.

20.4 OPTICAL ANTENNA PROBES FOR SUPER-RESOLUTION IMAGING

The subwavelength aperture probe as used in NSOM constitutes in fact one of the first examples of an optical antenna, since the aperture surrounded by the metal film indeed concentrates optical fields at the nanometer scale. However, metal nanoapertures can be considered as a primitive type of antennas since they lack field amplification. In recent years, more creative optical antenna designs using sharp metallic tips, metal nanoparticles, and complex geometrical nanostructures are being currently explored to localize and to boost the optical field to dimensions smaller than 30 nm in size.[34]

Although modest yet, first applications on the use of these antenna configurations for biological imaging are starting to appear. For instance, using a gold nanoparticle-based optical antenna excited in the far field, Höppener et al. imaged single Ca^{2+} channels on erythrocyte plasma membranes under aqueous conditions[37] (Figure 20.6a and b). The spatial resolution obtained was 50 nm, although improvements on the antenna geometry and illumination schemes that reduce the far-field surrounding background can in principle improve the resolution to 10 nm. Other geometries include the fabrication of monopole antennas carved around a subwavelength aperture as used in NSOM. This concept takes advantage of the local illumination properties of the aperture to drive the antenna to resonance, enhancing and confining the optical field at the antenna tip, without background contribution from the far field.[38,39] In the first demonstration of this approach, simultaneous topography and fluorescent imaging of labeled DNA with 10 nm resolution was convincingly demonstrated.[40] More recently, the dimensions of these antenna probes have been tuned to the wavelength of the excitation field and used to detect individual fluorescent molecules embedded in polymer layers.[38]

Our group has recently demonstrated the potential of optical antennas for nanobioimaging of individual receptors and nanodomains on intact cells of the immune system.[39] The probe-based monopole optical antennas were fabricated by carving of the antenna on the tip apex of conventional NSOM probes at the glass–metal interface using (Ga+)-FIB milling. The geometry, that is, length, width, and radius of curvature of the antennas, can be carefully controlled during FIB to maximize their response in liquid conditions. In our case, the dimensions of the fabricated antennas varied from 50 to 60 nm in width, ~20 nm of radius of curvature, and lengths between 90 and 135 nm (Figure 20.6c). These probes were then used under appropriate excitation antenna conditions to image individual antibodies in liquid conditions with an unprecedented resolution of 26 ± 4 nm and virtually no surrounding background (Figure 20.6d). On intact cell membranes in physiological conditions, the obtained resolution is currently 30 ± 6 nm. Importantly, the method allowed us to distinguish individual proteins from nanodomains and to quantify the degree of

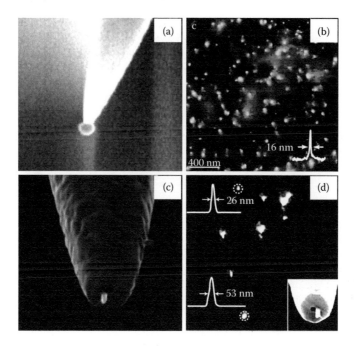

FIGURE 20.6   Super-resolution imaging using optical antennas. (a) Gold nanoparticle attached to a tapered optical fiber. The antenna is excited in the far field. (b) Near-field image of individual plasma membrane-bound Ca^{2+} pumps (PMCA4) on erythrocyte membranes as imaged with the gold nanoparticle antenna. (c) Monopole antenna carved at the apex of an aluminum-coated tapered optical fiber. Excitation of the antenna is performed through the NSOM probe. (d) Image of individual fluorescently labeled antibodies imaged by the antenna probe shown in (c). Cross sections of two encircled features show responses of 26 and 53 nm. (Panels a and b were kindly provided by L. Novotny; panel d was adapted from van Zanten, T.S. et al., *Small* 6, 270–275, 2010.)

clustering by directly measuring physical size and intensity of individual fluorescent spots.[39] Although true resolution down to the nanometer scale is achieved by means of monopole antenna probes, enhancement of the electromagnetic field is only modest and tightly coupled to the small dimensions of the antenna, which imposes high demands on the fabrication of these nanostructures.

Bowtie nanoaperture antennas (BNAs) carved at the end facet of tapered aluminum-coated optical fibers provide a more robust and alternative design to monopole antennas. These nanostructures consist of two triangle openings faced tip to tip and separated by a small opening gap providing a superconfined spot with an intense local field and broadband response in the visible regime.[41] Moreover, the effective confinement region of BNAs can be readily tuned by controlling the excitation polarization.[41,42] BNAs have been successfully used as nanometer-sized light sources for nanolithography[43] and as high-throughput near-field probes.[44,45] Recently, we showed single-molecule nanoimaging using a BNA scanning probe and revealed the full three-dimensional (3D) vectorial components of the optical near

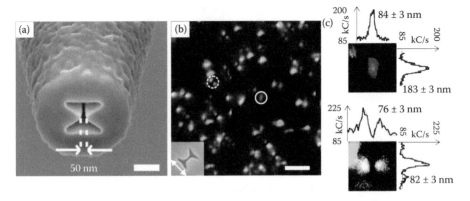

FIGURE 20.7 Single-molecule nanoimaging using a bowtie antenna probe. (a) Bowtie nanoaperture carved at the apex of a metal-coated tapered optical fiber. The gap region is 50 nm. The antenna is excited through the NSOM probe and the fluorescence emission collected in the far field using a polarization-detection scheme. (b) Single-molecule patterns as obtained from imaging individual molecules using the bowtie antenna excited with a field polarized along the antenna arms (see inset). Notice that the individual fluorescence patterns have different shapes, resulting from the 3D near-field components of the field emanating from the bowtie. (c) Intensity patterns and cross sections of two fluorescence features as encircled in (b). The upper pattern corresponds to an in-plane molecule while the two-lobe pattern (bottom) corresponds to a z-oriented molecule. The optical resolution is ~80 nm. (Adapted from Mivelle, M. et al., *Nano Lett.* 12, 5972–5978, 2012.)

field of BNAs using individual molecules as nanoscale optical sensors[42] (Figure 20.7). Furthermore, direct comparison of the response upon confocal and BNA probe excitation for each individual molecule allowed determination of the field enhancement provided by BNA probes. Our results showed an approximately sixfold enhancement on the fluorescence emission of individual molecules when the BNA is properly excited and aligned to the dipole emitter. In addition, fabrication of BNA probes on tapered optical fibers near the cutoff region provides approximately three orders of magnitude higher throughput than circular aperture probes of similar dimensions, making these bright nanostructures ideal candidates for a large number of highly sensitive applications, including biosensing, spectroscopy, and nanoimaging of biological samples.

20.5 NANOPHOTONIC APPROACHES FOR NANOSCALE DYNAMICS IN LIVING CELL MEMBRANES

One of the great advantages of light microscopy is the possibility to image living cells. However, the diffusion of most proteins and lipids on the cell membrane occurs in the millisecond time scale, posing a challenge to most optical imaging techniques. As a result, single-molecule fluorescence approaches that provide sufficient time resolution do not rely on imaging but rather on following a subset of labeled molecules as they laterally diffuse on the cell surface, as used in SPT[3,46] or in FCS.[47] Yet, the large illumination volume of the diffraction-limited confocal spot as used in FCS hides diffusion heterogeneities taking place at the nanoscopic length scale.[22] Recently, STED nanoscopy has been combined with FCS to detect nanoscopic anomalous diffusion, such as of single lipid or protein molecules in the plasma membrane of living cells. Combining a (tunable) resolution down to ~20 nm with FCS, Eggeling and coworkers showed that sphingolipids or "raft"-associated proteins were transiently (~10 ms) trapped at the nanoscale in cholesterol-mediated molecular complexes.[48] However, STED-FCS suffers from several drawbacks that require further technological developments before full implementation in living cells, including the high power density of the STED depletion beam (10–100 MW/cm[2]), the difficulty to extend the technique to multiple colors, and the still diffraction-limited axial resolution.

These limitations can in principle be all overcome by the use of metallic nano-structures, fabricated either on glass substrates as 2D arrays or at the apex of NSOM probes. 2D arrays rely on the fabrication of subwavelength apertures in a metal film deposited on a glass substrate (called ZMWs). The utility of 2D subwavelength apertures in live cell membrane research has been demonstrated using different aperture sizes uncovering a relationship between the transient times of the molecules travers-ing the illumination volume and the illumination area.[49,50] Using a similar approach, it was also shown that gangliosides partition in compartments of 60 nm in size consistent with their association in nanoscale lipid raft platforms.[50] More recently, ZMWs were used to determine the subunit stoichiometry of the pentameric neuronal nicotinic acetylcholine receptors on living cell membranes.[51] Unfortunately, despite its great potential for live cell membrane investigations, 2D subwavelength apertures do not, in general, exhibit optical enhancement, imposing a size limit of approxi-mately 50–70 nm to the useful structures that can be used for FCS-type applications. Moreover, an important limitation of this method is directly related to the need for cell membranes to adhere to the substrate, causing membrane invaginations, curva-ture effects, or nonspecific adhesion of the membrane close to the aperture edges.[52] To overcome these limitations, planarized apertures of 50 nm in diameter have been recently developed by means of filling the metal apertures with silicon oxide and used to record FCS data on supported lipid and plasma membranes without penetra-tion of the sample into the aperture.[53]

An alternative way to fully eliminate membrane interactions with the nanostruc-tures is by using self-standing apertures in combination with an NSOM approach. In this configuration, the nanoaperture is held stationary above the sample surface (with a distance separation of approximately 10 nm so that no interaction with the membrane occurs), and intensity fluctuations arising from the diffusing molecules are recorded in the far field using conventional optics. The first demonstration of NSOM-FCS was performed in 2008 by Vobornik et al. by measuring the mobility of fluorescent lipids in supported lipid bilayers[54] and then followed by Naber's group determining the diffu-sion of ligands transported axially through single nuclear pore complexes.[55] Recently, we demonstrated for the first time the feasibility of performing NSOM-FCS on living cells by stably maintaining the NSOM probe in proximity to the sample, obtaining vertical distance fluctuations below 1 nm.[56] We used this configuration to measure the diffusion of different lipids on living Chinese hamster ovary cells (Figure 20.8a and b). While the lipid analog phosphatidylethanolamine (PE) showed free, Brownian diffu-sion on the cell membrane, with transit times that linearly scaled with the illumination

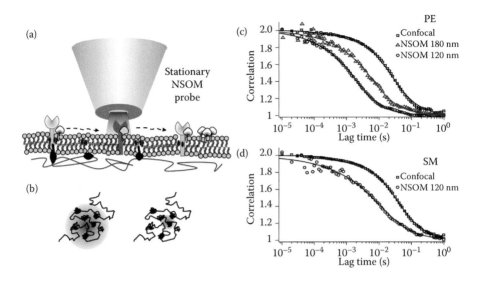

FIGURE 20.8 NSOM-based FCS in living cells. (a) In FCS mode, the NSOM probe is kept stationary over the membrane of the living cell so that only molecules that laterally diffuse through the small illumination area of NSOM are excited. (b) Schematics showing the comparison between confocal (left) and NSOM (right) illumination areas. Green denotes the illumination area in both cases, while the black curves illustrate the diffusion of individual molecules experiencing transient arrest and heterogeneity in their mobility. (c) Correlation curves as a function of lag time as obtained from the lipid PE for different illumination conditions: confocal and NSOM probes of 180 and 120 nm in diameter. (d) Correlation curves as a function of lag time for SM, obtained with confocal and with an NSOM probe of 120 nm in diameter. Symbols in (c) and (d) correspond to experimental data, while the lines are fittings to the curves using anomalous behavior.[56] (Reproduced from Dûfrene, Y.F., and Garcia-Parajo, M.F., *Nano Today* 7, 390–403, 2012.)

area (Figure 20.8c), the sphingolipid SM showed a clear deviation from Brownian diffusion when the illumination area was reduced from confocal to NSOM (Figure 20.8d), consistent with cholesterol-induced lateral confinement.[48]

There is a large potential for the use of NSOM-FCS since it combines membrane (proximal) specificity and high signal-to-noise ratios. The limitations of conventional NSOM probes in terms of light throughput can be easily overcome by the use of antenna probes, using geometries such as bowties. Indeed, as we already showed, BNA probes provide three-to-four orders of magnitude larger signal comparable to conventional NSOM apertures of the same size.[42] Moreover, BNAs have broadband emission allowing for multicolor excitation and dual-color cross-correlation spectroscopy in ultrasmall volumes. These devices in the future could be used to provide exquisite information on the coupling between the inner and outer leaflets of the membrane, signaling complex formation, and the intimate relation between membrane nanodomains and the actin cytoskeleton.

It should be also mentioned that 2D antenna configurations bear similar potential for studies on living cell membranes. So far, most efforts are being devoted to the fabrication of large arrays of antennas (necessary for inspection of multiple cells on a single substrate) and how to overcome unwanted interactions between the immediate cell membrane and the metal nanostructures. Recently, a combination of colloidal chemistry together with plasma processing has been developed to fabricate millions of bowtie antennas on a single substrate.[57] First proof-of-principle experiments were performed using model lipid bilayers and showed unhindered diffusion of individual proteins embedded in the bilayer. Although many technological challenges still lie ahead, it is clear that the field is moving forward driven by the exciting and unique possibilities offered by optical antennas.

20.6 OPTICAL ANTENNAS FOR IN VITRO SINGLE-BIOMOLECULE DETECTION

As already mentioned, subwavelength apertures on metallic films have been successfully used for single-molecule detection in solution at 10 μM sample concentrations.[24] Impressive in vitro studies include high-throughput fluorescence-based DNA sequencing,[58] protein–protein interactions at 5 μM concentrations,[59] and studies on the bacterial translation machinery.[60]

Because of the strong spatial confinement and field enhancement afforded by optical antennas, these devices are starting to emerge as superior alternatives for single-biomolecule detection at high concentrations. In 2009, Moerner and colleagues demonstrated fluorescence intensity enhancement of more than three orders of magnitude using gold-bowtie antennas.[35] This large enhancement resulted from an effective increase of the excitation field on the gap region of the bowtie (10 nm gap) by two orders of magnitude, in combination with an enhancement of the quantum yield of the emitter by a factor of 10.[35] Yet, in order to achieve such signal enhancements, molecules have to be precisely positioned in the gap region of the antenna, imposing several practical constrains and restricting the utility of antennas for broad applications in life sciences. To circumvent this limitation, an extremely attractive strategy has been recently reported by Tinnefeld and coworkers.[61] The approach used DNA-based self-assemble structures (also known as DNA origamis) as scaffold on which two gold nanoparticles were placed to form dimer antennas. The main advantage of this method is that the structure offers handles to place the biomolecule of interest at the right position within the hotspot of the antenna.[61] Using this concept, fluorescence enhancement of more than two orders of magnitude was demonstrated on gap antennas of 23 nm in size, allowing at the same time single-molecule measurements at 500 nM.

Recently, we introduced a "nanoantenna-in-box" platform especially designed for enhanced single-molecule analysis in solution at high concentrations. The design consists of a nanoantenna dimer formed by two gold hemispheres placed in a rectangular nanoaperture[62] (Figure 20.9). The rationale behind this design is that in any nanoantenna experiment on molecules in solution, the observed fluorescence signal is a sum of two contributions: the enhanced fluorescence from the few molecules in the nanoantenna gap region (hotspot) and a fluorescence background from several thousands of molecules within the diffraction-limited confocal volume. As such, the different components of the "antenna-in-box" have complementary roles: a central

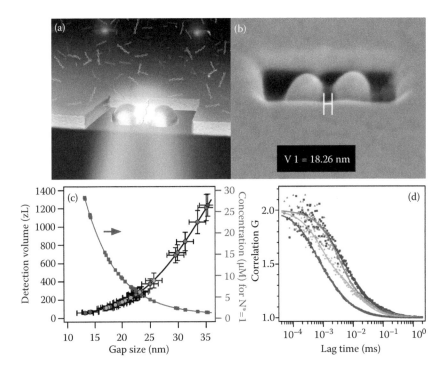

FIGURE 20.9 Antenna-in-box for single-molecule detection at micromolar concentrations. (a) Scheme of the antenna-in-box configuration. The dimer antenna is fabricated inside of a nanoaperture square carved in a gold film deposited on a glass substrate. (b) SEM image of the fabricated antenna-in-box. The gap region of the dimer antenna is ~19 nm. (c) Detection volume and concentration for which there is, on average, an individual molecule in the nano-antenna detection volume. (d) Normalized fluorescence correlation functions measured on an antenna-in-box of 15 nm gap size, with excitation polarization parallel to the antenna axis. The samples are Alexa Fluor 647 free dye (red), Annexin 5b (orange), 51 bp double-stranded DNA (green), and protein A (blue). The points correspond to experimental data and the solid lines correspond to a numerical fit. (Adapted from Punj, D. et al., *Nat. Nanotechnol.* 8, 512–516, 2013.)

gap antenna creates the hotspot for enhancement, while the surrounding nanoaperture screens the background by preventing direct excitation of molecules diffusing away from the central gap region. This configuration maximizes the signal-to-background discrimination by singling out the fluorescence signal from the hotspot while several thousands of nonexcited molecules are present in the confocal volume. Using this approach, we reached fluorescence enhancement values up to 1100-fold.[62] Furthermore, we monitored the diffusion of different individual biomolecules (DNA and proteins) in detection volumes of zeptoliter dimensions, corresponding to single-molecule detection at concentrations higher than 15 µM (Figure 20.9). The combined huge fluorescence enhancement and ultrasmall detection volume renders these type of optical antenna devices ideal for the design of massively parallel sensing platforms for single-biomolecule analysis at micromolar concentrations.

20.7 CONCLUSIONS AND PERSPECTIVES

In this chapter, we have highlighted the first exciting results where optical antennas have been already extended to biological applications at the level of nanoimaging and detection of dynamic events in vitro and in living cells. Concepts from FCS implemented in ultraconfined volumes as afforded by optical antennas now allow measurements of ultrafast dynamics at the nanoscale in living cell membranes as well as detection of individual molecules at the micromolar range. While these exciting results convincingly demonstrate the potential of these nanostructures, they also show important technological challenges that need improvement before their routine application in life sciences. Self-standing optical antennas require the combination of an NSOM configuration for manipulating and positioning the antenna close to the sample. On the positive side, the method provides the flexibility of placing the antenna at the desired location for maximum coupling to the fluorescent emitter, while avoiding direct unwanted interactions with the sample. However, these antenna configurations are commonly placed at the apex of tapered optical fibers, which are fragile and require high technical skills for probe manipulation. 2D optical antennas, on the other hand, are much easier to handle but less flexible in terms of coupling the antenna to the fluorescent dye. Moreover, unwanted effects attributed to physicochemical interactions of the fluorescent molecules (for in vitro studies) or the cell membrane (for in vivo applications) with the antennas complicate the analysis of the data and the throughput of successful experiments. While for in vitro studies small arrays of antennas might be sufficient, live-cell research imperatively requires the use of large antennas arrays. Current efforts are therefore focused on implementing techniques that allow the fabrication of low-cost, large-throughput, and highly reproducible (down to the nanometer scale) antenna arrays. Driven by their enormous potential, we expect that current technological obstacles will soon be overcome and that biology-compatible antenna geometries will be readily available to the biological community in the coming years.

ACKNOWLEDGMENTS

We gratefully acknowledge financial support from the European Commission (FP-ICT-2011-7, under grant agreement no 288263), Laserlab-Europe (EU-FP7 284464), the Spanish Ministry of Science (MAT2011-22887), and Agencia de Gestion d'Ajuts Universitaris i de Recerca (2009 SGR 597).

REFERENCES

1. Lingwood, D., K. Simons. "Lipid rafts as a membrane-organizing principle." *Science* 327 no. 5961 (2010): 46–50.
2. Simons, K., M. J. Gerl. "Revitalizing membrane rafts: New tools and insights." *Nat. Rev. Mol. Cell Biol.* 11 no. 10 (2010): 688–99.
3. Kusumi, A., C. Nakada, K. Ritchie et al. "Paradigm shift of the plasma membrane concept from the two-dimensional continuum fluid to the partitioned fluid: High-speed single-molecule tracking of membrane molecules." *Annu. Rev. Biophys. Biomol. Struct.* 34 (2005): 351–78.

4. Goswami, D., K. Gowrishankar, S. Bilgrami et al. "Nanoclusters of GPI-anchored proteins are formed by cortical actin-driven activity." *Cell* 135 no. 6 (2008): 1085–97.

5. Hemler, M. E. "Tetraspanin functions and associated microdomains." *Nat. Rev. Mol. Cell Biol.* 6 no. 10 (2005): 801–11.

6. Yanez-Mo, M., O. Barreiro, M. Gordon-Alonso, M. Sala-Valdes, F. Sanchez-Madrid. "Tetraspanin-enriched microdomains: A functional unit in cell plasma membranes." *Trends Cell Biol.* 19 no. 9 (2009): 434–46.

7. Lajoie, P., J. G. Goetz, J. W. Dennis, I. R. Nabi. "Lattices, rafts, and scaffolds: Domain regulation of receptor signaling at the plasma membrane." *J. Cell Biol.* 185 no. 3 (2009): 381–5.

8. Cambi, A., F. de Lange, N. M. van Maarseveen et al. "Microdomains of the C-type lectin DC-SIGN are portals for virus entry into dendritic cells." *J. Cell. Biol.* 164 no. 1 (2004): 145–55.

9. Sieber, J. J., K. I. Willig, C. Kutzner et al. "Anatomy and dynamics of a supramolecular membrane protein cluster." *Science* 317 no. 5841 (2007): 1072–6.

10. van Zanten, T. S., A. Cambi, M. Koopman, B. Joosten, C. G. Figdor, M. F. Garcia-Parajo. "Hotspots of GPI-anchored proteins and integrin nanoclusters function as nucleation sites for cell adhesion." *Proc. Natl. Acad. Sci USA* 106 no. 44 (2009): 18557–62.

11. Manzo, C., J. A. Torreno-Pina, B. Joosten et al. "The neck region of the C-type lectin DC-SIGN regulates its surface spatiotemporal organization and virus-binding capacity on antigen-presenting cells." *J. Biol. Chem.* 287 no. 46 (2012): 38946–55.

12. Cambi, A., B. Joosten, M. Koopman et al. "Organization of the integrin LFA-1 in nanoclusters regulates its activity." *Mol. Biol. Cell.* 17 no. 10 (2006): 4270–81.

13. Mayor, S., R. E. Pagano. "Pathways of clathrin-independent endocytosis." *Nat. Rev. Mol. Cell Biol.* 8 no. 8 (2007): 603–12.

14. Manes, S., A. Viola. "Lipid rafts in lymphocyte activation and migration." *Mol. Membr. Biol.* 23 no. 1 (2006): 59–69.

15. Donnert, G., J. Keller, R. Medda et al. "Macromolecular-scale resolution in biological fluorescence microscopy." *Proc. Natl. Acad. Sci. USA* 103 no. 31 (2006): 11440–5.

16. Betzig, E., G. H. Patterson, R. Sougrat et al. "Imaging intracellular fluorescent proteins at nanometer resolution." *Science* 313 no. 5793 (2006): 1642–5.

17. Hess, S. T., T. P. K. Girirajan, M. D. Mason. "Ultra-high resolution imaging by fluorescence photoactivation localization microscopy." *Biophys. J.* 91 no. 11 (2006): 4258–72.

18. Rust, M. J., M. Bates, X. Zhuang. "Subdiffraction limit imaging by stochastic optical reconstruction microscopy (STORM)." *Nat. Methods* 3 no. 10 (2006): 793–6.

19. Chen, Y., B. C. Lagerholm, B. Yang, K. Jacobson. "Methods to measure the lateral diffusion of membrane lipids and proteins." *Methods* 39 no. 2 (2006): 147–53.

20. Jacobson, K., O. G. Mouritsen, R. G. W. Anderson. "Lipid rafts: At a crossroad between cell biology and physics." *Nat. Cell Biol.* 9 no. 1 (2007): 7–14.

21. Chiantia, S., J. Ries, P. Schwille. "Fluorescence correlation spectroscopy in membrane structure elucidation." *Biochim. Biophys. Acta* 1788 no. 1 (2009): 225–33.

22. He, H. T., D. Marguet. "Detecting nanodomains in living cell membrane by fluorescence correlation spectroscopy." *Annu. Rev. Phys. Chem.* 62 (2011): 417–36.

23. Holzmeister, P., G. P. Acuna, D. Grohmann, P. Tinnefeld. "Breaking the concentration limit of optical single-molecule detection." *Chem. Soc. Rev.* 43 no. 4 (2014): 1014–28.

24. Levene, M. J., J. Korlach, S. W. Turner, M. Foquet, H. G. Craighead, W. W. Webb. "Zero-mode waveguides for single-molecule analysis at high concentrations." *Science* 299 no. 5607 (2003): 682–6.

25. van Zanten, T. S., A. Cambi, M. F. Garcia-Parajo. "A nanometer scale optical view on the compartmentalization of cell membranes." *Biochim. Biophys. Acta (BBA)—Biomembranes* 1798 no. 4 (2010): 777–87.

26. Hinterdorfer, P., M. F. Garcia-Parajo, Y. F. Dûfrene. "Single-molecule imaging of cell surfaces using near-field nanoscopy." *Acc. Chem. Res.* 45 no. 3 (2012): 327–36.

27. Dûfrene, Y. F., M. F. Garcia-Parajo. "Recent progress in cell surface nanoscopy: Light and forces in the near-field." *Nano Today* 7 no. 5 (2012): 390–403.

28. Koopman, M., A. Cambi, B. I. de Bakker et al. "Near-field scanning optical microscopy in liquid for high resolution single molecule detection on dendritic cells." *FEBS Lett.* 573 no. 1–3 (2004): 6–10.

29. van Zanten, T. S., J. Gomez, C. Manzo et al. "Direct mapping of nanoscale compositional connectivity on intact cell membranes." *Proc. Natl. Acad. Sci. USA* 107 no. 35 (2010): 15437–42.

30. Ianoul, A., D. D. Grant, Y. Rouleau, M. Bani-Yaghoub, L. J. Johnston, J. P. Pezacki. "Imaging nanometer domains of β-adrenergic receptor complexes on the surface of cardiac myocytes." *Nat. Chem. Biol.* 1 no. 4 (2005): 196–202.

31. de Bakker, B. I., F. de Lange, A. Cambi et al. "Nanoscale organization of the pathogen receptor DC-SIGN mapped by single-molecule high-resolution fluorescence microscopy." *Chemphyschem* 8 no. 10 (2007): 1473–80.

32. de Bakker, B. I., A. Bodnar, E. P. van Dijk et al. "Nanometer-scale organization of the alpha subunits of the receptors for IL2 and IL15 in human T lymphoma cells." *J. Cell Sci.* 121 no. 5 (2008): 627–33.

33. Garcia-Parajo, M. F. "Optical antennas focus in on biology." *Nat. Photon.* 2 no. 4 (2008): 201–3.

34. Novotny, L., N. F. van Hulst. "Antennas for light." *Nat. Photon.* 5 no. 2 (2011): 83–90.

35. Kinkhabwala, A., Z. Yu, S. Fan, Y. Avlasevich, K. Mullen, W. E. Moerner. "Large single-molecule fluorescence enhancements produced by a bowtie nanoantenna." *Nat. Photon.* 3 no. 11 (2009): 654–57.

36. van Hulst, N. F., T. H. Taminiau, A. G. Curto. "Directionality, polarization and enhancement of optical antennas." In *Optical Antennas*. Edited by M. Agio and A. Alu, pp. 81–99. Cambridge: Cambridge University Press, 2013.

37. Höppener, C., L. Novotny. "Antenna-based optical imaging of single Ca^{2+} transmembrane proteins in liquids." *Nano Lett.* 8 no. 2 (2008): 642–6.

38. Taminiau, T. H., R. J. Moerland, F. B. Segerink, L. Kuipers, N. F. van Hulst. "λ/4 Resonance of an optical monopole antenna probed by single molecule fluorescence." *Nano Lett.* 7 no. 1 (2007): 28–33.

39. van Zanten, T. S., M. J. Lopez-Bosque, M. F. Garcia-Parajo. "Imaging individual proteins and nanodomains on intact cell membranes with a probe-based optical antenna." *Small* 6 no. 2 (2010): 270–5.

40. Frey, H. G., S. Witt, K. Felderer, R. Guckenberger. "High-resolution imaging of single fluorescent molecules with the optical near-field of a metal tip." *Phys. Rev. Lett.* 93 (2004): 200801–4.

41. Guo, R., E. C. Kinzel, Y. Li et al. "Three-dimensional mapping of optical near field of a nanoscale bowtie antenna." *Opt. Express* 18 no. 5 (2010): 4961–71.

42. Mivelle, M., T. S. van Zanten, L. Neumann, N. F. van Hulst, M. F. Garcia-Parajo. "Ultrabright bowtie nanoaperture antenna probes studied by single molecule fluorescence." *Nano Lett.* 12 no. 11 (2012): 5972–8.

43. Wang, L., S. M. Uppuluri, E. X. Jin, X. F. Xu. "Nanolithography using high transmission nanoscale bowtie apertures." *Nano Lett.* 6 no. 3 (2006): 361–4.

44. Onuta, T.-D., M. Waegele, C. C. DuFort, W. L. Schaich, B. Dragnea. "Optical enhancement at cups between adjacent nanoapertures." *Nano Lett.* 7 no. 3 (2007): 557–64.

45. Mivelle, M., I. A. Ibrahim, F. Baida et al. "Bowtie nano-aperture as interface between near-fields and a single-mode fiber." *Opt. Express* 18 no. 15 (2010): 15964–74.

46. Saxton, M. J., K. Jacobson. "Single-particle tracking: Applications to membrane dynamics." *Annu. Rev. Biophys. Biomol. Struct.* 26 (1997): 373–99.

47. Kim, S. A., K. G. Heinze, P. Schwille. "Fluorescence cross-correlation spectroscopy in living cells." *Nat. Methods* 4 no. 11 (2007): 963–73.

48. Eggeling, C., C. Ringemann, R. Medda et al. "Direct observation of the nanoscale dynamics of membrane lipids in a living cell." *Nature* 457 no. 7233 (2009): 1159–62.

49. Wawrezinieck, L., H. Rigneault, D. Marguet, P. F. Lenne. "Fluorescence correlation spectroscopy diffusion law to probe the submicron cell membrane organization." *Biophys. J.* 89 no. 6 (2005): 4029–42.

50. Wenger, J., F. Conchonaud, J. Dintinger et al. "Diffusion analysis within single nanometric apertures reveals the ultrafine cell membrane organization." *Biophys. J.* 92 no. 3 (2007): 913–9.

51. Richards, C. I., K. Luong, R. Srinivasan et al. "Live-cell imaging of single receptor composition using zero-mode waveguide nanostructures." *Nano Lett.* 12 no. 7 (2012): 3690–4.

52. Samiee, K. T., J. M. Moran-Mirabal, Y. K. Cheung, H. G. Craighead. "Zero mode waveguides for single molecule spectroscopy on lipid membranes." *Biophys. J.* 90 no. 9 (2006): 3288–99.

53. Kelly, C. V., B. A. Baird, H. G. Craighead. "An array of planar apertures for near-field fluorescence correlation spectroscopy." *Biophys. J.* 100 no. 7 (2011): L34–6.

54. Vobornik, D., D. S. Banks, Z. Lu, C. Fradin, R. Taylor, L. J. Johnston. "Fluorescence correlation spectroscopy with sub-diffraction-limited resolution using near-field optical probes." *Appl. Phys. Lett.* 93 no. 16 (2008): 163904–6.

55. Herrmann, M., N. Neuberth, J. Wissler et al. "Near-field optical study of protein transport kinetics at a single nuclear pore." *Nano Lett.* 9 no. 9 (2009): 3330–6.

56. Manzo, C., T. S. van Zanten, M. F. Garcia-Parajo. "Nanoscale fluorescence correlation spectroscopy on intact living cell membranes with NSOM probes." *Biophys. J.* 100 no. 2 (2011): L8–10.

57. Lohmüller, T., L. Iversen, M. Schmidt et al. "Single molecule tracking on supported membranes with arrays of optical nanoantennas." *Nano Lett.* 12 no. 3 (2012): 1717–21.

58. Eid, J., A. Fehr, J. Gray et al. "Real-time DNA sequencing from single polymerase molecules." *Science* 323 no. 5910 (2009): 133–8.

59. Miyake, T., T. Tanii, H. Sonobe et al. "Real-time imaging of single molecule fluorescence with a zero-mode waveguide for the analysis of protein–protein interaction." *Anal. Chem.* 80 no. 15 (2008): 6018–22.

60. Uemura, S., C. E. Aitken, J. Korlach, B. A. Flusberg, S. W. Turner, J. D. Puglisi. "Real-time tRNA transit on single translating ribosomes at codon resolution." *Nature* 464 no. 7291 (2010): 1012–7.

61. Acuna, G. P., F. M. Moller, P. Holzmeister, S. Beater, B. Lalkens, P. Tinnefeld. "Fluorescence enhancement at docking sites of DNA-directed self-assembled nanoantennas." *Science* 338 no. 6106 (2012): 506–10.

62. Punj, D., M. Mivelle, S. B. Moparthi et al. "A plasmonic 'antenna-in-box' platform for enhanced single-molecule analysis at micromolar concentrations." *Nat. Nanotechnol.* 8 no. 22 (2013): 512–6.

Index

Page numbers followed by f and t indicate figures and tables, respectively.